In Situ Tissue Regeneration

This book is dedicated to
Jong Hyun Lee, Myung Hee Park, Bae Hyun Choi, Soon Jin Jeong, and Jin San Choi

Sang Jin Lee

This book is dedicated to
Yook-IL, Kyung Whan, Kyung Jin, and Kyung Min

James J. Yoo

This book is dedicated to
Katherine, Christopher, and Zachary

Anthony Atala

In Situ Tissue Regeneration

Host Cell Recruitment and Biomaterial Design

Edited by

Sang Jin Lee
James J. Yoo
Anthony Atala

Wake Forest Institute for Regenerative Medicine,
Wake Forest School of Medicine, Winston-Salem, NC, United States

ELSEVIER

AMSTERDAM • BOSTON • HEIDELBERG • LONDON
NEW YORK • OXFORD • PARIS • SAN DIEGO
SAN FRANCISCO • SINGAPORE • SYDNEY • TOKYO

Academic Press is an imprint of Elsevier

Academic Press is an imprint of Elsevier
125 London Wall, London EC2Y 5AS, United Kingdom
525 B Street, Suite 1800, San Diego, CA 92101-4495, United States
50 Hampshire Street, 5th Floor, Cambridge, MA 02139, United States
The Boulevard, Langford Lane, Kidlington, Oxford OX5 1GB, United Kingdom

Library of Congress Cataloging-in-Publication Data
A catalog record for this book is available from the Library of Congress

British Library Cataloguing-in-Publication Data
A catalogue record for this book is available from the British Library

ISBN: 978-0-12-802225-2

For information on all Academic Press publications
visit our website at http://www.elsevier.com/

Publisher: Mica Haley
Acquisition Editor: Mica Haley
Editorial Project Manager: Lisa Eppich
Production Project Manager: Lucía Pérez
Designer: Victoria Pearson

Typeset by TNQ Books and Journals

Contents

PART 5 TISSUE-SPECIFIC APPLICATIONS

List of Contributors

Ahmed Abdelbaset-Ismail
Stem Cell Institute, James Graham Brown Cancer Center, University of Louisville, KY, United States

Julie Allickson
Wake Forest Institute for Regenerative Medicine, Wake Forest School of Medicine, Winston-Salem, NC, United States

Feras Alshomer
Division of Surgery and Interventional Science, University College London, London, United Kingdom

Noaf Salah Ali AlWahab
Biomedical Engineering Department, Khalifa University, Abu Dhabi, United Arab Emirates

Antony Atala
Wake Forest Institute for Regenerative Medicine, Wake Forest School of Medicine, Winston-Salem, NC, United States

Alexander Baume
Wake Forest Institute for Regenerative Medicine, Wake Forest School of Medicine, Winston-Salem, NC, United States

Selwa Mokhtar Boularaoui
Biomedical Engineering Department, Khalifa University, Abu Dhabi, United Arab Emirates

Nicolas Christoforou
Biomedical Engineering Department, Khalifa University, Abu Dhabi, United Arab Emirates; Biomedical Engineering Department, Duke University, Durham, NC, United States

Manuela E. Gomes
3B's Research Group, Department of Polymer Engineering, University of Minho, Guimarães, Portugal

Ana I. Gonçalves
3B's Research Group, Department of Polymer Engineering, University of Minho, Guimarães, Portugal

Hyun Sook Hong
East-West Medical Research Institute, Kyung Hee University, Seoul, Korea

John D. Jackson
Wake Forest Institute for Regenerative Medicine, Wake Forest School of Medicine, Winston-Salem, NC, United States

Katherine A. Joyner
Department of Pharmaceutical Sciences, University of Maryland, Baltimore, MD, United States

Deepak M. Kalaskar
Division of Surgery and Interventional Science, University College London, London, United Kingdom

Ji Hyun Kim
Wake Forest Institute for Regenerative Medicine, Wake Forest School of Medicine, Winston-Salem, NC, United States

Moon Suk Kim
Department of Molecular Science and Technology, Ajou University, Suwon, Korea

Na Jung Kim
Wake Forest Institute for Regenerative Medicine, Wake Forest School of Medicine, Winston-Salem, NC, United States

Suna Kim
Department of Genetic Engineering, Graduate School of Biotechnology, Kyung Hee University, Yong In, Korea

In Kap Ko
Wake Forest Institute for Regenerative Medicine, Wake Forest School of Medicine, Winston-Salem, NC, United States

Byron Lambert
Abbott Vascular, Santa Clara, CA, United States

Bo Keun Lee
Department of Molecular Science and Technology, Ajou University, Suwon, Korea

Chang H. Lee
Regenerative Engineering Laboratory, Columbia University Medical Center, New York, NY, United States

Sang Jin Lee
Wake Forest Institute for Regenerative Medicine, Wake Forest School of Medicine, Winston-Salem, NC, United States

Yuqi Li
Department of Pharmaceutical Sciences, University of Maryland, Baltimore, MD, United States

Baisong Lu
Wake Forest Institute for Regenerative Medicine, Wake Forest School of Medicine, Winston-Salem, NC, United States

Ashwin Nair
Bioengineering Department, University of Texas at Arlington, Arlington, TX, United States

Rei Ogawa
Department of Plastic, Reconstructive and Aesthetic Surgery, Nippon Medical School, Tokyo, Japan

Harald C. Ott
Harvard Stem Cell Institute, Harvard Medical School, Boston, MA, United States

Seung Hun Park
Department of Molecular Science and Technology, Ajou University, Suwon, Korea

Richard Payne
Wake Forest Institute for Regenerative Medicine, Wake Forest School of Medicine, Winston-Salem, NC, United States

T. Konrad Rajab
Harvard Stem Cell Institute, Harvard Medical School, Boston, MA, United States

Richard Rapoza
Abbott Vascular, Santa Clara, CA, United States

Mariusz Z. Ratajczak
Stem Cell Institute, James Graham Brown Cancer Center, University of Louisville, KY, United States

Rui L. Reis
3B's Research Group, Department of Polymer Engineering, University of Minho, Guimarães, Portugal

Márcia T. Rodrigues
3B's Research Group, Department of Polymer Engineering, University of Minho, Guimarães, Portugal

Lindsey E. Shapiro
Wake Forest Institute for Regenerative Medicine, Wake Forest School of Medicine, Winston-Salem, NC, United States

Alexander Sheehy
Abbott Vascular, Santa Clara, CA, United States

Youngsook Son
Department of Genetic Engineering, Graduate School of Biotechnology, Kyung Hee University, Yong In, Korea; East-West Medical Research Institute, Kyung Hee University, Seoul, Korea

Joseph P. Stains
Department of Orthopedics, University of Maryland, Baltimore, MD, United States

Zhaoli Sun
Department of Surgery, The Johns Hopkins University School of Medicine, Baltimore, MD, United States

Liping Tang
Bioengineering Department, University of Texas at Arlington, Arlington, TX, United States

Marc B. Taraban
Department of Pharmaceutical Sciences, University of Maryland, Baltimore, MD, United States

Solaiman Tarafder
Regenerative Engineering Laboratory, Columbia University Medical Center, New York, NY, United States

Jeremy Choon Meng Teo
Biomedical Engineering Department, Khalifa University, Abu Dhabi, United Arab Emirates

Hung-Jen Wang
Division of Urology, Chang Gung Memorial Hospital, Kaohsiung County, Taiwan

George M. Williams
Department of Surgery, The Johns Hopkins University School of Medicine, Baltimore, MD, United States

James J. Yoo
Wake Forest Institute for Regenerative Medicine, Wake Forest School of Medicine, Winston-Salem, NC, United States

Yihua B. Yu
Department of Pharmaceutical Sciences, University of Maryland, Baltimore, MD, United States

Nan Zhang
National Institutes for Health, Bethesda, MD, United States; Wake Forest Institute for Regenerative Medicine, Wake Forest School of Medicine, Winston-Salem, NC, United States

Preface

Over the past few decades, cell-based therapies have become a treatment option for repairing or replacing damaged tissues and organs. However, development of cell-based therapies using a stem- or tissue-specific cell source presents substantial complexity for clinical use, and these include tissue harvest and cell isolation and expansion ex vivo. To simplify this process, researchers have sought for a means to avoid ex vivo cell manipulation, thus saving time, effort, and resources. Recent studies show that endogenous tissue-specific stem/progenitor cells can be utilized by controlling the host microenvironment, and that if given the proper biological cues, these cells could be guided to differentiate into specific cell lineages. More importantly, the differentiated tissue-specific cells, combined with biomaterials or artificial microenvironments, can be effectively integrated with the host tissue for structural and functional tissue restoration in situ. To this end, "in situ tissue regeneration" aims to take advantage of the body's own regenerating capacity to activate endogenous stem cells or tissue-specific progenitors for tissue repair.

This book provides the most recent development strategies for in situ tissue regeneration in terms of mechanisms of host cell recruitment, cell sourcing, and cellular and molecular roles involved with cell differentiation, navigational cues and niche signals, and tissue-specific smart biomaterial systems, from the perspective of tissue engineering and regenerative medicine. This book is divided into four parts: (1) endogenous cell sources, (2) biochemical and physical cues, (3) smart biomaterial development, and (4) tissue-specific applications. We believe that the "in situ tissue regeneration" strategy has the potential to accelerate research and clinical translation of tissue engineering and regenerative medicine applications.

The editors acknowledge and extend our sincere gratitude to the experts who generously devoted valuable time and effort to share their knowledge and experience to this book. The professional support of the editorial and production team at Elsevier is also appreciated. We hope that this book will encourage readers to investigate the new paradigms in tissue engineering and regenerative medicine research.

Sang Jin Lee
James J. Yoo
Anthony Atala

PART

INTRODUCTION

1

CHAPTER

FUNDAMENTALS OF IN SITU TISSUE REGENERATION

1

S.J. Lee, J.J. Yoo, A. Atala

Wake Forest Institute for Regenerative Medicine, Wake Forest School of Medicine, Winston-Salem, NC, United States

CHAPTER OUTLINE

INTRODUCTION

One of the strategies in tissue engineering involves the use of biomaterial scaffolds made by naturally derived materials or synthetic polymers that provide a 3-D architecture and structural support with or without cells [1–3]. This strategy is dictated by the implantable tissue constructs and the availability of suitable cells, which allow the production of new extracellular matrix (ECM), resembling that of the native tissue to regenerate the injured tissues or organs. Using this approach, numerous preclinical and clinical studies performed in different tissue systems have shown to be effective in tissue repair or regeneration [4–8].

Although this strategy has made considerable advancements, the cell-based therapeutic approaches have proved to be limited by the donor tissue availability. Harvesting autologous tissue to obtain cells is often constrained by the anatomical access limitations and associated with donor site morbidity [9,10]. Allogeneic and xenogeneic cell sources, on the other hand, present risks of inducing immunologic responses due to genetic differences and potential bacterial and viral transmission from the donor to the host. Furthermore, this approach requires cell isolation and expansion, which involves labor-intensive cell manipulation [11]. An alternative cell source is the use of stem or progenitor cells; however, this approach also necessitates ex vivo procedures such as cell isolation, expansion, and/or differentiation of desired cell lineages and may result in loss of cellular function during expansion [12].

In Situ Tissue Regeneration. http://dx.doi.org/10.1016/B978-0-12-802225-2.00001-5

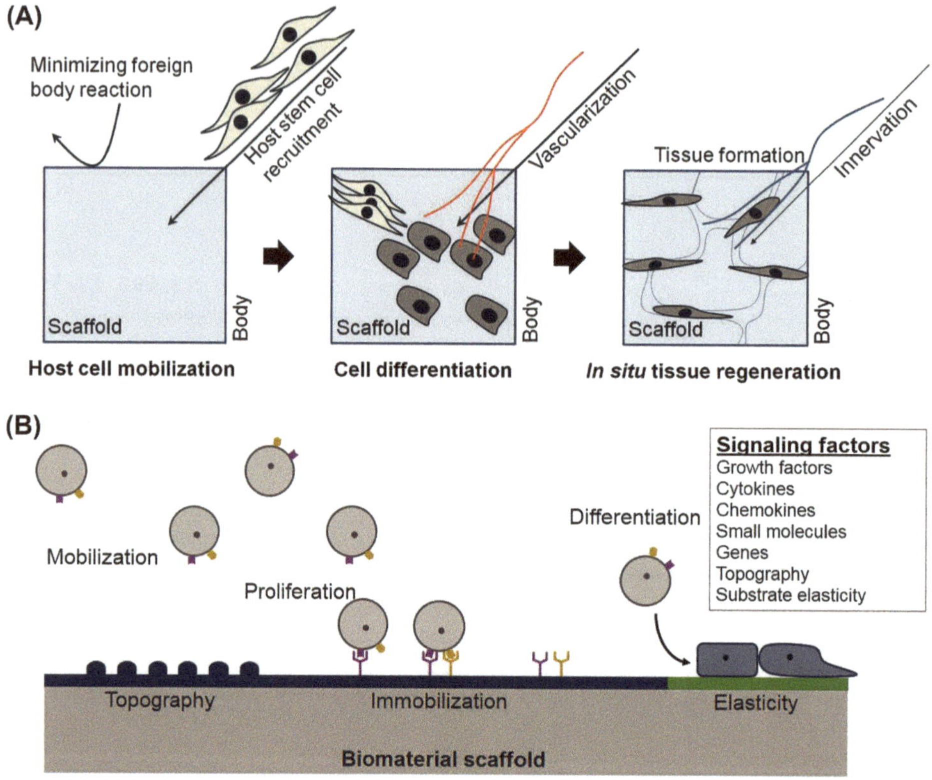

FIGURE 1.1

Schematic illustration of (A) strategy of in situ tissue regeneration and (B) interactions between endogenous stem cells and biomaterial scaffold. Stem cell fate in a particular microenvironment is regulated by intricate reciprocal molecular interactions with its surroundings.

Advanced strategies in tissue engineering and regenerative medicine have introduced the concept of recruiting host stem cell/progenitor cells to a target site of interest for in situ tissue regeneration 13–17]. The principle of in situ tissue regeneration is to take advantage of the body's own regenerative capability by utilizing endogenous stem cells or tissue-specific progenitor cells at the site of injury. This approach provides a more efficient means of therapy by eliminating ex vivo cell manipulation. Fig. 1.1 shows a strategy of in situ tissue regeneration. For instance, when scaffolds encapsulated with bioactive molecules are implanted, sustained release of these bioactive molecules unlocks the body's own regenerating capacity. In turn, this induces recruitment of stem/progenitor cells, drives differentiation of these cells into targeted cell types, and participates in the regeneration of functional tissues. This chapter reviews the recent development of strategies for in situ tissue regeneration, in terms of mechanism of recruitment, cell sources, cellular and molecular roles in cell differentiation, navigational cues and niche signals, and tissue-specific scaffolding systems from the perspective of regenerative medicine and tissue engineering.

STRATEGY: IN SITU TISSUE REGENERATION

Stem cells, whether derived from embryos, fetuses, or adults, possess an enormous capacity for the next frontier of tissue engineering and regenerative medicine. This is due to their remarkable potential to develop into many different tissues or organs in the body with specialized functions. Given their unique regenerative capabilities, stem cells offer new potentials for treating a broad range of diseases, such as diabetes and heart disease [18,19]. Because of the significant role of stem cells in the regenerative process, a readily available population of stem cells that are highly renewable and have an extensive ability to differentiate is critical for clinical success.

Due to the ethical concerns involved with the use of embryonic stem cells, adult stem cells have increasingly gained attention. Adult stem cells are undifferentiated cells found in almost every tissue or organ, which can self-renew and differentiate into tissue-specific cell types. Their primary role is to maintain and repair tissue in which they are found. The stem cells reside in a specialized microenvironment called stem cell niche. Tissue-specific stem cells remain quiescent for relatively long periods of time until they are activated by a need for tissue maintenance or by disease or tissue injury. The presence of an underlying regenerative mechanism in the form of tissue-specific stem or progenitor cells suggests that there could be a potential opportunity to bias the host response toward repair and reconstruction of tissue defects.

Indeed, it has been widely accepted that almost every tissue in the body contains various types of stem or progenitor cells, including brain, liver, circulating blood, heart, skin, fat, kidney, and muscle [20–26]. It would seem that these premature cells are part of underlying regenerative machinery that is responsible for daily maintenance activities, including repair of normal tissue wear and tear, as well as small injuries. However, when extensive tissue damage occurs and large tissue defects are present, the regenerative response is overwhelmed, and an immune-based reparative response takes over to maintain some level of function. While the immediate problem may be mitigated by these reparative processes, responses such as inflammation, which results in uncontrolled collagen deposition and fibrosis, are undesirable because they can lead to further complications and severe deficits in tissue and organ functionality. Therefore current research efforts have focused on the improvement of the regenerative capability by controlling the host microenvironment and stem cell mobilization for in situ tissue regeneration [16].

The concept of in situ tissue regeneration occurs via the recruitment of host stem cells into an injured tissue or other target niche. Currently, various functionalized biomaterial scaffolds have been used for the reconstruction of a large tissue defect with functional recovery. From a biomaterials perspective, placing a biomaterial in the in vivo microenvironment requires injection, insertion, or surgical implantation, all of which injure the tissues or organs involved. In such instances, various reconstructive measures are necessary to restore functionality of the affected tissues or organs. However, it is well known that a biomaterial implant will become populated with host cells that ultimately result in scar tissue. The host cell infiltrate has been assumed to be inflammatory and fibroblastic, as indirect evidence (ie, the presence of collagen) has suggested that fibroblasts are the predominant cell population present after the initial inflammation has subsided.

Even though inflammatory response and foreign body reaction have been well identified, the cell types that infiltrate the biomaterial have not been fully identified. Therefore the possibility of utilizing the body's biologic and environmental resources in situ for tissue regeneration has been investigated. As an initial step, the recruitment of host stem/progenitor cells into an implanted scaffold through the tissue repairing process has been examined. In our previous study [13], poly(glycolic acid) (PGA) nonwoven scaffold, a widely employed biocompatible, biodegradable, and implantable biomaterial, was used in a simple approach to address this dogma. The implant is highly porous and is designed to increase diffusion and accommodate host cell infiltrates. The results showed that the number of host cells continued to increase up to 3 weeks after implantation and began to decrease thereafter as collagen accumulates and fills the pores of the implanted scaffold. This is consistent with the normal inflammatory response seen in many tissue systems. However, we found that a small proportion of the infiltrated host cells within the biomaterial implants have multilineage potential (Fig. 1.2A) [13]. These results indicate that some of the host stem cells that can be mobilized into a biomaterial are multipotent, and given an optimal microenvironment, they can differentiate into specific cell types needed for functional regeneration at the implant site. One major concern is how sufficient stem cell populations can be migrated into the implanted scaffold, as the number of adult stem cells in the body is generally too low to have a significant effect on tissue regeneration in many cases. In this regard, we demonstrated effective recruitment of host stem cells into an implanted scaffold using a novel combined delivery system consisting of systemic injection of substance P and local release of stromal cell-derived factor-1α (SDF-1α) from the implanted scaffold (Fig. 1.2B) [16].

Based on these findings, a desirable paradigm in which a target-specific biomaterial system can be universally applied, without the need for ex vivo cell manipulation, may be attainable. Ideally, the patient's body would supply both the source of cells and the microenvironment for terminal differentiation, provided the appropriate cues can be mediated through the biomaterial scaffold. Therefore in contrast to current modalities that focus on in vitro manipulation of cells, it may be possible to control tissue morphogenesis in vivo by providing the appropriate cues to the infiltrating multipotent cells, leading to the production of functional tissues in situ.

DESIGN CONSIDERATIONS: BIOMATERIAL SCAFFOLDS

Creation of engineered tissue constructs requires a biomaterial scaffold that serves as an artificial microenvironment and provides structural support until native tissue forms. Although the requirements for biomaterial scaffolds may be different depending on the target tissues or organs, the general functions of scaffolds that need to be fulfilled include biodegradability, biocompatibility, and temporal structural integrity. In addition, the scaffold's internal architecture should facilitate the permeability of nutrients and neovascularization. The latter is particularly important, as this porous structure not only can provide space for the recruitment of cells to reside but also can encapsulate bioactive molecules and provide cues that enhance cell migration, proliferation, and differentiation, producing a biofunctional stem cell niche. To design a biomaterial scaffolding system for in situ tissue regeneration, it should: (1) minimize foreign body reaction and fibrosis; (2) utilize host microenvironment for activating/recruiting host stem/progenitor cells; and (3) control tissue-specific cell differentiation within the target tissue of interest.

As an initial step, sufficient numbers of adjacent stem cells must be recruited into the implanted scaffold for efficient and effective tissue regeneration. However, the number of stem cells present in the body is limited. Thus, several research teams have investigated chemotaxis of circulating mesenchymal stem cells (MSCs) using various chemokines. The interaction with chemokine and chemokine receptor induces a cellular reaction in response to a specific chemokine and β-actin filament rearrangement

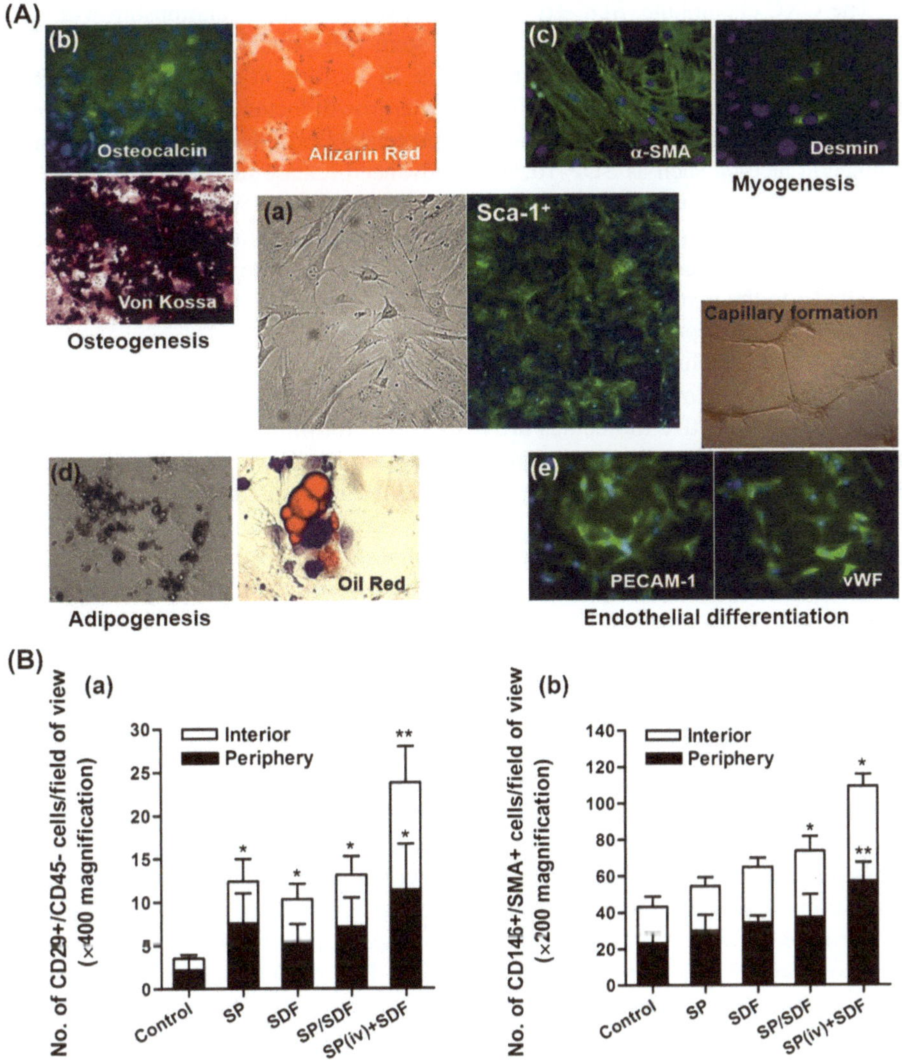

FIGURE 1.2

(A) The infiltrating cells (Sca-1 positive) that were induced into different cell lineages under specific conditions demonstrated the expression of their phenotypic and functional characteristics: (a) infiltrating host cells, (b) osteogenic differentiation, (c) myogenic differentiation, (d) adipogenic differentiation, and (e) endothelial differentiation as confirmed by specific marker expression. *(Reproduced with permission from Lee SJ, Van Dyke M, Atala A, Yoo JJ. Host cell mobilization for in situ tissue regeneration. Rejuvenation Res 2008;11:747–56.)* (B) Numbers of the recruited MSC-like cells: (a) $CD29^{+}CD45^{-}$ cells and (b) $CD146^{+}\alpha\text{-}SMA^{+}$ cells. *(Reproduced with permission from Ko IK, Ju YM, Chen T, Atala A, Yoo JJ, Lee SJ. Combined systemic and local delivery of stem cell inducing/recruiting factors for in situ tissue regeneration. FASEB J 2011;26:158–68.)*

(CXCL12). The CXC chemokine, SDF-1α (CXCL12), shows a close relationship with cell survival, migration, proliferation, and differentiation of host stem cell populations, including hematopoietic stem cells, tissue-specific progenitor cells, and MSCs. In addition, it is reported that MSCs respond in vivo to other bioactive molecules such as hepatocyte growth factor (HGF), matrix metalloproteinase-2 [27], galanin [28], and monocyte chemotactic protein-3 [29]. More directly, the sustained delivery of chemotactic factors, such as SDF-1α, using advanced release technology to drive endogenous stem cell recruitment to a tissue defect region represents a potentially novel approach to regeneration, eg, the encapsulation of these putative bioactive molecules into biodegradable polymeric scaffolds with sustained release kinetics. Furthermore, several research studies have demonstrated that delivery of exogenous SDF-1α to the myocardium prolongs the presence of SDF-1α after infarction, augmenting stem cell recruitment and improving cardiac function [30–33].

Bioactive molecules, including growth factors, cytokines, small molecules, and genes, for in situ tissue regeneration play an important role in the control of the microenvironment in vivo [15]. Chemotactic signals from bioactive molecules are responsible for directed cell migration. An anatomic destination is identified according to a certain concentration gradient of chemicals produced in the injured sites in their microenvironment. Therefore one of the significant criteria for developing biomaterial scaffolding systems, especially for in situ tissue regeneration purposes, is to deliver bioactive molecules and regulatory signals in a precise temporal and spatial manner [34]. Initially, it is critical to efficiently induce and direct recruitment of host stem cells to the targeted sites. To achieve this, identifying and understanding the roles of bioactive molecules that initiate the recruiting response of the cells is required. Ideal delivery of bioactive molecules requires sustained release to maintain effective concentrations in a local microenvironment. Additionally, it has been demonstrated that multiple factors need to be delivered to a target application due to the complexity of the microenvironment. Mooney et al. suggested a multiple protein delivery system for accelerating vascularization and tissue formation, as the development of tissues and organs is typically driven by the action of a number of growth factors [35]. They reported a new polymeric system that allows for the tissue-specific delivery of two or more growth factors, with controlled dose and rate of delivery. Controlling sustained release of bioactive molecules with different release kinetics enables effective tissue regeneration. Likewise, a recent study shows various methods of sustained release of bioactive molecules over time [36]. Multiple sustained release mimics actual in vivo tissue regeneration, and it contributes to effective and rapid tissue regeneration. In a recent study, a gelatin-based scaffold was delivered in vivo with chemical conjugations of four different bioactive molecules: vascular endothelial growth factor (VEGF), angiopoietin-1, keratinocyte growth factor (KGF), and platelet-derived growth factor-BB (PDGF-BB). This combined delivery of multiple bioactive molecules resulted in an increase in angiogenesis with a potential for enhanced tissue regeneration [37]. Another study in skeletal muscle regeneration shows effective and functional skeletal muscle regeneration using alginate, which simultaneously released insulin-like growth factor-1 (IGF-1) and VEGF [38]. This study is important because in addition to angiogenesis, a functional skeletal muscle tissue was created with activation of muscle satellite cells.

The mechanical and molecular information coded within the extracellular milieu is guiding the development of a new generation of biomaterials for future tissue regeneration. To this end, ECM-mimicking biomaterials may provide not only structural components for supporting cells but also contain a reservoir of cell-signaling motifs and sequestered growth factors that guide cellular anchorage and behavior, inspiring multiple examples of biomimetic design for biomaterial scaffolds. In vascular research, for example, the presence of endothelium-derived macromolecules or their cell interacting domains onto vascular grafts can mimic features of the ECM and thereby assist specific cell adhesion and promote endothelialization [39].

Another consideration for in situ regeneration is to provide cell attachment sites on the scaffold in conjunction with the release of bioactive molecules involved with target cell recruitment. One ECM peptide sequence that influences cell adhesion behavior is the integrin binding arginine–glycine–aspartic acid (RGD) sequence [40–47]. Together with the integrins, the cell surface receptors that recognize the sequence of various proteins, RGD constitutes a major recognition system for cell adhesion. The RGD motif may also enhance the recruitment and activation of endoneurial phagocytes (ie, phagocytes residing in *Lymnaea*'s nerves) in the injury response of the nervous system of the pond snail *Lymnaea stagnalis* and affect nerve regeneration [48]. In an in vitro study, a designer self-assembling peptide scaffold developed by Horii et al. significantly stimulated cell migration into the 3-D scaffold, suggesting that it would be possible to apply suitable and active biological scaffolds to stimulate and promote host stem cell recruitment, differentiation, and regeneration of tissues without introducing any foreign cells [49].

Cell–biomaterial interactions continue to be a principal source of inspiration for biomaterial functionalization and thus play a very important role in future cell recruiting device design [50]. This is a dynamic and rapidly evolving field that has gained considerable attention as a means of increasing scaffold potency and to improve their biological functionality [51]. Current research has identified many peptides/proteins, various factors, and numerous techniques that could be used for the functionalization of biomaterials. New biomaterials can adapt to the surrounding microenvironment and orchestrate the transport of ions, bioactive molecules, and information transfer between cells and their microenvironment [49,52–55]. However, less is known about how such biomaterials influence and control cell function, how much extrinsic physiochemical information is required to mobilize host stem cells into regenerating a complex tissue, and specifically, taking a combination of clinical performance, marketing, and cost-effectiveness into consideration, what minimum level of biomaterial complexity is required for a given task [50]. There is an ever-increasing demand for biomaterials that can match both the mechanical and biological properties of real tissue matrix, support vascularization, and recreate nanoscale topographical and cell-specific biochemical cues [56].

APPLICATIONS OF IN SITU TISSUE REGENERATION

The concept of in situ tissue regeneration has been well studied and documented in bone regeneration. The required property of biomaterial scaffolds to ensure successful treatment of bony defects is the temporary mechanical load bearing within the tissue defects. Moreover, it should minimize immune and/or inflammatory response. The biomaterials widely used for this purpose include calcium phosphate, calcium sulfate, and hydroxyapatite. Since native bone tissue consists of large amounts of such materials, they have been considered as the major component of scaffold material for bone tissue regeneration due to their chemical and crystal resemblance to the mineral phase of bone, demonstrating excellent biocompatibility and osteoconductivity [57]. As bioactive molecules for bone regeneration, bone morphogenetic protein-2 (BMP-2) [58–60] and basic fibroblast growth factor (bFGF) [61] are common and therefore vital growth factors that are introduced into the bone scaffolds [62–64]. Scaffolds made of natural polymers such as alginate, fibrin, or gelatin and synthetic biodegradable polymers such as polylactide (PLA) and poly(lactide-*co*-glycolide) (PLGA) incorporated with bioactive molecules alone, or in combination with calcium phosphate and/or hydroxyapatite, have been shown to be osteoinductive and osteoconductive. As such, these scaffolding systems have shown an ability to stimulate and induce neighboring bone marrow MSCs and enhance in situ bone tissue formation.

When injured, the success rate of cartilage regeneration is low compared to other types of tissues, which can lead to joint problems such as severe arthritis. In early studies, in vitro cartilage production from chondrocytes and specialized scaffolding systems has shown success. However, when the engineered cartilage was implanted, serious compatibility issues were noted in vivo. Recently, Erggelet et al. demonstrated the regeneration of cartilage using cell-free biomaterial scaffolds. They developed a biomaterial construct composed of PLGA scaffold incorporated with plasma and hyaluronic acid (HA) and implanted into a cartilage microfracture injury site [65]. The result showed that the implanted constructs induced the migration of bone marrow MSCs and the formation of neocartilage tissue. Mao and his team also demonstrated that the entire articular surface of the synovial joint can regenerate without cell transplantation using 3-D poly(ε-caprolactone) and hydroxyapatite composites fabricated by solid free-form technique. These fabricated scaffolds were coated with transforming growth factor β3 prior to implantation. This was shown to be effective in regenerating cartilage tissue by recruiting host stem cells to the site of implantation [66].

Loss of a large amount of skeletal muscle mass often results in incomplete recovery, with the development of scar tissue. If an injury is not properly treated, it will likely cause skeletal muscle weakness and atrophy [67]. As the target cell sources for in situ muscle regeneration, muscle satellite cells primarily play a significant role in muscle regeneration, owing to their self-renewal capabilities and muscle-specific differentiation [68,69]. Besides muscle satellite cells, several populations of other stem cells, such as muscle-derived stem cells (MDSCs) [70,71], pericytes [72], muscle resident macrophages [73], and bone marrow-derived MSCs [74] have been used in engineering muscle tissue, as they are closely involved in the muscle regeneration process. The roles of these cell populations are critical for efficient muscle regeneration by maturing blood vessels, secreting trophic factors, and reducing fibrotic tissue formation [71].

A novel approach that relies on the body's ability to repair itself has been developed by utilizing host stem cell recruitment and control of cell fate. This approach is based on the release of tissue-specific stem cell stimulating factors to utilize host stem cells, followed by effective tissue regeneration [38]. In our previous work [14], we demonstrated that host myogenic cells, expressing muscle satellite/progenitor cell markers, can be mobilized into biomaterial scaffolds and then differentiated to myogenic cells for in situ muscle regeneration. Mooney's team has also developed an injectable system based on alginate material that is able to deliver dual growth factors, IGF-1 and VEGF, for the enhancement of functional muscle regeneration. IGF-1 induces satellite cell mobilization to injured muscle tissue to proliferate and differentiate, and VEGF is a primary proangiogenic factor that recruits vessel-forming stem or progenitor cells. In another study, Kin et al. implanted a collagen scaffold into a rabbit hind limb muscle injury. Twenty-four weeks posttransplantation, implants without scaffold (control group) showed severe scar tissue formation and muscle contraction, whereas the collagen-based scaffold group showed focal tissue adhesion and new muscle tissue formation [75]. This study shows that it is possible to enrich the infiltrates with tissue-specific stem/progenitor cells to control their cell fate, provided the microenvironment imparts proper signaling to the implanted scaffold. Table 1.1 lists recent therapeutic applications of the biomaterial scaffolding systems for in situ tissue regeneration. While many technologies are at the early experimental stage, several technologies have been successfully performed in preclinical animal studies with satisfactory outcomes.

Table 1.1 Recent Therapeutic Applications of Biomaterial Scaffolds for In Situ Tissue Regeneration

	Biomaterials	Bioactive Factors	Animal Model	References
Bone	PLA	FGF-1/spraying	Rat calvarial bone defect	[76]
	Fibrin/PLGA	BMP-2/encapsulation	Rat calvarial bone defect	[58]
	Alginate	BMP-2/immobilization	Rat muscle	[60]
	Fibrin	Heparan sulfate	Rat cranial defect	[77]
	P(HEMA-VP) gel	FGF-2/immobilization	Rabbit femoral defect	[78]
	Gelatin	FGF-2	Mouse maxillae	[61]
	Fibrin/HA	BMP-2	Mouse calvarial bone defect	[59]
Bile duct	Collagen/PP mesh		Canine circumferential biliary defect	[79]
Heart and vessel	PGA/PLA/collagen		Porcine descending aorta, porcine pulmonary arterial trunk, canine ventricular outflow tract	[80]
	PGA/PLA/collagen		Canine carotid arteries	[81]
	Porcine SIS/collagen		Rabbit arterial bypass model	[82]
	PEUU		Rat myocardial infarction model	[83]
	Alginate		Rat myocardial infarction model	[84]
Cartilage	PGA	Autologous serum/HA/ microfracture	Sheep full-thickness cartilage defect	[65]
	Collagen		Rabbit articular cartilage	[85]
Esophagus	UBM		Rat abdominal esophagus	[86]
	Rat gastric acelluar matrix		Rat abdominal esophagus	[87]
Fat pad	Collagen/PP	FGF-2/gelatin microsphere	Rat	[88]
Muscle	Collagen		Rabbit muscle (vastus lateralis)	[75]
	Gelatin	SDF-1, HGF, IGF-1, or bFGF	Rat muscle (tibialis anterior)	[14]
Periodontal tissue	Collagen	FGF-2/gelatin microsphere	Canine periodontal	[89]
	PLGA	GDF-5	Canine periodontal	[90]
Skin	Chitosan		Porcine burned skin	[91]
Spine	PGA/HA	Blood serum	Rabbit disc defect	[92]
Stomach	Collagen/PGA		Canine stomach	[93]

BMP, *bone morphogenic protein;* FGF, *fibroblast growth factor;* GDF, *growth differentiation factor;* HA, *hyaluronic acid;* HGF, *hepatocyte growth factor;* PEUU, *polyester urethane urea;* PGA, *poly(glycolic acid);* PLA, *poly(lactic acid);* PLGA, *poly(lactide-*co*-glycolide);* PP, *polyprolene;* SDF-1, *stromal cell-derived factor 1α;* SIS, *small intestine submucosa;* UBM, *urinary bladder matrix.*

CONCLUSION AND FUTURE DIRECTIONS

The strategy of in situ tissue regeneration has become a promising approach to safer and more convenient translational tissue engineering by avoiding the need for ex vivo manipulation of autologous cell sources; therefore it holds a great promise for the future of translational medicine. To achieve successful tissue regeneration by host stem cell recruitment, it is indispensable to direct cells to the site of injury and provide the homed cells with a local microenvironment of artificial ECM where they can proliferate and differentiate. Advances in biomaterial scaffold design and engineering are converging to enable a new generation of instructive materials that bear complex information coded in their physical, biological, and chemical structures. Elucidating the molecular complexity of cell chemotaxis, identifying both the essential molecules that dictate stem cell trafficking and their dosing criteria, improving the pharmacokinetics and biodistribution of bioactive molecules released from an implanted biomaterial, and developing products tailored to different pathologies are but a few of the challenges in the design of medical devices that conduct sufficient stem cell recruitment and robust tissue regeneration, thereby improving the benefit to individuals suffering from severely injured tissues or organs. Addressing each of these issues will lead to a future medicine in which navigational cues will be delivered to the location where they are needed and only at the levels and time at which they are required, thereby creating an innovative, biologically-based generation of clinical treatments that utilize host stem cell recruitment to regenerate injured tissues or organs in situ. For a more efficient therapeutic outcome, a better understanding of the complex interactions and pathways of the molecules that are involved in the targeted tissue regeneration is necessary.

LIST OF ACRONYMS AND ABBREVIATIONS

Ang-1 Angiopoietin-1
bFGF Basic fibroblast growth factor
BMP-2 Bone morphogenetic protein-2
ECM Extracellular matrix
ESCs Embryonic stem cells
GDF Growth differentiation factor
HA Hyaluronic acid
HGF Hepatocyte growth factor
HSCs Hematopoietic stem cells
IGF-1 Insulin-like growth factor-1
KGF Keratinocyte growth factor
MCP-3 Monocyte chemotactic protein-3
MDSCs Muscle-derived stem cells
MMP-2 Matrix metalloproteinase-2
MSCs Mesenchymal stem cells
PCL Poly(ε-caprolactone)
PDGF-BB Platelet-derived growth factor-BB
PEUU Polyester urethane urea
PGA Poly(glycolic acid)
PLA Polylactide
PLGA Poly(lactide-*co*-glycolide)

PP Polyprolene
RGD Arginine-glycine-aspartic acid
SDF-1α Stromal cell-derived factor-1α
SIS Small intestine submucosa
SP Substance P
UBM Urinary bladder matrix
VEGF Vascular endothelial growth factor

ACKNOWLEDGMENTS

This work was supported in part by the Armed Forces Institute of Regenerative Medicine (W81XWH-08-2-0032) of the Department of Defense, and the Musculoskeletal Transplant Foundation (MTF).

REFERENCES

[1] Atala A. Recent developments in tissue engineering and regenerative medicine. Curr Opin Pediatr 2006; 18:167–71.
[2] Atala A, Murphy S. Regenerative medicine. JAMA 2015;313:1413–4.
[3] Langer R. Tissue engineering. Mol Ther 2000;1:12–5.
[4] Atala A, Bauer SB, Soker S, Yoo JJ, Retik AB. Tissue-engineered autologous bladders for patients needing cystoplasty. Lancet 2006;367:1241–6.
[5] Raya-Rivera A, Esquiliano DR, Yoo JJ, Lopez-Bayghen E, Soker S, Atala A. Tissue-engineered autologous urethras for patients who need reconstruction: an observational study. Lancet 2011;377:1175–82.
[6] Raya-Rivera AM, Esquiliano D, Fierro-Pastrana R, Lopez-Bayghen E, Valencia P, Ordorica-Flores R, et al. Tissue-engineered autologous vaginal organs in patients: a pilot cohort study. Lancet 2014;384:329–36.
[7] Ossendorf C, Kaps C, Kreuz PC, Burmester GR, Sittinger M, Erggelet C. Treatment of posttraumatic and focal osteoarthritic cartilage defects of the knee with autologous polymer-based three-dimensional chondrocyte grafts: 2-year clinical results. Arthritis Res Ther 2007;9:R41.
[8] Shin'oka T, Matsumura G, Hibino N, Naito Y, Watanabe M, Konuma T, et al. Midterm clinical result of tissue-engineered vascular autografts seeded with autologous bone marrow cells. J Thorac Cardiovasc Surg 2005;129:1330–8.
[9] Burg KJ, Porter S, Kellam JF. Biomaterial developments for bone tissue engineering. Biomaterials 2000;21:2347–59.
[10] Younger EM, Chapman MW. Morbidity at bone graft donor sites. J Orthop Trauma 1989;3:192–5.
[11] Langer R. Biomaterials in drug delivery and tissue engineering: one laboratory's experience. Acc Chem Res 2000;33:94–101.
[12] Guillot PV, Cui W, Fisk NM, Polak DJ. Stem cell differentiation and expansion for clinical applications of tissue engineering. J Cell Mol Med 2007;11:935–44.
[13] Lee SJ, Van Dyke M, Atala A, Yoo JJ. Host cell mobilization for in situ tissue regeneration. Rejuvenation Res 2008;11:747–56.
[14] Ju YM, Atala A, Yoo JJ, Lee SJ. In situ regeneration of skeletal muscle tissue through host cell recruitment. Acta Biomater 2014;10:4332–9.
[15] Ko IK, Lee SJ, Atala A, Yoo JJ. In situ tissue regeneration through host stem cell recruitment. Exp Mol Med 2013;45:e57.
[16] Ko IK, Ju YM, Chen T, Atala A, Yoo JJ, Lee SJ. Combined systemic and local delivery of stem cell inducing/recruiting factors for in situ tissue regeneration. FASEB J 2011;26:158–68.

[17] Zhao J, Zhang N, Prestwich GD, Wen X. Recruitment of endogenous stem cells for tissue repair. Macromol Biosci 2008;8:836–42.
[18] Wong SP, Rowley JE, Redpath AN, Tilman JD, Fellous TG, Johnson JR. Pericytes, mesenchymal stem cells and their contributions to tissue repair. Pharmacol Ther 2015;151:107–20.
[19] Joo S, Ko IK, Atala A, Yoo JJ, Lee SJ. Amniotic fluid-derived stem cells in regenerative medicine research. Arch Pharm Res 2012;35:271–80.
[20] Asahara T, Murohara T, Sullivan A, Silver M, van der Zee R, Li T, et al. Isolation of putative progenitor endothelial cells for angiogenesis. Science 1997;275:964–7.
[21] Bartsch G, Yoo JJ, De Coppi P, Siddiqui MM, Schuch G, Pohl HG, et al. Propagation, expansion, and multilineage differentiation of human somatic stem cells from dermal progenitors. Stem Cells Dev 2005;14:337–48.
[22] De Ugarte DA, Ashjian PH, Elbarbary A, Hedrick MH. Future of fat as raw material for tissue regeneration. Ann Plastic Surg 2003;50:215–9.
[23] Deasy BM, Huard J. Gene therapy and tissue engineering based on muscle-derived stem cells. Curr Opin Mol Ther 2002;4:382–9.
[24] Gage FH. Mammalian neural stem cells. Science 2000;287:1433–8.
[25] Pfister O, Mouquet F, Jain M, Summer R, Helmes M, Fine A, et al. $CD31^-$ but not $CD31^+$ cardiac side population cells exhibit functional cardiomyogenic differentiation. Circulation Res 2005;97:52–61.
[26] Zhang Y, Bai XF, Huang CX. Hepatic stem cells: existence and origin. World J Gastroenterol 2003;9:201–4.
[27] Ries C, Egea V, Karow M, Kolb H, Jochum M, Neth P. MMP-2, MT1-MMP, and TIMP-2 are essential for the invasive capacity of human mesenchymal stem cells: differential regulation by inflammatory cytokines. Blood 2007;109:4055–63.
[28] Louridas M, Letourneau S, Lautatzis ME, Vrontakis M. Galanin is highly expressed in bone marrow mesenchymal stem cells and facilitates migration of cells both in vitro and in vivo. Biochem Biophys Res Commun 2009;390:867–71.
[29] Schenk S, Mal N, Finan A, Zhang M, Kiedrowski M, Popovic Z, et al. Monocyte chemotactic protein-3 is a myocardial mesenchymal stem cell homing factor. Stem Cells 2007;25:245–51.
[30] Zaruba MM, Theiss HD, Vallaster M, Mehl U, Brunner S, David R, et al. Synergy between CD26/DPP-IV inhibition and G-CSF improves cardiac function after acute myocardial infarction. Cell Stem Cell 2009;4:313–23.
[31] Chen FM, Ma ZW, Wang QT, Wu ZF. Gene delivery for periodontal tissue engineering: current knowledge – future possibilities. Curr Gene Ther 2009;9:248–66.
[32] Zhang G, Nakamura Y, Wang X, Hu Q, Suggs LJ, Zhang J. Controlled release of stromal cell-derived factor-1 alpha in situ increases c-kit^+ cell homing to the infarcted heart. Tissue Eng 2007;13:2063–71.
[33] Sasaki T, Fukazawa R, Ogawa S, Kanno S, Nitta T, Ochi M, et al. Stromal cell-derived factor-1alpha improves infarcted heart function through angiogenesis in mice. Pediatr Int 2007;49:966–71.
[34] Lutolf MP, Gilbert PM, Blau HM. Designing materials to direct stem-cell fate. Nature 2009;462:433–41.
[35] Richardson TP, Peters MC, Ennett AB, Mooney DJ. Polymeric system for dual growth factor delivery. Nat Biotechnol 2001;19:1029–34.
[36] Chen FM, An Y, Zhang R, Zhang M. New insights into and novel applications of release technology for periodontal reconstructive therapies. J Control Release 2011;149:92–110.
[37] Elia R, Fuegy PW, VanDelden A, Firpo MA, Prestwich GD, Peattie RA. Stimulation of in vivo angiogenesis by in situ crosslinked, dual growth factor-loaded, glycosaminoglycan hydrogels. Biomaterials 2010;31:4630–8.
[38] Borselli C, Storrie H, Benesch-Lee F, Shvartsman D, Cezar C, Lichtman JW, et al. Functional muscle regeneration with combined delivery of angiogenesis and myogenesis factors. Proc Natl Acad Sci USA 2010;107:3287–92.
[39] Lutolf MP, Hubbell JA. Synthetic biomaterials as instructive extracellular microenvironments for morphogenesis in tissue engineering. Nat Biotechnol 2005;23:47–55.

[40] Benoit DS, Anseth KS. The effect on osteoblast function of colocalized RGD and PHSRN epitopes on PEG surfaces. Biomaterials 2005;26:5209–20.
[41] Fittkau MH, Zilla P, Bezuidenhout D, Lutolf MP, Human P, Hubbell JA, et al. The selective modulation of endothelial cell mobility on RGD peptide containing surfaces by YIGSR peptides. Biomaterials 2005;26:167–74.
[42] Kurihara H, Nagamune T. Cell adhesion ability of artificial extracellular matrix proteins containing a long repetitive Arg-Gly-Asp sequence. J Biosci Bioeng 2005;100:82–7.
[43] Marletta G, Ciapetti G, Satriano C, Pagani S, Baldini N. The effect of irradiation modification and RGD sequence adsorption on the response of human osteoblasts to polycaprolactone. Biomaterials 2005;26:4793–804.
[44] Martino MM, Mochizuki M, Rothenfluh DA, Rempel SA, Hubbell JA, Barker TH. Controlling integrin specificity and stem cell differentiation in 2D and 3D environments through regulation of fibronectin domain stability. Biomaterials 2009;30:1089–97.
[45] Oharazawa H, Ibaraki N, Ohara K, Reddy VN. Inhibitory effects of Arg-Gly-Asp (RGD) peptide on cell attachment and migration in a human lens epithelial cell line. Ophthalmic Res 2005;37:191–6.
[46] Sagnella S, Anderson E, Sanabria N, Marchant RE, Kottke-Marchant K. Human endothelial cell interaction with biomimetic surfactant polymers containing peptide ligands from the heparin binding domain of fibronectin. Tissue Eng 2005;11:226–36.
[47] Salinas CN, Anseth KS. Decorin moieties tethered into PEG networks induce chondrogenesis of human mesenchymal stem cells. J Biomed Mater Res Part A 2009;90:456–64.
[48] Hermann PM, Nicol JJ, Bulloch AG, Wildering WC. RGD-dependent mechanisms in the endoneurial phagocyte response and axonal regeneration in the nervous system of the snail *Lymnaea stagnalis*. J Exp Biol 2008;211:491–501.
[49] Horii A, Wang X, Gelain F, Zhang S. Biological designer self-assembling peptide nanofiber scaffolds significantly enhance osteoblast proliferation, differentiation and 3-D migration. PLoS One 2007;2:e190.
[50] Dutta RC, Dutta AK. Cell-interactive 3D-scaffold; advances and applications. Biotechnol Adv 2009;27:334–9.
[51] Place ES, Evans ND, Stevens MM. Complexity in biomaterials for tissue engineering. Nat Mater 2009;8:457–70.
[52] Zhang L, Rakotondradany F, Myles AJ, Fenniri H, Webster TJ. Arginine-glycine-aspartic acid modified rosette nanotube-hydrogel composites for bone tissue engineering. Biomaterials 2009;30:1309–20.
[53] Galler KM, Cavender A, Yuwono V, Dong H, Shi S, Schmalz G, et al. Self-assembling peptide amphiphile nanofibers as a scaffold for dental stem cells. Tissue Eng Part A 2008;14:2051–8.
[54] Kim KL, Han DK, Park K, Song SH, Kim JY, Kim JM, et al. Enhanced dermal wound neovascularization by targeted delivery of endothelial progenitor cells using an RGD-g-PLLA scaffold. Biomaterials 2009;30:3742–8.
[55] Re'em T, Tsur-Gang O, Cohen S. The effect of immobilized RGD peptide in macroporous alginate scaffolds on TGFbeta1-induced chondrogenesis of human mesenchymal stem cells. Biomaterials 2010;31:6746–55.
[56] Chen FM, Zhang J, Zhang M, An Y, Chen F, Wu ZF. A review on endogenous regenerative technology in periodontal regenerative medicine. Biomaterials 2010;31:7892–927.
[57] Jarcho M, Kay JF, Gumaer KI, Doremus RH, Drobeck HP. Tissue, cellular and subcellular events at a bone-ceramic hydroxylapatite interface. J Bioeng 1977;1:79–92.
[58] Chung YI, Ahn KM, Jeon SH, Lee SY, Lee JH, Tae G. Enhanced bone regeneration with BMP-2 loaded functional nanoparticle-hydrogel complex. J Control Release 2007;121:91–9.
[59] Osathanon T, Linnes ML, Rajachar RM, Ratner BD, Somerman MJ, Giachelli CM. Microporous nanofibrous fibrin-based scaffolds for bone tissue engineering. Biomaterials 2008;29:4091–9.
[60] Suzuki Y, Tanihara M, Suzuki K, Saitou A, Sufan W, Nishimura Y. Alginate hydrogel linked with synthetic oligopeptide derived from BMP-2 allows ectopic osteoinduction in vivo. J Biomed Mater Res 2000;50: 405–9.

[61] Kodama N, Nagata M, Tabata Y, Ozeki M, Ninomiya T, Takagi R. A local bone anabolic effect of rhFGF2-impregnated gelatin hydrogel by promoting cell proliferation and coordinating osteoblastic differentiation. Bone 2009;44:699–707.
[62] Ginebra MP, Traykova T, Planell JA. Calcium phosphate cements as bone drug delivery systems: a review. J Control Release 2006;113:102–10.
[63] Jansen JA, Vehof JW, Ruhe PQ, Kroeze-Deutman H, Kuboki Y, Takita H, et al. Growth factor-loaded scaffolds for bone engineering. J Control Release 2005;101:127–36.
[64] Seeherman H, Wozney JM. Delivery of bone morphogenetic proteins for orthopedic tissue regeneration. Cytokine Growth Factor Rev 2005;16:329–45.
[65] Erggelet C, Endres M, Neumann K, Morawietz L, Ringe J, Haberstroh K, et al. Formation of cartilage repair tissue in articular cartilage defects pretreated with microfracture and covered with cell-free polymer-based implants. J Orthop Res 2009;27:1353–60.
[66] Lee CH, Cook JL, Mendelson A, Moioli EK, Yao H, Mao JJ. Regeneration of the articular surface of the rabbit synovial joint by cell homing: a proof of concept study. Lancet 2010;376:440–8.
[67] Huard J, Li Y, Fu FH. Muscle injuries and repair: current trends in research. J Bone Joint Surg Am 2002;84-A:822–32.
[68] Le Grand F, Rudnicki M. Satellite and stem cells in muscle growth and repair. Development 2007;134:3953–7.
[69] Sacco A, Doyonnas R, Kraft P, Vitorovic S, Blau HM. Self-renewal and expansion of single transplanted muscle stem cells. Nature 2008;456:502–6.
[70] Qu-Petersen Z, Deasy B, Jankowski R, Ikezawa M, Cummins J, Pruchnic R, et al. Identification of a novel population of muscle stem cells in mice: potential for muscle regeneration. J Cell Biol 2002;157:851–64.
[71] Sun D, Martinez CO, Ochoa O, Ruiz-Willhite L, Bonilla JR, Centonze VE, et al. Bone marrow-derived cell regulation of skeletal muscle regeneration. FASEB J 2009;23:382–95.
[72] Crisan M, Yap S, Casteilla L, Chen CW, Corselli M, Park TS, et al. A perivascular origin for mesenchymal stem cells in multiple human organs. Cell Stem Cell 2008;3:301–13.
[73] Polesskaya A, Seale P, Rudnicki MA. Wnt signaling induces the myogenic specification of resident $CD45^+$ adult stem cells during muscle regeneration. Cell 2003;113:841–52.
[74] LaBarge MA, Blau HM. Biological progression from adult bone marrow to mononucleate muscle stem cell to multinucleate muscle fiber in response to injury. Cell 2002;111:589–601.
[75] Kin S, Hagiwara A, Nakase Y, Kuriu Y, Nakashima S, Yoshikawa T, et al. Regeneration of skeletal muscle using in situ tissue engineering on an acellular collagen sponge scaffold in a rabbit model. ASAIO J 2007;53:506–13.
[76] Gomez G, Korkiakoski S, Gonzalez MM, Lansman S, Ella V, Salo T, et al. Effect of FGF and polylactide scaffolds on calvarial bone healing with growth factor on biodegradable polymer scaffolds. J Craniofac Surg 2006;17:935–42.
[77] Woodruff MA, Rath SN, Susanto E, Haupt LM, Hutmacher DW, Nurcombe V, et al. Sustained release and osteogenic potential of heparan sulfate-doped fibrin glue scaffolds within a rat cranial model. J Mol Histol 2007;38:425–33.
[78] Mabilleau G, Aguado E, Stancu IC, Cincu C, Basle MF, Chappard D. Effects of FGF-2 release from a hydrogel polymer on bone mass and microarchitecture. Biomaterials 2008;29:1593–600.
[79] Nakashima S, Nakamura T, Han L, Miyagawa K, Yoshikawa T, Sakakura C, et al. Experimental biliary reconstruction with an artificial bile duct using in situ tissue engineering technique. Inflamm Regen 2007;27:579–85.
[80] Iwai S, Sawa Y, Taketani S, Torikai K, Hirakawa K, Matsuda H. Novel tissue-engineered biodegradable material for reconstruction of vascular wall. Ann Thorac Surg 2005;80:1821–7.
[81] Yokota T, Ichikawa H, Matsumiya G, Kuratani T, Sakaguchi T, Iwai S, et al. In situ tissue regeneration using a novel tissue-engineered, small-caliber vascular graft without cell seeding. J Thorac Cardiovasc Surg 2008;136:900–7.

[82] Huynh T, Abraham G, Murray J, Brockbank K, Hagen PO, Sullivan S. Remodeling of an acellular collagen graft into a physiologically responsive neovessel. Nat Biotechnol 1999;17:1083–6.
[83] Fujimoto KL, Guan J, Oshima H, Sakai T, Wagner WR. In vivo evaluation of a porous, elastic, biodegradable patch for reconstructive cardiac procedures. Ann Thorac Surg 2007;83:648–54.
[84] Landa N, Miller L, Feinberg MS, Holbova R, Shachar M, Freeman I, et al. Effect of injectable alginate implant on cardiac remodeling and function after recent and old infarcts in rat. Circulation 2008;117:1388–96.
[85] Kubo M, Imai S, Fujimiya M, Isoya E, Ando K, Mimura T, et al. Exogenous collagen-enhanced recruitment of mesenchymal stem cells during rabbit articular cartilage repair. Acta Orthop 2007;78:845–55.
[86] Dahms SE, Piechota HJ, Dahiya R, Gleason CA, Hohenfellner M, Tanagho EA. Bladder acellular matrix graft in rats: its neurophysiologic properties and mRNA expression of growth factors TGF-alpha and TGF-beta. Neurourol Urodyn 1998;17:37–54.
[87] Urita Y, Komuro H, Chen G, Shinya M, Kaneko S, Kaneko M, et al. Regeneration of the esophagus using gastric acellular matrix: an experimental study in a rat model. Pediatr Surg Int 2007;23:21–6.
[88] Hiraoka Y, Yamashiro H, Yasuda K, Kimura Y, Inamoto T, Tabata Y. In situ regeneration of adipose tissue in rat fat pad by combining a collagen scaffold with gelatin microspheres containing basic fibroblast growth factor. Tissue Eng 2006;12:1475–87.
[89] Nakahara T, Nakamura T, Kobayashi E, Inoue M, Shigeno K, Tabata Y, et al. Novel approach to regeneration of periodontal tissues based on in situ tissue engineering: effects of controlled release of basic fibroblast growth factor from a sandwich membrane. Tissue Eng 2003;9:153–62.
[90] Herberg S, Siedler M, Pippig S, Schuetz A, Dony C, Kim C-K, et al. Development of an injectable composite as a carrier for growth factor-enhanced periodeontal regeneration. J Clin Periodontol 2008;35:976–84.
[91] Boucard N, Viton C, Agay D, Mari E, Roger T, Chancerelle Y, et al. The use of physical hydrogels of chitosan for skin regeneration following third-degree burns. Biomaterials 2007;28:3478–88.
[92] Abbushi A, Endres M, Cabraja M, Kroppenstedt SN, Thomale UW, Sittinger M, et al. Regeneration of intervertebral disc tissue by resorbable cell-free polyglycolic acid-based implants in a rabbit model of disc degeneration. Spine 2008;33:1527–32.
[93] Hori Y, Nakamura T, Matsumoto K, Kurokawa Y, Satomi S, Shimizu Y. Experimental study on in situ tissue engineering of the stomach by an acellular collagen sponge scaffold graft. ASAIO J 2001;47:206–10.

PART 2

ENDOGENOUS CELL SOURCES

CHAPTER

STEM CELL HOMING

2

M.Z. Ratajczak, A. Abdelbaset-Ismail
Stem Cell Institute, James Graham Brown Cancer Center

CHAPTER OUTLINE

INTRODUCTION

Stem cell homing is a process whereby stem cells respond to gradients of chemoattractants by migrating up these gradients and lodging within specific tissue areas [1–3]. This process was initially described for hematopoietic stem cells (HSCs), which migrate after transplantation from peripheral blood (PB) to stem cell niches located in the bone marrow (BM) microenvironment. Stem cell niches provide HSCs with the optimal microenvironment for their biological functions. In BM niches, HSCs are retained, remain quiescent, respond to external cues, and, if necessary, undergo symmetric or asymmetric cell divisions [1,4–6].

Generally, two types of stem cell niches are distinguishable in the BM microenvironment: the osteoblastic niche, located close to the trabecular bone, and the vascular niche, which is associated with the endothelium lining BM sinusoids [7–11]. It has been postulated that, while osteoblastic niches are populated by HSCs that are more quiescent, endothelial niches contain stem cells that are more advanced in the cell cycle. On the other hand, recent morphological studies on the BM microenvironment suggest that often both types of niches overlap anatomically, and it is difficult to treat them as separate niches.

The major mechanism that retains HSCs in their niches in the BM microenvironment involves interaction of the CXCR4 receptor with α-chemokine stromal-derived factor 1 (SDF-1) and the α1β4 integrin receptor (VLA-4) with vascular adhesion molecule 1 (VCAM-1) [4,5,12–22]. While CXCR4 and VLA-4 receptors are expressed on the surface of HSCs, SDF-1 and VCAM-1 are expressed on the

In Situ Tissue Regeneration. http://dx.doi.org/10.1016/B978-0-12-802225-2.00002-7

surface of cells lining the osteoblastic and endothelial niches. Evidence has accumulated that retention of HSCs in BM is an active process that counteracts the chemotactic gradient of sphingosine-1-phosphate (S1P), which is already very steep between PB and BM under steady-state conditions and pulls these cells in the opposite direction [3,23–25].

In a broader sense of this term, homing mechanisms are also involved in migration of other types of circulating non-HSCs, such as mesenchymal stem cells (MSCs), endothelial progenitors (EPCs), or very small embryonic-like stem cells (VSELs), to damaged tissues, where these cells may play some role in local repair [26–32].

Homing is orchestrated by gradients of chemotactic factors that chemoattract stem cells via activation of receptors for these factors that are expressed on the surface of migrating cells. The list of chemoattractants for HSCs is limited, and so far it has been demonstrated that HSCs respond only to gradients of SDF-1, S1P, ceramide-1-phosphate (C1P), certain extracellular nucleotides, such as adenosine triphosphate (ATP) and uridine triphosphate (UTP), as well as certain ions, such as Ca^{2+} and H^{+} [26,33–45].

Other types of stem cells, such as MSCs, EPCs, and VSELs, respond also to other factors, such as hepatocyte growth factor (HGF) or vascular endothelial growth factor (VEGF), and to a broader repertoire of bioactive lipids, including lysophosphatidylcholine (LPC) and its derivative, lysophosphatidic acid (LPA) [26,32].

HOMING OF HEMATOPOIETIC STEM CELLS TO BONE MARROW NICHES

As mentioned above, migration and BM homing of HSCs after transplantation precedes their final engraftment and is a key factor in successful outcomes for hematopoietic transplantation. The major role in homing to BM has been assigned to gradients of the α-chemokine SDF-1, which, from a historical point of view, was reported as the first potent chemotactic factor for HSCs. However, the activity of this chemokine against HSCs has always been demonstrated in assays in vitro at very high, unphysiological doses [46–48]. It has been reported that SDF-1 mRNA increases in the BM microenvironment after myeloablative conditioning for transplantation in an hypoxia inducible factor-1 alpha-dependent manner [48]. On the other hand, myeloablative conditioning for transplant by radiochemotherapy induces a proteolytic microenvironment in this tissue [48–51]. As a peptide, SDF-1 is susceptible to proteolytic digestion by several enzymes released from myeloid cells that become damaged in BM during myeloablative conditioning [48,51,52].

This potential decrease in SDF-1 protein level in the BM microenvironment after conditioning for transplantation is somewhat mitigated by the release of several factors, such as ComC cleavage fragments (C3a and $_{desArg}$C3a), cathelicidin (LL-37), and β2-defensin released by BM stromal cells, as well as other molecules, such as hyaluronic acid, fibronectin, and soluble vascular cell adhesion molecule 1 (VCAM-1), intercellular cell adhesion molecule 1, and urokinase receptor (uPAR), which in toto may enhance the responsiveness of hematopoietic stem/progenitor cells (HSPCs)to a shallow SDF-1 gradient [1,4,9,19,37,48,50,51,53–62]. This phenomenon is known in the literature as a priming effect on an SDF-1 gradient and significantly compensates for any potential decreases in SDF-1 homing gradient due to the induction of a proteolytic microenvironment in BM (Fig. 2.1).

While there is no doubt that the SDF-1–CXCR4 axis plays an important role in retention of HSCs in BM niches, and that disruption of this interaction, as seen, for example, after administration of small molecules that block the CXCR4 receptor (eg, AMD3100 or plerixafor) results in the egress of HSCs

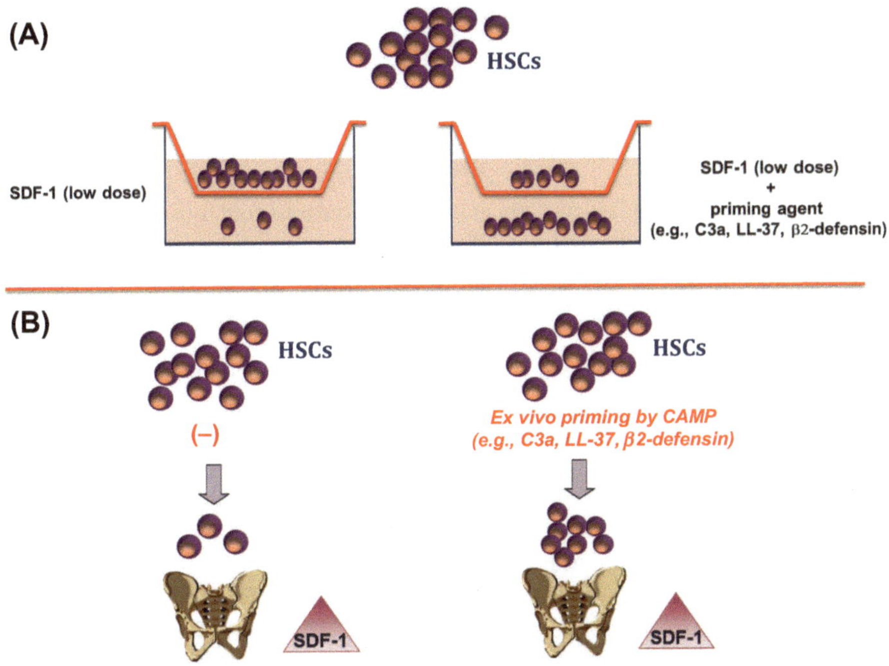

FIGURE 2.1 A priming effect increases the responsiveness of HSCs to shallow SDF-1 gradients.

The overall scheme of chemotactic assays performed in the Transwell system to evaluate the HSPC priming phenomenon (Panel A). In the presence of a priming agent [eg, cationic antimicrobial peptides (CAMPs), such as C3a, cathelicidin (LL-37), or β2-defensin], HSPCs respond more robustly to low doses of SDF-1. The same priming phenomenon enhances HSC homing in vivo (Panel B).

from BM into PB (mobilization), its role in homing is more complicated [12,63]. Specifically, evidence has accumulated that HSCs also home to the BM in an SDF-1–CXCR4 axis-independent manner. In support of this notion, (1) CXCR4$^{-/-}$ fetal liver HSCs may still home to BM despite the lack of CXCR4 receptor on these cells [4]; (2) homing of murine HSCs made refractory to SDF-1 by incubation and coinjection with a CXCR4 receptor antagonist is normal or only mildly reduced [47]; and (3) HSCs in which CXCR4 has been knocked down by means of an SDF-1 intrakine strategy are still able to engraft after transplantation in a myeloablated host [64]. All of these observations prompt us to look for other homing factors that could compensate for an SDF-1 deficiency.

As mentioned above, the list of homing factors for HSCs is very short. So far, only a few factors besides SDF-1 have been identified that induce chemotactic activity against human and murine HSCs, and SDF-1 as a chemokine is unique in this respect [65–69]. Specifically, while more than 25 different cytokines endowed with chemotactic activity (chemokines) have been described, SDF-1 is the only member of the chemokine family that chemoattracts HSCs [46,47,67,70]. All other chemokines are potent chemoattractants for more differentiated cells from hematopoietic and lymphatic lineages but are unable to chemoattract HSCs. Moreover, to demonstrate SDF-1 chemotactic activity in routine chemotactic assays in vitro, this chemokine has to be employed at 100-fold higher doses than under physiological conditions in compartments such as PB [46–48,71]. However, its biological effects are enhanced by certain factors, due to the abovementioned priming phenomenon (Fig. 2.1).

In contrast to SDF-1, bioactive phosphosphingolipids such as S1P and C1P are already potent chemoattractants for HSCs at physiological concentrations, such as those measured in PB [23,25,28,48,49,72–75]. Interestingly, in contrast to S1P and C1P, other bioactive lipids, including LPA and LPC, do not exhibit chemotactic activity against HSCs. In fact, HSCs freshly isolated from BM respond much better to an S1P or C1P gradient at the concentrations found in PB plasma than to SDF-1 at its physiological PB plasma concentrations [28,49].

Nevertheless, the responsiveness of HSCs to S1P and C1P gradients depends on the functional state of the corresponding receptors. While there are five S1P-binding receptors ($S1P_{1\text{-}5}R$) described, the receptor/s for C1P are not yet identified [76]. It is well known that S1P receptors and, most likely, putative C1P receptors are rapidly internalized from the cell surface after ligand binding [28,77,78]. This phenomenon renders HSCs unresponsive to S1P and C1P gradients and is important because S1P and C1P are already present at high concentrations in PB plasma. Therefore HSCs isolated from murine or human PB or human HSCs isolated from umbilical cord blood (UCB) are desensitized in their responsiveness to S1P and C1P gradients because the corresponding receptors are internalized [3].

Another group of factors besides SDF-1, S1P, and C1P that have been shown to be able to chemoattract HSCs are extracellular nucleotides (eg, ATP and UTP). This group of potential chemoattractants, like S1P and C1P, is very active against HSCs freshly isolated from the BM and displays significantly lower chemotactic activity for HSCs isolated from PB or UCB [39,43,79]. Again, this decrease in responsiveness of HSCs could be explained by desensitization and internalization of specific receptors on HSCs because these cells are exposed to high concentrations of extracellular nucleotides present in PB or UCB plasma.

CHANGES IN THE BONE MARROW LEVEL OF CHEMOATTRACTANTS FOR HEMATOPOIETIC STEM CELLS

The major role of myeloablative radio and/or chemotherapy conditioning before transplantation of HSCs is to destroy pathological hematopoiesis and prepare the BM microenvironment for colonization by transplanted HSCs. Therefore one of the important mechanisms in the homing process is local upregulation of homing chemotactic factors for these cells.

Since myeloablative treatment inflicts damage on the BM microenvironment, several factors emerge as a response to injury in BM [42,73,80–83]. First, damage to BM-residing myeloid cells results in the release of several proteolytic enzymes, including metalloproteinases 2 and 9, cathepsins G and K, as well as elastase, which digest peptide-based molecules in the BM microenvironment [84]. As mentioned above, this is one of the factors limiting an increase in SDF-1 protein level, despite its upregulation at the mRNA level. Tissue injury by conditioning for transplantation leads not only to release of proteolytic enzymes from damaged monocytes and granulocytes, but also exposure of the neoepitope on the surface of damaged cells activates in the BM microenvironment three developmentally ancient proteolytic cascades: the complement cascade (ComC), the coagulation cascade (CoaC), and the fibrynolytic cascade (FibC) [85,86]. Some cleavage fragments of these cascades, such as ComC-derived C3a, $_{desArg}$C3a, and C5bC9; CoaC-derived thrombin; and FibC-derived soluble uPAR have been described as modulating the migration of HSCs [19,31,48,87–93]. However, the more detailed role of these factors in HSC homing and the mutual interactions of these cascades in this process require further study.

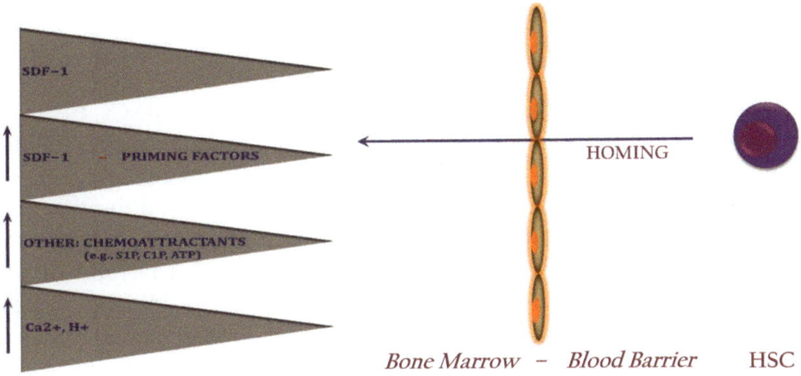

FIGURE 2.2 The proposed major mechanism underlying the processes of homing of HSCs.

HSCs infused into blood respond to a gradient of SDF-1 between bone marrow and blood; however, conditioning for transplantation by chemoradiotherapy may also upregulate other homing factors, such as S1P and C1P, and increase the levels of extracellular nucleotides (ATP and UTP). In addition, LL-37 and β2-defensin released from BM stromal cells and osteoblasts increase the responsiveness of HSCs to an SDF-1 gradient by a priming mechanism. Homing is also regulated by Ca^{2+} and H^+ gradients in the BM microenvironment. Most likely, there are other unidentified factors involved in the homing process.

Exposure of the hematopoietic microenvironment to radiochemotherapy also upregulates the expression of certain priming factors, such as LL-37 and β2-defensin, in BM [50,61,94]. It has been demonstrated that these factors are released from irradiated BM stromal cells. Moreover, the proteolytic microenvironment in BM induced by conditioning therapy leads to the release of phosphosphingolipids (S1P and C1P) and nucleotides (ATP and UTP) from the damaged and leaky cells. All these factors, together with SDF-1 and SDF-1 priming factors (eg, C3a, $_{desArg}$C3a, LL-37, and β2-defensin), provide a homing gradient for HSCs (Fig. 2.2). However, in addition to these known factors, it is very likely that other not-yet-identified factors also exist. To find support for the involvement of these other factors in homing, we performed transplants of CXCR4-deficient HSCs into sphingosine phosphate kinase 1-deficient (Sphk1-KO) mice [95]. In addition, before transplantation, these cells were desensitized in their responsiveness to high doses of ATP and UTP by preincubation in a medium containing high concentrations of both nucleotides. By employing this strategy, we targeted all three potential homing axes, including SDF-1–CXCR4, S1P–$S1P_{1-5}$R, and ATP–P2Y receptor axes. We observed that HSCs transplanted in this model had a lower engraftment and homing efficiency but were still able to establish chimerism in transplanted animals. Further studies are needed to identify these potential new factors facilitating homing as well as to better address the role of $C2a^+$- and H^+-sensing receptors in this model of engraftment [33,41].

HOMING OF NONHEMATOPOIETIC STEM CELLS TO DAMAGED ORGANS

As mentioned at the beginning of this chapter, the term "stem cell homing" was initially coined for the homing of HSCs to BM niches. However, it has also been recently employed in a much broader context to describe a similar process when other types of normal stem cells navigate in the tissues by sensing chemotactic gradients that direct them to lodge in new locations. The best example is the homing of stem cells injected intravenously as therapy for damaged organs (eg, heart, kidney, or liver) [96–100].

Several different types of stem cells have been described, including MSCs, EPCs, amniotic fluid-derived stem cells, adipose tissue-derived stem cells, and VSELs that are employed intravenously to treat damaged organs [96,97,101–105]. Like HSCs, all of these stem cells respond to SDF-1, S1P, C1P, ATP, and UTP gradients [26]. However, some of them may respond to other chemoattractants that do not attract HSCs (eg, VEGF, HGF, or LIF) [106]. MSCs and EPCs, as well as adipose tissue-derived stem cells, respond also to a broader panel of chemokines [32,107,108]. All of these chemotactic factors can be upregulated in damaged hypoxic tissues [26]. Additional strategies have also been developed to upregulate their expression in various organs for the optimal recruitment and homing of stem cells.

To enhance the homing of circulating stem cells to myocardium, injectable hydrogels containing SDF-1 and angiogenic peptides, which are injected directly into damaged heart tissue, have been employed [109]. This strategy was found to be efficient, as this combination injected into myocardium established new vessels, decreased fibrosis, and improved the function of heart damaged by chronic infarction. A similar strategy of controlled local delivery of fibroblast growth factor 1 and neuregulin 1 was effective in inducing heart tissue remodeling following rat myocardial infarction, a process that involved recruitment and homing of stem cells [110]. To enhance homing of MSCs to damaged myocardium, injectable microrods releasing proteins of the insulin-like growth factor family have also been employed with good results [111].

On the other hand, to enhance the homing of MSCs injected intravenously into kidney, a strategy of nondestructive pulsed focused ultrasound (pFUS) exposure, which mimics the mechanical effect of the ultrasound influence on tissues and leads to transient upregulation of the cytokines, integrins, and growth factors involved in homing, has been developed. Such a pFUS-induced microenvironment in the kidney recruited more MSC cells than the collateral kidney unexposed to pFUS [112].

A similar strategy has also been employed in a model of kidney damage using ultrasound contrast agent microbubbles that produce intense echoes and enhance blood-to-tissue contrast in clinical ultrasonography [113]. Ultrasound destruction of these microbubbles under ultrasonic irradiation induced a pro-homing environment in the kidney exposed to this procedure compared with the collateral kidney. In another approach, SDF-1-loaded microbubbles were developed that, after intravenous injection, were exposed to ultrasound destruction that locally increased the SDF-1 homing gradient for MSCs [114]. On the other hand, homing of MSCs into liver damaged by partial hepatectomy in rats was improved by preoperative administration of resveratrol [115].

In order to improve the homing of stem cells to damaged tissues, other strategies based on direct manipulation of transplanted cells have also been employed. For example, it has been demonstrated that overexpression of CXCR4 in MSCs enhances their homing to damaged myocardium or kidney [13,16,38]. Similarly, preconditioning of MSCs before infusion by exposing them to hypoxia has a beneficial effect on subsequent homing to infracted myocardium [116,117].

The most important strategies to enhance homing of non-HSCs in damaged myocardium kidney or liver are depicted in Fig. 2.3.

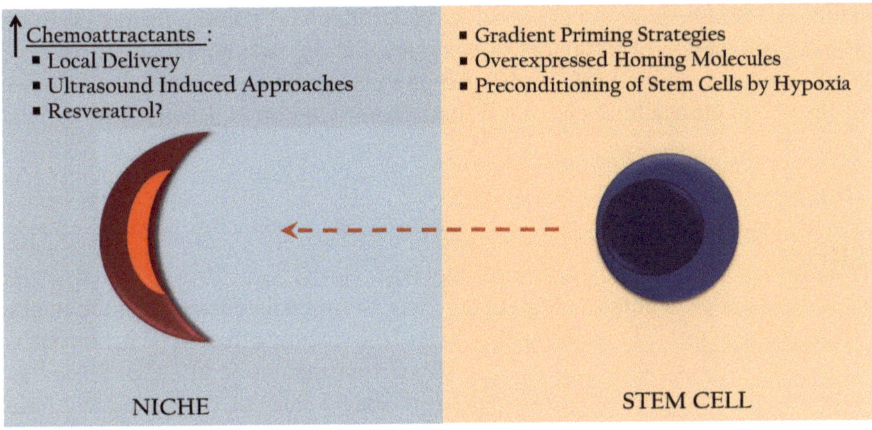

FIGURE 2.3 Proposed strategies to enhance homing of stem cells to damaged organs.

Right panel. Stem cell homing may be enhanced by overexpression of homing molecules on the surface of stem cells (eg, CXCR4), preconditioning with hypoxia, or exposure to priming factors that increase chemotactic responsiveness to an SDF-1 gradient. **Left panel**. Homing of stem cells could also be enhanced by modulating the stem cell niche by local delivery of chemoattractants, ultrasound-induced upregulation of chemotactic factors, or pharmacological modulation of stem cell niche biology (eg, with resveratrol).

TO MODULATE HOMING GRADIENTS AS A STRATEGY TO DELIVER THERAPEUTIC STEM CELLS TO THE DAMAGED ORGANS

One of the problems in regenerative medicine is delivery of cells that are employed as therapeutics to the injured organs (eg, heart). One of the possible routes is cell infusion into PB (eg, into coronary arteries) with hope that infused cells will find their way home and lodge in the damaged tissues and subsequently resume a proper role in restoration of function and perhaps even structure of affected by pathological process organ. Another possibility is a delivery of therapeutic cells directly to the tissue by using special catheters or needles (eg, by employing NOGA catheter for infarcted myocardium). It is obvious that in both of these cases, homing factors are playing a crucial role in attraction and retention of cells employed for therapeutic purposes.

However, the ideal situation would be to maintain a proper microenvironment in the damaged areas so that cells will not only efficiently settle down in response to homing/retention signals but also would be able to show their full regenerative potential [26,33–45]. Therefore another important therapeutic step would be to modify the pro-homing microenvironment so that it will also maintain its pro-regenerative potential.

To support this notion, infarcted myocardium in addition to homing signals may be enriched, for example, in: (1) enzymes that may degrade homing peptides (eg, metalloproteinases that would affect integrity of peptide-based homing factors, such as chemokines and growth factors); (2) some lipolytic enzymes that may affect gradient of pro-homing bioactive lipids; and (3) ectonucleosidases that may process pro-homing gradients of extracellular nucleotides.

Based on this, it would be important to consider upregulation of homing factors in damaged tissues in parallel with a combination of inhibitors of enzymes that degrade peptides-, bioactive lipids-, and extracellular nucleotides-degrading [26,38–40]. An interesting strategy, would also be downregulation of heme-oxyganse-1, an intracellular enzyme that, as recently reported, is a negative regulator of stem cell migration [118].

CONCLUSIONS

Efficient homing of stem cells employed in therapy has an immediate impact on the final outcome of the therapy. Efficient homing will also allow the desired therapeutic effect to be achieved using a lower number of stem cells. This is important, for example, in transplantation of UCB. Since the number of HSCs in UCB is limited and often insufficient to transplant into an adult recipient, strategies that enhance homing (seeding efficiency of HSCs to BM) and subsequent engraftment of UCB-derived HSCs are vital for positive clinical outcomes [48]. In the near future, we can expect that novel and more powerful strategies will be developed to enhance stem cell homing that target both the local niche and the stem cells employed for treatment.

ACKNOWLEDGMENTS

This work was supported by NIH grants 2R01 DK074720 and R01HL112788 and the Stella and Henry Endowment to MZR.

REFERENCES

[1] Bonig H, Priestley GV, Oehler V, Papayannopoulou T. Hematopoietic progenitor cells (HPC) from mobilized peripheral blood display enhanced migration and marrow homing compared to steady-state bone marrow HPC. Exp Hematol 2007;35(2):326–34.

[2] Li L, Xie T. Stem cell niche: structure and function. Annu Rev Cell Dev Biol 2005;21:605–31.

[3] Ratajczak MZ, Suszynska M, Borkowska S, Ratajczak J, Schneider G. The role of sphingosine-1 phosphate and ceramide-1 phosphate in trafficking of normal stem cells and cancer cells. Expert Opin Ther Targets 2014;18(1):95–107.

[4] Ma Q, Jones D, Springer TA. The chemokine receptor CXCR4 is required for the retention of B lineage and granulocytic precursors within the bone marrow microenvironment. Immunity 1999;10(4):463–71.

[5] Ratajczak MZ, Kim C, Janowska-Wieczorek A, Ratajczak J. The expanding family of bone marrow homing factors for hematopoietic stem cells: stromal derived factor 1 is not the only player in the game. The Scientific World Journal 2012;2012:758512.

[6] Ratajczak MZ, Kim C, Ratajczak J, Janowska-Wieczorek A. Innate immunity as orchestrator of bone marrow homing for hematopoietic stem/progenitor cells. Adv Exp Med Biol 2013;735:219–32.

[7] Arai F, Hirao A, Ohmura M, Sato H, Matsuoka S, Takubo K, et al. Tie2/angiopoietin-1 signaling regulates hematopoietic stem cell quiescence in the bone marrow niche. Cell 2004;118(2):149–61.

[8] Guerrouahen BS, Al-Hijji I, Tabrizi AR. Osteoblastic and vascular endothelial niches, their control on normal hematopoietic stem cells, and their consequences on the development of leukemia. Stem Cells Int 2011;2011:375857.

[9] Levesque JP, Helwani FM, Winkler IG. The endosteal 'osteoblastic' niche and its role in hematopoietic stem cell homing and mobilization. Leukemia 2010;24(12):1979–92.

[10] Wilson A, Oser GM, Jaworski M, Blanco-Bose WE, Laurenti E, Adolphe C, et al. Dormant and self-renewing hematopoietic stem cells and their niches. Ann NY Acad Sci 2007;1106:64–75.

[11] Zhang J, Li L. Stem cell niche: microenvironment and beyond. J Biol Chem 2008;283(15):9499–503.

[12] Broxmeyer HE, Orschell CM, Clapp DW, Hangoc G, Cooper S, Plett PA, et al. Rapid mobilization of murine and human hematopoietic stem and progenitor cells with AMD3100, a CXCR4 antagonist. J Exp Med 2005;201(8):1307–18.

[13] Cao Z, Zhang G, Wang F, Liu H, Liu L, Han Y, et al. Protective effects of mesenchymal stem cells with CXCR4 up-regulation in a rat renal transplantation model. PLoS One 2013;8(12):e82949.

[14] Kortesidis A, Zannettino A, Isenmann S, Shi S, Lapidot T, Gronthos S. Stromal-derived factor-1 promotes the growth, survival, and development of human bone marrow stromal stem cells. Blood 2005;105(10):3793–801.

[15] Levesque JP, Takamatsu Y, Nilsson SK, Haylock DN, Simmons PJ. Vascular cell adhesion molecule-1 (CD106) is cleaved by neutrophil proteases in the bone marrow following hematopoietic progenitor cell mobilization by granulocyte colony-stimulating factor. Blood 2001;98(5):1289–97.

[16] Liu N, Patzak A, Zhang J. CXCR4-overexpressing bone marrow-derived mesenchymal stem cells improve repair of acute kidney injury. Am J Physiol Renal Physiol 2013;305(7):F1064–73.

[17] Neiva K, Sun YX, Taichman RS. The role of osteoblasts in regulating hematopoietic stem cell activity and tumor metastasis. Braz J Med Biol Res 2005;38(10):1449–54.

[18] Peled A, Grabovsky V, Habler L, Sandbank J, Arenzana-Seisdedos F, Petit I, et al. The chemokine SDF-1 stimulates integrin-mediated arrest of CD34(+) cells on vascular endothelium under shear flow. J Clin Invest 1999;104(9):1199–211.

[19] Ratajczak MZ, Reca R, Wysoczynski M, Yan J, Ratajczak J. Modulation of the SDF-1-CXCR4 axis by the third complement component (C3)–implications for trafficking of CXCR4+ stem cells. Exp Hematol 2006;34(8):986–95.

[20] Ratajczak MZ, Serwin K, Schneider G. Innate immunity derived factors as external modulators of the CXCL12-CXCR4 axis and their role in stem cell homing and mobilization. Theranostics 2013;3(1):3–10.

[21] Rettig MP, Ansstas G, DiPersio JF. Mobilization of hematopoietic stem and progenitor cells using inhibitors of CXCR4 and VLA-4. Leukemia 2012;26(1):34–53.

[22] Sharma M, Afrin F, Satija N, Tripathi RP, Gangenahalli GU. Stromal-derived factor-1/CXCR4 signaling: indispensable role in homing and engraftment of hematopoietic stem cells in bone marrow. Stem Cells Dev 2011;20(6):933–46.

[23] Fyrst H, Saba JD. An update on sphingosine-1-phosphate and other sphingolipid mediators. Nat Chem Biol 2010;6(7):489–97.

[24] Mierzejewska K, Klyachkin YM, Ratajczak J, Abdel-Latif A, Kucia M, Ratajczak MZ. Sphingosine-1-phosphate-mediated mobilization of hematopoietic stem/progenitor cells during intravascular hemolysis requires attenuation of SDF-1-CXCR4 retention signaling in bone marrow. Biomed Res Int 2013;2013 :814549.

[25] Ratajczak MZ, Lee H, Wysoczynski M, Wan W, Marlicz W, Laughlin MJ, et al. Novel insight into stem cell mobilization-plasma sphingosine-1-phosphate is a major chemoattractant that directs the egress of hematopoietic stem progenitor cells from the bone marrow and its level in peripheral blood increases during mobilization due to activation of complement cascade/membrane attack complex. Leukemia 2010;24(5):976–85.

[26] Kim C, Schneider G, Abdel-Latif A, Mierzejewska K, Sunkara M, Borkowska S, et al. Ceramide-1-phosphate regulates migration of multipotent stromal cells and endothelial progenitor cells–implications for tissue regeneration. Stem Cells 2013;31(3):500–10.

[27] Kucia M, Zhang YP, Reca R, Wysoczynski M, Machalinski B, Majka M, et al. Cells enriched in markers of neural tissue-committed stem cells reside in the bone marrow and are mobilized into the peripheral blood following stroke. Leukemia 2006;20(1):18–28.

[28] Ratajczak MZ, Kim CH, Abdel-Latif A, Schneider G, Kucia M, Morris AJ, et al. A novel perspective on stem cell homing and mobilization: review on bioactive lipids as potent chemoattractants and cationic peptides as underappreciated modulators of responsiveness to SDF-1 gradients. Leukemia 2012;26(1):63–72.

[29] Ratajczak MZ, Shin DM, Liu R, Mierzejewska K, Ratajczak J, Kucia M, et al. Very small embryonic/epiblast-like stem cells (VSELs) and their potential role in aging and organ rejuvenation–an update and comparison to other primitive small stem cells isolated from adult tissues. Aging 2012;4(4):235–46.

[30] Wojakowski W, Landmesser U, Bachowski R, Jadczyk T, Tendera M. Mobilization of stem and progenitor cells in cardiovascular diseases. Leukemia 2012;26(1):23–33.

[31] Wojakowski W, Tendera M, Kucia M, Zuba-Surma E, Paczkowska E, Ciosek J, et al. Mobilization of bone marrow-derived Oct-4+ SSEA-4+ very small embryonic-like stem cells in patients with acute myocardial infarction. J Am Coll Cardiol 2009;53(1):1–9.

[32] Kim C, Liu R, Kucia M, Ratajczak MZ. New evidence that the bioactive lipid ceramide-1-phosphate (C1P) is a potent chemoattractant for mesenchymal stromal cells (MSC), endothelial progenitor cells (EPCs.) and very small embryonic-like stem cells (VSELs), demonstrating its potential involvement in tissue/organ repair and angiogenesis. Blood 2011;118:1028.

[33] Adams GB, Chabner KT, Alley IR, Olson DP, Szczepiorkowski ZM, Poznansky MC, et al. Stem cell engraftment at the endosteal niche is specified by the calcium-sensing receptor. Nature 2006;439(7076):599–603.

[34] Arana L, Gangoiti P, Ouro A, Trueba M, Gomez-Munoz A. Ceramide and ceramide 1-phosphate in health and disease. Lipids Health Dis 2010;9:15.

[35] Golan K, Vagima Y, Ludin A, Itkin T, Cohen-Gur S, Kalinkovich A, et al. S1P promotes murine progenitor cell egress and mobilization via S1P1-mediated ROS signaling and SDF-1 release. Blood 2012;119(11):2478–88.

[36] Granado MH, Gangoiti P, Ouro A, Arana L, Gonzalez M, Trueba M, et al. Ceramide 1-phosphate (C1P) promotes cell migration involvement of a specific C1P receptor. Cell Signal 2009;21(3):405–12.

[37] Karapetyan AV, Klyachkin YM, Selim S, Sunkara M, Ziada KM, Cohen DA, et al. Bioactive lipids and cationic antimicrobial peptides as new potential regulators for trafficking of bone marrow-derived stem cells in patients with acute myocardial infarction. Stem Cells Dev 2013;22(11):1645–56.

[38] Klyachkin YM, Karapetyan AV, Ratajczak MZ, Abdel-Latif A. The role of bioactive lipids in stem cell mobilization and homing: novel therapeutics for myocardial ischemia. Biomed Res Int 2014;2014:653543. Epub 2014/03/29.

[39] Kronlage M, Song J, Sorokin L, Isfort K, Schwerdtle T, Leipziger J, et al. Autocrine purinergic receptor signaling is essential for macrophage chemotaxis. Sci Signal 2010;3(132):ra55.

[40] Lemoli RM, Ferrari D, Fogli M, Rossi L, Pizzirani C, Forchap S, et al. Extracellular nucleotides are potent stimulators of human hematopoietic stem cells in vitro and in vivo. Blood 2004;104(6):1662–70.

[41] Okajima F. Regulation of inflammation by extracellular acidification and proton-sensing GPCRs. Sci Signal 2013;25(11):2263–71.

[42] Ratajczak MZ, Kim C. Bioactive sphingolipids and complement cascade as new emerging regulators of stem cell mobilization and homing. J Stem Cell Res Ther 2011;1(2).

[43] Rossi L, Manfredini R, Bertolini F, Ferrari D, Fogli M, Zini R, et al. The extracellular nucleotide UTP is a potent inducer of hematopoietic stem cell migration. Blood 2007;109(2):533–42.

[44] Salvestrini V, Zini R, Rossi L, Gulinelli S, Manfredini R, Bianchi E, et al. Purinergic signaling inhibits human acute myeloblastic leukemia cell proliferation, migration, and engraftment in immunodeficient mice. Blood 2012;119(1):217–26.

[45] Yang L, Wang L, Geiger H, Cancelas JA, Mo J, Zheng Y. Rho GTPase Cdc42 coordinates hematopoietic stem cell quiescence and niche interaction in the bone marrow. Proc Natl Acad Sci USA 2007;104(12):5091–6.

[46] Basu S, Ray NT, Atkinson SJ, Broxmeyer HE. Protein phosphatase 2A plays an important role in stromal cell-derived factor-1/CXC chemokine ligand 12-mediated migration and adhesion of CD34+ cells. J Immunol 2007;179(5):3075–85.

[47] Christopherson 2nd KW, Hangoc G, Mantel CR, Broxmeyer HE. Modulation of hematopoietic stem cell homing and engraftment by CD26. Science 2004;305(5686):1000–3.
[48] Kim CH, Wu W, Wysoczynski M, Abdel-Latif A, Sunkara M, Morris A, et al. Conditioning for hematopoietic transplantation activates the complement cascade and induces a proteolytic environment in bone marrow: a novel role for bioactive lipids and soluble C5b-C9 as homing factors. Leukemia 2012;26(1):106–16.
[49] Kim C, Wan W, Liu R, Kucia M, Laughlin MJ, Ratajczak J, et al. A novel paradigm in stem cell trafficking: the ratio of peripheral blood sphingosine-1 phosphate (S1P) to bone marrow ceramide-1 phosphate (C1P) regulates mobilization and homing of hematopoietic stem cells. Blood 2010;116:246.
[50] Lee HM, Wu W, Wysoczynski M, Liu R, Zuba-Surma EK, Kucia M, et al. Impaired mobilization of hematopoietic stem/progenitor cells in C5-deficient mice supports the pivotal involvement of innate immunity in this process and reveals novel promobilization effects of granulocytes. Leukemia 2009;23(11):2052–62.
[51] Levesque JP, Hendy J, Takamatsu Y, Simmons PJ, Bendall LJ. Disruption of the CXCR4/CXCL12 chemotactic interaction during hematopoietic stem cell mobilization induced by GCSF or cyclophosphamide. J Clin Invest 2003;111(2):187–96.
[52] Pelus LM, Bian H, King AG, Fukuda S. Neutrophil-derived MMP-9 mediates synergistic mobilization of hematopoietic stem and progenitor cells by the combination of G-CSF and the chemokines GRObeta/CXCL2 and GRObetaT/CXCL2delta4. Blood 2004;103(1):110–9.
[53] Avigdor A, Goichberg P, Shivtiel S, Dar A, Peled A, Samira S, et al. CD44 and hyaluronic acid cooperate with SDF-1 in the trafficking of human CD34+ stem/progenitor cells to bone marrow. Blood 2004;103(8):2981–9.
[54] Delaney C, Ratajczak MZ, Laughlin MJ. Strategies to enhance umbilical cord blood stem cell engraftment in adult patients. Expert Rev Hematol 2010;3(3):273–83.
[55] Ganz T. Defensins: antimicrobial peptides of innate immunity. Nat Rev Immunol 2003;3(9):710–20.
[56] Greenbaum AM, Link DC. Mechanisms of G-CSF-mediated hematopoietic stem and progenitor mobilization. Leukemia 2011;25(2):211–7.
[57] Lee H, Ratajczak MZ. Innate immunity: a key player in the mobilization of hematopoietic stem/progenitor cells. Arch Immunol Ther Exp Warsz 2009;57(4):269–78.
[58] Levesque JP, Hendy J, Takamatsu Y, Williams B, Winkler IG, Simmons PJ. Mobilization by either cyclophosphamide or granulocyte colony-stimulating factor transforms the bone marrow into a highly proteolytic environment. Exp Hematol 2002;30(5):440–9.
[59] Ratajczak MZ, Reca R, Wysoczynski M, Kucia M, Baran JT, Allendorf DJ, et al. Transplantation studies in C3-deficient animals reveal a novel role of the third complement component (C3) in engraftment of bone marrow cells. Leukemia 2004;18(9):1482–90.
[60] Shirvaikar N, Marquez-Curtis LA, Ratajczak MZ, Janowska-Wieczorek A. Hyaluronic acid and thrombin upregulate MT1-MMP through PI3K and Rac-1 signaling and prime the homing-related responses of cord blood hematopoietic stem/progenitor cells. Stem Cells Dev 2011;20(1):19–30.
[61] Wu W, Kim CH, Liu R, Kucia M, Marlicz W, Greco N, et al. The bone marrow-expressed antimicrobial cationic peptide LL-37 enhances the responsiveness of hematopoietic stem progenitor cells to an SDF-1 gradient and accelerates their engraftment after transplantation. Leukemia 2012;26(4):736–45.
[62] Wysoczynski M, Reca R, Lee H, Wu W, Ratajczak J, Ratajczak MZ. Defective engraftment of C3aR-/- hematopoietic stem progenitor cells shows a novel role of the C3a-C3aR axis in bone marrow homing. Leukemia 2009;23(8):1455–61.
[63] Ratajczak MZ, Kim C. The use of chemokine receptor agonists in stem cell mobilization. Expert Opin Biol Ther 2012;12(3):287–97.
[64] Onai N, Zhang Y, Yoneyama H, Kitamura T, Ishikawa S, Matsushima K. Impairment of lymphopoiesis and myelopoiesis in mice reconstituted with bone marrow-hematopoietic progenitor cells expressing SDF-1-intrakine. Blood 2000;96(6):2074–80.

[65] Ara T, Tokoyoda K, Sugiyama T, Egawa T, Kawabata K, Nagasawa T. Long-term hematopoietic stem cells require stromal cell-derived factor-1 for colonizing bone marrow during ontogeny. Immunity 2003;19(2):257–67.
[66] Lapidot T. Mechanism of human stem cell migration and repopulation of NOD/SCID and B2mnull NOD/SCID mice. The role of SDF-1/CXCR4 interactions. Ann NY Acad Sci 2001;938:83–95.
[67] Lapidot T, Dar A, Kollet O. How do stem cells find their way home? Blood 2005;106(6):1901–10.
[68] Nagasawa T. A chemokine, SDF-1/PBSF, and its receptor, CXC chemokine receptor 4, as mediators of hematopoiesis. Int J Hematol 2000;72(4):408–11.
[69] Vagima Y, Lapid K, Kollet O, Goichberg P, Alon R, Lapidot T. Pathways implicated in stem cell migration: the SDF-1/CXCR4 axis. Methods Mol Biol 2011;750:277–89.
[70] Wright DE, Bowman EP, Wagers AJ, Butcher EC, Weissman IL. Hematopoietic stem cells are uniquely selective in their migratory response to chemokines. J Exp Med 2002;195(9):1145–54.
[71] Gazitt Y, Liu Q. Plasma levels of SDF-1 and expression of SDF-1 receptor on CD34+ cells in mobilized peripheral blood of non-Hodgkin's lymphoma patients. Stem Cells 2001;19(1):37–45.
[72] Boath A, Graf C, Lidome E, Ullrich T, Nussbaumer P, Bornancin F. Regulation and traffic of ceramide 1-phosphate produced by ceramide kinase: comparative analysis to glucosylceramide and sphingomyelin. J Biol Chem 2008;283(13):8517–26.
[73] Durand EM, Zon LI. Newly emerging roles for prostaglandin E2 regulation of hematopoiesis and hematopoietic stem cell engraftment. Curr Opin Hematol 2010;17(4):308–12.
[74] Ratajczak MZ, Kim CH, Wojakowski W, Janowska-Wieczorek A, Kucia M, Ratajczak J. Innate immunity as orchestrator of stem cell mobilization. Leukemia 2010;24(10):1667–75.
[75] Seitz G, Boehmler AM, Kanz L, Mohle R. The role of sphingosine 1-phosphate receptors in the trafficking of hematopoietic progenitor cells. Ann NY Acad Sci 2005;1044:84–9.
[76] Rivera J, Proia RL, Olivera A. The alliance of sphingosine-1-phosphate and its receptors in immunity. Nat Rev Immunol 2008;8(10):753–63.
[77] Graler MH, Goetzl EJ. The immunosuppressant FTY720 down-regulates sphingosine 1-phosphate G-protein-coupled receptors. FASEB J 2004;18(3):551–3.
[78] Sciorra VA, Morris AJ. Roles for lipid phosphate phosphatases in regulation of cellular signaling. Biochim Biophys Acta 2002;1582(1–3):45–51.
[79] Rauvala H, Prieels JP, Finne J. Cell adhesion mediated by a purified fucosyltransferase. Proc Natl Acad Sci USA 1983;80(13):3991–5.
[80] Eirin A, Gloviczki ML, Tang H, Gossl M, Jordan KL, Woollard JR, et al. Inflammatory and injury signals released from the post-stenotic human kidney. Eur Heart J 2013;34(7):540–8a.
[81] Hoggatt J, Singh P, Sampath J, Pelus LM. Prostaglandin E2 enhances hematopoietic stem cell homing, survival, and proliferation. Blood 2009;113(22):5444–55.
[82] Ratajczak MZ, Borkowska S, Ratajczak J. An emerging link in stem cell mobilization between activation of the complement cascade and the chemotactic gradient of sphingosine-1-phosphate. Prostagl Other Lipid Mediat 2013;104–105:122–9.
[83] Zughaier SM, Svoboda P, Pohl J, Stephens DS, Shafer WM. The human host defense peptide LL-37 interacts with Neisseria meningitidis capsular polysaccharides and inhibits inflammatory mediators release. PLoS One 2010;5(10):e13627.
[84] McQuibban GA, Butler GS, Gong JH, Bendall L, Power C, Clark-Lewis I, et al. Matrix metalloproteinase activity inactivates the CXC chemokine stromal cell-derived factor-1. J Biol Chem 2001;276(47):43503–8.
[85] Borkowska S, Suszynska M, Mierzejewska K, Ismail A, Budkowska M, Salata D, et al. Novel evidence that crosstalk between the complement, coagulation and fibrinolysis proteolytic cascades is involved in mobilization of hematopoietic stem/progenitor cells (HSPCs). Leukemia 2014;28(11):2148–54.
[86] Gong Y, Zhao Y, Li Y, Fan Y, Hoover-Plow J. Plasminogen regulates cardiac repair after myocardial infarction through its noncanonical function in stem cell homing to the infarcted heart. J Am Coll Cardiol 2014;63(25 Pt A):2862–72.

[87] Bene MC, Castoldi G, Knapp W, Rigolin GM, Escribano L, Lemez P, et al. CD87 (urokinase-type plasminogen activator receptor), function and pathology in hematological disorders: a review. Leukemia 2004;18(3):394–400.
[88] Degryse B. The urokinase receptor system as strategic therapeutic target: challenges for the 21st century. Curr Pharm Des 2011;17(19):1872–3.
[89] Mizukami IF, Todd 3rd RF. A soluble form of the urokinase plasminogen activator receptor (suPAR) can bind to hematopoietic cells. J Leukoc Biol 1998;64(2):203–13.
[90] Plesner T, Behrendt N, Ploug M. Structure, function and expression on blood and bone marrow cells of the urokinase-type plasminogen activator receptor, uPAR. Stem Cells 1997;15(6):398–408.
[91] Selleri C, Montuori N, Ricci P, Visconte V, Baiano A, Carriero MV, et al. In vivo activity of the cleaved form of soluble urokinase receptor: a new hematopoietic stem/progenitor cell mobilizer. Cancer Res 2006;66(22):10885–90.
[92] Selleri C, Montuori N, Ricci P, Visconte V, Carriero MV, Sidenius N, et al. Involvement of the urokinase-type plasminogen activator receptor in hematopoietic stem cell mobilization. Blood 2005;105(5):2198–205.
[93] Sloand EM, Pfannes L, Scheinberg P, More K, Wu CO, Horne M, et al. Increased soluble urokinase plasminogen activator receptor (suPAR) is associated with thrombosis and inhibition of plasmin generation in paroxysmal nocturnal hemoglobinuria (PNH) patients. Exp Hematol 2008;36(12):1616–24.
[94] Lehrer RI. Primate defensins. Nat Rev Microbiol 2004;2(9):727–38.
[95] Adamiak M, Borkowska S, Wysoczynski M, Suszynska M, Kucia M, Rokosh G, et al. Evidence for the involvement of sphingosine-1-phosphate in the homing and engraftment of hematopoietic stem cells to bone marrow. Oncotarget 2015;6(22):18819–28.
[96] Chen J, Li Y, Wang L, Zhang Z, Lu D, Lu M, et al. Therapeutic benefit of intravenous administration of bone marrow stromal cells after cerebral ischemia in rats. Stroke 2001;32(4):1005–11.
[97] Forrester JS, Price MJ, Makkar RR. Stem cell repair of infarcted myocardium: an overview for clinicians. Circulation 2003;108(9):1139–45.
[98] Kang SK, Shin IS, Ko MS, Jo JY, Ra JC. Journey of mesenchymal stem cells for homing: strategies to enhance efficacy and safety of stem cell therapy. Stem Cells Int 2012;2012:342968.
[99] Kirpatovskii VI, Kazachenko AV, Plotnikov EY, Marei MV, Musina RA, Nadtochii ON, et al. Experimental intravenous cell therapy of acute and chronic renal failure. Bull Exp Biol Med 2007;143(1):160–5.
[100] Sakaida I, Terai S, Yamamoto N, Aoyama K, Ishikawa T, Nishina H, et al. Transplantation of bone marrow cells reduces CCl4-induced liver fibrosis in mice. Hepatology 2004;40(6):1304–11.
[101] Gutierrez-Fernandez M, Rodriguez-Frutos B, Ramos-Cejudo J, Teresa Vallejo-Cremades M, Fuentes B, Cerdan S, et al. Effects of intravenous administration of allogenic bone marrow- and adipose tissue-derived mesenchymal stem cells on functional recovery and brain repair markers in experimental ischemic stroke. Stem Cell Res Ther 2013;4(1):11.
[102] Kucia M, Halasa M, Wysoczynski M, Baskiewicz-Masiuk M, Moldenhawer S, Zuba-Surma E, et al. Morphological and molecular characterization of novel population of CXCR4+ SSEA-4+ Oct-4+ very small embryonic-like cells purified from human cord blood: preliminary report. Leukemia 2007;21(2):297–303.
[103] Kucia M, Reca R, Campbell FR, Zuba-Surma E, Majka M, Ratajczak J, et al. A population of very small embryonic-like (VSEL) CXCR4(+)SSEA-1(+)Oct-4+ stem cells identified in adult bone marrow. Leukemia 2006;20(5):857–69.
[104] Ratajczak MZ, Jadczyk T, Pedziwiatr D, Wojakowski W. New advances in stem cell research: practical implications for regenerative medicine. Pol Arch Med Wewn 2014;124(7–8):417–26.
[105] Schwarz S, Huss R, Schulz-Siegmund M, Vogel B, Brandau S, Lang S, et al. Bone marrow-derived mesenchymal stem cells migrate to healthy and damaged salivary glands following stem cell infusion. Int J Oral Sci 2014;6(3):154–61.
[106] Ratajczak MZ. A novel view of the adult bone marrow stem cell hierarchy and stem cell trafficking. Leukemia 2015;29(4):776–82.

[107] Kanzler I, Tuchscheerer N, Steffens G, Simsekyilmaz S, Konschalla S, Kroh A, et al. Differential roles of angiogenic chemokines in endothelial progenitor cell-induced angiogenesis. Basic Res Cardiol 2013;108(1):310.

[108] Zhang H, Albersen M, Jin X, Lin G. Stem cells: novel players in the treatment of erectile dysfunction. Asian J Androl 2012;14(1):145–55.

[109] Song M, Jang H, Lee J, Kim JH, Kim SH, Sun K, et al. Regeneration of chronic myocardial infarction by injectable hydrogels containing stem cell homing factor SDF-1 and angiogenic peptide Ac-SDKP. Biomaterials 2014;35(8):2436–45.

[110] Formiga FR, Pelacho B, Garbayo E, Imbuluzqueta I, Diaz-Herraez P, Abizanda G, et al. Controlled delivery of fibroblast growth factor-1 and neuregulin-1 from biodegradable microparticles promotes cardiac repair in a rat myocardial infarction model through activation of endogenous regeneration. J Control Release 2014;173:132–9.

[111] Doroudian G, Pinney J, Ayala P, Los T, Desai TA, Russell B. Sustained delivery of MGF peptide from microrods attracts stem cells and reduces apoptosis of myocytes. Biomed Microdevices 2014;16(5):705–15.

[112] Ziadloo A, Burks SR, Gold EM, Lewis BK, Chaudhry A, Merino MJ, et al. Enhanced homing permeability and retention of bone marrow stromal cells by noninvasive pulsed focused ultrasound. Stem Cells 2012;30(6):1216–27.

[113] Zhang Y, Ye C, Wang G, Gao Y, Tan K, Zhuo Z, et al. Kidney-targeted transplantation of mesenchymal stem cells by ultrasound-targeted microbubble destruction promotes kidney repair in diabetic nephropathy rats. Biomed Res Int 2013;2013:526367.

[114] Wu S, Li L, Wang G, Shen W, Xu Y, Liu Z, et al. Ultrasound-targeted stromal cell-derived factor-1-loaded microbubble destruction promotes mesenchymal stem cell homing to kidneys in diabetic nephropathy rats. Int J Nanomed 2014;9:5639–51.

[115] Okay E, Simsek T, Subasi C, Gunes A, Duruksu G, Gurbuz Y, et al. Cross effects of resveratrol and mesenchymal stem cells on liver regeneration and homing in partially hepatectomized rats. Stem Cell Rev 2015;11(2):322–31.

[116] Rota C, Imberti B, Pozzobon M, Piccoli M, De Coppi P, Atala A, et al. Human amniotic fluid stem cell preconditioning improves their regenerative potential. Stem Cells Dev 2012;21(11):1911–23.

[117] Yu SP, Wei Z, Wei L. Preconditioning strategy in stem cell transplantation therapy. Transl Stroke Res 2013;4(1):76–88.

[118] Adamiak M, Iv JB, Zhao J, Abdelbaset-Ismail A, Grubczak K, Borkowska S, et al. Downregulation of heme oxygenase 1 (HO-1) activity in hematopoietic cells enhances their engraftment after transplantation. Cell Transpl 2015.

CHAPTER

IMMUNOLOGY: HOST RESPONSES TO BIOMATERIALS

3

J.D. Jackson

Wake Forest Institute for Regenerative Medicine, Wake Forest School of Medicine, Winston-Salem, NC, United States

CHAPTER OUTLINE

INTRODUCTION

The immune system has evolved in vertebrates to protect the individual from pathogens. Innate and adaptive immune responses combine to define the overall immune response to an infection. Innate immunity is the first line of defense against pathogens and occurs rapidly following an infection. Following the innate response, adaptive immunity adds specificity and memory to eliminate any residue pathogens and adds long-term protection to subsequent exposure to the pathogens. The function of antigen presenting cells directly links the innate and adaptive immune responses. Bone marrow resident hematopoietic stem cells give rise to the many types of cells comprising the immune system. This

In Situ Tissue Regeneration. http://dx.doi.org/10.1016/B978-0-12-802225-2.00003-9

chapter will define the components of an immune response and describe the current understanding of the interaction of the immune system with biomaterials.

INNATE IMMUNITY

CELL TYPES

The initial response to an infection is mediated by the innate immune system. The cellular component of innate immunity contains macrophages, dendritic cells, neutrophils, eosinophils, basophils, mast cells, and natural killer (NK) cells. These cells use receptors to recognize repeating structural patterns on microorganisms. These repetitive structures are called pathogen-associated molecular patterns (PAMPS). The receptors that recognize PAMPS are termed pattern recognition receptors (PRRs) [1]. PAMPS are expressed on many pathogens but are not expressed on mammalians cells, which results in discrimination of self and nonself. Toll-like receptors (TLRs) are one class of PRRs that recognize PAMPS expressed on virus, bacteria, fungus, and protozoa [2]. Other PRRs include nucleotide-binding oligomerization domain-like receptors, C-type lectin receptors, and scavenger receptors [3–5]. PRRs are fixed in the genome; therefore all cells of a specific cell type (ie, neutrophils) express the same receptor (nonclonal), unlike cells of the adaptive system, which rearrange their antigen receptor genes, resulting in clonal distribution of the receptors.

Neutrophils and macrophages are the predominant cell types that initially respond to an infection. Tissue cells and endothelial cells at a site of injury or infection secrete chemokines and other cytokines to direct responding immune cells to the site as well as upregulate specific cell surface adhesion molecules such as selectins and integrins to aid in the migration of the leukocytes. A small number of macrophages are the first to encounter pathogens, since they reside in tissues but are quickly joined by a large number of neutrophils via the circulatory system. The primary role of neutrophils and macrophages is to phagocytize microorganisms and to release bactericidal products that aid in the killing of the pathogens. In addition to clearing pathogens, macrophages also perform another important immune function by processing and presenting antigens to T cells. This initiates the adaptive response. Dendritic cells are professional antigen presenting cells and are critical in linking the innate response to the adaptive response by engulfing, processing, and presenting antigens to T cells.

Eosinophils and basophils circulate in the blood and are involved in parasitic and allergy responses. Mast cells are similar to basophils but are tissue resident and are involved in parasitic and allergy responses as well as inflammatory responses.

NK cells are important effector cells in the elimination of viral infected cells and have some role in antitumor responses.

COMPLEMENT

Another component of the innate immune response is the complement system. Complement is a series of plasma proteins that undergo a cascade of enzymatic degradation that results in products that aid in elimination of microorganisms. There are three main pathways to complement activation. The classical pathway involves C1q binding directly to the surface of pathogens, binding of C1q to pathogen bound C-reactive protein (an acute phase protein), and binding of C1q to antigen–antibody complexes on the surface of pathogens. The alternative pathway involves the binding of hydrolysis-activated C3 to the surface of a pathogen. The lectin pathway involves the binding of lectins to patterns of carbohydrates on the surface of pathogens. The primary complement effector molecule is C3b, which binds to the surface of microorganisms, enhancing phagocytosis by leukocytes. C3b also participates in the further production of a membrane attack complex that forms a pore in the membrane of pathogens, resulting in the lysis of the microorganism. The cleavage of C3 and C5 results in C3a and C5a peptides that are potent chemoattractants and activators of leukocytes.

ADAPTIVE IMMUNITY

Adaptive immune responses add specificity and memory to eliminate pathogens. The antigen specificity is a result of random recombination of several gene segments that gives a large number of possible combinations resulting in diversity of the receptor repertoire with the ability to recognize a wide range of antigens. After stimulation of naive lymphocytes with antigen (primary response), the cells undergo proliferation (clonal expansion) and maturation (production of effector molecules or effector cells). Once the infection is eliminated, the majority of the responding lymphocytes undergo apoptosis and are removed. However, some of the effector cells remain and become memory cells that can respond to a reinfection with a much shorter period than the initial (primary) response. These properties are responsible for the success of vaccines.

T CELL DEVELOPMENT

The thymus is the site of T cell production. Bone marrow-derived progenitor cells seed the thymus and proceed through a series of maturation stages. The thymus has two distinct regions with an outer cortical region and an inner medulla. The cortex contains cortical epithelial cells and immature thymocytes. The medulla contains medullary epithelial cells, dendritic cells, and macrophages. The cortex and medulla perform different functions during the maturation of the thymocytes. Bone marrow-derived T precursor cells enter the thymus at the cortico-medulary junction. The developing thymocytes move through the cortex in a defined pattern undergoing specific maturation steps. Cells entering the thymus express few cell surface markers characteristic of T cells and are known as double negative (absence of CD4 and CD8). Their receptor genes are germline and not rearranged. The thymocytes migrate toward the outer cortex and then migrate back through the cortex toward the medulla. During this time, the thymocytes mature to the double positive stage (CD4 and CD8 positive), rearrange their receptor genes, and express the T cell receptor (TCR) on their membrane surface. These maturation steps occur in close association with the cortical epithelial cells. At this point, the thymocytes must interact with self-peptides presented in the context of self-major histocompatibility complex (MHC) and undergo positive selection. If this interaction is unsuccessful, the thymocytes undergo apoptosis. If the interaction of the TCR with self-peptide and self-MHC is successful, the thymocytes continue on the maturation pathway to a single positive phenotype (CD4 or CD8) and migrate to the medulla. The outcome of positive selection is the identification of functional TCRs that can bind with self-MHC. The majority (greater than 90%) of thymocytes do not progress beyond positive selection and die in the thymus via apoptosis. After migrating to the medulla, thymocytes undergo negative selection. Negative selection can also occur in the cortex. The Negative selection process identifies T cells that activate when their TCR recognizes self-peptides in the context of self-MHC. These T cells represent autoreactive clones and have the potential to participate in autoimmunity. The elimination of the self-reactive T cells represents the process of central tolerance. The negatively selected single positive T cells (helper T cells expressing CD4 and cytotoxic T cells expressing CD8) leave the thymus and populate the peripheral lymphoid tissues.

HELPER T CELLS

CD4 cells are helper T cells. Naive CD4 cells activate via the recognition of foreign peptide presented in the context of MHC class II by antigen presenting cells. The primary effector function of activate CD4 T cells is the production of cytokines that add help to other cell populations. Helper T cells provide signals to other cell populations, such as B cells, to mature and produce antibodies, and macrophages to enhance phagocytosis and killing of microorganisms. Activated CD4 T cells differentiate into several subsets of T cell helper effector cells, Th1, Th2, Th17, and regulatory T cells (Treg). These subsets of CD4 helper T cells are defined by their specific cytokine secretion patterns.

Th1 and Th2 subsets were the first to be described [6] (see Figs. 3.1 and 3.2). Th1 cells produce IL-2, IFN-γ, and lymphotoxin, and Th2 cells produce IL-4 and IL-5, IL-6, IL-10, and IL-13 [7]. The cytokine secretion patterns direct specific types of immune responses. IL-2 and IFN-γ secreted by Th1 cells drive a cell-mediated immune response such as delayed hypersensitivity, macrophage activation, and antibody-dependent cell-mediated cytotoxicity to eliminate intracellular pathogens (bacteria,

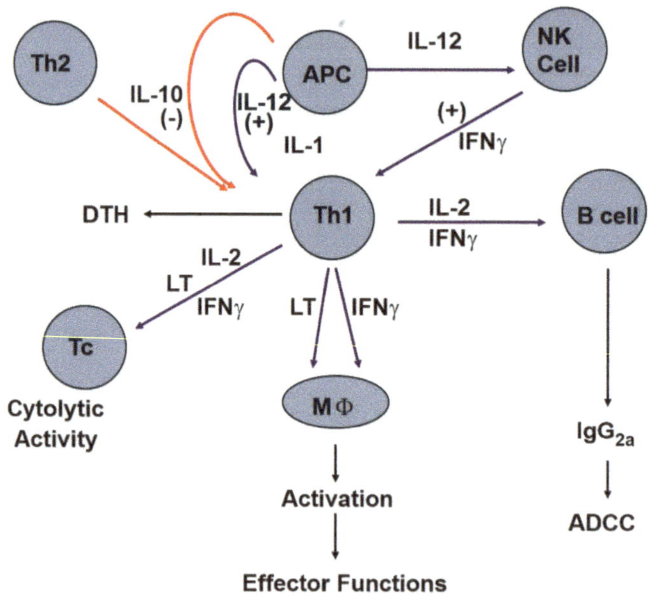

FIGURE 3.1

Regulation of Th1 response. IL-12 produced by antigen presenting cells drives a Th1 response. Th1 cells produce a cytokine profile that supports a cell-mediated immune response. IL-10 produced by antigen presenting cells and Th2 cells inhibit the secretion of cytokines by Th1 cells.

viruses, and protozoa). Cytokines produced by Th2 cells direct humoral immune responses biased to IgG1 and IgE to eradicate parasitic infections (helminths). Dysregulated Th1 responses result in chronic inflammation and tissue damage, whereas dysregulation of Th2 responses results in allergy and asthma. TH1 and Th2 cells cross-regulate their production. IFN-γ produced by Th1 cells decreases the proliferation of Th2 cells. IL10 inhibits cytokine production by Th1 cells. The environment during the initiation of an immune response helps determine the direction of the T helper cell subset production. IL-12 and IFN-are major drivers of Th1 differentiation, whereas IL-4 and IL-10 are dominant initiators for Th2 differentiation.

TGF-β and IL-6 induce the differentiation of CD4 helper T cells to the Th17 subset, which produces IL-17. Although TGF-β and IL-6 are responsible for the differentiation of CD4 helper cells to the Th17 lineage, IL-23 is necessary for expansion and maintenance of the Th17 response [8]. Th17 cells are important in responses to eliminate extracellular bacterial infections [9]. To this end, some of the defined activities of IL-17 are the mobilization of neutrophils in vivo and the stimulation of neutrophil production from hematopoietic progenitors in vitro [10]. Dysregulation of Th17 response may play a role in autoimmune diseases [9,11].

The role of Treg cells is to suppress T cell responses. Treg cells are produced directly from the thymus and are also induced from peripheral T cells in the presence of TGF-β. Treg cells are identified by the expression of CD4, CD25, and Foxp3. Treg cells can exert antigen-specific

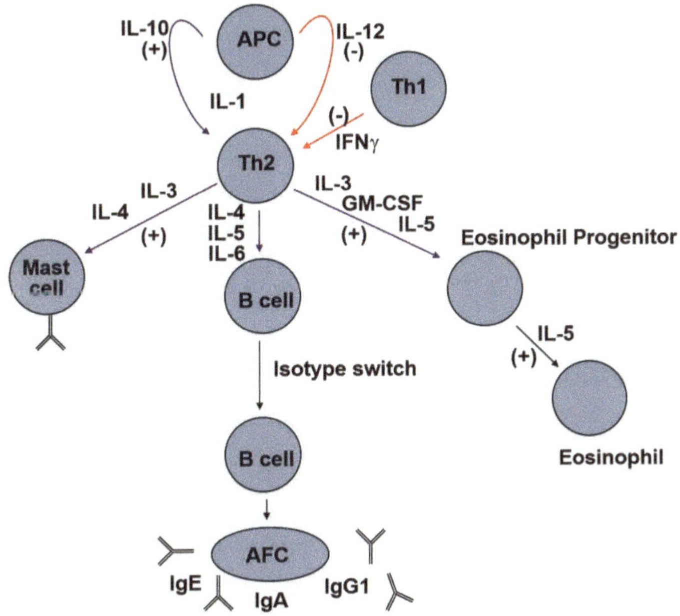

FIGURE 3.2

Regulation of Th2 Response: IL-10 produced by antigen presenting cells drives a Th2 response. Th2 cells produce a cytokine profile that supports a humoral immune response as well as supports the production of mast cells and eosinophils, which, in combination with IgE, provides a response to parasites and allergy responses. IL-12 produced by antigen presenting cells and IFN-γ produced by Th1 cells inhibit the proliferation of Th2 cells.

suppressive active by direct cell contact, modulation of dendritic cell function, and secretion of suppressive cytokines (IL-10 and TGF-β).

B CELLS

B cells are produced in the bone marrow from hematopoietic stem cells. Maturation proceeds through specific steps associated with the rearrangement of the B cell receptor genes. At the immature B cell stage, the newly expressed B cell receptor is assessed for reactivity to self-antigens. If reactivity to self-antigens is present, the B cell undergoes apoptosis, receptor editing, or anergy. If no self-reactivity is present, the immature B cell undergoes maturation, exits the bone marrow, and resides in peripheral tissues. Once the naïve B cell encounters an antigen via binding to its B cell receptor, the B cell activates, proliferates, and differentiates into a plasma cell that secretes immunoglobulin molecules with the same specificity as the B cell receptor. The initial immunoglobulin secreted is IgM. Class switching of the antibody is directed by cytokines. The most abundant antibody in plasma is IgG. Each class of antibodies has specific functions. IgM is a pentamer and is effective in activating complement. Because of the multivalent binding of the IgM pentamer, it is efficient at clearing antigens. IgG is the most abundant antibody in plasma and is important in optimization of antigens for clearance by phagocytes and activates complement. IgA is a dimer, is found primarily in mucosal areas, and is important in neutralization pathogens such as viruses. IgE is found at low concentrations in plasma but binds to receptors on mast cells and is important in responses to parasites and allergy.

BIOMATERIALS

As medical treatments have advanced over the years, many types of materials are used to repair tissues. Implant materials include metals, ceramics, plastics, and nature scaffolds. The immune system has evolved to recognize and eliminate any invading organisms; however, any foreign material implanted in vivo will elicit an immune response. The challenge for tissue engineering and regenerative medicine is to develop biomaterials that provide the appropriate environment for healing.

ACUTE RESPONSE TO BIOMATERIALS

On implantation, a biomaterial encounters body fluids, including blood plasma and interstitial fluid. Immediately, proteins in the plasma begin to adhere to the surface of the biomaterial [12]. These bound proteins include albumin, IgG, C3, fibrinogen, and factor XII [13]. Factor XII is part of the coagulation system and can activate on the surface of biomaterials. This cascade leads to thrombin formation, cleavage of fibrinogen to form fibrin that coats the biomaterial surface. Platelets can activate when contacting damaged endothelium, collagen, and artificial surfaces [14]. Plasma proteins such as thrombin and fibrinogen also can activate platelets. Platelets release a number of growth factors and cytokines that are involved in proinflammatory responses, antiinflammatory responses, and wound healing.

Complement is another component of the innate immune response. The surface properties of the biomaterial can affect the activation of complement. Hydrophilic surfaces are less activating than hydrophobic surfaces [15]. Surfaces that have free hydroxyl and amide groups on the biomaterial surface offer a more activating substrate for complement, due to the binding of C3b [16]. Binding of immunoglobulin (IgG) to the surface of biomaterials can activate complement via the classical pathway [17]. In addition, C3 can absorb to the surface of biomaterials, initiating the complement cascaded via the alternative pathway [15]. One consequence of complement activation is the production of cleaved peptide fragments of C3 and C5 termed C3a and C5a. C3a and C5a are known as anaphylatoxins, which can induce systemic anaphylactic shock when produced in large quantities. Both peptides induce smooth muscle contraction, increase vascular permeability, and are potent activators and chemoattractants for neutrophils, macrophages, basophils, and tissue mast cells [18,19]. Therefore these peptides play an important role in the induction and regulation of the initial inflammatory response.

Neutrophils are the first cell population to migrate to the site of biomaterial implantation. At sites of injury or infection, damaged tissue cells and endothelial cells lining adjacent blood vessels recruit neutrophils from the peripheral circulation by secreting chemokines and upregulating adhesion molecules such as selectins and integrins on the endothelial cells. Receptors on the surface of neutrophils interact with selectins on the endothelial cells. This causes the neutrophils to roll along the vessel lumen and slows their movement in the blood. Integrins expressed on neutrophils bind to receptors on endothelial cells to anchor the neutrophil and allow the migration of neutrophils through the endothelial barrier to the site of injury or infection directed by a chemokine gradient of IL-8 and C5a. The main function of neutrophils is to phagocytize pathogens. In the case of implanted biomaterials, the neutrophils cannot engulf the material because of the large surface area; however, neutrophils can activate via binding of integrins (primarily β2 integrins) and PRRs (such as TLR) expressed on their surface to proteins coating the biomaterial. The neutrophil activation results in the release of granules containing bioactive molecules that enhance the acute inflammatory response as well as damage surrounding normal tissue. Activated neutrophils also secrete chemokines that attract and activate macrophages, dendritic cells, and lymphocytes [20]. The neutrophil response is transient, and in a few days, the neutrophil response ends [12].

Mast cells recruited to the site of an implanted biomaterial can adhere to the surface of biomaterials through interaction of integrin expression, bind to absorbed proteins (fibronectin) on the surface of the biomaterial, and activate and release histamine and cytokines that continue the acute inflammatory response [21,22].

Macrophages are the next cell population to migrate to the site of a biomaterial implant because of factors produced by complement and neutrophils. C5a is a potent chemoattractant of monocytes and macrophages as well as the chemokine IL-8, which is produced by neutrophils. Macrophages use PRR and integrins to recognize the serum protein-coated surface of the biomaterials. Once activated, macrophages are potent producers of cytokines and chemokines that continue the inflammatory response. Similar to the subsets of T helper cells, two subsets of macrophages, M1 (classically activated macrophages) and M2 (alternatively activated macrophages), have been described [23]. Functionally, M1 macrophages are proinflammatory and exhibit antimicrobial activity, whereas M2 macrophages are immunomodulatory and participate in tissue repair [24]. Phenotypically, M1 macrophages are characterized by the expression of CD80, CD68, and CCR7, and M2 macrophages expressed CD163 [25,26]. The M2 macrophage subset has been further divided into three subpopulations based on phenotype (M2a, M2b, and M2c) [23].

Macrophages primed in the presence of IFN-γ and LPS or TNF-α polarized the macrophages into an M1 phenotype that secretes proinflammatory cytokines (IL-12, TNF-α, IL-1, and IL-23) and are responsible for the development of a Th1 cell-mediated response directed to the elimination of intracellular pathogens and antitumor responses [23,24,27]. Chronic stimulation of an M1 response results in tissue damage. Macrophages primed in the presence of IL-4, IL-13, or IL-10 polarized the macrophages into an M2 phenotype that secretes antiinflammatory cytokines (IL-10, IL-1ra, TGF-β) and are responsible for the development of Th2 and Treg responses that are directed to antiparasitic activity, allergy, B cell help, and immune regulation [23,24,27].

CHRONIC IMMUNE RESPONSE TO BIOMATERIALS

Adhesion of macrophages

Chronic inflammation directed to biomaterials is confined to the site of implantation and is usually limited to several weeks [12]. The presence of macrophages and T lymphocytes at the site of inflammation signals the beginning of a chronic immune response [28]. Signals from the injured tissue as well as chemokines produced by neutrophils direct increased numbers of macrophages to the site of the biomaterial implant. A primary role for macrophages is the phagocytosis and degradation of foreign material. Binding of macrophages to biomaterials can occur through several mechanisms. Integrin, primarily B2 integrin, recognition of ligands associated with the serum protein coat covering the surface of an implanted biomaterial is the primary route for the adhesion and activation of macrophages [29]. PRRs on the macrophage can also recognize PAMPS on the surface of the biomaterial. There is evidence that direct TLR binding to biomaterial surface can activate macrophages [30]. Biomaterial surface characteristics have been shown to direct the specific cytokine profile that is then produced by the macrophage [31]. This differential expression of cytokines by the macrophage can contribute to the type of response, proinflammatory or antiinflammatory, produced in response to the biomaterial.

Foreign body response

Macrophages adherent to biomaterials can undergo fusion to form multinucleated giant cells termed foreign body giant cells. The local presence of certain cytokines can induce cell fusion. IL-4 was the first cytokine identified to induce fusion of macrophages [32]. Subsequently, IL-13 was identified as a macrophage fusion cytokine [33]. Early in the immune response, mast cells are recruited to the site of inflammation and activate and release numerous factors and cytokines, including IL-4 and IL-13. Later in the immune response, recruitment of T cells to the site of inflammation also may be involved in the production of IL-4 and IL-13, particularly Th2 cells. The presence of these cytokines in the localized site surrounding the implanted biomaterial provides an inductive environment for macrophage fusion. The foreign body giant cells cover the biomaterial and deposit a fibrous layer around the material to wall off the implant from the surrounding tissue. Foreign body giant cells produce reactive products associated with phagocytosis and respiratory burst that can degrade the surface of the biomaterial, resulting in the potential failure of the implanted biomaterial [34].

ADAPTIVE IMMUNE RESPONSE TO BIOMATERIALS

In a classical adaptive response, macrophage and dendritic cells take up, process, and present antigen in the context of MHC to T cells. However, implantation of synthetic biomaterials is not considered to be classically immunogenic for an adaptive response.

These synthetic biomaterial constructs tend to be large and cannot be engulfed by macrophages. The local environment containing IL-4 and IL-13 supports the fusion of macrophages into multinucleated giant cells. The activated macrophages and fused giant cells secrete chemokines that recruit T cells to the site of implantation and secrete cytokines that activate the T cells. These T cells contribute to the overall chronic immune response to the biomaterial. The classical adaptive immune response is not seen as directed toward the biomaterial. However, other methods of T cell interaction with biomaterials have been described. In an in vitro coculture system containing macrophages and T cells, the majority of the T cells were found to bind to the adhered macrophages and fused giant cells rather than to the biomaterial surface [35]. This binding can occur by TCR interaction with the MHC expressed on the macrophages. This type of interaction should not activate the T cell unless there is a foreign (nonself) peptide bound to the macrophage MHC. If there is an infection (bacterial or viral) associated with the implantation of the biomaterial, then a classical adaptive immune response can be observed. Although macrophages cannot take up, process, or present synthetic biomaterial from a large implant to activate an adaptive response, the macrophages bound to the biomaterial are activated through the interaction of their PRR and TLR to serum proteins coating the surface of the biomaterial. These activated macrophages produce cytokines, IL-1β, IL-6, and TNF-α, that can induce the proliferation of T cells [36]. This idea of a nonclassical activation of T cells is supported by the finding that following a secondary exposure of biomaterials in vivo did show an increase in total cells at the implantation site; however, there was no increase in memory T cells, suggesting no adaptive response to biomaterials [37]. There is evidence that T cells can bind to biomaterials. T cells express TLR, which can be used to recognize PAMPS on biomaterial surfaces; however, the T cell response to TLR modulates the TCR, suggesting that a direct activating response from TLR signaling is not present [38].

BIOMATERIAL COMPOSITION INFLUENCES THE IMMUNE RESPONSE

Biomaterials for implantation can consist of natural or synthetic material. Natural materials include fibrin, alginate, collagen, and hyaluronan as well as decellularized scaffolds [39–43]. Synthetic materials include poly(ε-caprolactone), poly(glycolic acid), poly(lactic-co-glycolic acid), and poly(ethylene glycol) [44–46].

Hydrophobic surfaces tend to bind higher levels of proteins than hydrophilic surfaces [47]. Since neutrophils and macrophages attach more readily to protein-coated surfaces, a hydrophilic biomaterial surface is expected to exhibit less macrophage adhesion as well as less cytokine secretion, resulting in a reduced inflammatory response [48,49]. Surface charge also influences cytokine production from adherent macrophages. A negatively charged hydrophilic surface decreased the adhesion of macrophages, increased the expression of IL-10, and inhibited the IL-4 induced fusion into multinucleated giant cells, thereby promoting an antiinflammatory and prohealing response [31].

Decellularization of tissues and organs offers an excellent technique to produce scaffolds that maintain the structure of the tissue or organ with many of the extracellular matrix (ECM) components as well as growth factors and cytokines specific to that tissue or organ. The decellularized scaffold also lends itself to remodeling after implantation in vivo. Although the decellularized scaffold contains natural components, an innate immune response is seen when implanted in vivo. Modifications to the ECM can modulate the macrophage response. Porcine small intestinal submucosa ECM induced an M2 macrophage response when implanted in a rat model of body wall repair; however, cross-linking of the ECM using carbodiimide induced a switch from an M2 to an M1 response [25]. M2 profiles encourage a remodeling and healing response, whereas an M1 response is associated with chronic inflammation.

The cross-linking of the ECM also decreased the ability of the macrophages to degrade the scaffold, which may influence the overall remodeling and healing of the implanted construct [50].

A natural IgG antibody was identified in humans that recognizes the Galα1→3Gal epitope [51,52]. The α-gal antigen is expressed on glycolipids and glycoproteins in nonprimate mammals and in new world monkeys [53]. Old world monkeys, apes, and humans lack the expression of α-1,3galactosyltransferase, which results in the absence of expression of the α-gal epitope on their cell membranes [54]. In humans, antigal antibodies are produced in response to cell wall carbohydrate antigens on bacterial residing in the gastrointestinal track [55]. The natural antibodies are produced continuously throughout the life of the individual and make up about 1% of the circulating IgG antibodies [51,56]. The use of xenogeneic decellularized scaffolds from nonprimate mammals presents problems associated with the host immune response. Decellularized porcine scaffolds retain the α-gal epitopes [57]. On implantation of the porcine scaffolds, the natural antibodies can bind to the epitopes and may initiate an inflammatory response related to the activation of complement, which can accelerate the degradation of the ECM and can drive the response to fibrosis rather than remodeling [57]. The tissue source of the ECM scaffold also plays a role in the severity of the immune response from the circulating anti-α-gal antibodies. This may reflect the concentration of the α-gal epitopes on the ECM. Swine intestinal submucosa (SIS) ECM has a lower α-gal expression than porcine cartilage ECM [58]. Implantation of SIS ECM in wild-type and α-1,3-galactosyltransferase gene knockout mice showed anti-α gal antibodies delayed but did not inhibit the remodeling of the implant [59]. However, the implantation of porcine cartilage into cynomolgus monkeys resulted in significant inflammatory response associated with the α-gal epitope [60]. To overcome this problem, scaffolds can be treated with α-galactosidase to remove α-gal epitope, or the scaffold can be obtained from α-1,3-galactosyltransferase knockout pigs [61].

CONCLUSION

The understanding of the immune response to the implantation of biomaterials is critical for the design and development of new materials for tissue engineering and regenerative medicine. The implantation of a biomaterial in vivo initiates a series of events that involves an acute inflammatory response that leads to either a chronic inflammatory response with potential adjacent tissue damage and fibrosis formation or to an antiinflammatory response with a healing response. A better understating of surface chemistry and how the biomaterial surface characteristics influence and direct the immune response will be critical in the identification and manufacturing of novel biomaterials for tissue engineering applications in the future.

LIST OF ACRONYMS AND ABBREVIATIONS

Ig Immunoglobulin
MHC Major histocompatibility complex
NK cells Natural killer cells
NOD Nucleotide-binding oligomerization domain
PAMPS Pathogen-associated molecular patterns
PRRs Pattern recognition receptors

REFERENCES

[1] Newton K, Dixit VM. Signaling in innate immunity and inflammation. Cold Spring Harb Perspect Biol 2012;4(3).

[2] Kumar H, Kawai T, Akira S. Toll-like receptors and innate immunity. Biochem Biophys Res Commun 2009;388(4):621–5.

[3] Weis WI, Taylor ME, Drickamer K. The C-type lectin superfamily in the immune system. Immunol Rev 1998;163:19–34.

[4] Janeway Jr CA, Medzhitov R. Innate immune recognition. Annu Rev Immunol 2002;20:197–216.

[5] Inohara N, Nunez G. NODs: intracellular proteins involved in inflammation and apoptosis. Nat Rev Immunol 2003;3(5):371–82.

[6] Mosmann TR, Cherwinski H, Bond MW, Giedlin MA, Coffman RL. Two types of murine helper *Immunol* T cell clone. I. Definition according to profiles of lymphokine activities and secreted proteins. J Immunol 1986;136(7):2348–57.

[7] Mosmann TR, Coffman RL. TH1 and TH2 cells: different patterns of lymphokine secretion lead to different functional properties. Annu Rev Immunol 1989;7:145–73.

[8] Mangan PR, Harrington LE, O'Quinn DB, et al. Transforming growth factor-beta induces development of the T(H)17 lineage. Nature 2006;441(7090):231–4.

[9] Stokinger B, Veldhoen M. Differentiation and function of Th17 T cells. Curr Opin Immunol 2007;19(3):281–6.

[10] Fossiez F, Banchereau J, Murray R, Van Kooten C, Garrone P, Lebecque S. Interleukin-17. Int Rev Immunol 1998;16(5–6):541–51.

[11] Harrington LE, Mangan PR, Weaver CT. Expanding the effector CD4 T-cell repertoire: the Th17 lineage. Curr Opin Immunol 2006;18(3):349–56.

[12] Anderson JM, Rodriguez A, Chang DT. Foreign body reaction to biomaterials. Semin Immunol 2008;20(2):86–100.

[13] Nilsson B, Korsgren O, Lambris JD, Ekdahl KN. Can cells and biomaterials in therapeutic medicine be shielded off from innate immune recognition? Trends Immunol 2010;31(1):32.

[14] Gorbet MB, Sefton MV. Biomaterial-associated thrombosis: roles of coagulation factors, complement, platelets and leukocytes. Biomaterials 2004;25(26):5681–703.

[15] Andersson J, Ekdahl KN, Larsson R, Nilsson UR, Nilsson B. C3 adsorbed to a polymer surface can form an initiating alternative pathway convertase. J Immunol 2002;168(11):5786–91.

[16] Chenoweth DE. Complement activation in extracorporeal circuits. Ann NY Acad Sci 1987;516:306–13.

[17] Wettero J, Bengtsson T, Tengvall P. Complement activation on immunoglobulin G-coated hydrophobic surfaces enhances the release of oxygen radicals from neutrophils through an actin-dependent mechanism. J Biomed Mater Res 2000;51(4):742–51.

[18] Erdei A, Andrásfalvy M, Péterfy H, Tóth G, Pecht I. Regulation of mast cell activation by complement-derived peptides. Immunol Lett 2004;92(1–2):39–42.

[19] Zhou W. The new face of anaphylatoxins in immune regulation. Immunobiology 2012;217(2):225–34.

[20] Yamashiro S, Kamohara H, Wang J-M, Yang D, Gong W-H, Yoshimura T. Phenotypic and functional change of cytokine-activated neutrophils: inflammatory neutrophils are heterogeneous and enhance adaptive immune responses. J Leukoc Biol 2001;69(5):698–704.

[21] Garg K, Ryan JJ, Bowlin GL. Modulation of mast cell adhesion, proliferation, and cytokine secretion on electrospun bioresorbable vascular grafts. J Biomed Mater Res Part A 2011;97(4):405–13.

[22] Tang L, Jennings TA, Eaton JW. Mast cells mediate acute inflammatory responses to implanted biomaterials. Proc Natl Acad Sci 1998;95(15):8841–6.

[23] Mantovani A, Sica A, Sozzani S, Allavena P, Vecchi A, Locati M. The chemokine system in diverse forms of macrophage activation and polarization. Trends Immunol 2004;25(12):677–86.

[24] Kou PM, Babensee JE. Macrophage and dendritic cell phenotypic diversity in the context of biomaterials. J Biomed Mater Res Part A 2011;96A(1):239–60.
[25] Badylak SF, Valentin JE, Ravindra AK, McCabe GP, Stewart-Akers AM. Macrophage phenotype as a determinant of biologic scaffold remodeling. Tissue Eng Part A 2008;14(11):1835–42.
[26] Brown BN, Valentin JE, Stewart-Akers AM, McCabe GP, Badylak SF. Macrophage phenotype and remodeling outcomes in response to biologic scaffolds with and without a cellular component. Biomaterials 2009;30(8):1482–91.
[27] Verreck FA, de Boer T, Langenberg DM, et al. Human IL-23-producing type 1 macrophages promote but IL-10-producing type 2 macrophages subvert immunity to (myco)bacteria. Proc Natl Acad Sci USA 2004;101(13):4560–5.
[28] Anderson J, McNally A. Biocompatibility of implants: lymphocyte/macrophage interactions. Semin Immunopathol 2011;33(3):221–33.
[29] McNally AK, Anderson JM. Complement C3 participation in monocyte adhesion to different surfaces. Proc Natl Acad Sci USA 1994;91(21):10119–23.
[30] Flo TH, Ryan L, Latz E, et al. Involvement of toll-like receptor (TLR) 2 and TLR4 in cell activation by mannuronic acid polymers. J Biol Chem 2002;277(38):35489–95.
[31] Brodbeck WG, Nakayama Y, Matsuda T, Colton E, Ziats NP, Anderson JM. Biomaterial surface chemistry dictates adherent monocyte/macrophage cytokine expression in vitro. Cytokine 2002;18(6):311–9.
[32] McInnes A, Rennick DM. Interleukin 4 induces cultured monocytes/macrophages to form giant multinucleated cells. J Exp Med 1988;167(2):598–611.
[33] DeFife KM, Jenney CR, McNally AK, Colton E, Anderson JM. Interleukin-13 induces human monocyte/macrophage fusion and macrophage mannose receptor expression. J Immunol 1997;158(7):3385–90.
[34] Kalbacova M, Roessler S, Hempel U, et al. The effect of electrochemically simulated titanium cathodic corrosion products on ROS production and metabolic activity of osteoblasts and monocytes/macrophages. Biomaterials 2007;28(22):3263–72.
[35] Brodbeck WG, MacEwan M, Colton E, Meyerson H, Anderson JM. Lymphocytes and the foreign body response: lymphocyte enhancement of macrophage adhesion and fusion. J Biomed Mater Res Part A 2005;74A(2):222–9.
[36] Rodriguez A, Meyerson H, Anderson JM. Quantitative in vivo cytokine analysis at synthetic biomaterial implant sites. J Biomed Mater Res Part A 2009;89(1):152–9.
[37] Rodriguez A, Voskerician G, Meyerson H, MacEwan SR, Anderson JM. T cell subset distributions following primary and secondary implantation at subcutaneous biomaterial implant sites. J Biomed Mater Res Part A 2008;85(2):556–65.
[38] Kabelitz D. Expression and function of Toll-like receptors in T lymphocytes. Curr Opin Immunol 2007;19(1):39–45.
[39] Li Y, Meng H, Liu Y, Lee BP. Fibrin gel as an injectable biodegradable scaffold and cell carrier for tissue engineering. Sci World J 2015;2015:685690.
[40] Lee KY, Mooney DJ. Alginate: properties and biomedical applications. Prog Polym Sci 2012;37(1):106–26.
[41] Lee CH, Singla A, Lee Y. Biomedical applications of collagen. Int J Pharm 2001;221(1–2):1–22.
[42] Xu X, Jha AK, Harrington DA, Farach-Carson MC, Jia X. Hyaluronic acid-based hydrogels: from a natural polysaccharide to complex networks. Soft Matter 2012;8(12):3280–94.
[43] Arenas-Herrera JE, Ko IK, Atala A, Yoo JJ. Decellularization for whole organ bioengineering. Biomed Mater 2013;8(1):014106.
[44] Hutmacher DW, Goh JC, Teoh SH. An introduction to biodegradable materials for tissue engineering applications. Ann Acad Med Singap 2001;30(2):183–91.
[45] Webb AR, Yang J, Ameer GA. Biodegradable polyester elastomers in tissue engineering. Expert Opin Biol Ther 2004;4(6):801–12.

[46] Zhu J. Bioactive modification of poly(ethylene glycol) hydrogels for tissue engineering. Biomaterials 2010;31(17):4639–56.
[47] Wang YX, Robertson JL, Spillman Jr WB, Claus RO. Effects of the chemical structure and the surface properties of polymeric biomaterials on their biocompatibility. Pharm Res 2004;21(8):1362–73.
[48] Jenney CR, Anderson JM. Adsorbed serum proteins responsible for surface dependent human macrophage behavior. J Biomed Mater Res 2000;49(4):435–47.
[49] Brodbeck WG, Voskerician G, Ziats NP, Nakayama Y, Matsuda T, Anderson JM. In vivo leukocyte cytokine mRNA responses to biomaterials are dependent on surface chemistry. J Biomed Mater Res Part A 2003;64(2):320–9.
[50] Valentin JE, Stewart-Akers AM, Gilbert TW, Badylak SF. Macrophage participation in the degradation and remodeling of extracellular matrix scaffolds. Tissue Eng Part A 2009;15(7):1687–94.
[51] Galili U, Rachmilewitz EA, Peleg A, Flechner I. A unique natural human IgG antibody with anti-alpha-galactosyl specificity. J Exp Med 1984;160(5):1519–31.
[52] Galili U, Macher BA, Buehler J, Shohet SB. Human natural anti-alpha-galactosyl IgG. II. The specific recognition of alpha (1----3)-linked galactose residues. J Exp Med 1985;162(2):573–82.
[53] Galili U, Shohet SB, Kobrin E, Stults CL, Macher BA. Man, apes, and Old World monkeys differ from other mammals in the expression of alpha-galactosyl epitopes on nucleated cells. J Biol Chem 1988;263(33):17755–62.
[54] Galili U. Evolution and pathophysiology of the human natural anti-alpha-galactosyl IgG (anti-Gal) antibody. Springer Semin Immunopathol 1993;15(2–3):155–71.
[55] Galili U, Mandrell RE, Hamadeh RM, Shohet SB, Griffiss JM. Interaction between human natural anti-alpha-galactosyl immunoglobulin G and bacteria of the human flora. Infect Immun 1988;56(7):1730–7.
[56] Galili U, Buehler J, Shohet SB, Macher BA. The human natural anti-Gal IgG. III. The subtlety of immune tolerance in man as demonstrated by crossreactivity between natural anti-Gal and anti-B antibodies. J Exp Med 1987;165(3):693–704.
[57] Galili U. Avoiding detrimental human immune response against mammalian extracellular matrix implants. Tissue Eng Part B Rev 2014;21(2):231–41.
[58] McPherson TB, Liang H, Record RD, Badylak SF. Galalpha(1,3)Gal epitope in porcine small intestinal submucosa. Tissue Eng 2000;6(3):233–9.
[59] Raeder RH, Badylak SF, Sheehan C, Kallakury B, Metzger DW. Natural anti-galactose alpha1,3 galactose antibodies delay, but do not prevent the acceptance of extracellular matrix xenografts. Transpl Immunol 2002;10(1):15–24.
[60] Stone KR, Ayala G, Goldstein J, Hurst R, Walgenbach A, Galili U. Porcine cartilage transplants in the cynomolgus monkey. III. Transplantation of alpha-galactosidase-treated porcine cartilage. Transplantation 1998;65(12):1577–83.
[61] Phelps CJ, Koike C, Vaught TD, et al. Production of alpha 1,3-galactosyltransferase-deficient pigs. Science 2003;299(5605):411–4.

CHAPTER

FOREIGN BODY REACTION AND STEM CELL RESPONSES

4

A. Nair, L. Tang

University of Texas at Arlington, Arlington, TX, United States

CHAPTER OUTLINE

INTRODUCTION

Stem cells have been shown to be an integral part of tissue engineering. Stem cells, both mesenchymal and hematopoietic, have been shown to facilitate tissue regeneration and alter adverse inflammatory responses. Most commonly, porous and degradable scaffolds are seeded with stem cells prior to implantation. Despite improvements in tissue regeneration, the implementation of this approach is hindered by limited cell sources, extensive time consumption, high expenses, and poor shelf-life. Therefore there is a need for the development of novel methods for incorporating stem cells into tissue engineering design. Interestingly, many of our damaged tissues can be regenerated via the recruitment and differentiation of autologous stem cells into specialized tissues. Also, studies have shown that autologous stem cells

In Situ Tissue Regeneration. http://dx.doi.org/10.1016/B978-0-12-802225-2.00004-0

are found at the implant tissue interface. A number of factors that include implant surface chemistry, inflammatory cells, and various cytokines are responsible for this phenomenon. Going forward, this phenomenon can be harnessed to yield more successful tissue engineering outcomes using biomaterials and autologous stem cells. It is likely that with proper microenvironment and localized biological stimulation to injured tissue, such as fractured bone, specific tissue scaffolds can be fabricated to trigger normal tissue regeneration via autologous stem cells without the need for cell isolation, seeding, and prolonged in vitro culture. To achieve this goal, it is important to find answers to the following questions. First, how do host cells respond to scaffold implants? Will biomaterial-mediated inflammatory responses elicit autologous stem cell reactions? What is the role of stem cells in foreign body reactions? How can we alter localized stem cell responses? How will altered stem cell responses affect subsequent tissue regeneration? This chapter summarizes scientific understanding and findings in addressing the above questions. It also recapitulates key aspects of biomaterial-mediated inflammatory and fibrotic responses, elucidates the spontaneous recruitment of autologous stem cells, and explains how this phenomenon can be harnessed to successfully regenerate tissues and organs.

IMPLANT-MEDIATED INFLAMMATORY RESPONSES AND STEM CELL RECRUITMENT

All biomaterial and scaffold implants prompt different extents of tissue responses, starting with inflammatory responses and ending with fibrotic tissue formation. Such reactions are generally considered as adverse responses, since extensive inflammatory and fibrotic reactions to biomaterials have been thought to contribute to the failure of many implants, including temporomandibular joint implants [1], breast implants [2], neural electrodes [3], eye implants [4], and other joint implants [5]. Extensive research efforts have been placed on answering the questions – "How does the immune system recognize medical implants?" and "Do foreign body reactions differ from normal wound healing responses?".

FOREIGN BODY REACTIONS VERSUS WOUND HEALING RESPONSES

Placement of a biomaterial implant, such as tissue scaffolds, is usually accomplished by injection, insertion, or surgical placement that causes varying levels of tissue and cell injury. The implantation procedure often elicits mast cell activation [6,7] followed by an influx of plasma proteins and blood clot formation at the implantation sites [8]. This is similar to the responses seen in wound sites. In normal wounds, fibrin clots prompt the accumulation and activation of neutrophils and then macrophages. With the degradation of fibrin clots, inflammatory responses retreat and are replaced by fibrotic cells, which subsequently leads to scar formation. However, a fibrin clot has a different fate when it is near medical implants. Possibly due to hydrophobic interactions, plasma proteins that are initially loosely bound to biomaterial surfaces bind tightly via conformational changes of the proteins [9]. Medical implants are often surrounded by both enzymatically formed fibrin clots and surface-denatured fibrin(ogen). Unlike fibrin clots in "normal" wounds, biomaterial-associated fibrin clots cannot be fully degraded by inflammatory cells via enzymatic digestion and/or phagocytosis. Thus medical devices and scaffold implants are recognized as undissolvable fibrin clots, which cause chronic inflammatory and then fibrotic responses [9]. The chronic immune responses to scaffolds and biomaterial implants lead to fibrotic tissue or scar formations, which isolate the implants from surrounding host tissues.

Extensive studies have revealed the complexity of foreign body reactions, which are orchestrated by a wide variety of inflammatory cytokines and chemokines. Briefly, mast cell activation and degranulation release many inflammatory mediators, including histamine, monocyte chemoattractant protein-1 (MCP-1), and tumor necrosis factor-α (TNF-α) [6,9]. These inflammatory mediators open the vasculature for immigration of neutrophils and monocytes/macrophages into the biomaterial implantation sites. Once they exit the blood vessels, inflammatory cells migrate toward the implants guided by the gradient of chemokines, like macrophage inflammatory protein-1α (MIP-1α) and MCP-1 [9]. Upon arriving at the implant surface, immigrated inflammatory cells produce different inflammatory cytokines, such as TNF-α, interleukine-1β (IL-1β), IL-6, IL-8, keratinocyte chemoattractant (KC), MIP-1α/γ, MCP-1, platelet factor-4 (PF-4), tissue inhibitor of metalloproteinases-1 (TIMP1), and vascular endothelial growth factor (VEGF) [10–12]. It is generally believed that release of inflammatory cytokines prompts inflammatory cell responses to biomaterial implants. However, there are many gaps in our understanding of how biomaterial implants prompt the recruitment and responses of regenerative cells, such as stem cells and fibroblasts.

IMPLANT-MEDIATED STEM AND PROGENITOR CELL RECRUITMENT

We have found many spindle-shaped cells in the culture of tissue fluids isolated from poly-L lactic acid (PLLA) tubes implanted in subcutaneous cavities. Interestingly, many of these cells were found to have markers resembling mesenchymal stem cells (MSCs, CD90+/CD105+/CD73+/CD45-), hematopoietic stem cells (HSCs, Sca1+/ckit+/Lin-), and fibrocytes [CD45+/Collagen-1+/ α-smooth muscle actin- (α-SMA-)] in addition to inflammatory cells [11,13]. Many of these cells could proliferate and be differentiated into various lineages in vitro, including osteogenic, neurogenic, adipogenic, etc. In addition, immunofluorescence analysis using the same markers confirmed the presence of MSC [with different sets of markers, including CD105+/CD45-/CD34-/CD56-, Stro-1+/CD45-/CD34-, and stage specific embryonic antigen-4+ (SSEA4+)/CD45-] (Fig. 4.1A) and HSC (Lin-/Sca-1+/ckit+) (Fig. 4.1B) at the implantation sites of poly-l-lactic-co-glycolic acid (PLGA) and PLLA scaffolds [11,14–20].

INFLAMMATION-MEDIATED STEM CELL RECRUITMENT

Interestingly, when we studied the recruitment of inflammatory and stem cells around implantable microparticle biomaterials with varying inflammatory stimuli, a very interesting phenomenon unraveled. We found that inflammatory cell recruitment preceded stem cell recruitment with CD11b + inflammatory cell numbers increasing until day 4 following implantation (~35%), after which they declined (to ~10%). However, stem cell numbers peaked only by day 7, almost 3 days after maximal inflammatory cell accumulation was observed (Fig. 4.1C). This phenomenon suggests that inflammatory responses influence the extent of stem cell recruitment. Indeed, by administering an antiinflammatory drug, dexamethasone, around the implants, inflammatory as well as stem cell numbers reduced dramatically (Fig. 4.1D) [11]. In support of these observations, there have been numerous studies that have shown reduced MSC recruitment as well as neural stem cell proliferation following administration of antiinflammatory drugs [21,22].

The effect of foreign body reactions on stem cell recruitment could also be visualized using near infrared (NIR) labeled MSCs. It should be noted that to reduce trauma associated with biomaterial implantation, microparticles made of different biomaterials were used to provide maximal cell:material interactions. We found that shortly after implantation, large numbers of MSCs accumulated in the areas with

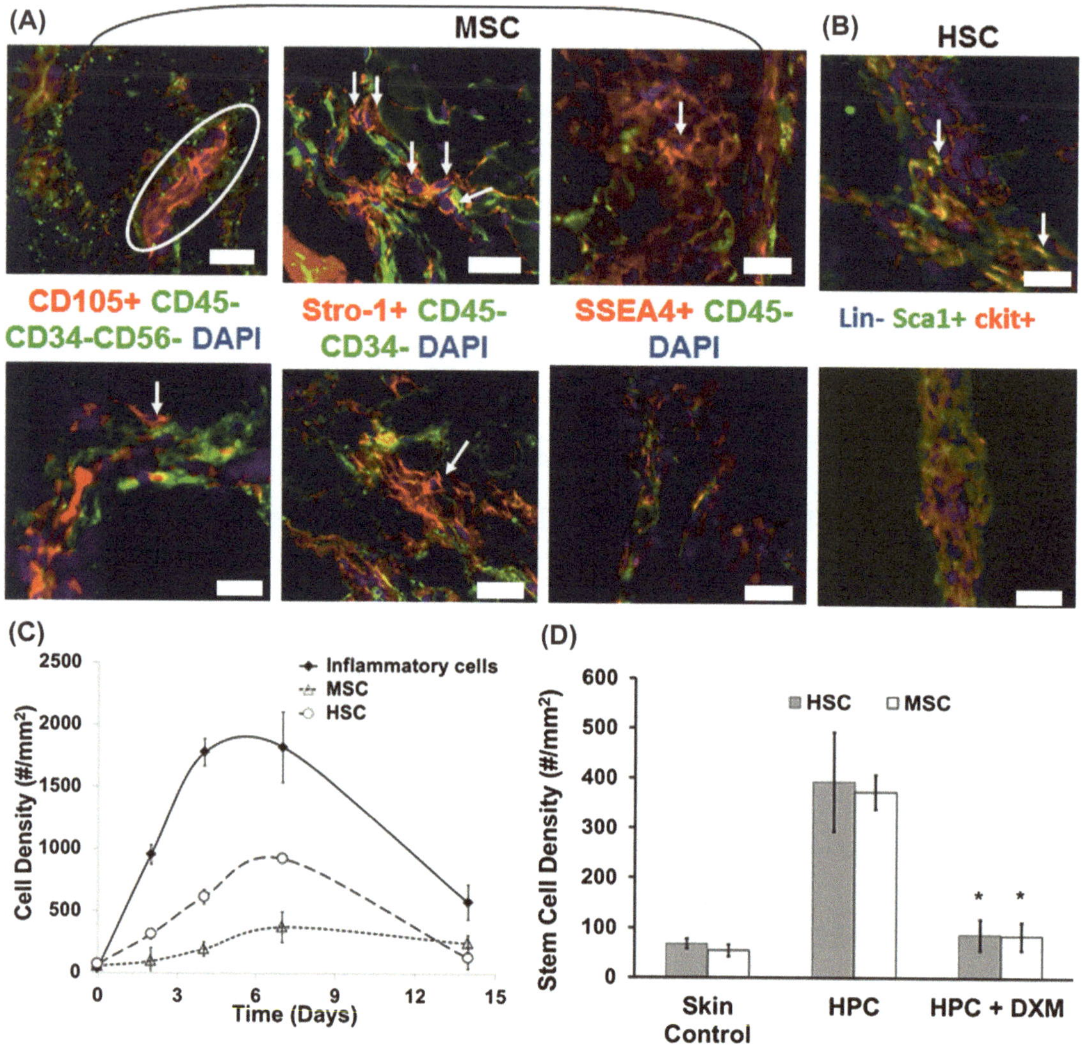

FIGURE 4.1

Accumulation of autologous stem cells, both MSCs and HSCs, was greater around the proinflammatory materials (top panel) as compared to the least inflammatory materials (lower panel) (A–B). Stem cells, as well as inflammatory cells, were quantified to reveal that inflammatory cell numbers peaked by day 4, while stem cell numbers peaked around day 7 (C). Administration of the antiinflammatory drug dexamethasone resulted in stem cell numbers (D).

Adapted from Nair A, Shen J, Lotfi P, Ko CY, Zhang CC, Tang L. Biomaterial implants mediate autologous stem cell recruitment in mice. Acta Biomater November 2011;7(11):3887–95.

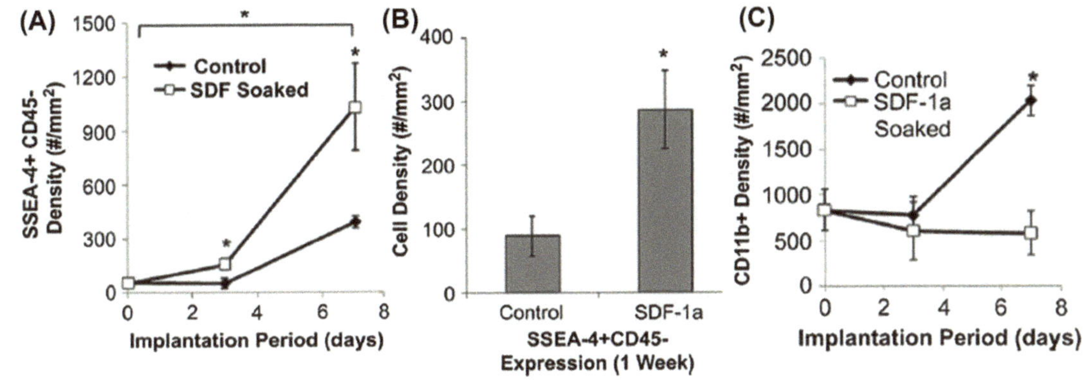

FIGURE 4.2

Engraftment of MSCs increased following CXCL12 (SDF-1α) release from scaffolds (A) with an almost threefold increase in cell numbers by 1 week (B). At the same time, inflammatory cell density decreased by day 3 and remained at those levels until a week following CXCL12 release (C).

Adapted from Thevenot PT, Nair AM, Shen J, Lotfi P, Ko CY, Tang L. The effect of incorporation of SDF-1alpha into PLGA scaffolds on stem cell recruitment and the inflammatory response. Biomaterials May 2010;31(14):3997–4008.

microsphere implants (Fig. 4.2A), and the numbers of recruited MSCs increased with time (Fig. 4.2B). Since there was no surgical trauma associated with microparticle implants, the accumulation of MSCs was most likely mediated by the inflammatory signals released as a result of foreign body reactions.

The extent of stem cell recruitment is likely controlled by the degree of foreign body reactions. To test this hypothesis, we used a series of biomaterial microparticles known to elicit different extents of inflammatory responses. Specifically, we tested microparticles made of PLLA (used for tissue engineering scaffolds), N-isopropyl acrylamide (NIPAm, used for drug delivery applications) [23], polypropylene (PP), and hydroxypropyl cellulose (HPC) (both PP and HPC used for drug delivery). All microparticles were implanted for 7 days (sufficient time for both inflammatory cell and stem cell responses) and then recovered for histological analyses. We found significant recruitment of MSC (with different sets of markers, including CD105+/CD45-/CD34-/CD56-, Stro-1+/CD45-/CD34-, and SSEA4+/CD45-) and HSCs (Lin-/Sca-1+/ckit+) at the sites of microparticles made of HPC, PLLA, and PP. On the other hand, NIPAm microsphere implants were found to have statistically lesser (>4x) numbers of stem and progenitor cells [11].

There is overwhelming evidence to support that stem cells assist in wound healing through angiogenesis, paracrine production, and cell differentiation [24,25]. It is generally believed that recruited stem cells participate in tissue repair and regeneration and scar tissue formation [11]. However, the function and activities of recruited stem cells at the biomaterial implant sites have yet to be determined.

INFLAMMATORY CYTOKINES AND STEM CELL RECRUITMENT

The notion that something in the milieu around the implants could be triggering the recruitment of autologous stem cells has become increasingly credible, and delivering these specific biomolecules in

Table 4.1 Relative Expression of Inflammatory Cytokines in Tissue Space Surrounding Proinflammatory Implants (HPC) Versus Normal Skin and Least Inflammatory (NIPAm) After Implantation for 7 days

Protein	Expression	
	HPC Versus Normal Skin Control	HPC Versus NIPAm
CXCL1/KC	*3.62*	*3.24*
CCL2/MCP-1	*11.47*	*6.63*
CCL3/MIP-1α	*19.75*	*13.42*
CCF18/MIP-1γ	*7.52*	*2.62*
CXCL2/MIP-2	*23.49*	*14.35*
CCL4/PF-4	*4.17*	*Not significant*
TIMP-1	*41.26*	*11.42*
CCLS/RANTES; CXCL5/LIX; Fas Ligand; GM-CSF; G-CSF, IGFBP-3, 5, 6; IL-2, 3, 4, 5, 6, 9; IFN-γ, TNF-α; TPO; VCAM-1; VEGF; SCF; SDF-1	*Not significant*	*Not significant*

Adapted from Nair A, Shen J, Lotfi P, Ko CY, Zhang CC, Tang L. Biomaterial implants mediate autologous stem cell recruitment in mice. Acta Biomater November 2011;7(11):3887–95.

high concentrations over stipulated time periods has been the focus of many strategies. However, it is imperative to identify and understand some of these biomolecules. A number of in vitro studies have pointed toward the involvement of numerous cytokines like CC chemokine ligand-2 (CCL2), CCL3, CCL5, CCL7, CCL17, CCL19, CCL20, CCL21, CCL22, CCL25, CCL28, C-X-C motif ligand 8 (CXCL8), CXCL10, CXCL11, CXCL12, CXCL13, CXCL16, and C-X3-C motif ligand 1 in MSC chemotaxis [26–31].

In an attempt to understand the mechanism behind the recruitment of autologous stem cells in response to inflammatory stimuli, we compared the expression of various cytokines around a proinflammatory subcutaneous implant (HPC microparticles) with that around the least inflammatory implants (NIPAm microparticles) [11]. While it was not surprising to see the overexpression of several inflammatory cytokines like CXCL1/KC, CCL2/MCP-1, CCL3/MIP-1α, MIP-1γ, and TIMP1, it must be noted that some of these inflammatory cytokines like CCL3/MIP-1α and CCL2/MCP-1 have been associated with recruitment of hematopoietic progenitors and bone marrow cells like MSCs [32–34]. A reduction in the expression of interferon-γ (IFN-γ) was also observed and can be attributed to the anti-inflammatory nature of MSCs (Table 4.1) [35].

FIBROCYTES—PROGENITOR FIBROTIC CELLS—AND THEIR ROLE IN TISSUE REACTIONS TO MATERIALS

All biomaterial implants prompt varying degrees of fibrotic tissue reactions [9,36,37]. Biomaterial-mediated fibrotic responses are at least partially responsible for the failure of several medical implants, including a variety of biosensors, spine/joint implants, breast implants, encapsulated tissues/cells, drug delivery systems, neural electrodes, and eye implants [38–48]. However, the processes governing biomaterial-mediated fibrotic reactions are not totally understood. Fibroblasts and myofibroblasts are well established to participate in fibrotic tissue formation. However, the source of these fibrotic cells and the mediators responsible for the fibrotic cell reactions are not clear. Interestingly, for the longest time, the origin of these fibroblast-like cells was believed to be only mesenchymal. Based on several lines of evidence, we believe that fibroblast progenitor cells, fibrocytes, are responsible for fibrotic tissue reactions to biomaterial implants.

FIBROCYTES—FIBROBLAST PROGENITOR CELLS—AND THEIR ROLE IN TISSUE REACTIONS TO MATERIALS

Fibrocytes, a blood circulating $CD45^+/CD34^+$/collagen I^+/vimentin$^+$ leukocyte subpopulation, were first identified in 1994 and have been known to produce excessive extracellular matrix (ECM) proteins, such as collagens I and III and vimentin, both in vitro and in vivo [49]. Fibrocytes have been found to play a dominant role in fibrotic reactions and diseases including pulmonary fibrosis [50–54], hepatic fibrosis [55], renal fibrosis [56], and dermal wound healing [57,58]. These studies have also uncovered that certain inflammatory cytokines such as TGF-β, platelet derived growth factor, IL-10, TNF-α, IL-1β, etc., trigger the migration, proliferation, and differentiation of fibrocytes, which lead to various stages of healing or fibrosis [58–62]. Specifically, the fibrocytes typically arrive at injury sites within approximately 4days after injury, possibly through the same stromal cell-derived factor-1α (SDF-1α)/C-X-C chemokine receptor type 4 axis, which has been linked with peripheral stem cell mobilization [63]. After arrival at the wound site, fibrocytes participate in fibrotic reactions through differentiation to myofibroblasts (α-SMA$^+$) and secretion of collagen I, vimentin, and other proteins, which influence the development of fibrotic matrix [51,57,64–66].

Fibrocytes and fibrocyte-associated cellular responses are found to be essential to the fibrotic tissue reactions elicited by medical implants [13]. Studies have shown that in addition to macrophages/monocytes and polymorphonuclear neutrophils, a large number of fibroblast-like cells were recruited to biomaterial implant sites [13,67]. These fibroblast-like cells possess surface markers CD45+/collagen-1+/α-SMA-resembling fibrocytes [50,55,60]. Interestingly, we have found that fibrocytes migrate to the implant following the inflammatory cell influx and may be directly related to the degree of collagen production around the implant (Fig. 4.3). Interestingly, one study has shown that there are good correlations between the number of implant-associated fibrocytes, but not resident fibroblasts (α-SMA+), and the extent of fibrotic reactions [67].

Histological results also found that fibrocytes reach a maximal accumulation at 10days after implantation and then begin to decrease in number [13]. The reduction of implant-associated fibrocytes is likely caused by their differentiation to myofibroblasts. It is well established that as this occurs, the expression of identifying leukocyte CD34 and CD45 markers on fibrocytes diminishes while expression of α-SMA increases [50,63,68]. The fibrocyte–myofibroblast differentiation is most likely caused by the presence of inflammatory cytokines such as IL-1β and TGF-β as shown in previous work [51,69]. The differentiation of fibrocytes to myofibroblasts (α-SMA$^+$) leads to the overwhelming secretion of different ECM proteins, including collagen I, vimentin, and other ECM proteins, and then fibrotic tissue/scar formation [51,57,64–66].

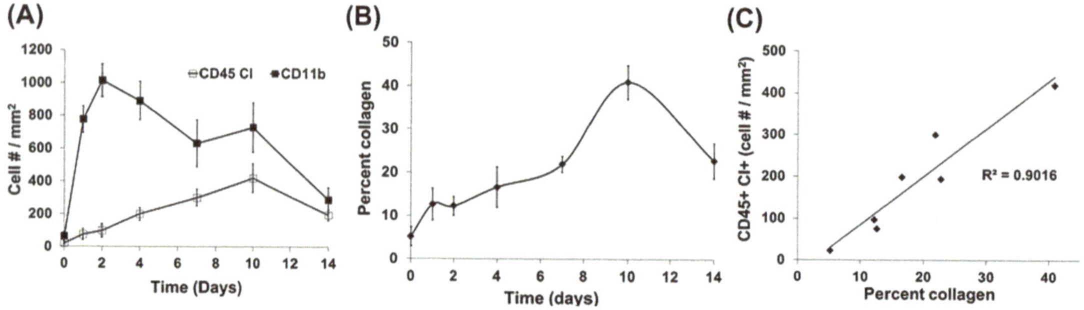

FIGURE 4.3

(A) Histological analysis of an implant surrounding tissue shows early arrival of inflammatory CD11b cells followed by an influx of fibrocytes. (B) Collagen percentage is observed to gradually increase with time around the implants. (C) Correlation reveals strong connection between recruited fibrocytes and subsequent collagen formation around the biomaterial implant.

Adapted from Thevenot PT, Baker DW, Weng H, Sun MW, Tang L. The pivotal role of fibrocytes and mast cells in mediating fibrotic reactions to biomaterials. Biomaterials November 2011;32(33):8394–403.

INFLUENCE OF INFLAMMATORY RESPONSES ON FIBROCYTES RECRUITMENT

It is well established that biomaterial-mediated inflammatory responses are initiated via mast cell activation [6,7]. Coincidentally, studies have determined that mast cell-deficient mice failed to trigger fibrotic tissue formation surrounding subcutaneous implants. Such defects can be corrected with localized replenishment of mast cells [13]. These results concur with earlier observations that highlighted the role played by mast cells in the fibrotic response of liver, lung, and many inflammatory diseases [70–74].

Mast cell and fibrocyte responses are essential to biomaterial-mediated fibrotic tissue reactions. It is likely that the products of activated mast cells are responsible for fibrocyte responses. It is well established that activated mast cells secrete a number of mediating cytokines, chemokines, growth factors, and granules, such as SDF-1α, TGF-β, IL-1β, secondary lymphoid-tissue chemokine, and MCPs [58,75]. Some of these mast cell products, including histamine, TGF-β, TNF-α, MCP-1, and SDF-1α, have been shown to promote inflammatory cells and fibrocyte immigration in vivo [6,50,58,60,76]. It should be noted that extensive research studies have demonstrated that inflammatory signals play a critical role in fibrocyte migration [50,63,68,77].

SOURCE OF FIBROCYTES

Many studies have found that fibrocytes are blood-borne, migratory, and progenitor cells [49,59,76,78]. To determine whether implant-associated fibrocytes are recruited from the blood stream, a chimeric study was carried out using bone marrow stem cells from green fluorescent protein (GFP)-transgene mice and then transplanted in radiated congenic control animals. After transplantation for 6 weeks, the chimeric animals were subcutaneously implanted with catheter tubes, as described earlier [11,49,79]. Using flow cytometry analyses, we found that biomaterial implantation substantially increased the numbers of circulating fibrocytes in blood. In addition, the numbers of implant-associated fibrocytes also increased with time (Fig. 4.4).

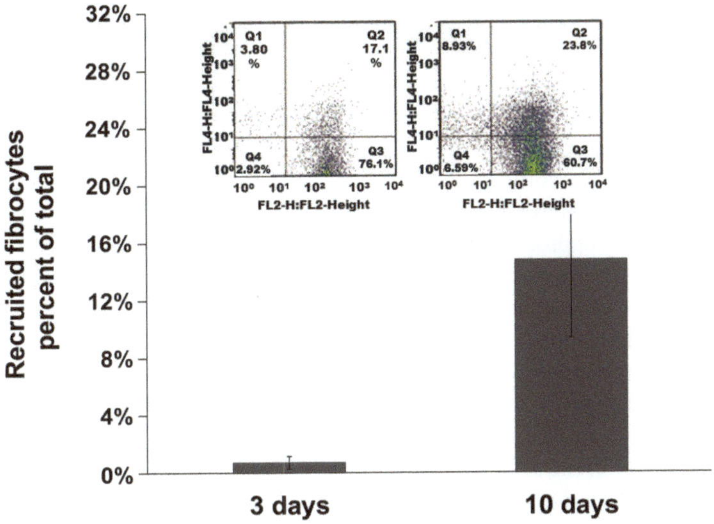

FIGURE 4.4

Implant-associated fibrocytes identified by fluorescence activate cell sorting migrate from the chimeric bone marrow (GFP+) and increase with time.

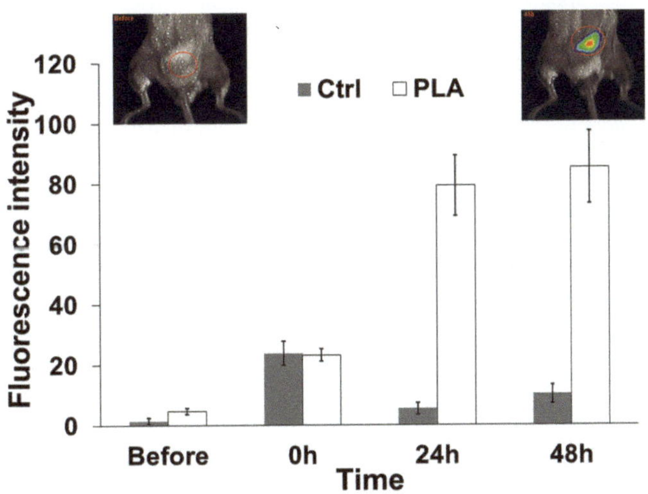

FIGURE 4.5

NIR-labeled fibrocyte migration to the site of biomaterial implantation was monitored over time at the implant sites.

Using an in vivo imaging approach [79,80], studies were carried out to examine the effect of biomaterial implants on fibrocyte recruitment. Fibrocytes harvested from the spleen were labeled with an NIR probe prior to cell transplantation [11]. As anticipated, shortly after transplantation, a substantial number of fibrocytes was found to accumulate at the implant site and was found to increase with time (Fig. 4.5). These results support our hypothesis that foreign body reactions are responsible for fibrocyte recruitment.

NEW STRATEGIES TO ENGINEER STEM CELL RESPONSES FOR TISSUE REGENERATIONS

Tissue engineering has emerged as a promising technology to replace lost, damaged, or diseased tissues. Due to their potent regenerative property and plasticity, stem cells have been widely used in tissue engineering applications. Most commonly, porous and degradable scaffolds were seeded with stem cells isolated from different sources prior to implantation. Despite improved tissue regeneration, the implementation of such an approach is hindered by limited cell sources, time consumption, high expenses, and poor shelf-life. Therefore there is a need for the development of novel methods for incorporating stem cells into tissue engineering design.

Our studies have shown that the implantation of biomaterials or tissue engineering scaffolds prompts the recruitment of the stem cells, MSCs, HSCs, fibrocytes, etc. [11,13,81] Stem cells were attracted to the implant sites by inflammatory chemokines and cytokines [11]. Without further manipulation, the recruited stem cells can turn into fibrotic and scar tissue. With the stimulation provided by inflammatory signals, these cells differentiated into myofibroblasts and fibroblasts. Such implant-surrounding myofibroblasts and fibroblasts are responsible for fibrotic tissue formation [13]. These observations suggest that spontaneously recruited and activated stem cells are programmed for scar and fibrotic tissue formations. Different strategies are needed to reprogram stem cell responses for tissue regeneration.

Under normal conditions, many of our tissues regenerate via the recruitment and differentiation of autologous stem cells into specialized tissues, such as bone, skin, muscles, etc. It is possible that with proper microenvironment and localized biological stimulation similar to damaged or diseased tissue, tissue-specific scaffolds can be made to trigger normal and specialized tissue regeneration via autologous stem cells without the need for cell isolation and in vitro manipulation. Based on this assumption, several new strategies have been explored to develop tissue engineering scaffolds capable of directing the responses of autologous stem cells. Some of these approaches are summarized in the following sections.

TISSUE ENGINEERING SCAFFOLDS FOR DIRECTING AUTOLOGOUS STEM CELL RESPONSES

To program cell responses, it is essential that scaffolds be engineered with proper regenerative microenvironment and localized biological stimulation. Many procedures have been developed for the preparation of porous matrices, such as solvent casting/particulate leaching, emulsion freeze drying, gas foaming, and thermally induced phase separation. These methods are very effective in producing scaffolds with different porosities and physical and mechanical properties. However, to facilitate optimum compatibility with cells and maintain reactivity, these scaffolds often require further processing like biomolecule coating or conjugation. Physical adsorption has been used in many studies to create growth factor-releasing scaffolds by immersing the scaffolds in growth factor-containing solution. However, this method could permit the release of growth factors for only 1–2 days. To extend the duration of release, chemical conjugation processes have been developed to produce growth factor conjugated scaffolds. Unfortunately, the chemical reactions that are part of the conjugation process often alter the bioactivity of incorporated protein. In addition, many conjugation techniques require additional complex chemical reactions. To overcome these challenges, a novel two-step porous scaffold fabrication procedure has been created in which albumin and gelatin microbubbles (MB) were used as porogens and growth factor carriers [82,83]. These MBs were added to PLGA polymer solution, which was frozen and lyophilized to yield porous scaffolds. This method was able to create porous scaffolds with pore sizes ranging from 100 to 150 μm with good interconnectivity. In addition, we found that MBs were able to protect the bioactivity (~85%) of growth factor, such as insulin-like growth factor-1, SDF-1α, and erythropoietin (Epo) [82,84].

To direct stem cell responses, scaffolds should be able to enhance stem cell recruitment and then direct specific stem cell differentiation. Many inflammatory chemokines have been shown to increase stem cell migration. Unfortunately, the release of inflammatory chemokines also promotes inflammatory responses at the implant sites. The presence of inflammatory cells and their products forces fibrotic differentiation and impedes cell-specific differentiation of the stem cells [11]. To overcome this challenge, biomolecule(s) should be selected to only react with stem cells and not inflammatory cells. For example, since SDF-1α has been shown to trigger MSC migration without proinflammatory property [79,85,86], we hypothesized that scaffolds releasing exogenous SDF-1α could prompt a substantial increase of autologous stem cell recruitment. As expected, we found that localized release of SDF-1α treated scaffolds (Fig. 4.6A and B) showed an almost three times increase in MSC engraftment [79]. In addition, by imaging the migration of intravenously administered MSCs tagged with an NIR dye, we found that SDF-1α scaffolds had a greater tendency to attract MSCs (Fig. 4.6C) [79]. In addition, we

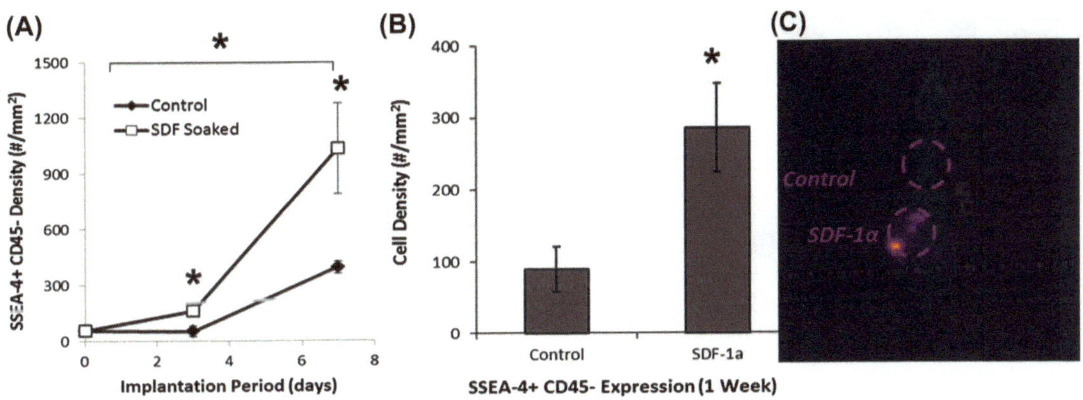

FIGURE 4.6

SDF-1α increases engraftment of MSC (SSEA-4þ CD45-cells) to subcutaneously implanted PLGA scaffolds (SSEA-4 *green*, CD45 *red*). At day 7, control untreated PLGA scaffolds have very low engraftment of MSC, while SDF-1α treated scaffolds have enhanced MSC engraftment. The density of engrafted MSC was quantified at days 3 and 7 and compared between treatment groups (A). At both time points, we observe a significant, roughly threefold increase in engrafted MSC in the SDF-1α scaffold group, Bonferroni test ($p<.05$). The density of MSC in the scaffold interior was also quantified between groups (B) and reveals again a roughly threefold increase in MSC density, Student *t*-test ($p<.05$). SDF-1α induced engraftment of tail vein injected MSC to the site of scaffold implantation 48 hrs after injection was visualized using an animal whole body imaging system (C).

Adapted from Thevenot PT, Nair AM, Shen J, Lotfi P, Ko CY, Tang L. The effect of incorporation of SDF-1alpha into PLGA scaffolds on stem cell recruitment and the inflammatory response. Biomaterials May 2010;31(14):3997–4008.

found that the localized delivery of SDF-1α could not only enhance MSC migration but also HSC and endothelial progenitor cell (EPC) ($CD34^+$ $CD133^+$) engraftment near the scaffolds [79].

Rather surprisingly, we found that localized release of SDF-1α substantially reduced the recruitment of activated mast cells and inflammatory cells in the subcutaneous space around the implant. In addition, SDF-1α treatment reduced the thickness of tissue capsule surrounding the scaffold implants. The mechanism of SDF-1α-associated antiinflammatory and antifibrotic responses is yet to be determined. It is, however, possible that increased stem cell recruitment at the implant site alleviates inflammatory responses and release of inflammatory products, as suggested in an early work [87]. Furthermore, scaffolds releasing SDF-1α were found to promote angiogenesis in the tissue surrounding scaffold implants.

Overall, our results provide a novel strategy to recruit autologous stem cells for tissue regeneration and also create an angiogenic environment favoring later tissue ingrowth inside scaffolds. The hypothetical mechanism governing preferential recruitment of stem cells leading to healthy and regenerative tissue environment has been investigated between untreated and SDF-1α treated implants (Fig. 4.7).

PROGRAMMED STEM CELL DIFFERENTIATION TO ALTER FIBROCYTE REACTIONS

The stem cells recruited by biomaterial-mediated inflammatory responses undergo fibrotic cell differentiation, which leads to fibrotic tissue formations. Since adult stem cells are multipotent and can be

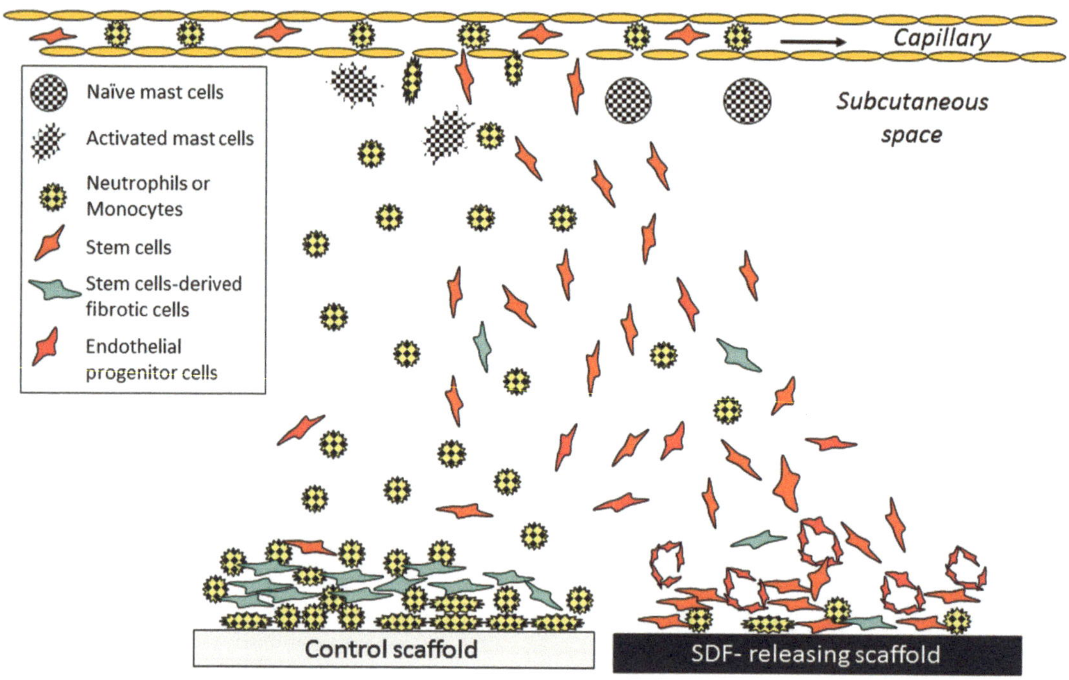

FIGURE 4.7

Hypothetical mechanism of SDF-directed stem cell responses with reduced inflammatory responses and improved angiogenesis.

differentiated into specialized cells such as osteoblasts, neuronal cells, adipocytes, etc., it is possible that with localized exogenous stimulation, recruited stem cells can be differentiated into nonfibrotic cells and lead to reduced fibrotic tissue responses. To test this hypothesis, we first confirmed that 65–70% of fibrocytes can be differentiated into adipocytes with the stimulation of an adipogenic medium in vitro [81]. Fibrocytes have spindle-shaped morphology. On the other hand, the fibrocyte-derived adipocytes are larger and stained positive with Oil Red O. These findings are in agreement with previous reports indicating that adipocyte and myofibroblast differentiation pathways of fibrocytes show reciprocal inhibition of each other [88,89].

Subsequent studies were carried out to assess the effect of adipogenic differentiation of fibrocytes on fibrotic tissue responses to biomaterial implants. Indeed, with adipogenic cocktail stimulation, we found a substantial increase in the lipid droplet accumulation (2.8-fold) throughout the developing tissue surrounding scaffold implants, thereby supporting an increase in adipogenesis. On the other hand, collagen staining results showed significantly lesser collagen productions (2.3-fold) compared to untreated controls. These results suggest that adipogenic treatment forced fibrocytes to differentiate into adipocytes and indirectly reduce fibrocytes' myofibroblast differentiations. To test this hypothesis, we quantified the numbers of adipocytes and myofibroblasts surrounding variously treated implants at days 5 and 14 (Fig. 4.8). At day 5 (acute phase), we found no difference between fibrocyte numbers in both untreated versus adipogenic cocktail-treated scaffolds (Fig. 4.8A). These results suggest that the release of adipogenic cocktail has little or no influence

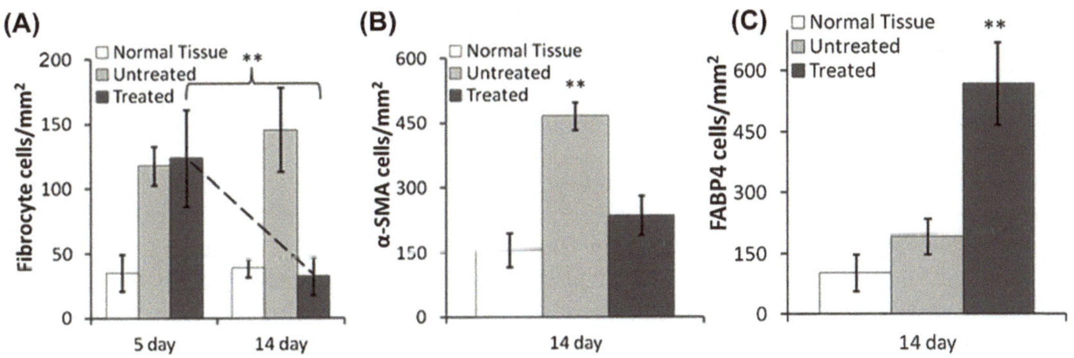

FIGURE 4.8

Quantification of fibrocytes, myofibroblasts expression (α-SMA), and adipocyte expression (FABP4) during adipogenic differentiation. (A) The acute fibrocyte response shows approximately equal recruitment to both the untreated and treated scaffold samples, where the 14-day response shows a drastic reduction in the fibrocyte numbers surrounding the treated scaffold implants. (B) After 14 days, the α-SMA expression levels are significantly reduced during treatment from the untreated scaffold samples and remain within the range of the normal tissue response. (C) As anticipated, after 14 days, the adipogenic marker FABP4 expression levels are significantly increased on the treated samples. Statistics are performed with ANOVA using Bonferroni comparisons and taken to be significant at $^{**}p<.01$.

Adapted from Baker DW, Tsai YT, Weng H, Tang L. Alternative strategies to manipulate fibrocyte involvement in the fibrotic tissue response: pharmacokinetic inhibition and the feasibility of directed-adipogenic differentiation. Acta Biomater July 2014;10(7):3108–16.

on fibrocyte recruitment. However, after 14 days (middle to chronic state), a significantly lesser number of fibrocytes (4.5-fold) was found throughout the capsule in adipogenic cocktail-treated scaffolds than untreated controls (Fig. 4.8A). Coincidentally, we also observed a 51% decrease in the α-SMA + myofibroblasts in capsules surrounding adipogenic cocktail-treated scaffolds in comparison with controls (Fig. 4.8B). Furthermore, the fatty acid binding protein 4 (FABP4) positive mature adipocytes showed a 66% increase in treated samples as compared with untreated controls (Fig. 4.8C). These results support our hypothesis that by forcing nonfibrotic differentiation of stem cells, including fibrocytes, we can change the course of "normal" wound healing responses to substantially increase specialized cell formation at the implant sites and, rather indirectly, reduce undesirable tissue responses, such as fibrotic tissue scar formation surrounding tissue scaffold implants.

CYTOKINE-MEDIATED STEM CELL RECRUITMENT AND TISSUE REGENERATION

The results from the previous two approaches support the possibility that chemokines/growth factor-loaded tissue engineering scaffolds can be fabricated to enhance the recruitment of autologous stem cells and promote the specialized cell differentiation of immigrated progenitor/stem cells. To regenerate specialized tissue using autologous stem cells, we then explored the possibility of using chemokines/growth factors to simultaneously direct stem cell recruitment and differentiation. Specifically, we are interested in Epo and SDF-1α, which have been shown to be a potent chemokine for both MSC and HSC recruitment as well as angiogenesis [79,90–92]. In addition, it has been suggested that Epo triggers the osteogenic differentiation of MSCs [93]. Based on these reports and our own results, we focused our investigation on the proosteogenic effects of Epo. On the other hand, bone morphogenetic protein-2 (BMP-2) was used as an osteogenic agent, since the incorporation of BMP-2 in tissue engineering scaffolds has been shown to promote bone mineralization both in vitro and in vivo [94,95].

A series of studies were carried out to test the hypothesis that tissue scaffolds can be fabricated to simultaneously recruit and then differentiate autologous stem cells into bone forming cells in an effort to regenerate bone tissue. Specifically, Epo and SDF-1α were used to fabricate chemokine-releasing scaffolds. Our studies first identified greater migration of injected MSCs to Epo loaded scaffolds followed by SDF-1α scaffolds. The results led to the use of Epo as a stem cell chemoattractant in later studies. Both Epo and BMP-2 were used as osteogenic agents to fabricate a series of scaffolds, including scaffolds loaded with Epo alone, BMP-2 alone, or a combination of Epo + BMP-2. The osteogenic capability of these scaffolds was then tested using a murine calvarial defect model. As expected, we found that the release of Epo significantly increased the presence of osteoblasts and osteogenic products, such as osteocalcin and osteopontin, as compared with BMP-2 treatment. Furthermore, as seen in the computerized tomography scan images, we found that Epo-loaded scaffolds and Epo + BMP-2-loaded scaffolds had the highest ectopic bone formation with almost complete (>80%) bridging than BMP-2-loaded scaffolds (Fig. 4.9A). These observations were confirmed with quantitative measurement of bone volumes (Fig. 4.9B) [96]. These results support the idea that incorporation of combined stem cell chemoattractant and differentiation agents can create suitable microenvironment to significantly improve regeneration of specialized tissue, such as bone.

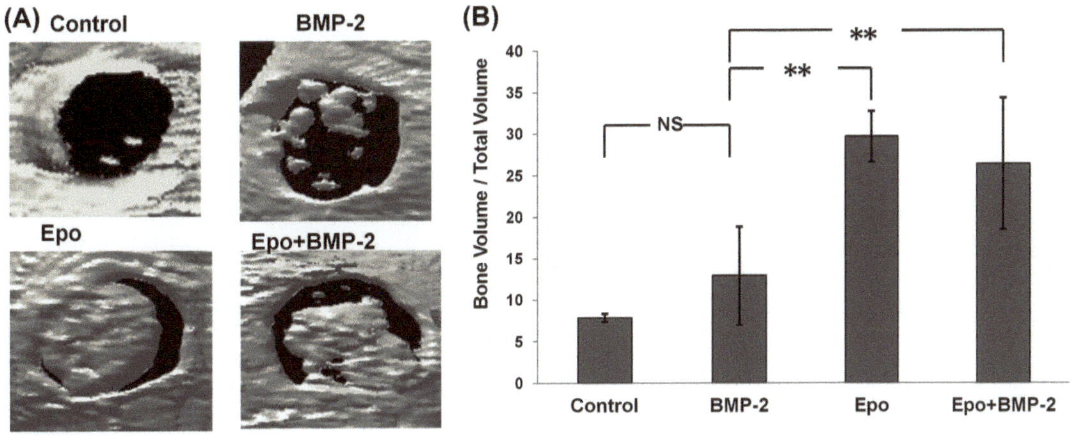

FIGURE 4.9

Bridging calvarial defect using cytokine scaffolds after 8 weeks. (A) CT scan images show incomplete to almost complete bridging of the defect in various treatment groups. (B) Bone mineral density was quantified (n=6 per group; significance of mean values versus control tested at $p<.01$, **).

Adapted from Nair AM, Tsai YT, Shah KM, Shen J, Weng H, Zhou J, et al. The effect of erythropoietin on autologous stem cell-mediated bone regeneration. Biomaterials October 2013;34(30):7364–71.

CONCLUSIONS

Implantation of biomaterials and tissue scaffolds often triggers the recruitment of stem and progenitor cells, including MSCs, HSCs, fibrocytes, EPCs, etc. Nevertheless, in light of the current results, our findings bring forth a plethora of opportunities to harness the proosteogenic effect of Epo for biomaterial and bone tissue engineering research and product development.

Although still in the nascent stages, the exploration of combinatorial cytokine delivery might hold the key to the future of tissue engineering. Significant effort must be expended in the identification of the molecular mechanisms at play and the interactions between the cytokines and the tissue space to successfully facilitate autologous stem cell-mediated in vivo tissue regeneration.

LIST OF ACRONYMS AND ABBREVIATIONS

BMP-2 Bone morphogenetic protein-2
CCL CC chemokine ligand
CT Computerized tomography
CXCL C-X-C motif ligand
CX_3CL1 C-X3-C motif ligand 1
CXCR4 C-X-C chemokine receptor type 4
ECM Extracellular matrix
EPCs Endothelial progenitor cells

Epo Erythropoietin
FABP4 Fatty acid binding protein 4
HPC Hydroxypropyl cellulose
HSCs Hematopoietic stem cells
IFN-γ Interferon-γ
IGF-1 Insulin-like growth factor-1
IL-1 β Interleukin-1β
KC Keratinocyte chemoattractant
MΦ Macrophages/monocytes
MCP-1 Monocyte chemoattractant protein-1
MIP-1α Macrophage inflammatory protein-1α
MSCs Mesenchymal stem cells
NIPAm N-Isopropyl acrylamide
NIR Near infrared
PDGF Platelet-derived growth factor
PF-4 Platelet factor-4
PLGA Poly-l-lactic-co-glycolic acid
PLLA poly-L lactic acid
PMN Polymorphonuclear neutrophils
PP Polypropylene
SDF-1α Stromal cell-derived factor-1α
SLC Secondary lymphoid-tissue chemokine
α-SMA α-Smooth muscle actin
TIMP1 Tissue inhibitor of metalloproteinases-1
TNF-α Tumor necrosis factor-α
VEGF Vascular endothelial growth factor

REFERENCES

[1] Giannakopoulos HE, Sinn DP, Quinn PD. Biomet microfixation temporomandibular joint replacement system: a 3-year follow-up study of patients treated during 1995 to 2005. J Oral Maxillofac Surg April 2012;70(4):787–94. discussion 95–6.

[2] Orciani M, Bolletta E, Campanati A, Di Benedetto G, Di Primio R. The response of breast cancer cells to mesenchymal stem cells: a possible role of inflammation by breast implants. Plast Reconstr Surg December 2013;134(6):899e–910e.

[3] Groothuis J, Ramsey NF, Ramakers GM, van der Plasse G. Physiological challenges for intracortical electrodes. Brain Stimul January–February 2014;7(1):1–6.

[4] Wertheimer C, Siedlecki J, Kook D, Mayer WJ, Wolf A, Klingenstein A, et al. EGFR inhibitor Gefitinib attenuates posterior capsule opacification in vitro and in the ex vivo human capsular bag model. Graefes Arch Clin Exp Ophthalmol March 2015;253(3):409–17.

[5] Gallo J, Goodman SB, Konttinen YT, Wimmer MA, Holinka M. Osteolysis around total knee arthroplasty: a review of pathogenetic mechanisms. Acta Biomater September 2013;9(9):8046–58.

[6] Tang L, Jennings TA, Eaton JW. Mast cells mediate acute inflammatory responses to implanted biomaterials. Proc Natl Acad Sci USA July 21, 1998;95(15):8841–6.

[7] Zdolsek J, Eaton JW, Tang L. Histamine release and fibrinogen adsorption mediate acute inflammatory responses to biomaterial implants in humans. J Transl Med 2007;5:31.

[8] Tsai YT, Zhou J, Weng H, Tang EN, Baker DW, Tang L. Optical imaging of fibrin deposition to elucidate participation of mast cells in foreign body responses. Biomaterials February 2014;35(7):2089–96.
[9] Tang L, Eaton JW. Natural responses to unnatural materials: a molecular mechanism for foreign body reactions. Mol Med June 1999;5(6):351–8.
[10] Tang L, editor. Molecular mechanism of biomaterial-mediated phagocyte responses. The Humana Press; 2000.
[11] Nair A, Shen J, Lotfi P, Ko CY, Zhang CC, Tang L. Biomaterial implants mediate autologous stem cell recruitment in mice. Acta Biomater November 2011;7(11):3887–95.
[12] Rokstad AM, Brekke OL, Steinkjer B, Ryan L, Kollarikova G, Strand BL, et al. The induction of cytokines by polycation containing microspheres by a complement dependent mechanism. Biomaterials January 2013;34(3):621–30.
[13] Thevenot PT, Baker DW, Weng H, Sun MW, Tang L. The pivotal role of fibrocytes and mast cells in mediating fibrotic reactions to biomaterials. Biomaterials November 2011;32(33):8394–403.
[14] Chamberlain G, Fox J, Ashton B, Middleton J. Concise review: mesenchymal stem cells: their phenotype, differentiation capacity, immunological features, and potential for homing. Stem Cells November 2007;25(11):2739–49.
[15] da Silva Meirelles L, Caplan AI, Nardi NB. In search of the in vivo identity of mesenchymal stem cells. Stem Cells September 2008;26(9):2287–99.
[16] Dominici M, Le Blanc K, Mueller I, Slaper-Cortenbach I, Marini F, Krause D, et al. Minimal criteria for defining multipotent mesenchymal stromal cells. The International Society for Cellular Therapy position statement. Cytotherapy 2006;8(4):315–7.
[17] Gang EJ, Bosnakovski D, Figueiredo CA, Visser JW, Perlingeiro RC. SSEA-4 identifies mesenchymal stem cells from bone marrow. Blood February 15, 2007;109(4):1743–51.
[18] Vranken I, De Visscher G, Lebacq A, Verbeken E, Flameng W. The recruitment of primitive Lin(−) Sca-1(+), CD34(+), c-kit(+) and CD271(+) cells during the early intraperitoneal foreign body reaction. Biomaterials March 2008;29(7):797–808.
[19] Weissman IL, Shizuru JA. The origins of the identification and isolation of hematopoietic stem cells, and their capability to induce donor-specific transplantation tolerance and treat autoimmune diseases. Blood November 1, 2008;112(9):3543–53.
[20] Wong SH, Lowes KN, Bertoncello I, Quigley AF, Simmons PJ, Cook MJ, et al. Evaluation of Sca-1 and c-Kit as selective markers for muscle remodelling by nonhemopoietic bone marrow cells. Stem Cells June 2007;25(6):1364–74.
[21] Chang JK, Li CJ, Wu SC, Yeh CH, Chen CH, Fu YC, et al. Effects of anti-inflammatory drugs on proliferation, cytotoxicity and osteogenesis in bone marrow mesenchymal stem cells. Biochem Pharmacol November 1, 2007;74(9):1371–82.
[22] Schroter A, Lustenberger RM, Obermair FJ, Thallmair M. High-dose corticosteroids after spinal cord injury reduce neural progenitor cell proliferation. Neuroscience July 7, 2009;161(3):753–63.
[23] Weng H, Zhou J, Tang L, Hu Z. Tissue responses to thermally-responsive hydrogel nanoparticles. J Biomater Sci Polym Edn 2004;15(9):1167–80.
[24] Wu Y, Chen L, Scott PG, Tredget EE. Mesenchymal stem cells enhance wound healing through differentiation and angiogenesis. Stem Cells October 2007;25(10):2648–59.
[25] Wu Y, Wang J, Scott PG, Tredget EE. Bone marrow-derived stem cells in wound healing: a review. Wound Repair Regen September–October 2007;15(Suppl. 1):S18–26.
[26] Honczarenko M, Le Y, Swierkowski M, Ghiran I, Glodek AM, Silberstein LE. Human bone marrow stromal cells express a distinct set of biologically functional chemokine receptors. Stem Cells April 2006;24(4):1030–41.
[27] Kalwitz G, Andreas K, Endres M, Neumann K, Notter M, Ringe J, et al. Chemokine profile of human serum from whole blood: migratory effects of CXCL-10 and CXCL-11 on human mesenchymal stem cells. Connect Tissue Res April 2010;51(2):113–22.

[28] Ponte AL, Marais E, Gallay N, Langonne A, Delorme B, Herault O, et al. The in vitro migration capacity of human bone marrow mesenchymal stem cells: comparison of chemokine and growth factor chemotactic activities. Stem Cells July 2007;25(7):1737–45.
[29] Ringe J, Strassburg S, Neumann K, Endres M, Notter M, Burmester GR, et al. Towards in situ tissue repair: human mesenchymal stem cells express chemokine receptors CXCR1, CXCR2 and CCR2, and migrate upon stimulation with CXCL8 but not CCL2. J Cell Biochem May 1, 2007;101(1):135–46.
[30] Sordi V, Malosio ML, Marchesi F, Mercalli A, Melzi R, Giordano T, et al. Bone marrow mesenchymal stem cells express a restricted set of functionally active chemokine receptors capable of promoting migration to pancreatic islets. Blood July 15, 2005;106(2):419–27.
[31] Von Luttichau I, Notohamiprodjo M, Wechselberger A, Peters C, Henger A, Seliger C, et al. Human adult CD34- progenitor cells functionally express the chemokine receptors CCR1, CCR4, CCR7, CXCR5, and CCR10 but not CXCR4. Stem Cells Dev June 2005;14(3):329–36.
[32] Lord BI, Woolford LB, Wood LM, Czaplewski LG, McCourt M, Hunter MG, et al. Mobilization of early hematopoietic progenitor cells with BB-10010: a genetically engineered variant of human macrophage inflammatory protein-1 alpha. Blood June 15, 1995;85(12):3412–5.
[33] Pelus LM, Fukuda S. Peripheral blood stem cell mobilization: the CXCR2 ligand GRObeta rapidly mobilizes hematopoietic stem cells with enhanced engraftment properties. Exp Hematol August 2006;34(8):1010–20.
[34] Zhang F, Tsai S, Kato K, Yamanouchi D, Wang C, Rafii S, et al. Transforming growth factor-beta promotes recruitment of bone marrow cells and bone marrow-derived mesenchymal stem cells through stimulation of MCP-1 production in vascular smooth muscle cells. J Biol Chem June 26, 2009;284(26):17564–74.
[35] Glennie S, Soeiro I, Dyson PJ, Lam EW, Dazzi F. Bone marrow mesenchymal stem cells induce division arrest anergy of activated T cells. Blood April 1, 2005;105(7):2821–7.
[36] Tang L, Eaton JW. Inflammatory responses to biomaterials. Am J Clin Pathol April 1995;103(4):466–71.
[37] Franz S, Rammelt S, Scharnweber D, Simon JC. Immune responses to implants - a review of the implications for the design of immunomodulatory biomaterials. Biomaterials October 2011;32(28):6692–709.
[38] Chegini N. Peritoneal molecular environment, adhesion formation and clinical implication. Front Biosci April 1, 2002;7:e91–115.
[39] Backovic A, Wolfram D. Silicone mammary implants–can we turn back the time? Exp Gerontol August 2007;42(8):713–8.
[40] Patil SD, Papadimitrakopoulos F, Burgess DJ. Dexamethasone-loaded poly(lactic-co-glycolic) acid microspheres/poly(vinyl alcohol) hydrogel composite coatings for inflammation control. Diabetes Technol Ther December 2004;6(6):887–97.
[41] Giurgiutiu V, Friedman H, Bender J, Borg T, Yost M, Newcomb W, et al. Electromechanical impedance sensor for in vivo monitoring the body reaction to implants. J Invest Surg September–October 2004;17(5):257–70.
[42] Sargeant A, Goswami T. Pathophysiological aspects of hip implants. J Surg Orthop Adv Summer 2006;15(2):111–2.
[43] Adams Jr WP, Haydon MS, Raniere Jr J, Trott S, Marques M, Feliciano M, et al. A rabbit model for capsular contracture: development and clinical implications. Plast Reconstr Surg April 2006;117(4):1214–9. discussion 20–1.
[44] Cutroneo KR, White SL, Chiu JF, Ehrlich HP. Tissue fibrosis and carcinogenesis: divergent or successive pathways dictate multiple molecular therapeutic targets for oligo decoy therapies. J Cell Biochem April 15, 2006;97(6):1161–74.
[45] Prantl L, Schreml S, Fichtner-Feigl S, Poppl N, Eisenmann-Klein M, Schwarze H, et al. Clinical and morphological conditions in capsular contracture formed around silicone breast implants. Plast Reconstr Surg July 2007;120(1):275–84.
[46] Seymour JP, Kipke DR. Neural probe design for reduced tissue encapsulation in CNS. Biomaterials September 2007;28(25):3594–607.

[47] Shirai K, Saika S, Okada Y, Oda S, Ohnishi Y. Histology and immunohistochemistry of fibrous posterior capsule opacification in an infant. J Cataract Refract Surg February 2004;30(2):523–6.
[48] Polikov VS, Tresco PA, Reichert WM. Response of brain tissue to chronically implanted neural electrodes. J Neurosci Methods October 15, 2005;148(1):1–18.
[49] Bucala R, Spiegel LA, Chesney J, Hogan M, Cerami A. Circulating fibrocytes define a new leukocyte subpopulation that mediates tissue repair. Mol Med November 1994;1(1):71–81.
[50] Phillips RJ, Burdick MD, Hong K, Lutz MA, Murray LA, Xue YY, et al. Circulating fibrocytes traffic to the lungs in response to CXCL12 and mediate fibrosis. J Clin Invest August 2004;114(3):438–46.
[51] Schmidt M, Sun G, Stacey MA, Mori L, Mattoli S. Identification of circulating fibrocytes as precursors of bronchial myofibroblasts in asthma. J Immunol July 1, 2003;171(1):380–9.
[52] Mehrad B, Burdick MD, Strieter RM. Fibrocyte CXCR4 regulation as a therapeutic target in pulmonary fibrosis. Int J Biochem Cell Biol August–September 2009;41(8–9):1708–18.
[53] Andersson-Sjoland A, de Alba CG, Nihlberg K, Becerril C, Ramirez R, Pardo A, et al. Fibrocytes are a potential source of lung fibroblasts in idiopathic pulmonary fibrosis. Int J Biochem Cell Biol 2008;40(10):2129–40.
[54] Ishida Y, Kimura A, Kondo T, Hayashi T, Ueno M, Takakura N, et al. Essential roles of the CC chemokine ligand 3-CC chemokine receptor 5 axis in bleomycin-induced pulmonary fibrosis through regulation of macrophage and fibrocyte infiltration. Am J Pathol March 2007;170(3):843–54.
[55] Scholten D, Reichart D, Paik YH, Lindert J, Bhattacharya J, Glass CK, et al. Migration of fibrocytes in fibrogenic liver injury. Am J Pathol July 2011;179(1):189–98.
[56] Sakai N, Wada T, Yokoyama H, Lipp M, Ueha S, Matsushima K, et al. Secondary lymphoid tissue chemokine (SLC/CCL21)/CCR7 signaling regulates fibrocytes in renal fibrosis. Proc Natl Acad Sci USA September 19, 2006;103(38):14098–103.
[57] Mori L, Bellini A, Stacey MA, Schmidt M, Mattoli S. Fibrocytes contribute to the myofibroblast population in wounded skin and originate from the bone marrow. Exp Cell Res March 10, 2005;304(1):81–90.
[58] Metz CN. Fibrocytes: a unique cell population implicated in wound healing. Cell Mol Life Sci July 2003;60(7):1342–50.
[59] Chesney J, Bucala R. Peripheral blood fibrocytes: mesenchymal precursor cells and the pathogenesis of fibrosis. Curr Rheumatol Rep December 2000;2(6):501–5.
[60] Herzog EL, Bucala R. Fibrocytes in health and disease. Exp Hematol July 2010;38(7):548–56.
[61] Bellini A, Mattoli S. The role of the fibrocyte, a bone marrow-derived mesenchymal progenitor, in reactive and reparative fibroses. Lab Invest September 2007;87(9):858–70.
[62] Shao DD, Suresh R, Vakil V, Gomer RH, Pilling D. Pivotal Advance: Th-1 cytokines inhibit, and Th-2 cytokines promote fibrocyte differentiation. J Leukoc Biol June 2008;83(6):1323–33.
[63] Quan TE, Cowper S, Wu S-P, Bockenstedt LK, Bucala R. Circulating fibrocytes: collagen-secreting cells of the peripheral blood. Int J Biochem Cell Biol 2004;36(4):598–606.
[64] El-Asrar AMA, Struyf S, Van Damme J, Geboes K. Circulating fibrocytes contribute to the myofibroblast population in proliferative vitreoretinopathy epiretinal membranes. Br J Ophthalmol May 2008;92(5): 699–704.
[65] Quan TE, Cowper SE, Bucala R. The role of circulating fibrocytes in fibrosis. Curr Rheumatol Rep April 2006;8(2):145–50.
[66] Strieter RM, Keeley EC, Hughes MA, Burdick MD, Mehrad B. The role of circulating mesenchymal progenitor cells (fibrocytes) in the pathogenesis of pulmonary fibrosis. J Leukoc Biol November 2009;86(5):1111–8.
[67] Baker DW, Liu X, Weng H, Luo C, Tang L. Fibroblast/fibrocyte: surface interaction dictates tissue reactions to micropillar implants. Biomacromolecules April 11, 2011;12(4):997–1005.
[68] Moore BB, Kolodsick JE, Thannickal VJ, Cooke K, Moore TA, Hogaboam C, et al. CCR2-mediated recruitment of fibrocytes to the alveolar space after fibrotic injury. Am J Pathol March 1, 2005;166(3):675–84.
[69] Chesney J, Metz C, Stavitsky AB, Bacher M, Bucala R. Regulated production of type I collagen and inflammatory cytokines by peripheral blood fibrocytes. J Immunol January 1, 1998;160(1):419–25.

[70] Masuda T, Tanaka H, Komai M, Nagao K, Ishizaki M, Kajiwara D, et al. Mast cells play a partial role in allergen-induced subepithelial fibrosis in a murine model of allergic asthma. Clin Exp Allergy 2003;33(5):705–13.
[71] Mori H, Kawada K, Zhang P, Uesugi Y, Sakamoto O, Koda A. Bleomycin-induced pulmonary fibrosis in genetically mast cell-deficient WBB6F1-W/Wv mice and mechanism of the suppressive effect of tranilast, an antiallergic drug inhibiting mediator release from mast cells, on fibrosis. Int Arch Allergy Appl Immunol 1991;95(2–3):195–201.
[72] Ayako S, Tohru T, Yukihisa F, Yasuo N, Nobuyuki T. Evaluation of role of mast cells in the development of liver fibrosis using mast cell-deficient rats and mice. J Hepatol 1999;30(5):859–67.
[73] Fairweather D, Frisancho-Kiss S, Yusung SA, Barrett MA, Davis SE, Gatewood SJL, et al. Interferon-{gamma} protects against chronic viral myocarditis by reducing mast cell degranulation, fibrosis, and the profibrotic cytokines transforming frowth vactor-{beta}1, interleukin-1{beta}, and interleukin-4 in the heart. Am J Pathol December 1, 2004;165(6):1883–94.
[74] Tcacencu I, Wendel M. Collagen-hydroxyapatite composite enhances regeneration of calvaria bone defects in young rats but postpones the regeneration of calvaria bone in aged rats. J Mater Sci Mater Med 2008;19(5):2015–21.
[75] Brightling CE, Bradding P, Pavord ID, Wardlaw AJ. New insights into the role of the mast cell in asthma. Clin Exp Allergy May 2003;33(5):550–6.
[76] Abe R, Donnelly SC, Peng T, Bucala R, Metz CN. Peripheral blood fibrocytes: differentiation pathway and migration to wound sites. J Immunol June 15, 2001;166(12):7556–62.
[77] Moore BB, Murray L, Das A, Wilke CA, Herrygers AB, Toews GB. The role of CCL12 in the recruitment of fibrocytes and lung fibrosis. Am J Respir Cell Mol Biol August 2006;35(2):175–81.
[78] Chesney J, Bucala R. Peripheral blood fibrocytes: novel fibroblast-like cells that present antigen and mediate tissue repair. Biochem Soc Trans May 1997;25(2):520–4.
[79] Thevenot PT, Nair AM, Shen J, Lotfi P, Ko CY, Tang L. The effect of incorporation of SDF-1alpha into PLGA scaffolds on stem cell recruitment and the inflammatory response. Biomaterials May 2010;31(14):3997–4008.
[80] Zhou J, Tsai YT, Weng H, Baker DW, Tang L. Real time monitoring of biomaterial-mediated inflammatory responses via macrophage-targeting NIR nanoprobes. Biomaterials December 2011;32(35):9383–90.
[81] Baker DW, Tsai YT, Weng H, Tang L. Alternative strategies to manipulate fibrocyte involvement in the fibrotic tissue response: pharmacokinetic inhibition and the feasibility of directed-adipogenic differentiation. Acta Biomater July 2014;10(7):3108–16.
[82] Nair A, Yang J, Tang L. Novel porous scaffold for releasing bioactive biomolecules. San Antonio, Texas: Transactions of the Society for BIomaterials; 2009. p. 58.
[83] Nair A, Thevenot P, Dey J, Shen J, Sun MW, Yang J, et al. Novel polymeric scaffolds using protein microbubbles as porogen and growth factor carriers. Tissue Eng Part C Methods February 2010;16(1):23–32.
[84] Nair A, Thevenot PT, Dey J, Shen J, Sun MW, Yang J, et al. Novel polymeric scaffolds using protein microbubbles as porogen and growth factor carriers. Tissue Eng Part C Methods March 27, 2009;16(1):23–32.
[85] Ceradini DJ, Kulkarni AR, Callaghan MJ, Tepper OM, Bastidas N, Kleinman ME, et al. Progenitor cell trafficking is regulated by hypoxic gradients through HIF-1 induction of SDF-1. Nat Med August 2004;10(8):858–64.
[86] Zemani F, Silvestre JS, Fauvel-Lafeve F, Bruel A, Vilar J, Bieche I, et al. Ex vivo priming of endothelial progenitor cells with SDF-1 before transplantation could increase their proangiogenic potential. Arterioscler Thromb Vasc Biol April 2008;28(4):644–50.
[87] Lee RH, Pulin AA, Seo MJ, Kota DJ, Ylostalo J, Larson BL, et al. Intravenous hMSCs improve myocardial infarction in mice because cells embolized in lung are activated to secrete the anti-inflammatory protein TSG-6. Cell Stem Cell July 2, 2009;5(1):54–63.
[88] Hong KM, Belperio JA, Keane MP, Burdick MD, Strieter RM. Differentiation of human circulating fibrocytes as mediated by transforming growth factor-beta and peroxisome proliferator-activated receptor gamma. J Biol Chem August 3, 2007;282(31):22910–20.

[89] Burgess HA, Daugherty LE, Thatcher TH, Lakatos HF, Ray DM, Redonnet M, et al. PPAR gamma agonists inhibit TGF-beta induced pulmonary myofibroblast differentiation and collagen production: implications for therapy of lung fibrosis. Am J Physiol-Lung C June 2005;288(6):L1146–53.
[90] Kato S, Amano H, Ito Y, Eshima K, Aoyama N, Tamaki H, et al. Effect of erythropoietin on angiogenesis with the increased adhesion of platelets to the microvessels in the hind-limb ischemia model in mice. J Pharmacol Sci February 2010;112(2):167–75.
[91] Liu N, Tian J, Wang W, Cheng J, Hu D, Zhang J. Effect and mechanism of erythropoietin on mesenchymal stem cell proliferation in vitro under the acute kidney injury microenvironment. Exp Biol Med (Maywood) September 1, 2011;236(9):1093–9.
[92] Copland IB, Jolicoeur EM, Gillis MA, Cuerquis J, Eliopoulos N, Annabi B, et al. Coupling erythropoietin secretion to mesenchymal stromal cells enhances their regenerative properties. Cardiovasc Res August 1, 2008;79(3):405–15.
[93] Shiozawa Y, Jung Y, Ziegler AM, Pedersen EA, Wang J, Wang Z, et al. Erythropoietin couples hematopoiesis with bone formation. PLoS One 2010;5(5):e10853.
[94] Bessa PC, Casal M, Reis RL. Bone morphogenetic proteins in tissue engineering: the road from laboratory to clinic, part II (BMP delivery). J Tissue Eng Regen Med Mar-Apr 2008;2(2–3):81–96.
[95] Bessa PC, Casal M, Reis RL. Bone morphogenetic proteins in tissue engineering: the road from the laboratory to the clinic, part I (basic concepts). J Tissue Eng Regen Med January 2008;2(1):1–13.
[96] Nair AM, Tsai YT, Shah KM, Shen J, Weng H, Zhou J, et al. The effect of erythropoietin on autologous stem cell-mediated bone regeneration. Biomaterials October 2013;34(30):7364–71.

PART

BIOCHEMICAL AND PHYSICAL CUES

3

CHAPTER

5

ROLES OF ENDOGENOUS GROWTH FACTORS AND SMALL PEPTIDES IN IN SITU TISSUE REGENERATION

S. Kim[1], H.S. Hong[2], Y. Son[1,2]

[1]Kyung Hee University, Yong In, Korea; [2]Kyung Hee University, Seoul, Korea

CHAPTER OUTLINE

INTRODUCTION

Wound healing and tissue repair require concerted actions of a variety of immune cells, neighboring tissue resident cells, and systemically summoned reparative progenitor or stem cells from bone marrow (BM). Accordingly, in situ tissue regeneration will start with the input signals from the injury-created specific microenvironment, which is highly enriched with a variety of growth factors, chemokines, proinflammatory cytokines, antiinflammatory cytokines and factors, neurohormone, neuropeptide, extracellular matrix (ECM), and their degraded functional fragments from damaged cells, sensory neurons, resident tissue cells, provisional matrix, and blood clots (Fig. 5.1). If those molecules are induced to the concentration high enough to diffuse into the circulation, they immediately reach to the highly perfused remote organs such as the BM, liver, lung, and kidney, where they may be interpreted as an injury-inducible messenger. Especially in the BM, as a reservoir of adult stem and progenitor cells, reparative stem cells such as hematopoietic stem cells (HSCs), BM stromal cells (BMSCs), also generally known as mesenchymal stem cells (MSCs), and endothelial precursor cells (EPCs) may sense these injury signals and respond to stimulate cell proliferation and migration for access to the circulation.

In Situ Tissue Regeneration. http://dx.doi.org/10.1016/B978-0-12-802225-2.00005-2

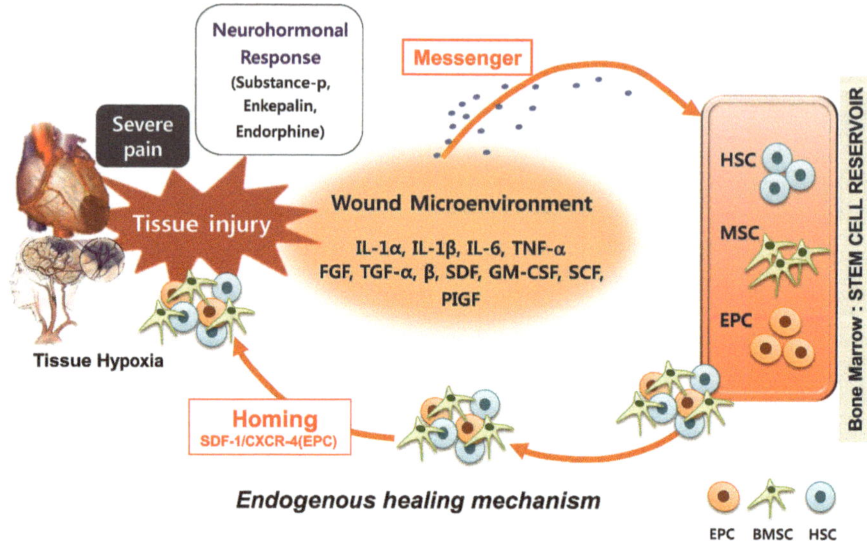

FIGURE 5.1 Tissue injury may signal stem cell mobilization from the BM.

A specific wound microenvironment is created immediately after the tissue injury, which is enriched with growth factors, cytokines, chemokines, and neurohormones. Some of these molecules may diffuse out to the circulation, reach to the BM stem cell reservoir of HSC, EPC, and BMSC, stimulate stem cell proliferation and mobilization to the peripheral blood, reroute to the injure tissue, and finally be engaged in the tissue repair, such as stroke and AMI. This may be one of the endogenous healing mechanisms, which are possibly triggered by the action of the injury-inducible messenger, but are yet not fully demonstrated.

Those mobilized cells are then recruited into the injury site and engaged directly in the wound healing process through a tissue-specific homing mechanism. Those sequential events of endogenous healing mechanisms were not fully elucidated, but several studies are strongly supporting participation of mobilized EPCs and BMSCs directly or indirectly to the tissue regeneration in situ. [1–7].

Adult stem cells, embryonic stem cells, and induced pluripotent stem cells are expected to replace tissue loss and repair the injured tissue for functional recovery in a variety of degenerative diseases and trauma. Currently, several critical issues, such as well-controlled lineage-specific differentiation, mass production of stem cells, the high cost of ex vivo cell culture, low engraftment at transplantation site, and short half-life of the therapeutic cells have to be resolved for the advancement of clinical application. On the other hand, endogenous adult or tissue stem cells reserved in the tissue and organs of the body may be utilized for the purpose of tissue repair without elaborate ex vivo cell culture if small molecules or growth factors regulating stem cell self-renewal and trafficking are identified. This will be a new paradigm of stem cell therapy (Fig. 5.2). Those small molecules or biologics may be more efficiently and immediately treated to the patients with emergency care, such as strokes and acute myocardial infarction (AMI), by utilizing patients' own stem cells through stem cell mobilization and homing.

Several factors have been identified to stimulate cell proliferation and mobilization of endogenous stem or progenitor cells from the in vivo reservoir, such as BM. Among recombinant growth factors produced in clinical grade, granulocyte-colony stimulating factor (G-CSF), granulocyte-macrophage

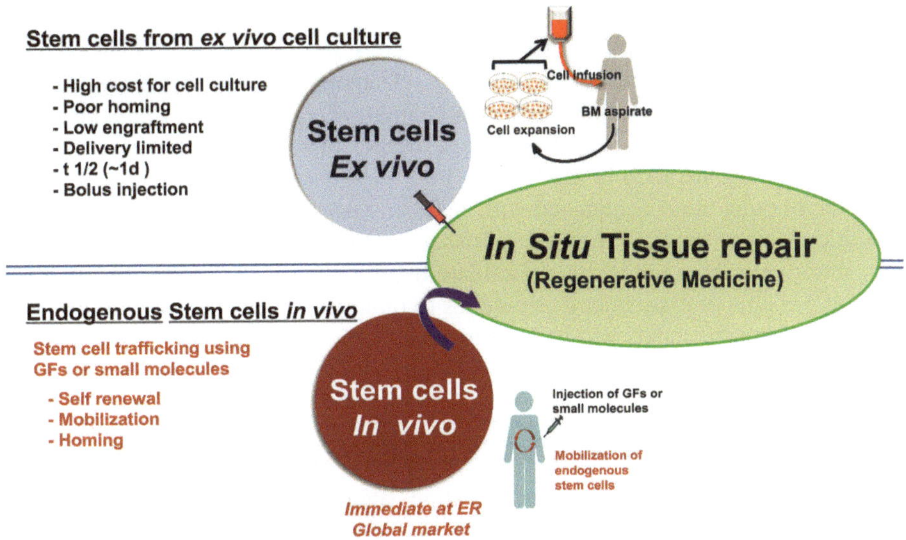

FIGURE 5.2 A new paradigm of stem cell therapy.

Stem cells expanded from ex vivo culture may be infused or directly transplanted to the injury or disease tissue for tissue regeneration. However, those stem cells require high cell culture cost for mass production and may change their phenotype during cell expansion. Numerous clinical studies showed poor homing, low engraftment, and less effect than preclinical expectations. Also, those viable therapeutic cells are only viable approximately for 1 day in the refrigerator. Bolus injection of numerous cells may also reduce cell survival under hypoxic high cell density and preclude natural cell alignment along with host cellular components and architecture. On the other hand, endogenous stem cells reserved in the BM may also be utilized for tissue regeneration in situ without ex vivo cell culture through stem cell trafficking mechanisms. Those factors may work like a remote controller to mobilize BM stem cells to the injured tissue. If efficiency of those molecules is proved, it can be efficiently and immediately used in the ER and may have a better chance to grow in the global market.

colony-stimulating factor, vascular endothelial growth factor (VEGF), erythropoietin, stromal cell-derived factor 1 alpha (SDF-1α), and their combinations, based on their EPC and HSC mobilizing capacities, are actively translated to find therapeutic modality in ischemic vascular disease such as AMI, ischemic limb disease, diabetic ulcer, and stroke. Other candidate new molecules such as substance-P (SP), retaining BMSC mobilization capacity, are also actively studied in the specific injury- and disease-animal models such as AMI, stroke, diabetic ulcer, ischemic limb disease, rheumatoid arthritis, spinal cord injury, radiation-induced gastrointestinal damages, and corneal injury [2,3,8–10].

Some clinical studies showed variable outcomes and more limited effects than expected. Their differential responses may lie on the fundamental issue of tissue regeneration in the adult, since tissue regeneration in situ requires recapitulation of developmental organogenesis to some extent. Thus strategies for fine tuning and regulation of complex factors and cells spatially as well as temporally, based on organogenesis and traits of tissue injury and patients, need to be designed. Especially, critical threshold concentrations of factors, locally as well as systemically, to initiate the trafficking of progenitor and stem cells from the origin to the target organ are largely unknown, except a few factors. In addition, other accessory cellular components, such as myeloid cells and lymphocytes, may secrete auxiliary factors to control a burning inflammatory environment, clean up dead cells to prepare a receptive tissue environment for incoming reparative stem cells, and facilitate specific local recruitment and positioning of circulating cells to reconstruct well-defined tissue architecture, whose roles have not been considered well for the tissue regeneration in situ.

In this chapter, in order to get acquainted with endogenous growth factors and small peptides found in the wound microenvironment at the aspect of tissue repair in situ, several growth factors known to mobilize progenitor cells from the BM and facilitate tissue repair in well-defined animal models will be reviewed, and a couple of experimental examples to monitor kinetics of stem cell mobilization and homing using animal injury models will be introduced.

STEM CELL MOBILIZATION AND VASCULOGENESIS

The majority of the adult vasculature consists of mature, stable, nonleaky vessels encircled by perivascular cells such as pericytes, smooth muscle cells, and specialized hematopoietic cells. During the wound healing, regeneration of blood vessels is required to revascularize the wounded tissue. Accordingly, injured tissues release proangiogenic factors such as VEGF, basic fibroblast growth factor, and angiopoietins (Ang), which support assembly of the neo-vessels. In contrast to developmental vascularization, adult neo-vascularization may utilize circulating EPC mobilized from BM and eventually incorporated within the forming vasculature in a distant organ [11–13].

The stem cell mobilization is initiated by stress-induced activation of neutrophils and osteoclasts and repeated stimulation with cytokines such as G-CSF, resulting in the release of membrane-bound stem cell factor, proliferation of progenitor cells, and activation and/or degradation of adhesion molecules such as very late antigen-4 and P/E selectins. The dynamic secretion and inactivation of the chemokines SDF-1α and interleukin-8 and multiple cycles of inactivation and degradation of BM components by proteolytic enzymes, such as elastase, cathepsin G, proteinase 3, CD26, and various matrix metalloproteinases (MMPs), all are implicated as major players in progenitor mobilization [14].

STROMAL CELL-DERIVED FACTOR 1 ALPHA

Chemokine SDF-1α is a constitutively expressed and inducible chemokine that regulates multiple physiological responses. This pleiotropic chemokine is expressed in several organs including lung, liver, and BM. CXCR4, the receptor for SDF-1α, is expressed by numerous tissues, including hematopoietic and endothelial cells. SDF-1α is degraded to a nonfunctional chemokine by lymphocyte-associated cathepsin G, NE (neutrophil elastase), and MMPs [15,16]. Expression of SDF-1α is upregulated in damaged tissue, such as liver [17], arteries [18], or irradiated BM [19]. Especially, SDF-1α expression in ischemic sites is directly correlated with the amplitude hypoxia [20], and SDF-1α upregulation involves the recruitment of integrin-linked kinase and hypoxia-inducible factor-1. As early as 1 h after induction of hypoxia in the myocardium or hind limbs, SDF-1α expression was increased, suggesting a role in the initiation of tissue repair and revascularization [21–23].

Experimental data with mice deficient in SDF-1α and CXCR4 have shown that the SDF-1α–CXCR4 pathway has a crucial role in modulating trafficking and proper engraftment of HSCs and reconstitution of hematopoiesis. Several studies have demonstrated that SDF-1α expression is sufficient to induce cell mobilization, enhancing angiogenesis and tissue recovery. Enforced release of SDF-1α, locally in ischemic tissue, increases EPC mobilization and neo-angiogenesis.

SDF-1α in the intravascular compartment is translocated to the BM compartment through a complex vesicular transport system, a process referred to as transcytosis [24]. When SDF-1α enters the BM microenvironment, it induces the activation of MMP-9 and the release of soluble kit-ligand (sKitL). Subsequently, sKitL induces the release of more SDF-1α, enhancing mobilization of the CXCR4+ and c-Kit+ cells to the circulation [25]. Another pathway participating in amplifying the SDF-1α response is the nitric oxide (NO) pathway. SDF-1α induces the release of NO by endothelial cells, resulting in the upregulation of MMP-9 and subsequent release of sKitL. Similarly, mobilization of proangiogenic cells is impaired in eNOS–/– mice, supporting the NO signaling pathway in SDF-1α-induced BM cell mobilization [26].

Either CXCR4 inhibition or activation promotes mobilization, which seems to be driven by two different cellular pathways. A single injection of the CXCR4 antagonist, AMD3100, efficiently induces rapid mobilization of HSCs, proangiogenic cells, and EPCs into the circulation [27]. On the other hand, plasma elevation of SDF-1α also provokes mobilization of BM cells over a period of several days. This rapid mobilization of the HSCs induced by the AMD3100, suggests that cells in close apposition to vascular cells were forced to enter the circulation, appearing in the peripheral blood within an hour by interfering with SDF-1α binding to CXCR4. By contrast, SDF-1α or its agonists [28] need several days to allow the recruitment of quiescent tethered HSCs from the BM, delaying the entry of the cells to the peripheral circulation. Indeed, acute treatment with AMD3100 induces a rapid displacement and release of SDF-1α, which peaks at 6 h, into the plasma, resulting in the mobilization of CXCR4+ hematopoietic stem or progenitor cells. Once mobilized into the circulation, CXCR4+ cells must extravasate into the ischemic site through the blood vessel wall. Collectively, SDF-1α seems to be a master player in the angiogenic switch and de novo adult revascularization by recruiting and entrapping diverse proangiogenic cells, including EPCs, CXCR4+VEGFR1+ hemangiocytes, and CXCR4+ platelet-derived growth factor receptor (PDGFR) + cKit+ pericytes, and by promoting in situ neo-angiogenesis. In other cases, SDF-1α exerts a more potent proangiogenic effect when delivered in combination with VEGF-A, providing a possibility that these two factors may augment angiogenesis by reciprocal mutually exclusive pathways in the ischemic limb model [29].

VASCULAR ENDOTHELIAL GROWTH FACTOR

The VEGF family consists of five members that bind to and activate three distinct receptors. VEGF-A binds to VEGFR1, VEGFR2, and placental growth factor, and VEGF-B bind only to VEGFR1. VEGF-C and VEGF-D binds to VEGFR2 and VEGFR3 [30–32]. It is well known that VEGF-A plays essential roles in vascular and lymphatic growth, whose deficiency has been shown in experimental and clinical diabetic wounds [33]. VEGF acts through receptors, expressed primarily on endothelial cells, along with other vascular cytokines as PDGF to induce and maintain the vasculature [34]. VEGF facilitates tissue repair by increasing vascular permeability, allowing the efflux of inflammatory cells into the injury, and increasing the migration and proliferation of preexisting endothelial cells [35,36]. Under steady state of physiological conditions, VEGFR2+ EPCs represent only less than 0.01% of circulating mononuclear cells. Vascular trauma results in plasma elevation of VEGF, which induces mobilization of BM cells into the bloodstream and promotes recruitment of endothelial cells to the site of active angiogenesis [37]. Rapid recruitment of endothelial cells accelerates vascular repair and prevents the vascular complications due to thrombosis or hypoxia.

Proangiogenic myeloid cells may be equivalently important for neovascularization in the adult with distinct function from EPC. Using a tissue-specific VEGF expression system in the liver and heart, it was shown that VEGF led massive infiltration of circulating cells, specifically into the respective target organ, which was evident shortly after the onset of VEGF induction, clearly visible within the first 4 days, and notably, preceding emergence of new vessels [29]. Those BM-derived infiltrated cells, mobilized by VEGF, were confirmed to be mainly BM derived proangiogenic myeloid cells, serving a distinct function from EPCs. VEGF, in addition to EPC mobilization, locally stimulates activated pericytes to secrete SDF-1 and then recruits circulating mononuclear myeloid cells to the perivascular position to exert their unique proangiogenic activity [29].

VEGF regulates mobilization of HPC and EPC differentially, which seems to be mediated via distinct VEGF receptors, VEGFR1 on HPCs and VEGFR2 on EPCs, respectively [1]. Administration of the CXCR4 antagonist alone increased circulating numbers of HPCs and EPCs within 1 h. However, VEGF pretreatment profoundly suppressed circulating numbers of HPCs (77% reduction) mobilized by the CXCR4 antagonist but did not disrupt the CXCR4/SDF1α chemokine axis. Meanwhile, VEGF pretreatment stimulates mobilization of EPC via VEGFR2 in response to CXCR4 antagonism [1].

GRANULOCYTE-COLONY STIMULATING FACTOR

G-CSF, widely used to induce HSC/EPC mobilization, is also a candidate to promote BM cell recruitment for tissue regeneration in situ. G-CSF induces the mobilization of angiogenic BM cells, including $CD34^+CD133^+VEGFR2^+$ EPCs and, in addition, directly promotes angiogenesis, in part by upregulating SDF-1α [38]. Administration of G-CSF induces functional changes within the BM microenvironment, as enzymes released from myeloid cells cleave adhesion molecules and disrupt the interactions between chemokines, their receptors, and the ECM. In the presence of G-CSF, the number of myeloid cells committed to the granulocytic lineage increases, which causes the release of active neutrophil serine proteases cathepsin G and NE, along with MMP-9, into the extracellular fluid of the BM. This results in enhanced cleavage of the adhesion molecules, vascular cell adhesion molecule-1, c-kit, CXCR4, and SDF-1α [16,25,39–41].

G-CSF is able to mobilize EPC to the blood and then to the injured tissue in myocardial infarction [42,43], although there is only a narrow window for the extravasation of those mobilized EPC to the infarcted zone. However, G-CSF evokes a strong inflammatory response, which further aggravates the inflammatory burden in the injured tissue and may limit its general use for EPC mobilization in myocardial infarction and other ischemic tissue damages. Furthermore, G-CSF seems to be not a specific mobilizer for EPC in the BM but rather to create an elastase-rich microenvironment favorable for EPC dislodgement.

SUBSTANCE-P

SP is an 11 amino acid neuropeptide secreted from the peripheral terminals of sensory nerve fibers, where it acts as a neurotransmitter or hormone. Subsets of neurons in the central and peripheral nervous systems [44–46], nonneuronal cells, including macrophages and T lymphocytes, immune cells, and BM stroma [47–49], and some cells involved at the earliest stages of preosseous fracture repair [50,51] express SP and other structurally related peptides [52], all of which are encoded by the same gene, preprotachykinin-1. Moreover, the SP receptor, neurokinin 1 receptor (NK-1R), is expressed on a variety of nonneuronal cells such as BMSC, chondrocytes, osteocytes, osteoblasts, osteoclasts, and mast cells [53–56].

SP mediates neuroimmune modulation, cell proliferation, and differentiation, all of which are expected from its local action, direct nerve innervation, and direct cellular contacts [57–59]. In addition to its local action, intravenously injected SP also works systemically to mobilize CD29+ stromal-like cells (namely BMSC) from the BM to the periphery blood, resulting in accelerated wound healing [2,3,8–10]. This new function of SP was initially identified as an injury-inducible messenger to trigger the endogenous wound healing mechanism, which recalls BMSCs mobilization and homing to the injured tissue. Using this role of SP, Ko IK et al. developed a delivery method, which was used to enhance recruitment of endogenous stem cells, such as MSCs and HSCs, into implanted scaffolds, and to subsequently increase angiogenesis [60]. Kohara H et al. confirmed that the local release of SP also achieves the recruitment of circulating cells from blood flow around the site released, resulting in enhanced angiogenesis [57]. Taken together, SP is one of the candidate factors, which can induce angiogenesis and tissue repair through an enhanced mobilization and recruitment of endogenous stem cells.

EXPERIMENTAL STRATEGIES TO IDENTIFY STEM CELL TRAFFICKING AND HOMING USING CANDIDATE MOLECULES

The injury-inducible molecules in the wound microenvironment are produced immediately postinjury. The first step to identify the candidate injury-inducible molecules would be to analyze the expression patterns of cytokines/growth factors at different time points in the wound tissue and wound fluids, which can be performed by various bioassays, including cytokine array, reverse transcription polymerase chain reaction, proteomics analysis, and enzyme-linked immunosorbent assay .

Then, to explore whether any candidate molecule may have function to bring up systemic action like stem cell trafficking or not, those have to be kinetically monitored in the peripheral blood. Thus a more sensitive detection system and multiple blood sampling, if possible, in the same animal is essential in order not to miss the optimal time point for the peak level. If it is a small animal, it may be more difficult to measure kinetic pattern due to the difficulty in multiple blood samplings without sacrificing. Contrary, if it is a large animal like a rabbit, it may be much easier to take multiple blood samplings in the same animal, but only shortlists of detecting tools for cytokine and growth factors are available.

If a candidate molecule is detected at the injured tissue as well as in the blood, the functional capacity of this molecule to stimulate stem cell trafficking has to be evaluated in a noninjured animal in order to estimate this candidate, regardless of other injury-induced molecules, by injecting a similar peak level of the candidate molecule [2]. If recombinant molecules or synthetic peptides are available, it may be easier. If not, this may have to be prepared. For stem cell trafficking, mobilized stem cells may be detected in the

Table 5.1 List of Specific Cell Surface Markers for HSC, EPC, BMSC in Human and Mouse

Cell Type	Species	Expression	Specific Marker
BMSC	Human	+	CD29, CD44, CD73, CD90, CD105, CD106, CD146, CD166, Stro-1
		–	CD45, CD34, CD14, and CD11b
	Mouse	+	CD29, CD44, CD73, CD90, CD105, CD106, CD166, Sca-1
		–	CD45, CD34, CD14, and CD11b
HSC	Human	+	CD34+, CD59+, CD90/Thy1
		–	CD38, c-Kit$^-$, Lin- (–) or low
	Mouse	+	SCA-1, CD90, CD38, c-kit
		–	CD34low/-, Lin- (–) or low
EPC	Human	+	CD34, CD31, CD133, CD309, VE-cadherin
		–	CD45, CD11b, CD19
	Mouse	+	eNOS, CD31, CD309, VE-cadherin
		–	CD45, CD11b, CD19

peripheral blood by FACS analysis with multiple surface markers for HSC, EPC, and BMSC, which are listed as shown in Table 5.1. Again, different strategies may be designed for the small animal and large animal, considering kinetic analysis as well as availability of antibodies. However, many surface markers are redundantly expressed in a variety of cells. Therefore the colony forming unit (CFU), CFU-f for BMSC, CFU-c for HSC, and CFU-e for EPC, may have to adopt unless antibodies is available. For a clear definition of BMSC mobilized from BM, the capacity to form ectopic bone and BM may be tested in the nude mice by subcutaneously implanting mobilized cells along with tricalcium phosphate and hydroxyapatite for at least more than 6weeks [2]. For identification of EPC, vascular tubule formation on the matrigel in vitro or its transplantation into nude mice may be performed [61].

As a last step to prove stem cell trafficking to the target injured tissue, BM transplantation with whole BM cells derived from GFP transgenic mice of the same genetic background or using two different mouse strains with a congenic marker, such as CD45.1 versus CD45.2, may be adopted to monitor stem cell mobilization from the BM, as well as homing to the target tissue in the same animal. If it is a large animal like a rabbit, autologous cell transplantation may be designed to trace back the homing and fate of infused cells labeled with PKH red or green (or both colors if two cell types are used). The mobilized cells may be harvested from 3 mL of peripheral blood of a noninjured rabbit at the expected mobilizing time points (in the case of SP, it is approximately 3–5 days postinjection); magnetic-activated cell sorting (MACS) -sorted cells (for example, NK-1R+, Cd29+, CD45-cells for BMSC) may be labeled directly with PKH (or may be cultured before transfusion back to the same animal) and transfused to the same animal after the injury at their expected peripheral mobilization time point (3 days in the case of SP) (see Fig. 5.3). The labeled cells may be monitored in the injured tissue as well as BM, lung, and liver by fluorescence observation of frozen sections along immunofluorescence staining with different color antibodies of other surface markers. If MRI imaging tools are available, transfusing cells may be allowed to take up ferrous oxide particles such as Feridex or related compounds, and in vivo imaging of transfused cells may be monitored in a noninvasive way.

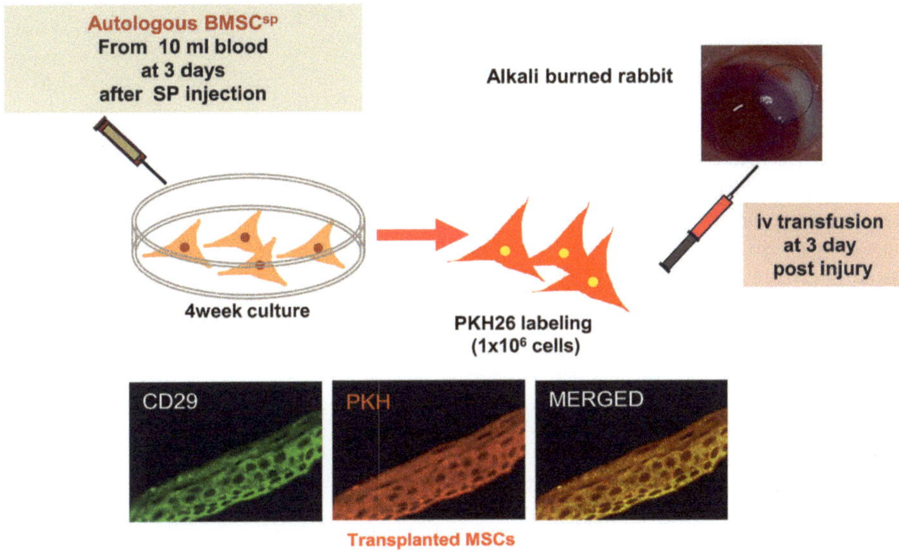

FIGURE 5.3 Autologous stem cell transplantation scheme and cell tracking method.

Mobilized BMSCs can be harvested in the blood at 3 days post-SP injection, and cells can be labeled with PKH 26 red, either after the cell culture or directly after MACS cell sorting. Those cells are transfused intravenously to the same rabbit at 3 days after the injury. Their arrival to the injure site and other remote organs can be monitored by fluorescence analysis of the frozen sections.

CONCLUSION

Several factors, such as SDF-1, VEGF, GCSF, and SP, have been identified to stimulate cell proliferation and mobilization of endogenous stem or progenitor cells such as HSCs, EPCs, and BMSCs from the in vivo reservoir, such as BM, and then final engagement in the tissue regeneration. However, several preclinical and clinical studies showed variable outcomes and less effect in the clinic than preclinical expectation. Those differential results may be further resolved by fine analysis of injury microenvironment in patients and their adjustment, combinations of multiple factors, maintenance of threshold concentrations using controlled drug delivery systems, and participation of axillary immune cells. Even though several limitations exist for active translation to the clinic, those small molecules are anticipated to provide a new paradigm of stem cell therapy for more efficient clinical application in a variety of emergent diseases and accidents.

LIST OF ACRONYMS AND ABBREVIATIONS

AMI Acute myocardial infarction
Ang Angiopoietin
b-FGF Basic fibroblast growth factor
BM Bone marrow
BMSC Bone marrow stromal cells
DLL4 Delta like ligand 4

ECM Extracellular matrix
EPC Endothelial progenitor cells
EPO Erythropoietin
ES cells Embryonic stem cells
G-CSF Granulocyte-colony stimulating factor
GM-CSF Granulocyte-macrophage colony-stimulating factor
HIF-1 Hypoxia-inducible factor-1
HPC Hematopoietic progenitor cells
HSC Hematopoietic stem cells
IL-8 Interleukin-8
iPS cells Induced pluripotent stem cells
MMPs Matrix metalloproteinases
MSC Mesenchymal stem cells
NE Neutrophil elastase
NK-1R Neurokinin one receptor
NO Nitric oxide
PDGFR Platelet-derived growth factor receptors
PlGF Placental growth factor
PPT-1 Preprotachykinin-1
SCF Stem cell factor
SDF-1α Stromal cell-derived factor one alpha
sKitL Soluble kit-ligand
SMC Smooth muscle cell
SP Substance-P
VEGF Vascular endothelial growth factor
VEGFR Vascular endothelial growth factor receptor

ACKNOWLEDGMENTS

This study was supported by the Bio and Medical Technology Development Program of the National Research Foundation (NRF) funded by the Korea Ministry of Science, ICT and Future Planning (NRF2010-0020405, NRF2012-050485), and a Korean Health Technology R&D Project Grant (HI13C1479) from the Ministry of Health and Welfare (Sejong, Republic of Korea).

REFERENCES

[1] Pitchford SC, Furze RC, Jones CP, Wengner AM, Rankin SM. Differential mobilization of subsets of progenitor cells from the bone marrow. Cell Stem Cell 2009;4(1):62–72.
[2] Hong HS, Lee J, Lee E, Kwon YS, Ahn W, Jiang MH, et al. A new role of substance P as an injury-inducible messenger for mobilization of CD29(+) stromal-like cells. Nat Med 2009;15(4):425–35.
[3] Kim JH, Jung Y, Kim BS, Kim SH. Stem cell recruitment and angiogenesis of neuropeptide substance P coupled with self-assembling peptide nanofiber in a mouse hind limb ischemia model. Biomaterials 2013;34(6):1657–68.
[4] Petit I, Szyper-Kravitz M, Nagler A, Lahav M, Peled A, Habler L, et al. G-CSF induces stem cell mobilization by decreasing bone marrow SDF-1 and up-regulating CXCR4. Nat Immunol 2002;3(7):687–94.

[5] Velders GA, Pruijt JF, Verzaal P, van Os R, van Kooyk Y, Figdor CG, et al. Enhancement of G-CSF-induced stem cell mobilization by antibodies against the beta 2 integrins LFA-1 and Mac-1. Blood 2002;100(1):327–33.

[6] Rafii S, Heissig B, Hattori K. Efficient mobilization and recruitment of marrow-derived endothelial and hematopoietic stem cells by adenoviral vectors expressing angiogenic factors. Gene Ther 2002;9(10):631–41.

[7] Galiano RD, Tepper OM, Pelo CR, Bhatt KA, Callaghan M, Bastidas N, et al. Topical vascular endothelial growth factor accelerates diabetic wound healing through increased angiogenesis and by mobilizing and recruiting bone marrow-derived cells. Am J Pathol 2004;164(6):1935–47.

[8] Hong HS, Son Y. Substance P ameliorates collagen II-induced arthritis in mice via suppression of the inflammatory response. Biochem Biophys Res Commun 2014;453(1):179–84.

[9] Jiang MH, Chung E, Chi GF, Ahn W, Lim JE, Hong HS, et al. Substance P induces M2-type macrophages after spinal cord injury. Neuroreport 2012;23(13):786–92.

[10] An YS, Lee E, Kang MH, Hong HS, Kim MR, Jang WS, et al. Substance P stimulates the recovery of bone marrow after the irradiation. J Cell Physiol 2011;226(5):1204–13.

[11] Asahara T, Murohara T, Sullivan A, Silver M, van der Zee R, Li T, et al. Isolation of putative progenitor endothelial cells for angiogenesis. Science 1997;275(5302):964–7.

[12] Asahara T, Takahashi T, Masuda H, Kalka C, Chen D, Iwaguro H, et al. VEGF contributes to postnatal neovascularization by mobilizing bone marrow-derived endothelial progenitor cells. EMBO J 1999;18(14):3964–72.

[13] Lyden D, Hattori K, Dias S, Costa C, Blaikie P, Butros L, et al. Impaired recruitment of bone-marrow-derived endothelial and hematopoietic precursor cells blocks tumor angiogenesis and growth. Nat Med 2001;7(11):1194–201.

[14] Cottler-Fox MH, Lapidot T, Petit I, Kollet O, DiPersio JF, Link D, et al. Stem cell mobilization. Hematol Am Soc Hematol Educ Program 2003:419–37.

[15] Delgado MB, Clark-Lewis I, Loetscher P, Langen H, Thelen M, Baggiolini M, et al. Rapid inactivation of stromal cell-derived factor-1 by cathepsin G associated with lymphocytes. Eur J Immunol 2001;31(3):699–707.

[16] Levesque JP, Takamatsu Y, Nilsson SK, Haylock DN, Simmons PJ. Vascular cell adhesion molecule-1 (CD106) is cleaved by neutrophil proteases in the bone marrow following hematopoietic progenitor cell mobilization by granulocyte colony-stimulating factor. Blood 2001;98(5):1289–97.

[17] Kollet O, Shivtiel S, Chen YQ, Suriawinata J, Thung SN, Dabeva MD, et al. HGF, SDF-1, and MMP-9 are involved in stress-induced human CD34+ stem cell recruitment to the liver. J Clin Invest 2003;112(2):160–9.

[18] Shiba Y, Takahashi M, Yoshioka T, Yajima N, Morimoto H, Izawa A, et al. M-CSF accelerates neointimal formation in the early phase after vascular injury in mice: the critical role of the SDF-1-CXCR4 system. Arterioscler Thromb Vasc Biol 2007;27(2):283–9.

[19] Ponomaryov T, Peled A, Petit I, Taichman RS, Habler L, Sandbank J, et al. Induction of the chemokine stromal-derived factor-1 following DNA damage improves human stem cell function. J Clin Invest 2000;106(11):1331–9.

[20] Ceradini DJ, Kulkarni AR, Callaghan MJ, Tepper OM, Bastidas N, Kleinman ME, et al. Progenitor cell trafficking is regulated by hypoxic gradients through HIF-1 induction of SDF-1. Nat Med 2004;10(8):858–64.

[21] Lee SP, Youn SW, Cho HJ, Li L, Kim TY, Yook HS, et al. Integrin-linked kinase, a hypoxia-responsive molecule, controls postnatal vasculogenesis by recruitment of endothelial progenitor cells to ischemic tissue. Circulation 2006;114(2):150–9.

[22] De Falco E, Porcelli D, Torella AR, Straino S, Iachininoto MG, Orlandi A, et al. SDF-1 involvement in endothelial phenotype and ischemia-induced recruitment of bone marrow progenitor cells. Blood 2004;104(12):3472–82.

[23] Yang C, Zhang ZH, Li ZJ, Yang RC, Qian GQ, Han ZC. Enhancement of neovascularization with cord blood CD133+ cell-derived endothelial progenitor cell transplantation. Thromb Haemost 2004;91(6):1202–12.

[24] Dar A, Goichberg P, Shinder V, Kalinkovich A, Kollet O, Netzer N, et al. Chemokine receptor CXCR4-dependent internalization and resecretion of functional chemokine SDF-1 by bone marrow endothelial and stromal cells. Nat Immunol 2005;6(10):1038–46.

[25] Heissig B, Hattori K, Dias S, Friedrich M, Ferris B, Hackett NR, et al. Recruitment of stem and progenitor cells from the bone marrow niche requires MMP-9 mediated release of kit-ligand. Cell 2002;109(5):625–37.
[26] Aicher A, Heeschen C, Mildner-Rihm C, Urbich C, Ihling C, Technau-Ihling K, et al. Essential role of endothelial nitric oxide synthase for mobilization of stem and progenitor cells. Nat Med 2003;9(11):1370–6.
[27] Shepherd RM, Capoccia BJ, Devine SM, Dipersio J, Trinkaus KM, Ingram D, et al. Angiogenic cells can be rapidly mobilized and efficiently harvested from the blood following treatment with AMD3100. Blood 2006;108(12):3662–7.
[28] Zhong R, Law P, Wong D, Merzouk A, Salari H, Ball ED. Small peptide analogs to stromal derived factor-1 enhance chemotactic migration of human and mouse hematopoietic cells. Exp Hematol 2004;32(5):470–5.
[29] Grunewald M, Avraham I, Dor Y, Bachar-Lustig E, Itin A, Jung S, et al. VEGF-induced adult neovascularization: recruitment, retention, and role of accessory cells. Cell 2006;124(1):175–89.
[30] Carmeliet P. Angiogenesis in health and disease. Nat Med 2003;9(6):653–60.
[31] Kerbel R, Folkman J. Clinical translation of angiogenesis inhibitors. Nat Rev Cancer 2002;2(10):727–39.
[32] Stacker SA, Achen MG, Jussila L, Baldwin ME, Alitalo K. Lymphangiogenesis and cancer metastasis. Nat Rev Cancer 2002;2(8):573–83.
[33] Frank S, Hubner G, Breier G, Longaker MT, Greenhalgh DG, Werner S. Regulation of vascular endothelial growth factor expression in cultured keratinocytes. Implications for normal and impaired wound healing. J Biol Chem 1995;270(21):12607–13.
[34] Carmeliet P, Ferreira V, Breier G, Pollefeyt S, Kieckens L, Gertsenstein M, et al. Abnormal blood vessel development and lethality in embryos lacking a single VEGF allele. Nature 1996;380(6573):435–9.
[35] Leung DW, Cachianes G, Kuang WJ, Goeddel DV, Ferrara N. Vascular endothelial growth factor is a secreted angiogenic mitogen. Science 1989;246(4935):1306–9.
[36] Flamme I, Breier G, Risau W. Vascular endothelial growth factor (VEGF) and VEGF receptor 2 (flk-1) are expressed during vasculogenesis and vascular differentiation in the quail embryo. Dev Biol 1995;169(2):699–712.
[37] Hattori K, Dias S, Heissig B, Hackett NR, Lyden D, Tateno M, et al. Vascular endothelial growth factor and angiopoietin-1 stimulate postnatal hematopoiesis by recruitment of vasculogenic and hematopoietic stem cells. J Exp Med 2001;193(9):1005–14.
[38] Ohki Y, Heissig B, Sato Y, Akiyama H, Zhu Z, Hicklin DJ, et al. Granulocyte colony-stimulating factor promotes neovascularization by releasing vascular endothelial growth factor from neutrophils. FASEB J 2005;19(14):2005–7.
[39] Vermeulen M, Le Pesteur F, Gagnerault MC, Mary JY, Sainteny F, Lepault F. Role of adhesion molecules in the homing and mobilization of murine hematopoietic stem and progenitor cells. Blood 1998;92(3):894–900.
[40] Levesque JP, Liu F, Simmons PJ, Betsuyaku T, Senior RM, Pham C, et al. Characterization of hematopoietic progenitor mobilization in protease-deficient mice. Blood 2004;104(1):65–72.
[41] Levesque JP, Hendy J, Takamatsu Y, Williams B, Winkler IG, Simmons PJ. Mobilization by either cyclophosphamide or granulocyte colony-stimulating factor transforms the bone marrow into a highly proteolytic environment. Exp Hematol 2002;30(5):440–9.
[42] Orlic D, Kajstura J, Chimenti S, Jakoniuk I, Anderson SM, Li B, et al. Bone marrow cells regenerate infarcted myocardium. Nature 2001;410(6829):701–5.
[43] Hong HS, Kim do Y, Yoon KJ, Son Y. A new paradigm for stem cell therapy: substance-P as a stem cell-stimulating agent. Arch Pharm Res 2011;34(12):2003–6.
[44] Barbut D, Polak JM, Wall PD. Substance P in spinal cord dorsal horn decreases following peripheral nerve injury. Brain Res 1981;205(2):289–98.
[45] Datar P, Srivastava S, Coutinho E, Govil G, Substance P. structure, function, and therapeutics. Curr Top Med Chem 2004;4(1):75–103.
[46] Zubrzycka M, Janecka A, Substance P. Transmitter of nociception (Minireview). Endocr Regul 2000;34(4):195–201.

[47] Bost KL, Pascual DW. Substance P: a late-acting B lymphocyte differentiation cofactor. Am J Physiol 1992;262(3 Pt 1):C537–45.
[48] Ho WZ, Lai JP, Zhu XH, Uvaydova M, Douglas SD. Human monocytes and macrophages express substance P and neurokinin-1 receptor. J Immunol 1997;159(11):5654–60.
[49] Rameshwar P. Substance P: a regulatory neuropeptide for hematopoiesis and immune functions. Clin Immunol Immunopathol 1997;85(2):129–33.
[50] Pinto FM, Almeida TA, Hernandez M, Devillier P, Advenier C, Candenas ML. mRNA expression of tachykinins and tachykinin receptors in different human tissues. Eur J Pharmacol 2004;494(2–3):233–9.
[51] Nelson DA, Bost KL. Non-neuronal mammalian tachykinin expression. Front Biosci 2004;9:2166–76.
[52] Quartara L, Maggi CA. The tachykinin NK1 receptor. Part I: ligands and mechanisms of cellular activation. Neuropeptides 1997;31(6):537–63.
[53] Millward-Sadler SJ, Mackenzie A, Wright MO, Lee HS, Elliot K, Gerrard L, et al. Tachykinin expression in cartilage and function in human articular chondrocyte mechanotransduction. Arthritis Rheum 2003;48(1):146–56.
[54] Goto T, Yamaza T, Kido MA, Tanaka T. Light- and electron-microscopic study of the distribution of axons containing substance P and the localization of neurokinin-1 receptor in bone. Cell Tissue Res 1998;293(1):87–93.
[55] Wang L, Zhao R, Shi X, Wei T, Halloran BP, Clark DJ, et al. Substance P stimulates bone marrow stromal cell osteogenic activity, osteoclast differentiation, and resorption activity in vitro. Bone 2009;45(2):309–20.
[56] Okada T, Hirayama Y, Kishi S, Miyayasu K, Hiroi J, Fujii T. Functional neurokinin NK-1 receptor expression in rat peritoneal mast cells. Inflamm Res 1999;48(5):274–9.
[57] Kohara H, Tajima S, Yamamoto M, Tabata Y. Angiogenesis induced by controlled release of neuropeptide substance P. Biomaterials 2010;31(33):8617–25.
[58] Rameshwar P, Joshi DD, Yadav P, Qian J, Gascon P, Chang VT, et al. Mimicry between neurokinin-1 and fibronectin may explain the transport and stability of increased substance P immunoreactivity in patients with bone marrow fibrosis. Blood 2001;97(10):3025–31.
[59] Castagliuolo I, Valenick L, Liu J, Pothoulakis C. Epidermal growth factor receptor transactivation mediates substance P-induced mitogenic responses in U-373 MG cells. J Biol Chem 2000;275(34):26545–50.
[60] Ko IK, Ju YM, Chen T, Atala A, Yoo JJ, Lee SJ. Combined systemic and local delivery of stem cell inducing/recruiting factors for in situ tissue regeneration. FASEB J 2012;26(1):158–68.
[61] Kim C, Yang H, Fukushima Y, Saw PE, Lee J, Park JS, et al. Vascular RhoJ is an effective and selective target for tumor angiogenesis and vascular disruption. Cancer Cell 2014;25(1):102–17.

CHAPTER

SMALL MOLECULES: CONTROLLING CELL FATE AND FUNCTION

6

B. Lu, A. Atala

Wake Forest School of Medicine, Winston-Salem, NC, United States

CHAPTER OUTLINE

INTRODUCTION

Unlike traditional molecular medicine, regenerative medicine restores normal function through the replacement or regeneration of human cells [1]. Regenerative medicine involves interdisciplinary research including (but not limited to) tissue engineering, cell therapy, gene therapy, and protein pharmaceutics. Drugs, which include small molecule drugs and biologics, have a great potential in regenerative medicine. Small molecule drugs have relative small molecular weights (typically below

In Situ Tissue Regeneration. http://dx.doi.org/10.1016/B978-0-12-802225-2.00006-4

1000 Da) and are typically manufactured through chemical synthesis, although some are also produced through fermentation. Biologics include peptides, proteins, nucleotides, and cells; these have larger molecular sizes and are typically produced through biological processes. To date, about 90% of drugs are small molecule drugs, and these have long been a focus of traditional molecular medicine. Clinical use of small molecule drugs in regenerative medicine is only beginning.

Compared with peptides and proteins, small molecules are inexpensive, have relatively simple storage or quality control requirements, and are easy to use. Small molecules provide reversible temporal control over protein function. Their actions on biological systems can be tuned by varying concentrations. They typically function across cell types and species. Although there may be off-target events, because of their advantages, interest in small molecules and small molecule drugs for tissue regeneration is increasing. A better understanding of signaling pathways to control cell fate (especially stem cell fate) and the development of technologies for high-throughput drug screening will make greater use of small molecules for tissue regeneration possible. Here, we discuss how small molecules can be used to regulate cell fate in vitro and in vivo and to boost tissue regeneration.

TARGET CELLS FOR SMALL MOLECULE REGULATION IN REGENERATIVE MEDICINE

Regardless of the nature of the cues used to restore normal organ function, they normally function through regulating the fates and functions of cells, the most important components of an organ. Several types of cells loom large in regenerative medicine. Our discussion will mainly focus on the interplay between small molecules with these cells.

HUMAN EMBRYONIC STEM CELLS

The establishment of pluripotent human embryonic stem cells (hESCs) in 1998 [2] provided a potential limitless cell source for regenerative medicine. Through different protocols, these cells have been differentiated into many cell types. In 2015, hESC-derived retinal-pigmented epithelial cells are being tested to treat Stargardt's macular dystrophy and dry age-related macular degeneration in clinical trials [3]. hESC-derived pancreatic progenitor cells are in clinical trials to treat type 1 diabetes.

HUMAN INDUCED PLURIPOTENT STEM CELLS

Human induced pluripotent stem cells (hiPSCs) were first generated by forced expression of the transcription factors octamer-binding transcription factor 4 (OCT4)/SRY (sex determining region Y)-box 2 (SOX2)/Kruppel-like factor 4 (KLF4)/myelocytomatosis oncogene (C-MYC) [4]. Now hiPSCs can be generated with mRNA or proteins without genetic modification. Generating hiPSCs using only small molecules has not yet been achieved, although using small molecules to induce iPSCs in mice is possible [5]. hiPSCs, like hESCs, are pluripotent and have an unlimited capacity for proliferation. They may not cause immune rejection if used in patents from whom hiPSCs are derived. hiPSCs have been induced to differentiate into essentially all of the same cell types as hESCs. The first clinical trial using integration-free hiPSC-derived cells to treat age-related macular degeneration has been approved.

ADULT STEM CELLS

Adult stem cells (somatic stem cells) are multipotent. They can self-renew and generate cell types constituting the organs wherein they reside. Adult stem cells have been described in the hematopoietic system (hematopoietic stem cells, HSCs), central nervous system (neural stem cells), liver (liver stem cells), skin (follicle and epidermal stem cells), cornea (the corneal stromal stem cells), gut (intestinal crypt stem cell), skeletal muscle (satellite cells), adipose tissue, and bone marrow (mesenchymal stem cells). HSCs and mesenchymal stem cells are widely used in cell therapy. Although adult stem cells have limited proliferation and differentiation capacity compared with hESCs and hiPSCs, they play important roles in tissue homeostasis and restoration and are a most important target for small molecule regulation in in vivo tissue regeneration.

TERMINALLY DIFFERENTIATED CELLS

Terminally differentiated cells normally do not transform into other types of cells, especially in vitro. However, in some organs, terminally differentiated cells can proliferate considerably. For example, during liver damage, hepatocytes proliferate. And beta cells proliferate and contribute to restoring beta cell mass [6]. Terminally differentiated fibroblasts are used in cell therapy in skin regeneration to treat burns and other ulcerations [7]. Chondrocytes have been tested to treat osteoarthritis and cartilage defects [8]. Terminally differentiated cells are another important target for small molecules in in vivo tissue regeneration.

In the following sections, we will describe the in vitro and in vivo uses of small molecules to regulate the fate of various cell types. Fig. 6.1 is an overview of the interactions of the small molecules with various cell types covered in this chapter.

IN VITRO/EX VIVO REGULATION OF HUMAN CELLS BY SMALL MOLECULES

Small molecules have been widely used in vitro to modulate cell fates. These include facilitating pluripotent stem cell maintenance, differentiation, and generation; eliminating pluripotent stem cells from differentiated cells before transplantation to enhance safety; and ex vivo treatment of adult stem cells to enhance cell proliferation and function.

SMALL MOLECULES FOR HESC/HIPSC CELL PROLIFERATION AND MAINTENANCE

Long-term maintenance of undifferentiated human pluripotent stem cells had been a challenge. With a better understanding of signaling pathways regulating pluripotent stem cell proliferation and differentiation, small molecules regulating these pathways have been used to facilitate pluripotent stem cell proliferation and maintenance (Table 6.1). Wingless and integration-1 (Wnt) signaling is very important for pluripotent stem cells to enable them to proliferate without differentiation. The Wnt-signaling activators bisindolylmaleimide 1i, CHIR99021, 6-bromoindirubin-3'-oxime (BIO), and ID-8 promote stem cell proliferation [9–12]. These small molecules activate Wnt signaling through inhibiting glycogen synthase kinase 3 (GSK-3) or dual-specificity tyrosine-(Y)-phosphorylation regulated kinase (DYRK).

hESCs and hiPSCs are vulnerable to apoptosis upon cellular detachment and dissociation. Upon complete dissociation, they undergo massive cell death. However, dissociation is normally important for clonal isolation following gene transfer and guided differentiation. After the discovery that Rho-associated kinase (ROCK) inhibitor Y-27632 can diminish dissociation-induced apoptosis and increase

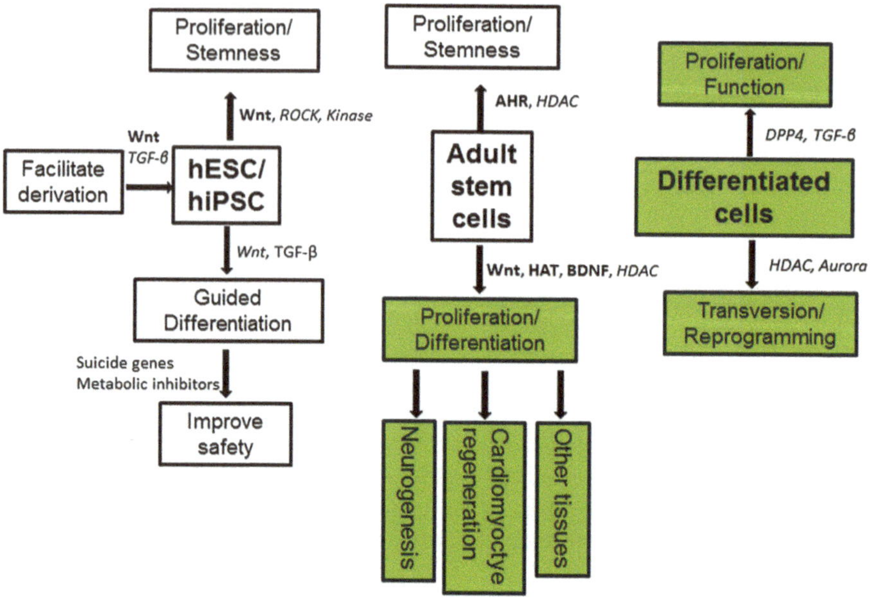

FIGURE 6.1 Overview of small molecular regulation of various cells in regenerative medicine

Green boxes indicate in vivo regulation and *white* boxes indicate in vitro/ex vivo applications. *Unboxed* texts indicate the pathways or the proteins that the small molecules regulate: *bold* font indicates that the small molecules activate the pathway/protein; *italic* font indicates that the small molecules inhibit the pathway/protein; *normal* font indicates that activation and inhibition are both possible. AHR, Aryl hydrocarbon receptor; DPP4, Dipeptidyl peptidase-4.*normal*

cloning efficiency [13], HA-1077, Thiazovivin, and Pinacidil were found to have similar activity through inhibiting ROCK [14–16].

Other small molecules (PD184352, pluripotin/SC1, PD0325901, and SB203580) enhance proliferation and inhibit differentiation through inhibiting one of the kinases in the rat sarcoma virus oncogene (Ras)–rapidly accelerated fibrosarcoma–MAPK/ERK kinase (MEK)–extracellular signal-regulated kinase (ERK)–mitogen-activated protein kinase (MAPK) pathway [10,17,18]. hESC and hiPSC depend on basic fibroblast growth factor (bFGF) to remain undifferentiated. Including bFGF in the medium raises the cost of maintaining human pluripotent stem cells. However, in a high content screening, trimipramine or ethopropazine are found to replace bFGF in the medium to maintain proliferation without differentiation [19]. The use of these chemicals in hESC/hiPSC culture will greatly reduce cost. Small molecules with different functional mechanisms have been used in combinations to formulate defined media for long-term maintenance of human pluripotent stem cells [20]. Erythro-9-(2-hydroxy-3- nonyl) adenine, IQ-1, and retinol (vitamin A) also improve maintenance of pluripotent stem cells in an undifferentiated state through various mechanisms [21–23].

SMALL MOLECULES FOR GUIDED PLURIPOTENT STEM CELL DIFFERENTIATION

The potential of pluripotent stem cells in regenerative medicine lies in their capability to differentiate into multiple cell fates. However, unguided differentiation is random and inefficient, and a sufficient number of target cells can only be obtained under guided differentiation. In addition, pluripotent stem cells pose the risk of tumor formation if directly transplanted to patients. Guided differentiation before transplantation both reduces the risk of tumor formation and enriches the target cells, thus facilitating downstream applications.

Protocols have been developed for differentiating various cell types, including neurons, skeletal muscle, and parenchymal cells of various organs. Many guided hESC/hiPSC differentiation protocols follow the embryonic developmental stages of the target cells through the stepwise use of signaling molecules, mostly growth factors and signaling protein ligands. With a better understanding of signaling pathways involved in stem cell differentiation, small molecules modulating various signaling pathways can be used to enhance differentiation of stem cells into certain lineages (see Table 6.2). Stauprimide promotes differentiation of pluripotent stem cells to all three germ layers through inhibiting MYC expression [24]. Other small molecules exert their effects during early specification to a certain germ layer. For example, the PI3K inhibitor LY294002 promotes mesoderm differentiation [25,26], whereas IDE1 and 2 promote differentiation to the endoderm layer [27].

Because Wnt and transforming growth factor-β (TGF-β) signaling are important in regulating pluripotent stem cell differentiation, many small molecules modulating these two signaling pathways were found to enhance guided differentiation. While small molecular Wnt activators enhance undifferentiated proliferation (see Wnt activators in Table 6.1) or promote neuronal differentiation (TWS119, a GSK-3 inhibitor) [28], small molecular Wnt inhibitors KY02111, XAV939, and IWR-1 promote differentiation of pluripotent stem cells to cardiac lineage [29–31]. Small molecules inhibiting TGF-β or bone morphogenetic protein (BMP) signaling (DMH1, SB-431542, and dorsomorphin) promote neural differentiation [32,33]. The sonic hedgehog activator purmorphamine promotes motor neuron differentiation from hESC [34]. X5050 and phenazopyridine (approved for relieving urinary tract pain) enhance neural differentiation through unspecified mechanisms [35,36]. Verapamil, cardiogenols (A–D), CW209E, and isoxazole enhance cardiomyocyte differentiation through different mechanisms [37–41]. Small molecules promoting the differentiation of pancreatic cells [(−) indolactam V] [42], hematopoietic cells (prostaglandin E2 and StemRegenin 1) [43], and epithelial cells (SU6656) [44,45] also have been described.

By combining small molecules that modulate different signaling pathways, the efficiency of guided differentiation can be greatly improved, and the yield of target cells can be increased. Based on these findings, small molecules have been used in protocols to obtain human neural progenitors and nociceptors [46–52], cardiomyocyte and cardiovascular progenitors [53,54], and insulin-producing cells [55] from human pluripotent stem cells. Neural progenitors differentiated from pluripotent stem cells with the help of small molecules can survive in vivo and are functional [48].

SMALL MOLECULES FOR HIPSC GENERATION

Forced expression of OCT4/SOX2/KLF4/MYC in fibroblasts can reprogram cells to a pluripotent stem cell fate [4]. Because these transcription factors can be carcinogenic, integration-free methods (for example, reprogramming with mRNA, protein, episomal plasmids, or nonintegrating virus) are being developed, but so far with unsatisfactory efficiency. Small molecules would be ideal tools, since many of them can change gene expression programming. In general, an open chromatin state particularly contributes to maintenance of pluripotency. Consistent with this notion, many small molecules favoring an open chromatin state improve the efficiency of iPSC generation (Table 6.3). These include the DNA methyltransferase inhibitors 5-aza-cytidine, RSC133, and RG108 [56–58]; the G9a histone methyltransferase inhibitor BIX-01,294 [59,60]; the lysine-specific demethylase 1 inhibitor tranylcypromine [61]; the lysine methyltransferase inhibitor 3-deazaneplanocin A [5]; the protein arginine

Table 6.1 Small Molecules Regulating Maintenance and Proliferation of Pluripotent Stem Cells

Name of Compound	Target Cell	Mode of Action	References
Bisindolylmaleimide 1i	mESC	GSK-3 inhibitor, enhances ESC self-renewal	[9]
CHIR99021	mESC	GSK-3 inhibitor, promotes self-renewal	[10]
6-Bromoindirubin-3'-oxime (BIO)	hESC, mESC	GSK-3 inhibitor and Wnt signaling activator, maintains ESC self-renewal	[11]
ID-8	hESC/hiPSC	DYRK inhibitor, activates Wnt signaling	[12]
Y-27632	hESC	ROCK inhibitor, diminishes dissociation-induced apoptosis, increases cloning efficiency	[13]
HA-1077	hESC	ROCK inhibitor	[14]
Thiazovivin	hESC	ROCK inhibitor, enhances ESC survival	[15]
Pinacidil	hESC	Kinase inhibitor (ROCK2, PRK2, and others), enhances ESC survival	[16]
PD184352	mESC	ERK kinase inhibitor, maintains self-renewal	[10]
Pluripotin/SC1	mESC	Inhibitor of RasGAP and ERK1, promotes self-renewal	[17]
PD0325901	mESC	MEK inhibitor	[10]
SU5402	mESC	FGFR receptor inhibitor, maintains self-renewal	[10]
SB203580	mESC	P38-MAPK inhibitor, promotes mESC survival	[18]
Pyrintegrin	hESC	Activates integrin signaling, improves survival of hESCs upon dissociation	[15]
Trimipramine	hESC	Replaces bFGF2	[19]
Ethopropazine	hESC	Replaces bFGF2	[19]
Y27632/CHIR99021/PD0325901	hESC	Inhibits ROCK, GSK-3, and MEK	[20]
Erythro-9-(2-hydroxy-3- nonyl) adenine	hESC	Inhibits adenosine deaminase and phosphodiesterase, allows hESC maintenance in chemically defined media	[21]
IQ-1	mESC	Binds to PP2A, decreases phosphorylation of p300, maintains mouse embryonic stem cells in the undifferentiated state	[22]
Retinol (vitamin A)	mESC	Activates PI3K, maintains feeder-independent self-renewal	[23]

methyltransferase inhibitor AMI-5 [62]; the histone deacetylase inhibitors (sodium butyrate, valproic acid, suberoylanilide hydroxamic acid (SAHA), and Trichostatin A) [63,64]; and the small molecule CYT296, which causes chromatin decondensation [65]. Not surprisingly, some small molecules that enhance undifferentiated proliferation of pluripotent stem cells also enhance iPSC generation. These include the Wnt activator CHIR99021 [10,61], the ROCK inhibitor Thiazovivin [15,66], and the MEK inhibitor PD0325901 [10,66].

Interestingly, inhibiting TGF-β signaling by SB431542 promotes the neural differentiation of pluripotent stem cells [33,52]. However, inhibiting TGF-β signaling also enhances iPSC generation when combined with small molecules that regulate other signaling pathways [66,67]. The environment and the balance between different signaling pathways dictate the cell fate. Simply reducing reactive oxygen species by vitamin C also improves the efficiency of reprogramming [68].

Table 6.2 Small Molecules Regulating Pluripotent Stem Cell Differentiation

Name of Compound	Target Cell	Mode of Action	References
KY02111	hiPSC	Wnt inhibitor; promotes cardiac differentiation	[29]
XAV939	mESC	Wnt inhibitor; cardiac induction	[31]
IWR-1	hESC	Wnt inhibitor; promotes ventricular cardiomyocyte differentiation	[30]
TWS119	mESC	GSK-3β inhibitor; directs neuronal differentiation	[28]
Purmorphamine	hESC	Shh signaling activator; promotes motor neuron differentiation	[34]
LY294002	hESC,	PI3K inhibitor; promotes differentiation to mesoderm	[25]
Verapamil	mESC	L-type Ca^{2+}channel blocker; promotes cardiomyocyte differentiation	[37]
Cardiogenols (A–D)	mESC	Action mode unspecified; induces efficient cardiogenesis	[38]
CW209E	mESC, hESC, hiPSC	Promotes cardiogenesis; mechanisms unknown	[39]
Isoxazoles	P19 carcinoma cells	MEF2 may be involved; promotes myocardial and neural differentiation	[40,41]
Stauprimide	mESC, hESC	Inhibitor of NME2 nuclear localization; downregulates c-Myc; enhances endoderm, ectoderm, and mesoderm differentiation	[24]
(–) indolactam V	hESC, mESC	Activates protein kinase C signaling; promotes pancreatic differentiation	[42]
DMH1	hiPSC	BMP inhibitor; promotes neurogenesis	[32]
X5050	hESC	Promotes expression of neuronal genes; mechanism unknown	[35]
Phenazopyridine	hESC	Action mode unspecified; enhances neuronal differentiation	[36]
SU6656	hESC	Promotes generation of epithelial cells; Src family kinase inhibitor	[44,45]
IDE1, IDE2	mESC	Activates TGF-β signaling; induces endoderm differentiation	[27]
Prostaglandin E2, StemRegenin 1	Primate iPSC	Promote hematopoietic progenitor generation and proliferation	[43]
SB431542, Dorsomorphin	hESC, iPSC	Nodal inhibitor; BMP inhibitor; induces neural specification	[33]
Dorsomorphin, all *trans*-retinoic acids, SAG	hESC, hiPSC, mESC	BMP inhibitor; retinoid acid receptor activator SHH agonist; promotes neural differentiation	[50]
SB-505124, IWP-2	hiPSC	TGF-β and Wnt inhibitors; promotes corneal epithelial cell differentiation	[51]
CKI-7, SB431542, Y27632	hESC, iPSC	Inhibit Wnt (blocks CKI), nodal and ROCK; Induce retinal specification	[52]
CHIR99021, AM580, TTNPB	hESC, hiPSC	Activate Wnt and retinoic acid receptor; promotes nephrogenic intermediate mesoderm	[132]
CCG143, LY294002, JAK1 inhibitor 1	mESC	Inhibit RhoA, PI3K and JAK1; enhances mesoderm differentiation	[26]

Table 6.3 Small Molecules Promoting iPSC Generation

Name of Compound	Target Cell	Mode of Action	References
CHIR99021[a], Tranylcypromine[a]	Rat liver progenitor, MEF, human IMR90	GSK-3β and lysine-specific demethylase 1 inhibitors; promotes reprogramming in the absence of SOX2	[61]
Forskolin[a]	MEF	Agonist of adenylate cyclase; enables reprogramming in the absence of OCT4	[5]
Valproic acid[a], SAHA, trichostatin A	MEF	HDAC inhibitors; increases reprogramming efficiency	[64]
E–616452 (RepSox)[a]	MEF	TGF-β signaling inhibitor; replaces Sox2 and c-Myc during reprogramming	[69]
3-Deazaneplanocin A (DZNep)[a]	MEF	Inhibits lysine methyltransferase EZH2; facilitates late reprogramming	[5]
TTNPB[a]	MEF	Retinoic acid receptor ligand; enhances chemical reprogramming efficiency	[5]
Sodium butyrate	Human IMR90 fibroblast	HDAC inhibitor; improves reprogramming efficiency	[63]
A-83-01, PD0325901 PS48	Human IMR90 fibroblast, rat liver progenitor cells	TGF-β and MEK inhibitors; PDK1 activators Promotes reprogramming of human and rat cells	[67]
SB431542, PD0325901, Thiazovivin	Rat liver progenitor, human IMR90	Inhibits TGF-β, MEK, ROCK; supports reprogramming	[66]
Kenpaullone	MEF	GSK-3β inhibitor; replaces Klf4	[70]
Vitamin C	miPSCs, hiPSCs	Enhances reprogramming efficiency	[68]
5-Aza-cytidine (AZA)	Partially reprogrammmed cells	Inhibits DNA methyltransferase; induces fully reprogrammed iPS state	[56]
BIX-01294	MEF, NPC	Inhibits G9a histone methyltransferase; increases reprogramming efficiency	[60]
RG108	IMR90 fibroblasts	Inhibits DNA MTase; facilitates fibroblast reprogramming	[57]
(+)Bayk 8644, BIX-01294	MEF	L-channel calcium agonists; inhibits G9a histone methyltransferase; enables omission of SOX2 and MYC	[59]
AMI-5, A-83-01	MEF	Inhibits protein arginine methyltransferase and TGF-β; enables reprogramming of MEFs with Oct4	[62]
Dasatinib, PP1, or iPYrazine	MEF	Inhibits Src family kinases; replaces Sox2 in MEF reprogramming	[71]
B6 compound	MEF	Inhibits aurora A kinase; increases reprogramming efficiency	[152]
DAPT	Human keratinocytes	Inhibits notch; enables iPSC generation without KLF4 and MYC	[72]
CYT296	MEF	Chromatin decondensation; facilitates induced pluripotent stem cell generation	[65]
RSC133	MEF, human foreskin fibroblasts	Inhibits Dnmt1; improves reprogramming and pluripotent state maintenance	[58]

[a]*Seven small molecules combined that can fully reprogram mouse fibroblasts [5].*

Many small molecules enable the generation of iPSC in the absence of one or two transcription factors. For example, the Wnt activator CHIR99021 and lysine-specific demethylase 1 inhibitor tranylcypromine promote hiPSC generation without SOX2 [61]; the adenylate cyclase agonist forskolin enables reprogramming in the absence of OCT4 [5]; the TGF-β signaling inhibitor E–616452 (RepSox), the L-channel calcium agonist (+)Bayk 8644, and the G9a histone methyltransferase inhibitor BIX-01294 enable reprogramming in the absence of SOX2 and MYC [59,69]; kenpaullone enables reprogramming without KLF4 [70]; the Src inhibitors dasatinib, PP1, or iPYrazine replace SOX2 in MEF reprogramming [71]; and the notch inhibitor *N*-[*N*-(3,5-difluorophenacetyl)-L-alanyl]-*S*-phenylglycine *t*-butyl ester (DAPT) enables iPSC generation from human keratinocytes without KLF4 and MYC [72]. Mouse iPSCs can be generated from fibroblasts using only these small molecule compounds: valproic acid, CHIR99021, 616452, tranylcypromine, forskolin, 3-deazaneplanocin A, and 4-[(E)-2-(5,6,7,8-Tetrahydro-5,5,8,8-tetramethyl-2-naphthalenyl)-1-propenyl]benzoic acid (TTNPB) [5]. hiPSCs have not been generated with only small molecules.

SMALL MOLECULES FOR IN VITRO ADULT STEM CELL REGULATION

Cell therapy often involves in vitro manipulation of adult stem cells, such as HSCs, mesenchymal stem cells, and cord blood cells. Specific conditions are required to preserve the differentiation potential of adult stem cells while expanding their cell number. Several small molecules have shown such activities (Table 6.4). Stemregenin1, eupalinilide E, the HDAC inhibitors (Trichostatin A, trapoxin, and chlamydocin), and 16,16-dimethyl prostaglandin E2 can promote proliferation of HSCs [73–76]. Stemregenin1 also promotes hematopoietic progenitor differentiation from primate iPSCs [43]. Purmorphamine analogs (Shh signaling activators) and decalpenic acid promote osteogenesis in mesenchymal stem cells [77–79]. The small molecule WS3 promotes the in vitro proliferation of retinal pigment epithelial cells. After WS3 withdrawal, the cells differentiate into a functional monolayer and can be transplanted [80].

Table 6.4 Small Molecules for In Vitro/Ex Vivo Adult Stem Cell Regulation

Name of Compound	Target Cell	Effects	References
Stemregenin1	HSC	Aryl hydrocarbon receptor antagonist; increases proliferation	[73]
Eupalinilide E	HSC	Promotes HSC expansion	[74]
Trichostatin A, trapoxin, chlamydocin	HSC	Inhibits HDAC; promotes self-renewal	[81]
16,16-Dimethyl prostaglandin E2	HSC	Increases numbers of multipotent HSC	[76]
Decalpenic acid	Pluripotent mesenchymal cells	Induces early osteogenesis	[77]
Purmorphamine analogs	Mesenchymal stem cells	Promotes osteogenic differentiation	[78,79]
Phosphoserine	Neural progenitors	Inhibits neural progenitor proliferation; promotes neural differentiation, upregulates mTOR	[133]
WS3	Retinal pigment epithelial cells	Enhances proliferation	[80]
Sulfonyl-hydrazone	Adult stem cells	Activates *NKX2.5*; promotes cardiogenesis	[134]

SMALL MOLECULES FOR IMPROVING SAFETY OF PLURIPOTENT STEM CELL-DERIVED CELLS

Since pluripotent stem cells carry the risk of tumor formation, target cells differentiated from pluripotent stem cells ideally should be free of pluripotent stem cells. Small molecules have been used to chemically eliminate pluripotent cells from differentiated cells to improve safety. Originally, the pluripotent stem cells were modified to express a "suicide" gene, which is controlled by a stem cell-specific promoter [81]. After differentiation, the cells were cultured in the presence of a nontoxic small molecule prodrug. In any residual pluripotent stem cells that express the suicide gene, the nontoxic prodrug will be transformed into a toxic metabolite that will kill pluripotent stem cells. The drawback of this strategy is that the pluripotent cells need to be genetically modified.

Alternatives are being sought to eliminate residual pluripotent stem cells from differentiated target cells. The isonicotinic acid N'-phenyl-hydrazine, an inhibitor of stearoyl-coA desaturase, can selectively eliminate human pluripotent stem cells from differentiated cells [82]. JC011 also showed high toxicity toward pluripotent stem cells but low toxicity toward differentiated cells [83]. Pluripotent stem cells treated with JC011 for 12 h before transplantation did not develop teratomas. Methyl 27-deoxy-27-oxookadaate was also toxic to pluripotent stem cells but not to differentiated cells. It may function, in part, through inhibiting the protein serine/threonine phosphatases, PP1 and PP2A [84]. Another strategy is to harness the dependence of pluripotent stem cells on survivin. For example, the survivin inhibitors quercetin and YM155 can efficiently kill undifferentiated pluripotent stem cells but leave differentiated cells undamaged [85]. Cardiomyocytes, but not other cell types, survive in glucose-depleted and lactate-enriched culture conditions; this culture condition can be used to enrich cardiomyocytes differentiated from human pluripotent stem cells [86].

USING SMALL MOLECULES TO ENHANCE IN VIVO TISSUE REGENERATION

Small molecules may be used in vivo to modulate signal transduction pathways and enhance tissue regeneration. They can be used to promote in situ tissue regeneration by means of at least three mechanisms: (1) promoting proliferation and differentiation of adult stem cells; (2) enhancing proliferation and function of differentiated cells; and (3) restoring missing cell types through changing the cell fate of existing cells in the damaged organ.

SMALL MOLECULES FACILITATING THE PROLIFERATION AND DIFFERENTIATION OF ADULT STEM CELLS

Tissues and organs contain adult stem cells in a microenvironment called the niche, which provides an anatomic space to regulate numbers of stem cells, instruct stem cells to self-renew or differentiate, and control stem cell motility [87]. Although cell therapy and tissue engineering are widely used to restore organ function, an attractive alternative is regulating activities of adult stem cells of the damaged organ and guiding these cells to restore the missing function. Transgenic animal models have helped to elucidate the signaling pathways that regulate various adult stem cells from lineage tracing studies. Small molecules that regulate these signaling pathways in adult stem cells are being explored to promote tissue regeneration in vivo.

Small molecules promoting neurogenesis

Neural stem cells are present in the dentate gyrus and the subventricular zone of adult human brain, and neurogenesis occurs throughout the lifetime. Small molecules promoting neurogenesis in vivo are greatly needed because cell therapy and tissue engineering are difficult to achieve in the nervous system. Many small molecules have neurogenesis-promoting activities (Table 6.5). For example, some antidepressants (eg, tranylcypromine, reboxetine, fluoxetine, and haloperidol) and the mood stabilizer valproate promote neuron proliferation and neurogenesis [88–91]; this property may account for their beneficiary clinical effects. Metformin (a drug to treat type 2 diabetes) and cilostazol (a medicine for

Table 6.5 Small Molecules Promoting Neurogenesis or Protecting the Nervous System

Name of Compound	Target Cell	Effects	References
Antidepressants[a]	Neural progenitors	Promotes neuron proliferation and neurogenesis	[88–90]
Valproate[a]	Neural progenitor cells	ERK activator; promotes cortical neuronal growth and neurogenesis	[91]
Metformin[a]	Neural stem cells	Activates PKC–CBP pathway; recruits neural stem cells; enhances neural function	[92]
Cilostazol[a]	Neural progenitor cells	Inhibits phosphodiesterase 3; promotes neurogenesis	[93]
Curcumin-loaded nanoparticles	Neural stem cells	Activates Wnt signaling; induces neuronal proliferation and differentiation	[94]
NP03112 (tideglusib)	Neural stem cells	Activates Wnt through GSK-3β inhibition; enhances neurogenesis	[95]
Kenpaullone	Motor neurons	Inhibits GSK-3β; promotes neuron survival	[96]
Valproic acid	Adult hippocampal neural progenitors	Inhibits HDAC; increases neural differentiation	[135]
CSP TTK21	Adult neuronal progenitors	HAT activator; promotes neurogenesis	[136]
Isoxazole 9	Neural stem cells	Induces neuronal proliferation and differentiation	[137]
7,8-Dihydroxyflavone and its derivatives	Neural stem cells	BDNF agonists, neurogenesis	[138,139]
P7C3A20	Neural progenitor cells	Promotes neurogenesis	[140]
17-Allylamino-17-demethoxygeldanamycin	Neural progenitor cells	Prevents apoptosis	[141]
CCX771	Oligodendrocyte progenitor cells	CXCR7 antagonist; promotes oligodendrocyte maturation	[142]
Benztropine	Oligodendrocytes	Antagonizes M1 and/or M3 muscarinic receptors; enhances remyelination	[143]
Compound 18b	Primary hippocampal neurons	Promotes neurite outgrowth	[144]

[a]*FDA approved medicines for other conditions.*

Table 6.6 Small Molecules Promoting Cardiomyocyte Regeneration

Name of Compound	Target Cell	Effects	References
Pyrvinium	Cardiomyocytes	Inhibits Wnt through activating casein kinase 1alpha; promotes wound repair and cardiac remodeling after myocardial infarction	[99]
ICG-001	Epicardium	Inhibits Wnt; promotes myocardial regeneration after myocardial infarction	[100]
BIO	Cardiomyocytes	Activates Wnt; promotes cardiomyocyte proliferation	[101]
SAG	Cardiomyocytes	Smoothened agonist; promotes cardiomyocyte proliferation	[102]
NBI-31772	Cardiomyocytes	IGF agonist; promotes cardiomyocyte proliferation	[102]

intermittent claudication) also promote neurogenesis [92,93]. These drugs are FDA approved for other purposes but may find new applications in promoting neurogenesis. Consistent with in vitro observations that activating Wnt signaling enhances neural differentiation, some Wnt activators also promote neurogenesis in vivo. These small molecules include curcumin and NP03112 (tideglusib) [94,95]; the latter drug has been tested in clinical trials for Alzheimer's disease. Another Wnt activator, kenpaullone, shows protective activities to motor neurons [96].

Small molecules promoting cardiomyocyte regeneration

Fewer than 50% of cardiomyocytes are exchanged during a lifetime in humans [97], suggesting that the regenerative capability of the heart is limited. However, changing gene expression programs can induce cardiomyocyte proliferation in adults [98]. Several small molecules have been found to promote heart regeneration (Table 6.6). Pyrvinium, a Wnt signaling inhibitor and a medicine for treating pinworms, was reported to promote cardiac remodeling after myocardial infarction [99]. ICG-001, another Wnt signaling inhibitor, showed similar activity [100]. BIO, a small molecule activating Wnt signaling, was reported to promote cardiomyocyte proliferation [101]. Smoothened agonist SAG and IGF1 agonist NBI-31772 both promote cardiomyocyte proliferation [102].

Small molecules promoting regeneration of other tissues

Mesenchymal stem cells are progenitor cells in bone marrow and fat tissues that can be differentiated into chondrocytes and osteoblasts. For example, kartogenin, a small molecule that binds filamin A, promotes chondrogenesis [103]. Purmorphamine [an agonist of the protein Smoothened) and CW008 (a cAMP/protein kinase A (PKA)/cAMP (cyclic adenosine monophosphate) response element binding protein (CREB) activator] promote osteogenesis through regulating mesenchymal stem cells [104,105]. Desferrioxamine accelerates bone regeneration through activating the hypoxia-inducible factor-1α (HIF-1α) pathway in osteoblasts [106].

Satellite cells are stem cells in the muscle tissue that are activated to regenerate muscle fibers after muscle injury. The TGF-β signaling inhibitor Ki26894, when orally delivered to normal mice or mice with muscle atrophy, can increase satellite cell numbers and increase myoblast differentiation [107]. FTY720 (fingolimod), used for relapsing multiple sclerosis, activates dural progenitor cells and macrophages and promotes local microvascular network formation and regeneration of cranial bone defects [108,109].

Table 6.7 Small Molecules Promoting Regeneration of Skeletal and Other Tissues

Name of Compound	Target Cell	Effects	References
Kartogenin	Mesenchymal stem cells	Binds filamin A; induces chondrogenesis	[103]
Purmorphamine	Mesenchymal progenitor cells	Smoothened agonist; induces osteogenesis; enhances bone generation	[104]
CW008	Mesenchymal stem cells	Activates cAMP/PKA/CREB; promotes osteogenesis	[105]
Desferrioxamine	Osteoblasts	Activates HIF-1α pathway; accelerates bone regeneration	[106]
Ki26894	Satellite cells	Inhibits TβRI kinase; ameliorates muscle atrophy	[107]
FTY720[a] (fingolimod)	Dural progenitor cells, macrophages	S1P agonist; promotes local microvascular network formation and regeneration of cranial bone defects	[108,109]
3α-aminocholestane	HSC, mesenchymal stem cells	Inhibits SHIP1; enhances allogeneic transplantation; boosts blood cell production	[110]
SB-497115 (eltrombopag)	HSC	TPO mimetic; increases platelet generation and hematopoiesis	[111–113]
Phenanthroline	Human mesenchymal stromal cells	Activates hypoxia-responsive genes; promotes angiogenesis	[145]
Metformin[a]	Pulmonary vascular endothelial cells	Activates AMPK; improves lung vascular endothelial cell regeneration	[146]
Plerixafor[a] (AMD3100)	Bone marrow progenitor cells	CXCR4 antagonist; improves skin regeneration and diabetic wound healing	[147–149]
Hh-Ag 1.8	Hair follicle cells	Hedgehog agonist; promotes hair regeneration	[150]
CG500354	Human primary glioblastoma	May act as a PDE4D inhibitor; induces growth arrest and differentiation	[151]

[a]*Approved drugs for other conditions.*

Src homology-2 domain-containing inositol 5-phosphatase 1 (SHIP1) plays an important role in limiting the size of the HSC compartment. 3α-aminocholestane, a SHIP1 inhibitor, can significantly increase the numbers of HSC and mesenchymal stem cells [110]. Another small molecule, SB-497115 (eltrombopag), stimulates proliferation and differentiation of megakaryocyte progenitors. This small molecule is FDA approved to treat chronic immune (idiopathic) thrombocytopenia [111–113]. In this regard, eltrombopag is a prototype regenerative medicine, since it acts through promoting production of the missing cells. Table 6.7 also listed small molecules enhancing angiogenesis, hair regeneration, and wound healing through various mechanisms.

ENHANCING THE PROLIFERATION/FUNCTION OF DIFFERENTIATED CELLS

Hepatocytes and beta cells, although terminally differentiated, preserve the capability of proliferation in vivo. It is believed that proliferation of these differentiated cells accounts for the restoring of tissue mass after injury. Efforts are being made to search for small molecules that can stimulate the proliferation of both hepatocytes and beta cells. Small molecule screening studies found that WS6,

Table 6.8 Small Molecules for Promoting Proliferation or Function of Differentiated Cells

Name of Compound	Target Cell	Effects	References
WS6	Pancreatic beta cell	May activate Erb3 binding protein-1 and the I kappa B kinase pathway; increase β cell proliferation	[114]
5-Iodotubercidin, ABT-702	Pancreatic beta cell	Inhibit adenosine kinase; promote β cell proliferation	[115]
DPP-4 inhibitors	Pancreatic beta cell	Inhibit DPP4; stimulate β cell proliferation	[116]
LY364947	Hepatocytes	Inhibit TGFβ type I receptor; promote hepatocyte regeneration	[117]
FPH1, FPH2, and FH1	Hepatocytes	Promote hepatocyte proliferation	[118]

5-iodotubercidin, and ABT-702 can stimulate beta cell proliferation (Table 6.8). WS6 may induce this effect through activating Erb3 and the I kappa B kinase pathway [114], whereas the other two small molecules promote beta cell proliferation through inhibiting adenosine kinase [115]. Glucagon-like peptide-1 (GLP-1)-derived peptides stimulate insulin secretion and promote beta cell regeneration. Dipeptidyl peptidase-4 (DPP-4) inactivates GLP-1 peptides, and DPP-4 inhibitors promote beta cell neogenesis through preserving active GLP-1 peptides [116]. The TGF-β family inhibitor LY364947 promotes hepatocyte regeneration through increasing cell proliferation [117]. High-throughput screening identified small molecules [FPH1 (functional proliferation hits 1) and FPH2 (functional proliferation hits 2)] that induce functional proliferation of hepatocytes and small molecule FH1 that enhances the function of cultured hepatocytes [118]. However, their mechanisms of actions were unspecified.

INDUCING REPROGRAMMING AND TRANSDIFFERENTIATION OF FIBROBLASTS TO TARGET CELLS

Fibroblasts can be induced to transdifferentiate into many other cell types through forced expression of lineage-specifying transcription factors (see [119]). Although most work on cell fate conversion was performed in vitro, exocrine cells can be transformed into β-cells, and cardiac fibroblasts can be reprogrammed into cardiomyocytes by virus-mediated transcription factor expression in vivo. Fibroblasts are abundant in many tissues. The ability to directly transform fibroblasts into the missing cell type important to the normal function of an organ (eg, myocytes in skeletal muscle, cardiomyocytes in the heart, neurons in the brain, hepatocytes in the liver, and beta cells in the pancreas) will facilitate the restoration of normal function. However, cell fate conversion through genetic approaches raises safety concerns. Small molecules are being explored to change the existing cells in situ into the cell types that are missing.

A chemically induced cell fate change was first observed after treating C3H/10T1/2CL8 and 3T3 cells with the DNA methylase inhibitor 5-azacytidine [120]. During the last few decades, many more examples of chemical-induced cell fate change have been reported. A 5-azacytidine analog, 5′-azadeoxycytidine, can convert ductal cells into islet cells [121]. Treating myotubes with myoseverin can change them into mononucleated myoblasts [122]. Treating C2C12 and annulus fibrosus cells with reversine could transform them into multipotent mesenchymal progenitors and skeletal progenitor cells, respectively [123,124]. C2C12 cells can also be changed into multipotent mesenchymal progenitors after being treated with hesperadin or VX-680 or MLN-8054, all aurora kinase inhibitors [125]. Oligodendrocyte precursor cells can be changed into multipotent neural

Table 6.9 Small Molecules for Cell Fate Transversion

Compound	Mode of Action	Start Cell	End Cell	References
5-azacytidine[a]	DNA methylase inhibitor	10T1/2 and 3T3 cells	Muscle, fat	[120]
5′-Azadeoxycytidine	Inhibits DNA methylation	Ductal cell	Islet cells	[121]
Myoseverin	Binds to microtubules	Myotubes	Mononucleated cells	[122]
Reversine	Inhibits MEK1/NMMII/Aurora	C2C12	Multipotent mesenchymal progenitors	[123]
Reversine	Inhibits MEK1/NMMII/Aurora	Annulus fibrosus cells	Skeletal progenitor cells	[124]
Dexamethasone[a] (organ culture)	Induces C/EBP beta	Pancreatic cells	Hepatocytes	[131]
Hesperadin or VX-680 or MLN-8054	Inhibits aurora	C2C12	Multipotent mesenchymal progenitors	[125]
Butyrate, Trichostatin A, MS-275, Apicidin	Inhibits HDAC	Oligodendrocyte precursor cells	Multipotent neural stem cells	[126,127]
BRD7389	Inhibits ribosomal S6 kinases	Mouse α-cell line, αTC1	β-cell	[128]
BRD7552	Mechanism unknown	Ductal cell	β-cell	[129]
5-Aza-2′-deoxycytidine, trichostatin A, retinoic acid	Inhibits DNA methylase and HDAC; retinoid acid receptor ligand	Hepatic stem-like WB cells	Insulin-producing cells	[130]

[a]*Approved drugs for other conditions.*

stem cells after being treated with histone deacetylase (HDAC) inhibitors [126,127]. The small molecules BRD7389 and BRD7552 can change other cell types into beta cells through different mechanisms [128,129]. In 2013, a combination of DNA methylase inhibitor 5-aza-2′-deoxycytidine, the HDAC inhibitor trichostatin A, and retinoic acid induced hepatic stem-like WB cells to transform into insulin-producing cells [130] (Table 6.9).

All the reported cell fate changes were observed in cell lines with one exception. Dexamethasone induced pancreatic cells to become hepatocytes in an organ culture system [131]. It is still unknown whether cell fate changes can be chemically induced in vivo and if so, how efficient the process is. The observations that transcription factor-induced transdifferentiation and reprogramming happen in vivo suggest that similar processes can be chemically induced in vivo.

CURRENT STATUS AND FUTURE DIRECTIONS

Small molecules find applications in pluripotent stem cell derivation, maintenance, production, and differentiation. They can be used in vitro to facilitate production and expansion of adult stem cells. They are also being applied to eliminate residual pluripotent stem cells in cell therapy products differentiated from pluripotent stem cells. In vivo, they are being explored for their ability to enhance proliferation and differentiation of tissue stem cells, improve proliferation and function of terminally differentiated cells, and ability to change existing cells into cell types that are missing in a damaged tissue or organ.

Although small molecules are widely used as research tools to regulate cell fates in vitro, only a few are being used for that purpose in clinical settings. A good example of a small molecule drug with regenerative activities is eltrombopag, which stimulates the proliferation and differentiation of megakaryocyte progenitors to produce platelets and is approved as a medicine for idiopathic thrombocytopenia. Antidepressants, long used clinically since 2000, have only been recognized for their promotion of neurogenesis, and that neurogenic activity may account for their mood elevating effects. Thus antidepressants may be considered as small molecule drugs that promote in situ tissue regeneration. Some approved small molecule drugs are found to have regenerative activities in organs other than their approved use. These drugs may be repurposed for regenerative medicine. Most of these small molecules function through regulating adult stem cells. DPP-4 inhibitors are used as drugs for diabetes; one of their mechanisms of action is stimulating beta cell neogenesis. From this regard, they can be regarded as regenerative medicine, functioning through regulation of proliferation and function of differentiated cells. In 2015, none of the small molecules capable of cell fate conversion is approved for clinical use for that purpose; this research is still in its early stage. Nevertheless, more small molecule drugs with tissue regenerative activities are certain to come in the near future.

Some issues remain to be solved when exploring the utility of small molecules for in situ tissue regeneration. One issue is how to enhance tissue regeneration in the damaged organ but not affect normal organs. The solution to this issue could be controlled release of small molecule drugs locally delivered via implanted scaffolds and injectable gels. Another issue is how to mimic the same signaling strength gradient as is observed in the stem cell niche. Again, this goal may need smart biomaterials to enable more precise drug release. For small molecules that function in the nervous system, brain bioavailability is another issue. Loading small molecules with nanoparticles improved brain bioavailability of the small molecule curcumin [94]. The ability of small molecules to regulate cell fate activities in vitro may not predict their in vivo performance. For example, isoxazole showed promising cardiogenic activity in vitro but had no beneficial effects in in vivo models of myocardial infarction. Several small molecules that promote neurogenesis are Wnt signaling activators; thus another issue is the risk of tumor formation associated with Wnt overactivation. Despite these challenges and unanswered questions, small molecules and small molecule drugs are certain to play an increasingly important role in regenerative medicine.

ACKNOWLEDGMENTS

The authors thank Ms. Karen Klein (Biomedical Research Services and Administration, Wake Forest University Health Sciences) for editing the manuscript.

REFERENCES

[1] Mason C, Dunnill P. A brief definition of regenerative medicine. Regen Med 2008;3(1):1–5.
[2] Thomson JA, Itskovitz-Eldor J, Shapiro SS, Waknitz MA, Swiergiel JJ, Marshall VS, et al. Embryonic stem cell lines derived from human blastocysts. Science 1998;282(5391):1145–7.
[3] Schwartz SD, Regillo CD, Lam BL, Eliott D, Rosenfeld PJ, Gregori NZ, et al. Human embryonic stem cell-derived retinal pigment epithelium in patients with age-related macular degeneration and Stargardt's macular dystrophy: follow-up of two open-label phase 1/2 studies. Lancet 2015;385(9967):509–16.

[4] Takahashi K, Tanabe K, Ohnuki M, Narita M, Ichisaka T, Tomoda K, et al. Induction of pluripotent stem cells from adult human fibroblasts by defined factors. Cell 2007;131(5):861–72.
[5] Hou P, Li Y, Zhang X, Liu C, Guan J, Li H, et al. Pluripotent stem cells induced from mouse somatic cells by small-molecule compounds. Science 2013;341(6146):651–4.
[6] Dor Y, Brown J, Martinez OI, Melton DA. Adult pancreatic beta-cells are formed by self-duplication rather than stem-cell differentiation. Nature 2004;429(6987):41–6.
[7] Wong T, McGrath JA, Navsaria H. The role of fibroblasts in tissue engineering and regeneration. Br J Dermatol 2007;156(6):1149–55.
[8] Oldershaw RA. Cell sources for the regeneration of articular cartilage: the past, the horizon and the future. Int J Exp Pathol 2012;93(6):389–400.
[9] Bone HK, Damiano T, Bartlett S, Perry A, Letchford J, Sanchez Y, et al. Involvement of GSK-3 in regulation of murine embryonic stem cell self-renewal revealed by a series of bisindolylmaleimides. Chem Biol 2009;16(1):15–27.
[10] Ying QL, Wray J, Nichols J, Batlle-Morera L, Doble B, Woodgett J, et al. The ground state of embryonic stem cell self-renewal. Nature 2008;453(7194):519–23.
[11] Sato N, Meijer L, Skaltsounis L, Greengard P, Brivanlou AH. Maintenance of pluripotency in human and mouse embryonic stem cells through activation of Wnt signaling by a pharmacological GSK-3-specific inhibitor. Nat Med 2004;10(1):55–63.
[12] Hasegawa K, Yasuda SY, Teo JL, Nguyen C, McMillan M, Hsieh CL, et al. Wnt signaling orchestration with a small molecule DYRK inhibitor provides long-term xeno-free human pluripotent cell expansion. Stem cells Transl Med 2012;1(1):18–28.
[13] Watanabe K, Ueno M, Kamiya D, Nishiyama A, Matsumura M, Wataya T, et al. A ROCK inhibitor permits survival of dissociated human embryonic stem cells. Nat Biotechnol 2007;25(6):681–6.
[14] Damoiseaux R, Sherman SP, Alva JA, Peterson C, Pyle AD. Integrated chemical genomics reveals modifiers of survival in human embryonic stem cells. Stem Cells 2009;27(3):533–42.
[15] Xu Y, Zhu X, Hahm HS, Wei W, Hao E, Hayek A, et al. Revealing a core signaling regulatory mechanism for pluripotent stem cell survival and self-renewal by small molecules. Proc Natl Acad Sci USA 2010;107(18):8129–34.
[16] Barbaric I, Gokhale PJ, Jones M, Glen A, Baker D, Andrews PW. Novel regulators of stem cell fates identified by a multivariate phenotype screen of small compounds on human embryonic stem cell colonies. Stem cell Res 2010;5(2):104–19.
[17] Chen S, Do JT, Zhang Q, Yao S, Yan F, Peters EC, et al. Self-renewal of embryonic stem cells by a small molecule. Proc Natl Acad Sci USA 2006;103(46):17266–71.
[18] Qi X, Li TG, Hao J, Hu J, Wang J, Simmons H, et al. BMP4 supports self-renewal of embryonic stem cells by inhibiting mitogen-activated protein kinase pathways. Proc Natl Acad Sci USA 2004;101(16):6027–32.
[19] Kumagai H, Suemori H, Uesugi M, Nakatsuji N, Kawase E. Identification of small molecules that promote human embryonic stem cell self-renewal. Biochem Biophys Res Commun 2013;434(4):710–6.
[20] Tsutsui H, Valamehr B, Hindoyan A, Qiao R, Ding X, Guo S, et al. An optimized small molecule inhibitor cocktail supports long-term maintenance of human embryonic stem cells. Nat Commun 2011;2:167.
[21] Burton P, Adams DR, Abraham A, Allcock RW, Jiang Z, McCahill A, et al. Erythro-9-(2-hydroxy-3-nonyl) adenine (EHNA) blocks differentiation and maintains the expression of pluripotency markers in human embryonic stem cells. Biochem J 2010;432(3):575–84.
[22] Miyabayashi T, Teo JL, Yamamoto M, McMillan M, Nguyen C, Kahn M. Wnt/beta-catenin/CBP signaling maintains long-term murine embryonic stem cell pluripotency. Proc Natl Acad Sci USA 2007;104(13):5668–73.
[23] Chen L, Khillan JS. A novel signaling by vitamin A/retinol promotes self renewal of mouse embryonic stem cells by activating PI3K/Akt signaling pathway via insulin-like growth factor-1 receptor. Stem Cells 2010;28(1):57–63.

[24] Zhu S, Wurdak H, Wang J, Lyssiotis CA, Peters EC, Cho CY, et al. A small molecule primes embryonic stem cells for differentiation. Cell Stem Cell 2009;4(5):416–26.
[25] McLean AB, D'Amour KA, Jones KL, Krishnamoorthy M, Kulik MJ, Reynolds DM, et al. Activin a efficiently specifies definitive endoderm from human embryonic stem cells only when phosphatidylinositol 3-kinase signaling is suppressed. Stem Cells 2007;25(1):29–38.
[26] Mae S, Shirasawa S, Yoshie S, Sato F, Kanoh Y, Ichikawa H, et al. Combination of small molecules enhances differentiation of mouse embryonic stem cells into intermediate mesoderm through BMP7-positive cells. Biochem Biophys Res Commun 2010;393(4):877–82.
[27] Borowiak M, Maehr R, Chen S, Chen AE, Tang W, Fox JL, et al. Small molecules efficiently direct endodermal differentiation of mouse and human embryonic stem cells. Cell Stem Cell 2009;4(4):348–58.
[28] Ding S, Wu TY, Brinker A, Peters EC, Hur W, Gray NS, et al. Synthetic small molecules that control stem cell fate. Proc Natl Acad Sci USA 2003;100(13):7632–7.
[29] Minami I, Yamada K, Otsuji TG, Yamamoto T, Shen Y, Otsuka S, et al. A small molecule that promotes cardiac differentiation of human pluripotent stem cells under defined, cytokine- and xeno-free conditions. Cell Rep 2012;2(5):1448–60.
[30] Karakikes I, Senyei GD, Hansen J, Kong CW, Azeloglu EU, Stilitano F, et al. Small molecule-mediated directed differentiation of human embryonic stem cells toward ventricular cardiomyocytes. Stem Cells Transl Med 2014;3(1):18–31.
[31] Wang H, Hao J, Hong CC. Cardiac induction of embryonic stem cells by a small molecule inhibitor of Wnt/beta-catenin signaling. ACS Chem Biol 2011;6(2):192–7.
[32] Neely MD, Litt MJ, Tidball AM, Li GG, Aboud AA, Hopkins CR, et al. DMH1, a highly selective small molecule BMP inhibitor promotes neurogenesis of hiPSCs: comparison of PAX6 and SOX1 expression during neural induction. ACS Chem Neurosci 2012;3(6):482–91.
[33] Morizane A, Doi D, Kikuchi T, Nishimura K, Takahashi J. Small-molecule inhibitors of bone morphogenic protein and activin/nodal signals promote highly efficient neural induction from human pluripotent stem cells. J Neurosci Res 2011;89(2):117–26.
[34] Li XJ, Hu BY, Jones SA, Zhang YS, Lavaute T, Du ZW, et al. Directed differentiation of ventral spinal progenitors and motor neurons from human embryonic stem cells by small molecules. Stem Cells 2008;26(4):886–93.
[35] Charbord J, Poydenot P, Bonnefond C, Feyeux M, Casagrande F, Brinon B, et al. High throughput screening for inhibitors of REST in neural derivatives of human embryonic stem cells reveals a chemical compound that promotes expression of neuronal genes. Stem Cells 2013;31(9):1816–28.
[36] Suter DM, Preynat-Seauve O, Tirefort D, Feki A, Krause KH. Phenazopyridine induces and synchronizes neuronal differentiation of embryonic stem cells. J Cell Mol Med 2009;13(9B):3517–27.
[37] Sachinidis A, Schwengberg S, Hippler-Altenburg R, Hippler-Altenburg R, Mariappan D, Kamisetti N, et al. Identification of small signalling molecules promoting cardiac-specific differentiation of mouse embryonic stem cells. Cell Physiol Biochem 2006;18(6):303–14.
[38] Wu X, Ding S, Ding Q, Gray NS, Schultz PG. Small molecules that induce cardiomyogenesis in embryonic stem cells. J Am Chem Soc 2004;126(6):1590–1.
[39] Oh SW, Lee JB, Kim B, Jeon S, Kim MK, Nam KH, et al. Peptidomimetic small-molecule compounds promoting cardiogenesis of stem cells. Arch Pharm Res 2012;35(11):1979–88.
[40] Schneider JW, Gao Z, Li S, Farooqi M, Tang TS, Bezprozvanny I, et al. Small-molecule activation of neuronal cell fate. Nat Chem Biol 2008;4(7):408–10.
[41] Russell JL, Goetsch SC, Aguilar HR, Frantz DE, Schneider JW. Targeting native adult heart progenitors with cardiogenic small molecules. ACS Chem Biol 2012;7(6):1067–76.
[42] Chen S, Borowiak M, Fox JL, Maehr R, Osafune K, Davidow L, et al. A small molecule that directs differentiation of human ESCs into the pancreatic lineage. Nat Chem Biol 2009;5(4):258–65.

[43] Gori JL, Chandrasekaran D, Kowalski JP, Adair JE, Beard BC, D'Souza SL, et al. Efficient generation, purification, and expansion of CD34(+) hematopoietic progenitor cells from nonhuman primate-induced pluripotent stem cells. Blood 2012;120(13):e35–44.
[44] Selekman JA, Lian X, Palecek SP. Generation of epithelial cell populations from human pluripotent stem cells using a small-molecule inhibitor of Src family kinases. Methods Mol Biol 2014;1307:319–27.
[45] Lian X, Selekman J, Bao X, Hsiao C, Zhu K, Palecek SP. A small molecule inhibitor of SRC family kinases promotes simple epithelial differentiation of human pluripotent stem cells. PLoS One 2013;8(3):e60016.
[46] Kirkeby A, Grealish S, Wolf DA, Nelander J, Wood J, Lundblad M, et al. Generation of regionally specified neural progenitors and functional neurons from human embryonic stem cells under defined conditions. Cell Rep 2012;1(6):703–14.
[47] Reinhardt P, Glatza M, Hemmer K, Tsytsyura Y, Thiel CS, Hoing S, et al. Derivation and expansion using only small molecules of human neural progenitors for neurodegenerative disease modeling. PLoS One 2013;8(3):e59252.
[48] Menendez L, Yatskievych TA, Antin PB, Dalton S. Wnt signaling and a Smad pathway blockade direct the differentiation of human pluripotent stem cells to multipotent neural crest cells. Proc Natl Acad Sci USA 2011;108(48):19240–5.
[49] Chambers SM, Qi Y, Mica Y, Lee G, Zhang XJ, Niu L, et al. Combined small-molecule inhibition accelerates developmental timing and converts human pluripotent stem cells into nociceptors. Nat Biotechnol 2012;30(7):715–20.
[50] Wada T, Honda M, Minami I, Tooi N, Amagai Y, Nakatsuji N, et al. Highly efficient differentiation and enrichment of spinal motor neurons derived from human and monkey embryonic stem cells. PLoS One 2009;4(8):e6722.
[51] Mikhailova A, Ilmarinen T, Uusitalo H, Skottman H. Small-molecule induction promotes corneal epithelial cell differentiation from human induced pluripotent stem cells. Stem Cell Rep 2014;2(2):219–31.
[52] Osakada F, Jin ZB, Hirami Y, Ikeda H, Danjyo T, Wantanabe K, et al. In vitro differentiation of retinal cells from human pluripotent stem cells by small-molecule induction. J Cell Sci 2009;122(Pt 17):3169–79.
[53] Cao N, Liang H, Huang J, Wang J, Chen Y, Chen Z, et al. Highly efficient induction and long-term maintenance of multipotent cardiovascular progenitors from human pluripotent stem cells under defined conditions. Cell Res 2013;23(9):1119–32.
[54] Parsons XH. Direct conversion of pluripotent human embryonic stem cells under defined culture conditions into human neuronal or cardiomyocyte cell therapy derivatives. Methods Mol Biol 2014;1307:299–318.
[55] Kunisada Y, Tsubooka-Yamazoe N, Shoji M, Hosoya M. Small molecules induce efficient differentiation into insulin-producing cells from human induced pluripotent stem cells. Stem Cell Res 2012;8(2):274–84.
[56] Mikkelsen TS, Hanna J, Zhang X, Ku M, Wernig M, Schorderet P, et al. Dissecting direct reprogramming through integrative genomic analysis. Nature 2008;454(7200):49–55.
[57] Pasha Z, Haider H, Ashraf M. Efficient non-viral reprogramming of myoblasts to stemness with a single small molecule to generate cardiac progenitor cells. PLoS One 2011;6(8):e23667.
[58] Lee J, Xia Y, Son MY, Jin G, Seol B, Kim MJ, et al. A novel small molecule facilitates the reprogramming of human somatic cells into a pluripotent state and supports the maintenance of an undifferentiated state of human pluripotent stem cells. Angew Chem Int Ed Engl 2012;51(50):12509–13.
[59] Shi Y, Desponts C, Do JT, Hahm HS, Scholer HR, Ding S. Induction of pluripotent stem cells from mouse embryonic fibroblasts by Oct4 and Klf4 with small-molecule compounds. Cell Stem Cell 2008;3(5):568–74.
[60] Shi Y, Do JT, Desponts C, Hahm HS, Scholer HR, Ding S. A combined chemical and genetic approach for the generation of induced pluripotent stem cells. Cell Stem Cell 2008;2(6):525–8.
[61] Li W, Zhou H, Abujarour R, Zhu S, Young Joo J, Lin T, et al. Generation of human-induced pluripotent stem cells in the absence of exogenous Sox2. Stem Cells 2009;27(12):2992–3000.

[62] Yuan X, Wan H, Zhao X, Zhu S, Zhou Q, Ding S. Brief report: combined chemical treatment enables Oct4-induced reprogramming from mouse embryonic fibroblasts. Stem Cells 2011;29(3):549–53.
[63] Mali P, Chou BK, Yen J, Ye Z, Zou J, Dowey S, et al. Butyrate greatly enhances derivation of human induced pluripotent stem cells by promoting epigenetic remodeling and the expression of pluripotency-associated genes. Stem Cells 2010;28(4):713–20.
[64] Huangfu D, Maehr R, Guo W, Eijkelenboom A, Snitow M, Chen AE, et al. Induction of pluripotent stem cells by defined factors is greatly improved by small-molecule compounds. Nat Biotechnol 2008;26(7):795–7.
[65] Wei X, Chen Y, Xu Y, Zhan Y, Zhang R, Wang M, et al. Small molecule compound induces chromatin de-condensation and facilitates induced pluripotent stem cell generation. J Mol Cell Biol 2014;6(5):409–20.
[66] Lin T, Ambasudhan R, Yuan X, Li W, Hilcove S, Abujarour R, et al. A chemical platform for improved induction of human iPSCs. Nat Methods 2009;6(11):805–8.
[67] Zhu S, Li W, Zhou H, Wei W, Ambasudhan R, Lin T, et al. Reprogramming of human primary somatic cells by OCT4 and chemical compounds. Cell Stem Cell 2010;7(6):651–5.
[68] Esteban MA, Wang T, Qin B, Yang J, Qin D, Cai J, et al. Vitamin C enhances the generation of mouse and human induced pluripotent stem cells. Cell Stem Cell 2010;6(1):71–9.
[69] Ichida JK, Blanchard J, Lam K, Son Ey, Chung JE, Egli D, et al. A small-molecule inhibitor of tgf-Beta signaling replaces sox2 in reprogramming by inducing nanog. Cell Stem Cell 2009;5(5):491–503.
[70] Lyssiotis CA, Foreman RK, Staerk J, Garcia M, Mathur D, Markoulaki S, et al. Reprogramming of murine fibroblasts to induced pluripotent stem cells with chemical complementation of Klf4. Proc Natl Acad Sci USA 2009;106(22):8912–7.
[71] Staerk J, Lyssiotis CA, Medeiro LA, Bollong M, Foreman RK, Zhu S, et al. Pan-Src family kinase inhibitors replace Sox2 during the direct reprogramming of somatic cells. Angew Chem Int Ed Engl 2011;50(25):5734–6.
[72] Ichida JK, Tcw J, Williams LA, Carter AC, Shi Y, Moura MT, et al. Notch inhibition allows oncogene-independent generation of iPS cells. Nat Chem Biol 2014;10(8):632–9.
[73] Boitano AE, Wang J, Romeo R, Bouchez LC, Parker AE, Sutton SE, et al. Aryl hydrocarbon receptor antagonists promote the expansion of human hematopoietic stem cells. Science 2010;329(5997):1345–8.
[74] de Lichtervelde L, Boitano AE, Wang Y, Krastel P, Petersen F, Cooke MP, et al. Eupalinilide E inhibits erythropoiesis and promotes the expansion of hematopoietic progenitor cells. ACS Chem Biol 2013;8(5):866–70.
[75] Young JC, Wu S, Hansteen G, Du C, Sambucetti L, Remiszewski S, et al. Inhibitors of histone deacetylases promote hematopoietic stem cell self-renewal. Cytotherapy 2004;6(4):328–36.
[76] North TE, Goessling W, Walkley CR, Lengerke C, Kopani KR, Lord AM, et al. Prostaglandin E2 regulates vertebrate haematopoietic stem cell homeostasis. Nature 2007;447(7147):1007–11.
[77] Sakamoto S, Kojima F, Igarashi M, Sawa R, Umekita M, Kubota Y, et al. Decalpenic acid, a novel small molecule from *Penicillium verruculosum* CR37010, induces early osteoblastic markers in pluripotent mesenchymal cells. J Antibiot 2010;63(12):703–8.
[78] Graneli C, Karlsson C, Lindahl A, Thomsen P. Virtual ligand-based screening reveals purmorphamine analogs with the capacity to induce the osteogenic differentiation of human mesenchymal stem cells. Cells Tissues Organs 2013;197(2):89–102.
[79] Wu X, Ding S, Ding Q, Gray NS, Schultz PG. A small molecule with osteogenesis-inducing activity in multipotent mesenchymal progenitor cells. J Am Chem Soc 2002;124(49):14520–1.
[80] Swoboda JG, Elliott J, Deshmukh V, de Lichtervelde L, Shen W, Tremblay MS, et al. Small molecule mediated proliferation of primary retinal pigment epithelial cells. ACS Chem Biol 2013;8(7):1407–11.
[81] Kiuru M, Boyer JL, O'Connor TP, Crystal RG. Genetic control of wayward pluripotent stem cells and their progeny after transplantation. Cell Stem Cell 2009;4(4):289–300.
[82] Ben-David U, Gan QF, Golan-Lev T, Arora P, Yanuka O, Oren YS, et al. Selective elimination of human pluripotent stem cells by an oleate synthesis inhibitor discovered in a high-throughput screen. Cell Stem Cell 2013;12(2):167–79.

[83] Richards M, Phoon CW, Goh GT, Seng EK, Guo XM, Tan CMF, et al. A new class of pluripotent stem cell cytotoxic small molecules. PLoS One 2014;9(3):e85039.
[84] Kuo TF, Mao D, Hirata N, Khambu B, Kimura Y, Kawase E, et al. Selective elimination of human pluripotent stem cells by a marine natural product derivative. J Am Chem Soc 2014;136(28):9798–801.
[85] Lee MO, Moon SH, Jeong HC, Yi JY, Lee TH, Shim SH, et al. Inhibition of pluripotent stem cell-derived teratoma formation by small molecules. Proc Natl Acad Sci USA 2013;110(35):E3281–90.
[86] Tohyama S, Hattori F, Sano M, Hishiki T, Nagahata Y, Matsuura T, et al. Distinct metabolic flow enables large-scale purification of mouse and human pluripotent stem cell-derived cardiomyocytes. Cell Stem Cell 2013;12(1):127–37.
[87] Morrison SJ, Spradling AC. Stem cells and niches: mechanisms that promote stem cell maintenance throughout life. Cell 2008;132(4):598–611.
[88] Malberg JE, Eisch AJ, Nestler EJ, Duman RS. Chronic antidepressant treatment increases neurogenesis in adult rat hippocampus. J Neurosci 2000;20(24):9104–10.
[89] Santarelli L, Saxe M, Gross C, Surget A, Battaglia F, Dulawa S, et al. Requirement of hippocampal neurogenesis for the behavioral effects of antidepressants. Science 2003;301(5634):805–9.
[90] Boldrini M, Underwood MD, Hen R, Rosoklija GB, Dwork AJ, Mann JJ, et al. Antidepressants increase neural progenitor cells in the human hippocampus. Neuropsychopharmacology 2009;34(11):2376–89.
[91] Hao Y, Creson T, Zhang L, Li P, Du F, Yuan P, et al. Mood stabilizer valproate promotes ERK pathway-dependent cortical neuronal growth and neurogenesis. J Neurosci 2004;24(29):6590–9.
[92] Wang J, Gallagher D, DeVito LM, Cancino GI, Tsui D, He L, et al. Metformin activates an atypical PKC-CBP pathway to promote neurogenesis and enhance spatial memory formation. Cell Stem Cell 2012;11(1):23–35.
[93] Tanaka Y, Tanaka R, Liu M, Hattori N, Urabe T. Cilostazol attenuates ischemic brain injury and enhances neurogenesis in the subventricular zone of adult mice after transient focal cerebral ischemia. Neuroscience 2010;171(4):1367–76.
[94] Tiwari SK, Agarwal S, Seth B, Yadav A, Nair S, Bhatnagar P, et al. Curcumin-loaded nanoparticles potently induce adult neurogenesis and reverse cognitive deficits in Alzheimer's disease model via canonical Wnt/beta-catenin pathway. ACS Nano 2014;8(1):76–103.
[95] Morales-Garcia JA, Luna-Medina R, Alonso-Gil S, Sanz-SanCristobal M, Palomo V, Gil C, et al. Glycogen synthase kinase 3 inhibition promotes adult hippocampal neurogenesis in vitro and in vivo. ACS Chem Neurosci 2012;3(11):963–71.
[96] Yang YM, Gupta SK, Kim KJ, Powers BE, Cerqueira A, Wainger BJ, et al. A small molecule screen in stem-cell-derived motor neurons identifies a kinase inhibitor as a candidate therapeutic for ALS. Cell Stem Cell 2013;12(6):713–26.
[97] Bergmann O, Bhardwaj RD, Bernard S, Zdunek S, Barnabe-Heider F, Walsh S, et al. Evidence for cardiomyocyte renewal in humans. Science 2009;324(5923):98–102.
[98] Eulalio A, Mano M, Dal Ferro M, Zentillin L, Sinagra G, Zacchigna S, et al. Functional screening identifies miRNAs inducing cardiac regeneration. Nature 2012;492(7429):376–81.
[99] Saraswati S, Alfaro MP, Thorne CA, Atkinson J, Lee E, Young PP. Pyrvinium, a potent small molecule Wnt inhibitor, promotes wound repair and post-MI cardiac remodeling. PLoS One 2010;5(11):e15521.
[100] Sasaki T, Hwang H, Nguyen C, Kloner RA, Kahn M. The small molecule Wnt signaling modulator ICG-001 improves contractile function in chronically infarcted rat myocardium. PLoS One 2013;8(9):e75010.
[101] Uosaki H, Magadum A, Seo K, Fukushima H, Takeuchi A, Nakagwa Y, et al. Identification of chemicals inducing cardiomyocyte proliferation in developmental stage-specific manner with pluripotent stem cells. Circ Cardiovasc Genet 2013;6(6):624–33.
[102] Choi WY, Gemberling M, Wang J, Holdway JE, Shen MC, Karlstrom RO, et al. In vivo monitoring of cardiomyocyte proliferation to identify chemical modifiers of heart regeneration. Development 2013;140(3):660–6.

[103] Johnson K, Zhu S, Tremblay MS, Payette JN, Wang J, Bouchez LC, et al. A stem cell-based approach to cartilage repair. Science 2012;336(6082):717–21.
[104] Gellynck K, Shah R, Parkar M, Young A, Buxton P, Brett P. Small molecule stimulation enhances bone regeneration but not titanium implant osseointegration. Bone 2013;57(2):405–12.
[105] Kim JM, Choi JS, Kim YH, Jin SH, Lim S, Jang HJ, et al. An activator of the cAMP/PKA/CREB pathway promotes osteogenesis from human mesenchymal stem cells. J Cell Physiol 2013;228(3):617–26.
[106] Wan C, Gilbert SR, Wang Y, Cao X, Shen X, Ramaswamy G, et al. Activation of the hypoxia-inducible factor-1alpha pathway accelerates bone regeneration. Proc Natl Acad Sci USA 2008;105(2):686–91.
[107] Ohsawa Y, Okada T, Nishimatsu S, Ishizaki M, Suga T, Fujino M, et al. An inhibitor of transforming growth factor beta type I receptor ameliorates muscle atrophy in a mouse model of caveolin 3-deficient muscular dystrophy. Lab Invest 2012;92(8):1100–14.
[108] Petrie Aronin CE, Sefcik LS, Tholpady SS, Tholpady A, Sadik KW, Macdonald TL, et al. FTY720 promotes local microvascular network formation and regeneration of cranial bone defects. Tissue Eng Part A 2010;16(6):1801–9.
[109] Das A, Segar CE, Hughley BB, Bowers DT, Botchwey EA. The promotion of mandibular defect healing by the targeting of S1P receptors and the recruitment of alternatively activated macrophages. Biomaterials 2013;34(38):9853–62.
[110] Brooks R, Iyer S, Akada H, Neelam S, Russo CM, Chisholm JD, et al. Coordinate expansion of murine hematopoietic and mesenchymal stem cell compartments by SHIPi. Stem Cells 2015;33(3):848–58.
[111] Duffy KJ, Darcy MG, Delorme E, Dillon SB, Eppley DF, Erickson-Miller C, et al. Hydrazinonaphthalene and azonaphthalene thrombopoietin mimics are nonpeptidyl promoters of megakaryocytopoiesis. J Med Chem 2001;44(22):3730–45.
[112] Bussel JB, Cheng G, Saleh MN, Psaila B, Kovaleva L, Meddeb B, et al. Eltrombopag for the treatment of chronic idiopathic thrombocytopenic purpura. N Engl J Med 2007;357(22):2237–47.
[113] Olnes MJ, Scheinberg P, Calvo KR, Desmond R, Tang Y, Dumitriu B, et al. Eltrombopag and improved hematopoiesis in refractory aplastic anemia. N Engl J Med 2012;367(1):11–9.
[114] Shen W, Tremblay MS, Deshmukh VA, Wang W, Filippi CM, Harb G, et al. Small-molecule inducer of beta cell proliferation identified by high-throughput screening. J Am Chem Soc 2013;135(5):1669–72.
[115] Annes JP, Ryu JH, Lam K, Carolan PJ, Utz K, Hollister-Lock J, et al. Adenosine kinase inhibition selectively promotes rodent and porcine islet beta-cell replication. Proc Natl Acad Sci USA 2012;109(10):3915–20.
[116] Mulvihill EE, Drucker DJ. Pharmacology, physiology, and mechanisms of action of dipeptidyl peptidase-4 inhibitors. Endocr Rev 2014;35(6):992–1019.
[117] Karkampouna S, Goumans MJ, Ten Dijke P, Dooley S, Kruithof-de Julio M. Inhibition of TGFbeta type I receptor activity facilitates liver regeneration upon acute CCl intoxication in mice. Arch Toxicol 2015;90(2):347–57.
[118] Shan J, Schwartz RE, Ross NT, Logan DJ, Thomas D, Duncan SA, et al. Identification of small molecules for human hepatocyte expansion and iPS differentiation. Nat Chem Biol 2013;9(8):514–20.
[119] Lu B, Atala A. Small molecules and small molecule drugs in regenerative medicine. Drug Discov Today 2014;19(6):801–8.
[120] Taylor SM, Jones PA. Multiple new phenotypes induced in 10T1/2 and 3T3 cells treated with 5-azacytidine. Cell 1979;17(4):771–9.
[121] Lefebvre B, Belaich S, Longue J, Vandewalle B, Oberholzer J, Gmyr V, et al. 5'-AZA induces Ngn3 expression and endocrine differentiation in the PANC-1 human ductal cell line. Biochem Biophys Res Commun 2010;391(1):305–9.
[122] Rosania GR, Chang YT, Perez O, Sutherlin D, Dong H, Lockhart DJ, et al. Myoseverin, a microtubule-binding molecule with novel cellular effects. Nat Biotechnol 2000;18(3):304–8.
[123] Anastasia L, Sampaolesi M, Papini N, Oleari D, Lamorte G, Tringali C, et al. Reversine-treated fibroblasts acquire myogenic competence in vitro and in regenerating skeletal muscle. Cell Death Differ 2006;13(12):2042–51.

[124] Saraiya M, Nasser R, Zeng Y, Addya S, Ponnappan RK, Fortina P, et al. Reversine enhances generation of progenitor-like cells by dedifferentiation of annulus fibrosus cells. Tissue Eng Part A 2010;16(4):1443–55.
[125] Amabile G, D'Alise AM, Iovino M, Jones P, Santaguida S, Musacchio A, et al. The Aurora B kinase activity is required for the maintenance of the differentiated state of murine myoblasts. Cell Death Differ 2009;16(2):321–30.
[126] Lyssiotis CA, Walker J, Wu C, Kondo T, Schultz PG, Wu X. Inhibition of histone deacetylase activity induces developmental plasticity in oligodendrocyte precursor cells. Proc Natl Acad Sci USA 2007;104(38):14982–7.
[127] Liu A, Han YR, Li J, Sun D, Ouyang M, Plummer MR, et al. The glial or neuronal fate choice of oligodendrocyte progenitors is modulated by their ability to acquire an epigenetic memory. J Neurosci 2007;27(27):7339–43.
[128] Fomina-Yadlin D, Kubicek S, Walpita D, Dancik V, Hecksher-Sorensen J, Bittker JA, et al. Small-molecule inducers of insulin expression in pancreatic alpha-cells. Proc Natl Acad Sci USA 2010;107(34):15099–104.
[129] Yuan Y, Hartland K, Boskovic Z, Wang Y, Walpita D, Lysy PA, et al. A small-molecule inducer of PDX1 expression identified by high-throughput screening. Chem Biol 2013;20(12):1513–22.
[130] Liu J, Liu Y, Wang H, Hao H, Han Q, Shen J, et al. Direct differentiation of hepatic stem-like WB cells into insulin-producing cells using small molecules. Sci Rep 2013;3:1185.
[131] Shen CN, Slack JM, Tosh D. Molecular basis of transdifferentiation of pancreas to liver. Nat Cell Biol 2000;2(12):879–87.
[132] Araoka T, Mae S, Kurose Y, Uesugi M, Ohta A, Yamanaka S, et al. Efficient and rapid induction of human iPSCs/ESCs into nephrogenic intermediate mesoderm using small molecule-based differentiation methods. PLoS One 2014;9(1):e84881.
[133] Saxe JP, Wu H, Kelly TK, et al. A phenotypic small-molecule screen identifies an orphan ligand-receptor pair that regulates neural stem cell differentiation. Chem Biol 2007;14(9):1019–30.
[134] Sadek H, Hannack B, Choe E, et al. Cardiogenic small molecules that enhance myocardial repair by stem cells. Proc Natl Acad Sci USA 2008;105(16):6063–8.
[135] Hsieh J, Nakashima K, Kuwabara T, Mejia E, Gage FH. Histone deacetylase inhibition-mediated neuronal differentiation of multipotent adult neural progenitor cells. Proc Natl Acad Sci USA 2004;101(47):16659–64.
[136] Chatterjee S, Mizar P, Cassel R, et al. A novel activator of CBP/p300 acetyltransferases promotes neurogenesis and extends memory duration in adult mice. J Neurosci 2013;33(26):10698–712.
[137] Petrik D, Jiang Y, Birnbaum SG, et al. Functional and mechanistic exploration of an adult neurogenesis-promoting small molecule. FASEB J 2012;26(8):3148–62.
[138] Jang SW, Liu X, Yepes M, et al. A selective TrkB agonist with potent neurotrophic activities by 7,8-dihydroxyflavone. Proc Natl Acad Sci USA 2010;107(6):2687–92.
[139] Liu X, Chan CB, Jang SW, et al. A synthetic 7,8-dihydroxyflavone derivative promotes neurogenesis and exhibits potent antidepressant effect. J Med Chem 2010;53(23):8274–86.
[140] Pieper AA, Xie S, Capota E, et al. Discovery of a proneurogenic, neuroprotective chemical. Cell 2010;142(1):39–51.
[141] Wang G, Krishnamurthy K, Tangpisuthipongsa D. Protection of murine neural progenitor cells by the Hsp90 inhibitor 17-allylamino-17-demethoxygeldanamycin in the low nanomolar concentration range. J Neurochem 2011;117(4):703–11.
[142] Williams JL, Patel JR, Daniels BP, Klein RS. Targeting CXCR7/ACKR3 as a therapeutic strategy to promote remyelination in the adult central nervous system. J Exp Med 2014;211(5):791–9.
[143] Deshmukh VA, Tardif V, Lyssiotis CA, et al. A regenerative approach to the treatment of multiple sclerosis. Nature 2013;502(7471):327–32.
[144] Dakas PY, Parga JA, Hoing S, et al. Discovery of neuritogenic compound classes inspired by natural products. Angew Chem Int Ed Engl 2013;52(36):9576–81.
[145] Doorn J, Fernandes HA, Le BQ, et al. A small molecule approach to engineering vascularized tissue. Biomaterials 2013;34(12):3053–63.

[146] Jian MY, Alexeyev MF, Wolkowicz PE, Zmijewski JW, Creighton JR. Metformin-stimulated AMPK-alpha1 promotes microvascular repair in acute lung injury. Am J Physiol Lung Cell Mol Physiol 2013;305(11):L844–55.
[147] Lin Q, Wesson RN, Maeda H, et al. Pharmacological mobilization of endogenous stem cells significantly promotes skin regeneration after full-thickness excision: the synergistic activity of AMD3100 and tacrolimus. J Invest Dermatol 2014;134(9):2458–68.
[148] Allen Jr RJ, Soares MA, Haberman ID, et al. Combination therapy accelerates diabetic wound closure. PLoS One 2014;9(3):e92667.
[149] Ruder C, Haase T, Krost A, et al. Combinatorial G-CSF/AMD3100 treatment in cardiac repair after myocardial infarction. PLoS One 2014;9(8):e104644.
[150] Paladini RD, Saleh J, Qian C, Xu GX, Rubin LL. Modulation of hair growth with small molecule agonists of the hedgehog signaling pathway. J Invest Dermatol 2005;125(4):638–46.
[151] Kang TW, Choi SW, Yang SR, et al. Growth arrest and forced differentiation of human primary glioblastoma multiforme by a novel small molecule. Sci Rep 2014;4:5546.
[152] Li Z, Rana TM. A kinase inhibitor screen identifies small-molecule enhancers of reprogramming and iPS cell generation. Nat Commun 2012;3:1085.

CHAPTER

SMALL RNA DELIVERY FOR IN SITU TISSUE REGENERATION

7

N.J. Kim, J.J. Yoo, A. Atala, S.J. Lee

Wake Forest School of Medicine, Winston-Salem, NC, United States

CHAPTER OUTLINE

INTRODUCTION

Modulating target gene expression has been of interest for decades in the field of biomedical research. It entails transfer of functional genes to control expression of target genes by replacing or silencing them. Especially, gene therapy using RNA interference (RNAi) has been significantly prospected in clinical applications [1]. RNAi is the mechanism by which gene expression is silenced by binding the

In Situ Tissue Regeneration. http://dx.doi.org/10.1016/B978-0-12-802225-2.00007-6

target mRNAs, leading to translational repression or destruction of specific mRNA molecules [2]. Using this mechanism, expression of specific proteins that are involved in blocking a desired function of proteins of interest can be suppressed. The delivery of synthetic small RNAs [small interfering RNA (siRNA) and/or microRNA (miRNA)] can play a vital role as a trigger of RNAi mechanism. Therefore it has been extensively studied for the treatment of various diseases, including cancers, neurologic disorders, and viral diseases [3]. This effort has advanced to clinical studies that can initiate medical applications of small RNAs [4]. However, the majority of small RNA studies have been limited to molecular biology in diseases, and few applications have concerned about regenerative medicine perspectives on tissue repair or regeneration [5].

The strategy of tissue engineering and regenerative medicine is to restore, maintain, or improve tissue function by combining concepts of engineering and life science [6,7]. Engineered tissue constructs composed of biomaterial scaffolds preseeded with patient-derived cells are one of the most promising approaches to generate functional replacement tissue constructs. In spite of considerable advancements, these cell-based approaches have limitations due to donor tissue availability. Harvesting autologous tissue to obtain cell sources is constrained by anatomic limitations and associated with significant donor site morbidity. Novel concept of recruiting host stem cells or tissue-specific progenitor cells has been introduced for in situ tissue regeneration [8–10]. The principle of this strategy is to take advantage of the body's own regenerating capacity by using the host's ability to mobilize endogenous stem cells to the site of injury. We believe that combined with RNAi mechanism, this strategy can be synergistically improved by enhancing the regenerative capacity of injured tissues or organs. Studies that attempted to combine small RNA therapy with regenerative medicine have recently demonstrated the potential of this strategy [11–13]. This chapter will outline the fundamentals of small RNA delivery in the biological system and their applications in current tissue regeneration and regenerative medicine.

STRATEGIES FOR SMALL RNAS IN TISSUE REGENERATION

RNA INTERFERENCE

Small RNAs have come forth as key players in gene modulation for eukaryotes. They are short (~20–30 nucleotides) double-stranded RNAs (dsRNAs) that are primarily associated with posttranscriptional gene regulations [4]. They predominantly repress gene expression by impeding mRNA translation to protein synthesis through the process called RNAi. RNAi is a naturally occurring cellular mechanism by which a target mRNA is degraded with the purpose of decreasing the expression of the encoded protein [14,15]. Since the first discovery of long dsRNAs in *Caenorhabditis elegans*, reducing the translation of the complementary endogenous mRNAs, RNAi mechanism has been utilized to exploit its natural regulatory function by inhibiting the expression of specific genes [2,16,17]. Due to the target-specific nature of the system, it has significant potential as a therapeutic tool and has been studied in various research fields for the treatment of gene-related diseases [1,18,19].

In addition to initiating RNAi, long dsRNAs trigger antiviral immune responses in higher organisms by stimulating interferon (IFN) release, which leads to a cascade of IFN-stimulated genes [20,21]. This will, in turn, stimulate nonspecific host antiviral immune response. Hence, on account of minimizing unwanted antiviral machinery, long dsRNAs are not a preferable RNAi induction material for mammalian studies. Fortunately, long dsRNAs are processed into short duplexes, small RNAs, inside the cells in order to mediate gene suppression. Small RNAs enter RNAi machinery at a later stage than long dsRNAs do, which enables triggering RNAi with reduced antiviral immune responses [22–27]. Encouraged by this low immunogenic property and the target-specific silencing potential, small RNAs have been increasingly explored in numerous biomedical research fields.

SMALL RNAS: SMALL INTERFERING RNAS AND MICRORNAS

Using small RNAs instead of long dsRNAs has less immunogenic response for inducing RNAi. Among many classes of small RNAs identified to date, two major categories are the most understood: siRNAs and miRNAs. They share similar function of gene modulation while having different biogenesis and primary purposes. First, siRNAs are 21–27 base-pair (bp) dsRNAs and essentially cellular defenders of host genome against viral nucleic acids. SiRNAs can be produced from plasmid DNA (pDNA), short-hairpin RNA (shRNA), or dsRNA. When introduced as an exogenous pDNA, it is transcribed into shRNA form. ShRNA or dsRNA can be cut by an endoribonuclease dicer into smaller siRNAs [28–30]. The target recognition of siRNA is such a sequence-specific process that only one mismatched nucleotide can disrupt the binding between siRNA and target mRNA [31]. Second, miRNAs are small endogenous noncoding RNAs (~22 bp) that are highly conserved from plants to mammals [32,33]. In particular, mammalian miRNAs mature through multiple-step processes. MiRNAs are first transcribed into a several kilobases-long primary miRNA (pri-miRNA) by RNA polymerase II in the nucleus. Then the pri-miRNA is cleaved at the one end into a ~60–70 bp stem loop intermediate miRNA precursor (pre-miRNA) by ribonuclease III endonuclease Drosha associated with Pasha (DGCR8) [33–36]. The pre-miRNA is now transported to cytoplasm by the export receptor Exportin-5 in ras-related nuclear protein-guanosine-5'-triphosphate (Ran-GTP)-dependent manner [37,38]. Once exported to the cytoplasm, Dicer cuts the other end of pre-miRNA to produce the mature miRNA [34]. Unlike siRNA, most mammalian miRNAs bind to target mRNAs with only a few complementary bp called seed sequence (2–7 bps) in the 3′ UTR (untranslated region) of target mRNAs [39]. This short-sequence specificity allows miRNAs to have multiple target genes, and each target can have multiple regulatory miRNAs [29]. Synthetic siRNAs and miRNAs are formulated to mimic natural ones and trigger RNAi in a consistent and predictable manner.

After being processed into siRNA or mature miRNA, they enter an intracellular multistep process of RNAi in a similar way. They are incorporated into the multiprotein cluster, RNA-induced silencing complex (RISC) forming siRISC and miRISC, respectively (Fig. 7.1) [40]. Recognizing the less stable 5′ end of the double strand, RNA helicase in the RISC unwinds double-stranded RNA into single strands. One strand of the duplex (the passenger strand) is discarded. The other strand (the guide strand) directs a sequence-specific hybridization to the target mRNA, which has the complementary sequence to the guide strand [41–43]. This process enables the target specificity of the RNAi silencing and also determines the degree of the specificity. From this point, different series of steps distinguish the action of siRISC from that of miRISC. The siRISC-targeted mRNA is cleaved by RISC and rapidly degraded due to its unprotected ends [44–46]. On the other hand, the target mRNA silencing by miRISC depends on the extent of complementarity. Perfect complementarity promotes mRNA cleavage as siRISC silencing, whereas central mismatches only lead to repression of mRNA translation. Since most animal miRNAs bind to target mRNAs with mismatches and bulges by recognizing multiple seed regions, it results in defective translational repression. For this reason, translational repression is suggested as the default mechanism of miRNA gene interference [47,48]. After the degradation of the target mRNA or repression of the mRNA translation, the RISC can be recycled for subsequent rounds, leading this process to the selective silencing in the target mRNA followed by decreased expression of the target gene.

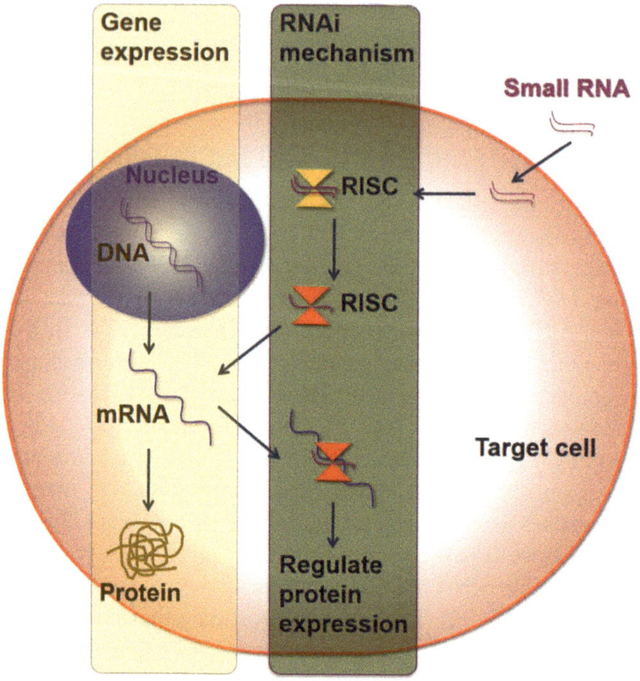

FIGURE 7.1

Schematic diagram of machinery of small RNA-induced gene regulation.

Selectively silencing posttranscriptional mRNA by RNAi offers a promising strategy for the inhibition of gene expression in vitro and in vivo [2]. Furthermore, it provides a foundation to advance the biomedical research for clinical applications. The most prominent potential of small RNAs in therapeutic use is that miRNA and siRNA silencing is readily reprogrammable. The silencing pathway can simply be modified by replacing old small RNA with a new one [47]. Moreover, many miRNAs are expressed with tissue specificity, implying their tissue-specific gene regulation. Their mechanisms are well established and readily applicable in tissue engineering and regenerative medicine strategy. Furthermore, researches on small RNA therapy have demonstrated the advantages of using small RNA instead of DNA, long RNA, or protein in terms of stability, reversibility, selectivity, and immunogenicity.

DESIGN CONSIDERATION FOR SMALL RNA DELIVERY

GENERAL DELIVERY STRATEGY OF SMALL RNAS

It has been well recognized that effective, controlled delivery of bioactive therapeutic molecules is the key in tissue engineering and regenerative medicine. A delivery system for small RNAs should provide therapeutic effects in a local and sustained manner. While small RNAs carry promising therapeutic potential in clinical applications, there are small hoops to be jumped through. One potential drawback in the therapeutic use of small RNAs is alteration of normal physiology in addition to target physiology, due to the many potential targets of a given small RNA. Endogenous small RNAs regulate hundreds of targets by mRNA degradation or translational repression of protein production [49–51]. Moreover, small RNAs are inherently unstable, unlike DNA, due to the hydroxyl group in their sticky overhangs that make them more vulnerable to hydrolysis by nucleases in serum and cytosol. This results in a shorter half-life of small RNAs [52]. Furthermore, they cannot passively diffuse through the cell membrane by themselves due to their large molecular weight (about 13 kDa) and polyanionic nature [14]. Native RNAs have low delivery efficiencies for these reasons. In order to deliver these molecules to cells, viral and nonviral carrier systems have been developed. The viral delivery vectors, including adenovirus and retrovirus, are efficient carriers for nucleic acids [53]. They capitalize on the molecular mechanism of virus to transport their genomes into the host cells [54]. Despite the fact that viral vectors are very effective tools in molecular biology owing to their infectious nature, concerns still remain for their immunogenicity, oncogenicity, and difficulty in large-scale production [55–57].

These concerns ask for the need of nonviral vector systems to deliver genes with reduced adverse effects. An ideal carrier is to protect RNA against enzymatic degradation to target cells, facilitate intracellular uptake, and promote efficient gene silencing. Several researches on small RNA delivery using nonviral carriers have successfully demonstrated the efficiency and target specificity [15,56,58]. Small RNAs, both siRNAs and miRNAs, have been systemically delivered by numerous viral and nonviral vectors; however, this approach may not meet the requirements for effective and controlled levels of small RNAs for in situ tissue regeneration. For in situ tissue regeneration using small RNA delivery, they should affect the adjacent cells for an extended period of time. Recently, nanofibrous scaffolds, solid porous scaffolds, and hydrogels have been developed to release small RNAs locally to the cells in the targeted sites. In this strategy, the incorporation of small RNA delivery into an implanted scaffold could provide not only a structural support but also proper microenvironment with effective bioactive signals.

POLYMERIC DELIVERY SYSTEM

Liposomes and polycations are two major nonviral gene delivery carriers. Liposome-based carriers such as Lipofectamine have been widely used as nonviral vectors to deliver numerous genes; however, safety and efficiency have yet to be achieved, due to their cytotoxicity, low transfection efficiency, and nonspecific uptake. Several cationic polymeric systems have been developed to deliver DNAs and RNAs for therapeutic prospective. These polymeric systems offer high versatility by controlling molecular weight, structure, and composition when compared with cationic liposome-based systems. The cationic polymers and genes (nucleic acids) form nanoscale complexes, called "polyplexes," via electrostatic interaction. Among many cationic polymers, polyethylenimine (PEI) is the most used carrier for gene delivery. PEI is a positively charged, linear, or branched polymer that is able to form polyplexes with small RNAs, leading to RNA protection, cellular delivery, and intracellular release [59]. However, it has been limited for the clinical uses due to their high cytotoxicity. Therefore modifications of the PEI system to improve efficacy, pharmacokinetic properties, and biocompatibility have been attempted. Liang et al. developed poly(lactide-*co*-glycolide) (PLGA)-based nanoparticles for gene delivery, which might be able to overcome the use of PEI or cationic liposome-based gene carriers [60]. The PLGA/PEI polyplexes showed improved delivery of miR-26a to induce cell cycle arrest in HepG2 cells with higher transfection efficiency and lower cytotoxicity. Chien et al. synthesized polyurethane-graft-short-branch PEI copolymer

(PU-PEI) that complexed with miR-122 to enhance the differentiation of induced pluripotent stem cells (iPSCs) into hepatocyte-like cells [61]. The PU-PEI delivery system showed higher transfection efficiency compared with Lipofectamine 2000-mediated transfection.

Naturally derived polymers, such as cationic polysaccharides, have also been used for delivering small RNAs. Chitosan is a linear disaccharide made of D-glucosamine and *N*-acetyl-D-glucosamine and has been widely used as a gene carrier material due to low toxicity, low immunogenicity, and biodegradability. The cationic charge density of chitosan to form polyplexes with negatively charged nucleotides can be adjustable. For instance, Louw et al. used chitosan/miR-124 polyplexes to specifically modulate macrophage/microglia activation and subsequently reduce neuroinflammation in a rat spinal hemisectional model [62]. The chitosan/miR-124 polyplexes were transfected into rat microglia, resulting in reduction of reactive oxygen species and tumor necrosis factor α and lower expression of major histocompatibility complex (MHC) class II. This approach offers a potential therapeutic method to reduce inflammation for a multitude of central nerve system neurodegenerative conditions.

ADVANCED CARRIER MATERIALS FOR SMALL RNA DELIVERY

The therapeutic applications of small RNAs have been hampered in the clinic due to poor stability, high cytotoxicity, and low cellular uptake in vivo. The main obstacle is the difficulty in delivering these molecules across the cell membrane to the cytoplasm, both in vitro and in vivo, where it can lead sequence-specific mRNA degradation or translational inhibition [63]. Recent advances in small RNA delivery using nanoscale complexes offer critical information for understanding the functional role of miRNAs in vivo and for supporting targeted gene therapy to treat miRNA-associated diseases. A promising novel approach employing cell-penetrating peptide (CPP) for small RNA delivery has been developed to overcome these limitations [63–65]. CPPs are short amphipathic peptides, which form stable nanoscale complexes with nucleic acids, and these complexes can enter cells independently of the endosomal pathway and efficiently deliver cargos [65]. Suh et al. developed an arginine-rich CPP (VSRRRRRRGGRRRR), which possesses cell translocating potential and effective delivery capacity of large protein molecules [63]. This CPP system has been used for delivering miR-29b to induce osteogenic differentiation of human MSCs. Osteogenic differentiation activity was enhanced by the suppression of intracellular inhibitory target gene expression. In order to improve the transfection efficiency using the CPP system, Li et al. developed a novel fusion protein system consisting of two CPPs (Hph1, YARVRRRGPRR) and one dsRBD [66]. The results demonstrated that this fusion protein system was capable of delivering siRNA in vitro and in vivo with high transfection efficiency (Fig. 7.2).

Functional hydrogels containing small RNAs could be used for the local delivery system for in situ tissue regeneration. The physicochemical properties of hydrogels can be tailored to improve the effectiveness of small RNA delivery. Nguyen et al. fabricated in situ forming poly(ethylene glycol) (PEG) hydrogels for controlled and localized delivery of small RNAs to differentiate stem cells encapsulated within the polymer network [67]. The results showed that small RNAs were released from the PEG hydrogels in a sustained manner over the course of 3–6 weeks with high bioactivity. Unlike the traditional gene delivery, prolonged delivery of small RNAs from the PEG hydrogel system provided extended regulation of cell behaviors. Recent examples using supramolecular hydrogels formed by self-assembled peptides have been reported as carriers to deliver small RNAs. Li et al. developed a dipeptide Gly–Ala linked with biphenyl-substituted tetrazole (Tet-GA) hydrogel that was used as an effective carrier to deliver miRNAs into living cells encapsulated inside the hydrogel construct [68].

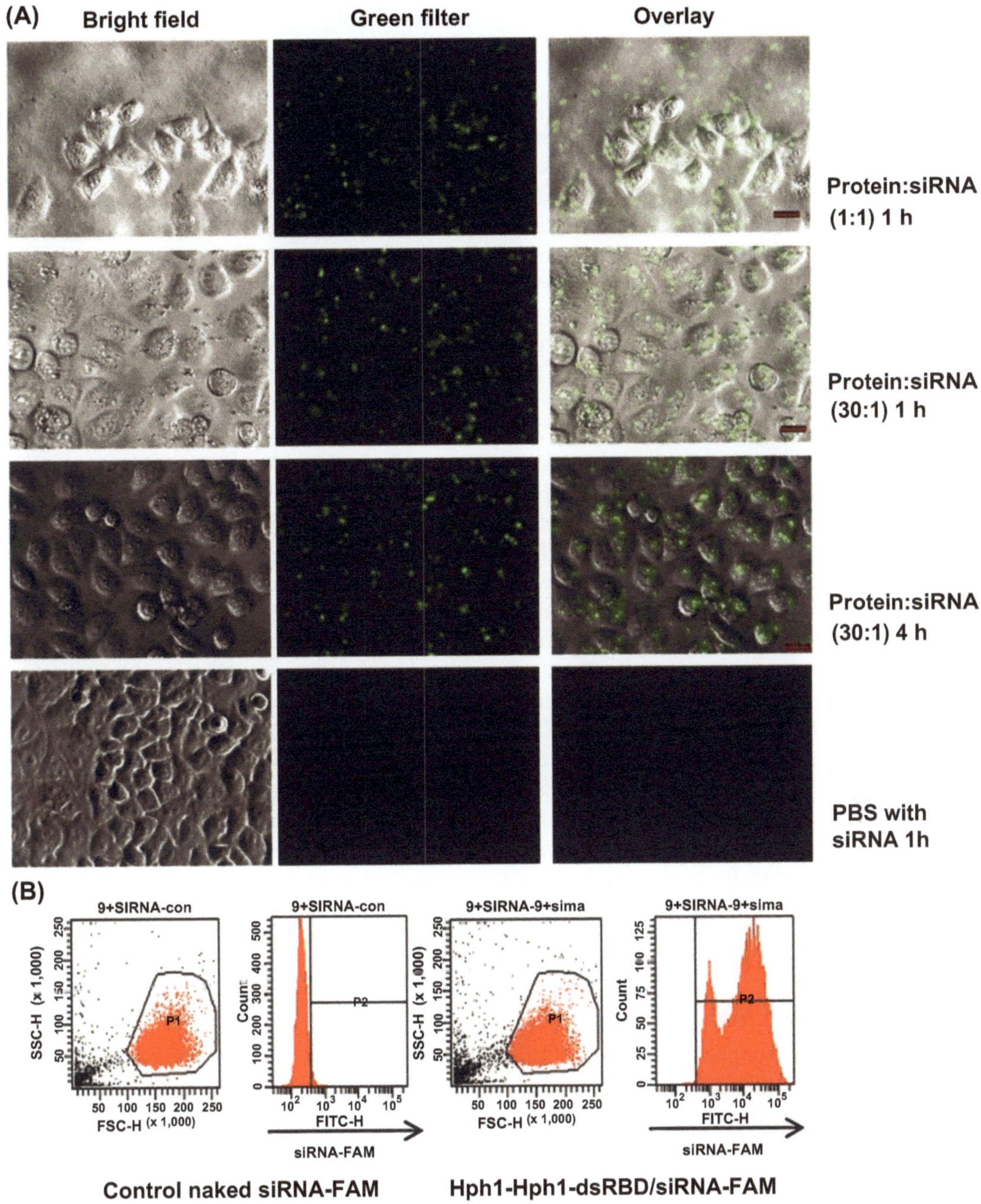

FIGURE 7.2

(A) Fluorescent microscope analysis concerning Hph1–Hph1–dsRBD delivery of siRNA into HeLa cells. Fluorescent images regarded to the Hph1–Hph1–dsRBD combined with FAM-siRNA (green) at a ratio of 30:1 for 1 h, 4 h, or with FAM-siRNA at a ratio of 30:1 for 1 h, 4 h, or with FAM-siRNA at a ratio of 1:1 condensed with 23.1 mM $CaCl_2$ for 1 h. HeLa cells were exposed to PBS–siRNA-FAM complex for 1 h as the control. From left to right: images were taken under bright field and green filter and then an overlay of above was presented. The scale bar was defined as 20 μm. (B) HeLa cells were exposed to naked siRNA or Hph1–Hph1–dsRBD/siRNA-FAM complex for 1 h, and the cell uptake was measured by the fluorescence-activated cell sorting.

Reprinted from Li H, Zheng X, Koren V, Vashist YK, Tsui TY. Highly efficient delivery of siRNA to a heart transplant model by a novel cell penetrating peptide-dsRNA binding domain. Int J Pharm 2014;469:206–13.

This Tet-Ga hydrogel system could provide not only a 3-D microenvironment for live cells but also gene delivery capacity to deliver miR-122 into the encapsulated cells [67].

Electrospinning technique can also be used to encapsulate small RNAs [69,70]. A combination of electrospun fibrous scaffold and small RNA delivery could provide a 3-D microenvironment with high surface area for cell adhesion and proliferation as well as target gene modulation for tissue development. For example, Cao et al. used the electrospinning technique to encapsulate siRNA within electrospun poly(ε-caprolactone) (PCL) nanofibers (300–400 nm in diameter) for the controlled release of intact siRNA [69]. Glyceraldehyde-3-phosphate dehydrogenase (GAPDH) siRNA released from PCL fibrous scaffolds was successfully transfected human embryonic kidney 293 cells at days 5, 15, and 30 and demonstrated that the encapsulated small RNAs remained bioactive throughout the period of sustained release, providing silencing efficiency of 61–81% that was comparable to conventional siRNA transfection. Direct seeding of cells on this siRNA-encapsulated PCL fibrous scaffold demonstrated enhanced cellular uptake and efficient GAPDH gene silencing. This approach demonstrated the potential of electrospun nanofibrous scaffold-mediated small RNA delivery. The combination of topographical features provided by nanofibrous scaffolds may provide synergistic contact guidance and biochemical signals to mediate and support cellular development for in situ tissue regeneration. For another example, Low et al. explored the feasibility of directing neuronal differentiation through synergistic integration of electrospun nanofibrous topographical cues and scaffold-mediated knockdown of RE-1 silencing transcription factor (REST) in mouse neural progenitor cells (NPCs) [71]. Electrospun PCL nanofibrous scaffold was prefabricated by mussel-inspired polydopamine (PD) coating to functionalize with REST siRNAs (denoted as siREST PD fiber). Sustained REST knockdown in NPCs was achieved for up to 5 days in vitro, and the silencing efficiency was significantly improved. The silencing of REST, together with nanofiber topographical effect, significantly enhanced NPC neuronal differentiation while reducing astrocytic and oligodendrocytic differentiation. This combination of scaffold-mediated REST knockdown and nanotopographical cues from PD-coated PCL nanofibrous scaffold may be a useful approach for generating functional neurons for therapeutic commitments.

SMALL RNAS FOR IN SITU TISSUE REGENERATION

REGULATION OF STEMNESS

Understanding the transcriptional regulatory factors of pluripotent stem cells and their early differentiation is fundamental for developing therapeutic approaches. It has been demonstrated that miRNAs have critical roles for an embryonic stem cell (ESC)'s self-renewal and differentiation capability [72–74]. Several studies showed that introduction of miRNAs targeted to ESCs could enhance the production of the iPSCs [75]. For instance, a combination of miRNAs, including miR-291-3p, miR-294, and miR-295, was used to increase the reprogramming efficiency by Oct4, Sox2, and Klf4. The results showed that introduction of miRNAs to standard transcription factors consistently increased the number of Oct4-GFP+colonies. In addition, Anokye-Danso et al. were able to achieve two orders of magnitude more efficient than standard transcription factor-mediated iPSCs using miR-302 and miR-367 [76]. MiRNAs also play an important role in the adult stem cells by regulating transcriptional factors for multiple lineages [77]. These outcomes indicate enormous future potential for the modulation of miRNA, signaling to direct stem cell differentiation in vivo [78].

Table 7.1 lists small RNAs involved in regulation of target-specific genes for in situ tissue regeneration.

Table 7.1 Small RNAs Involved in Regulation of Target-Specific Genes for Tissue Regeneration

Small RNAs	Functions	Outcomes	Applications	References
miR-1 miR-206 siGDF-8	Myostatin, myosin heavy chain (MyHC)	Muscle cell proliferation and differentiation	Myogenesis	[108]
miR-7	Klf4	Neural cell differentiation	Neurogenesis	[110]
miR-15a, miR-15b, miR-16–1, miR-16–2, miR-195, miR-497	Bcl2, Arl2	Cardiomyocytes resistant to hypoxia-induced cardiomyocyte cell death	Cardiac regeneration	[116]
miR-17, miR-20a, miR-106a	SIRPα	SIRPα-mediated macrophage inflammatory responses	Inflammation	[127]
miR-18a	CCN2/CTGF	Inhibition of the mature chondrogenic phenotype	Chondrogenesis	[86]
miR-20a siNoggin		Osteogenic differentiation of MSCs	Osteogenesis	[67]
miR-26a	CCND2 and CCNE2	Inhibition of hepatocyte proliferation	Liver regeneration	[128]
miR-26a	Runx2, ALP, OCN, Ang1	Osteogenesis–anginogeniss coupling	Osteogenesis	[124]
miR-27b	MMP-13	Inhibition of interleukin 1β (IL-1β) in human chondrocytes	Chondrogenesis	[85]
miR-29a/b	Sox9	Inhibition of collagen II production	Chondrogenesis	[89]
miR-29b	Collagen I/II	Regulation of ECM remodeling process after injury	Wound healing	[119]
miR-29b	HDAC4, CTNNBIP1, DUSP2, COL1A1, and COL5A3	Inhibition of antiosteogenic factors	Osteognesis	[63]
miR-31	Runx2, BMPR2	Inhibition of osteogenic differentiation of MSCs	Osteogenesis	[129]
miR-122	Sox17, HNF-3β, HNF-4a	Regulating hepatocyte metabolism and the differentiation process from hepatoblasts to matured hepatocytes	Liver regeneration	[61]
miR-124	Cdk6, Sox9	Differentiation of NSC into neurons or glial cells	Neurogenesis	[130]
miR-128a	IRS1/Akt insulin signaling	Inhibition of myoblast proliferation and myotube hypertrophy	Myogenesis	[131]
miR-132	RasGAP-1	Vessel maturation	Angiogenesis	[122]
miR-133b	RhoA	Spinal cord regeneration	Neurogenesis	[111]
miR-133 miR-135a	Runx2 Runx2 and Smad5	Inhibition of BMP-2 induced osteogenesis of C2C12 cells	Osteogenesis	[79]
miR-138	PTK2, FAK	Inhibition of osteogenic differentiation of hMSCs	Osteogenesis	[80]
miR-140 miR-27a	MMP-13, IGFBP-5	Inhibition of IGFBP-5 expression	Chondrogenesis	[81]
miR-140-5p	Sox9, TGF-beta	Chondrogenic differentiation of MSCs	Chondrogenesis	[132]

Continued

Table 7.1 Small RNAs Involved in Regulation of Target-Specific Genes for Tissue Regeneration—cont'd

Small RNAs	Functions	Outcomes	Applications	References
miR-145	Alpha-SMA	Enhancement of myofibroblast proliferation	Cardiac regeneration	[133]
miR-150	MMP-16	Inhibition of human cardiomyocyte progenitor cell proliferation	Cardiac regeneration	[134]
miR-199a	Smad1	Inhibition of cartilage olifomeric matrix protein (COMP), collagen II, and Sox9	Chondrogenesis	[84]
miR-200b	GATA2, VEGFR-2	Inhibition of wound angiogenesis	Angiogenesis	[135]
miR-206	Pax7, Notch3, and Igfbp5	satellite cell differentiation and fusion into muscle fibers	Myogenesis	[136]
miR-210	E2F3	Inhibition of keratinocyte proliferation	Wound healing	[120]
miR-221	Mdm2	Increase of chondrocyte proliferation by negatively regulating Mdm2	Chondrogenesis	[87]
miR-291-3p, miR-294, miR-295		Increase of the efficiency of reprogramming by Oct4, Sox2, and Klf4	Pluripotency	[75]
miR-302 miR-367	Oct4	Suppression of Hdac2	Pluripotency	[76]
miR-369-5p miR-371	FABP4, ADIPOQ	Adipogenic differentiation of MSCs is downregulated by miR-369-5p and unregulated by miR-371	Adipogenesis	[137]
miR-375	Wnt/β-catenin	Regulation of alveolar epithelial cell transdifferentiation	Lung regeneration	[138]
miR-375	Myotrophin	Insulin secretion	Pancreas regeneration	[125]
miR-590-3p and miR-199a-3p	MYH, DAB2, destrin, Runx1	Enhancement of cardiomyocyte proliferation	Cardiac regeneration	[117]
miR-675	Sox9	MMP-13 correlated with downregulation of miR-27b	Chondrogenesis	[88]
miR-1915 and miR-1225-5p	CD133, PAX-2, TRL2	Inhibition of renal progenitor markers	Kidney	[126]

BONE REGENERATION

Bone marrow-derived mesenchymal stem cells (MSCs), which are a population of self-renewing multipotent cells, are the most common cell source for bone tissue regeneration. The effects of miRNAs on osteogenic differentiation of MSCs have been investigated by targeting Runt-related transcription factor 2 (Runx2) gene. One approach to control osteogenic activity of Runx2 has been performed [79]. They observed that Runx2-targeting miRNAs, including miR-23a, miR-30c, miR-34c, miR-133a, miR-135a, miR-137, miR-204, miR-205, miR-217, miR-218, and miR-338, were inversely expressed relative to Runx2 during osteogenic and chondrogenic differentiation. Eskildsen et al. screened for differentially expressed miRNAs during osteogenic differentiation of human MSCs and identified inhibition of osteogenesis by miR-138 [80]. They

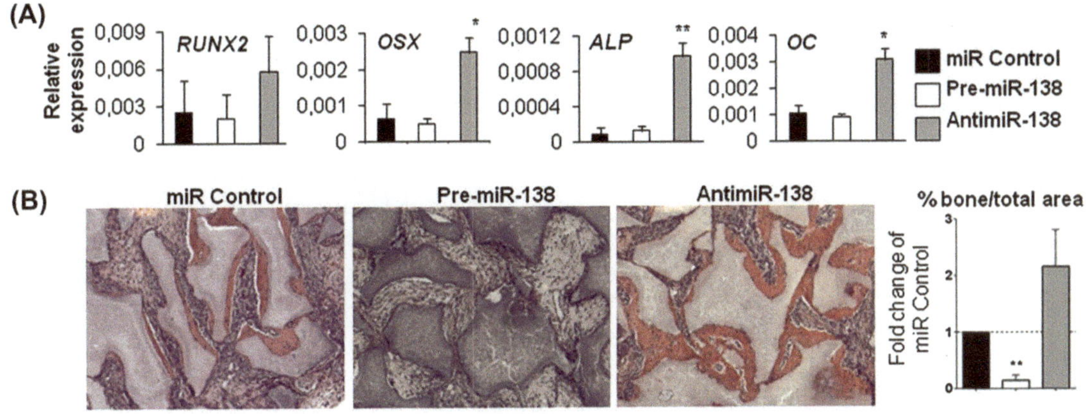

FIGURE 7.3

MiR-138 inhibits ectopic bone formation in vivo. Human MSCs were transfected with 25nM miR-C, premiR-138, or anti-miR-138 and implanted into nonobese diabetic (NOD)/severe combined immunodeficiency (SCID) mice. (A) qRT-PCR analysis of osteoblast marker genes (RUNX2, osterix, alkaline phosphatase (ALP), and OC normalized to β-actin) was performed after 1week of implantation. (B) Hematoxylin and eosin (H&E) staining was performed after 8weeks of implantation. Bone formation was quantified as total bone volume per total volume from H&E staining, and it was expressed as fold change of miR-C. Four implants per treatment were engrafted into mice, and three sections of each implant were quantified to minimize variations within the implants. $*p<.05$; $**p<.01$.

Reprinted from Eskildsen T, Taipaleenmaki H, Stenvang J, Abdallah BM, Ditzel N, Nossent AY, et al. MicroRNA-138 regulates osteogenic differentiation of human stromal (mesenchymal) stem cells in vivo. Proc Natl Acad Sci USA 2011;108:6139–44.

suggested that inhibition of miR-138 could lead to derepression of focal adhesion kinase (FAK) and its downstream signaling that coincides with increased bone formation (Fig. 7.3).

CARTILAGE REGENERATION

Numerous miRNAs play critical roles in the regulation of chondrogenesis. Among the miRNAs specific to cartilage tissue, several groups have demonstrated that miR-140 has important roles in tissue development and homeostasis by targeting insulin-like growth factor binding protein 5 (IGFBP-5), histone deacetylase 4 (HDAC4), and Smad3 [81–83]. Lin et al. investigated that miR-199a responds to bone morphogenic protein 2 (BMP-2)-induced chondrogenesis by direct targeting of Smad1 transcription factor [84]. In addition, miR-27b regulated matrix metallopeptidase 13 expression in human chondrocytes [85], miR-18a downregulated chondrogenic phenotype by targeting of chondrogenic transcription factors CCN family 2 (CCN2)/connective tissue growth factor (CTGF) [86], miR-221 promoted proteosomal degradation of Slug by targeting of Mdm2 transcription factor [87], and miR-675 regulated Sox9-mediated collagen type II expression in human chondrocytes [88]. Yan et al. identified miR-29a and miR-29b to directly target 3′ UTR of col2a1 encoding type II collagen by dualluciferase assay, and their activity was under the regulation of Sox9, the sex-determining region Y (SRY)-related high mobility group (HMG) box gene 9 [89]. The results explained the biological processes occurring between cell–substrate interface interactions via miRNAs (Fig. 7.4).

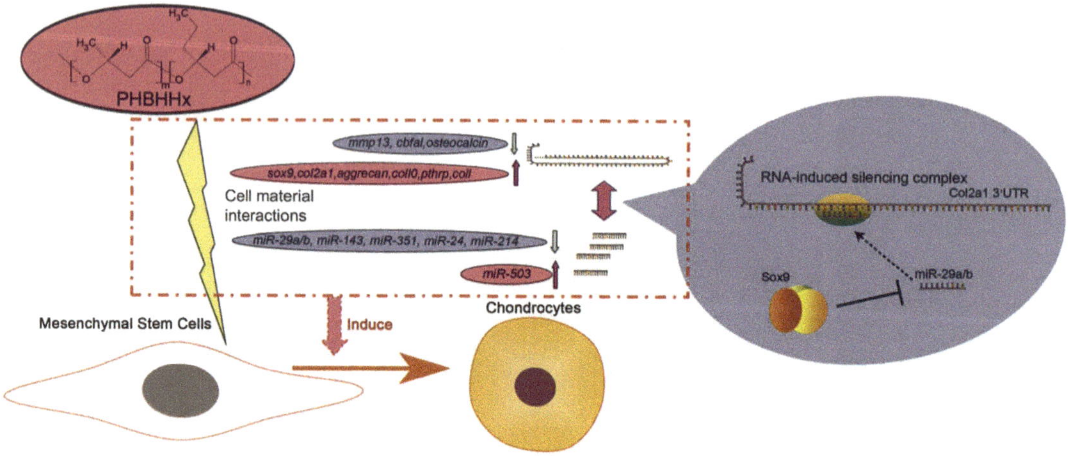

FIGURE 7.4

Schematic illustration of miRNA regulation-associated chondrogenesis of mouse MSCs grown on polyhydroxyalkanoates (PHA) mouse MSCs cultured on a poly(3-hydroxybutyrate-co-3-hydroxyhexanoate) (PHBHHx) film showed upregulated expression of chondrogenic marker genes including aggrecan, col2, sox9, col10, and pthrp. Among 44 miRNAs related to chondrogenesis, the seven most differentially expressed miRNAs were selected to study their target genes related to chondrogenesis. Two miRNAs out of the seven, namely, miR-29a and miR-29b, were revealed to directly target 3′ UTR of col2a1 encoding type II collagen, with their activity under the regulation of Sox9, the SRY-related high mobility group box gene 9. For the first time, miRNAs were discovered to regulate the stem cell differentiation processes mediated by cell–substrate interactions.

Reprinted from Yan C, Wang Y, Shen XY, Yang G, Jian J, Wang HS, et al. MicroRNA regulation associated chondrogenesis of mouse MSCs grown on polyhydroxyalkanoates. Biomaterials 2011;32:6435–44.

SKELETAL MUSCLE REGENERATION

Among the miRNAs associated with myogenic regulation, miR-1, miR-27, miR-133, miR-188, and miR-206 are major mediators. It has been reported that an miR-1, miR-133, and miR-206 are expressed in skeletal, smooth, and cardiac muscles [90–93]. miR-1 and miR-133 are transcriptionally regulated by the myogenic differentiation factors, including MyoD (a protein that regulate muscle differentiation), myocyte enhancer factor 2 (MEF2), and serum response factor, through negative feedback loops in skeletal muscles [90,94]. MyoD and MEF2 enhance the gene expression of miR-1-2/-133a-1 [95]. miR-27 down-regulates Pax3, promoting myogenesis in adult muscle regeneration, whereas its repression delays muscle regeneration in injured muscle in vivo [96]. In dystrophic tibialis anterior (TA) muscles of *mdx* mice, miR-206 expression was significantly elevated as compared to that in control TA muscles of age-matched B10 mice, whereas there were no differences in miR-1 or miR-133a expression between B10 and *mdx* TA muscles. Strong signals for miR-206 were found in newly formed myofibers with centralized nuclei, indicating active regeneration and efficient maturation of skeletal muscle tissue [97].

Satellite cells (SCs) are skeletal muscle progenitors that are responsible for muscle regeneration [11,13]. In mouse soleus muscle cardiotoxin injury model, Myf-5, MyoD, and MRF4 mRNAs were detected in satellite cell-derived myoblasts at 2–3 days after injury in the first stages of muscle regeneration. The Myf-5 transcript was decreased in young multinucleated myotubes, while MyoD and

MRF4 were maintained throughout regeneration. Myogenin mRNA was transiently expressed in forming myotubes. Muscle denervation accelerated the overexpression of Myf-5 and MRF4 mRNAs at 8 days after injury, followed by MyoD and myogenin overexpression in the late stages of regeneration at 30 days after injury [11]. Transforming growth factor-β (TGF-β) superfamily, consisting of myostatin, TGF-α, TGF-β1, and BMPs, are major inhibitory factors in development and postnatal regeneration of skeletal muscle [98,99]. TGF-β1 prevents myoblast differentiation and recruitment as well as SC proliferation and differentiation [100–102]. In SCs and myoblasts, myostatin maintains their quiescence through inhibiting expression of Pax3 and Myf5 in addition to silencing MyoD expression [103–105]. It stimulates fibroblast-induced remodeling and repair of the extracellular matrix (ECM) and the basal membrane. It also causes production of collagen and fibronectin, leading to scar tissue formation [106]. An inhibitor of TGF-β, decorin, reduced muscle fibrosis and enhanced skeletal muscle regeneration [107].

It has been demonstrated that single local injection of miR-1, miR-133, and miR-206 in combination could accelerate muscle regeneration in a rat skeletal muscle injury model [12]. One week after laceration of the rat TA muscle, miR-1, miR-133, and miR-206 mixture mediated atelocollagen injection-enhanced muscle regeneration morphologically and physiologically. Furthermore, the single injection effectively prevented TGF-β-induced fibrosis. Administrating three miRNAs in combination promoted myotube differentiation and the expression of MyoD1, myogenin, and Pax7 in C2C12 cells in vitro. Very recently, we employed this strategy to accelerate and enhance skeletal muscle regeneration for the treatment of muscular atrophy [108]. We selected myostatin-siRNA (siGDF-8), a major inhibitory factor in development and postnatal regeneration of skeletal muscle, and muscle-specific miRNAs (miR-1 and miR-206) to further accelerate muscle regeneration. The results showed that the combination of small RNAs significantly improved the gene expression of myogenic regulatory factors such as myoD, myogenin, Pax7, and MyHC1 in vitro, suggesting myogenic activation. Moreover, cell proliferation and myotube formation improved without compromising each other, which indicates the myogenic potential of this particular combination of small RNAs. The recovery of chemically injured TA muscles in rats was significantly accelerated both functionally and structurally (Fig. 7.5). This novel combination of siRNA and miRNAs has a promising therapeutic potential to improve in situ skeletal muscle regeneration.

NERVE REGENERATION

Understanding of the miRNAs involved in nerve regeneration can lead to an in situ nerve regeneration strategy [109]. For example, Cui et al. selected miR-7 to target Kruppel-like factor 4 (Klf4), which is a key transcription factor for self-renewal of neural stem cells (NSCs) [110]. Their outcomes indicate that miR-7 plays a critical role in maintaining the self-renewal capacity via Klf4-mediated pathway in 3-D cultured NSCs. More specifically, one study has shown upregulation of miR-133b expression in regenerating neurons of the brainstem after transection of the spinal cord in zebrafish [111]. The results showed that inhibition of miR-133b expression resulted in impaired locomotor recovery and reduced regeneration of axons from neurons because miR-133b could target the small GTPase RhoA, which is an inhibitor of axonal growth, as well as other neurite outgrowth-related molecules.

Peripheral nerve regeneration is directly correlated with skeletal muscle recovery, since conditions such as muscular atrophy are caused by denervation, as the recovery is promoted by reinnervation [112]. In Amyotrophic lateral sclerosis (ALS) mouse model, lack of miR-206 accelerates disease

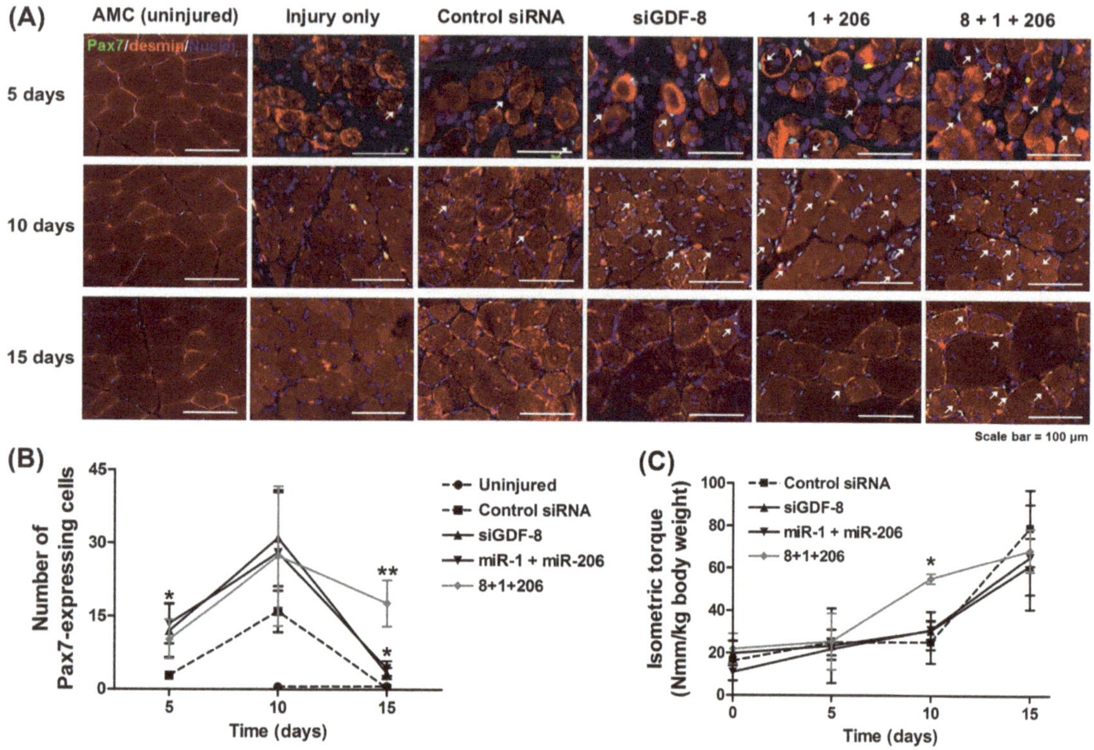

FIGURE 7.5

Pax7-expressinge cells were evaluated for the effect of RNA on muscle stem cell self-renewal. Myofibers were stained against desmin (shown in red), and SCs were stained against Pax7 (shown in green) with counter-stained nuclei (shown in blue). (A) Pax7-positive nuclei in myofibers are shown in light blue (indicated by *white arrows*). Scale bar = 100 μm. (B) Cell population was quantified by the number of Pax7-expressing cells in myofibers per field. The combination delivery of the three RNAs extended the increased number of cells to 15 days indicating prolonged self-renewal of muscle SCs. $*p<.05$ compared to control and $**p<.05$ compared to the others. (C) Muscle force of injured muscle showed significantly accelerated functional recovery in the combination RNA injected muscle at 10 days post-RNA injection, when the other groups showed similar muscle force recovery ($*p<.05$).

Reprinted from Kim N, Yoo JJ, Atala A, Lee SJ. Combination of small RNAs for skeletal muscle regeneration. FASEB J 2015;30(3):1198–206.

progression, suggesting the role of miR-206 for regeneration of neuromuscular synapses after acute nerve injury. Williams et al. showed that miR-206 could reduce ALS progression by sensing motor neuron injury and promoting the compensatory regeneration of neuromuscular synapses [113]. Successful activation of transcriptional regulatory pathways enables adult peripheral sensory neurons to functionally and anatomically recover after nerve injury. For example, it has been known that transcription factor Sox11 is highly expressed in developing sensory neurons. Jankowski et al. modified siRNA targeting to Sox11 to transiently prevent in vivo regeneration of mouse saphenous nerve [114]. The stress- and injury-associated activating transcription factor 3 was expressed in the majority of neurons in ganglia of crushed nerve, and it was downregulated followed by Sox11-siRNA treatment in vitro and in vivo. The result suggested that Sox11 could be used for successful regeneration following peripheral nerve injury.

CARDIAC TISSUE REGENERATION

Myocardial infarction is a leading cause of death in the world [115]. It has been demonstrated that miRNAs play important roles during different forms of heart diseases. Hullinger et al. showed that inhibition of miR-15 family could improve cardiomyocytes resistant to hypoxia-induced cell death [116]. Systemic delivery of anti-miR-15dose dependently repressed miR-15 family in both murine and porcine cardiac tissues. The results showed that anti-miR targeting to miR-15 family in mice reduced infarct size and enhanced cardiac function in response to ischemic injury. Very recently, Eulalio et al. selected miRNAs (I-miR-590 alhsa-miR-199a) to promote cell cycle reentry of adult cardiomyocytes ex vivo and to promote cardiomyocyte proliferation in both neonatal and adult animals [117]. After myocardial infarction in mice, these miRNAs stimulated marked cardiac regeneration and almost complete recovery of cardiac functional parameters (Fig. 7.6).

WOUND HEALING

Abnormally increasing production and deposition of collagen is a critical mechanism of fibrosis and scar formation. This can cause further issues by disrupting functional recovery and regeneration of neighboring tissues. A study showed that adenovirus-mediated transfer of heat shock protein 47 siRNA inhibited the expression of type I collagen and the formation of scar tissue in animal model [118]. In another approach to direct appropriate ECM remodeling, delivery of miR-29B has been suggested to modulate collagen types I and II expression [119]. Biswas et al. created a model of ischemic wounds to validate miR-210 function in limiting keratinocyte proliferation [120]. The results have demonstrated that the hypoxia component of ischemia may limit wound reepithelialization by stabilizing hypoxia-inducible factor 1α, which induces miR-210 expression, resulting in the downregulation of the cell cycle regulatory protein E2F transcription factor 3 (E2F3).

VASCULARIZATION

Vascularization is essential for cell and tissue survival and function. The ability to effectively induce vascularization into a region of interest should have a wide range of clinical applications. Among many small RNAs, miRNA-132 has been described as an angiogenic switch targeting p120RasGAP in the endothelium, permitting increased activation of Ras and leading to neovascularization in response to growth factor [121]. Devalliere et al. showed that transfection of endothelial cells (ECs) with miR-132 could enhance growth factor-mediated proliferation and migration [122]. Moreover, transplantation of the miR-132-transfected ECs resulted in a twofold increase in the microvessel number in immunodeficient mice (Fig. 7.7).

During the bone regeneration, angiogenic growth factors induce sprouting microvessels, facilitating the recruitment of osteogenic cells due to their highly vascularized nature [123]. Therefore the balance of the bone and vessel remodeling process should be critical to prevent excessive bone formation or vascular leakage. Li et al. identified miR-26a that positively regulates angiogenesis–osteogenesis

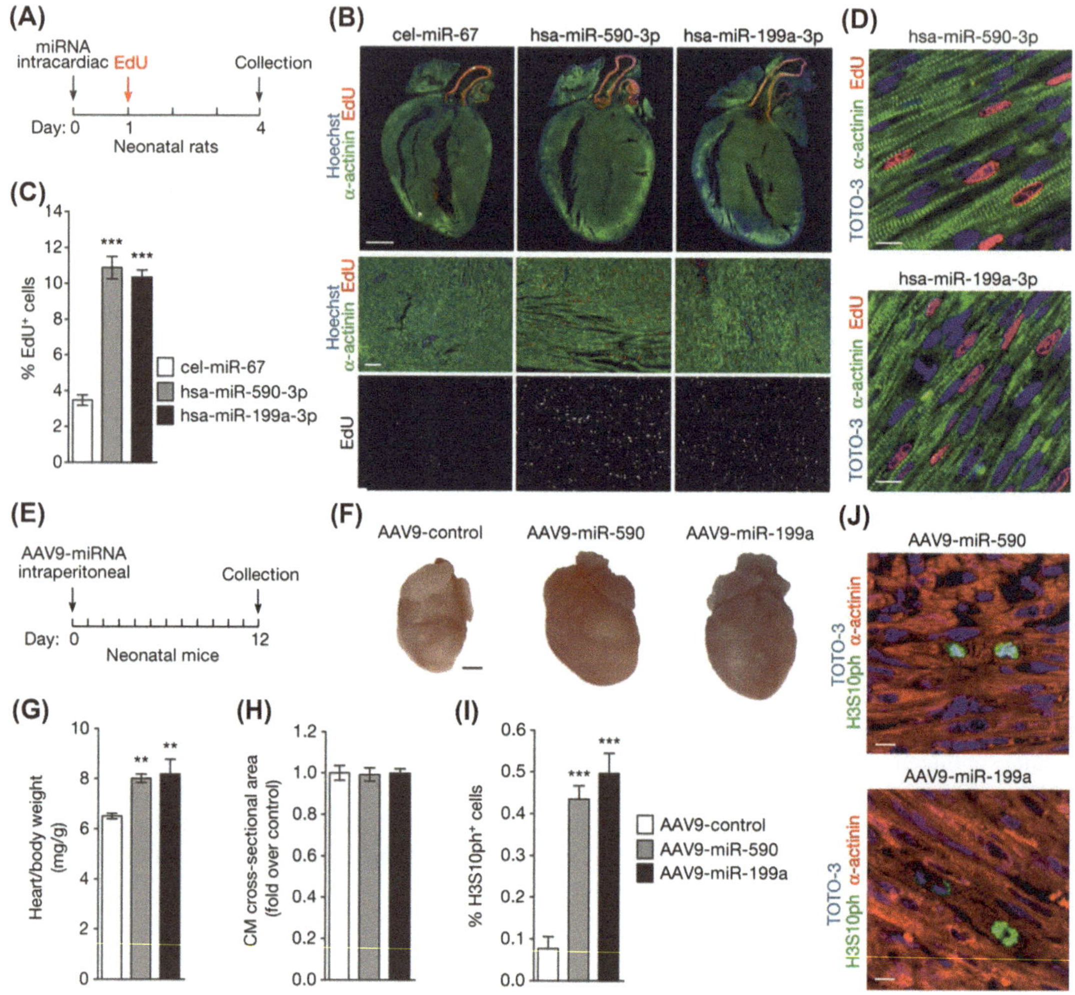

FIGURE 7.6

(A) Schematic of in vivo experiments using synthetic miRNAs. $n=8$ per group. (B) EdU and α-actinin staining of rat hearts injected with miRNAs. Scale bars, 1 mm (top), 100 μm (bottom). (C) Percentage of proliferating cells. (D) Confocal microscopy of rat hearts injected with hsa-miR-590-3p and hsa-miR-199a-3p. Scale bar, 10 μm. (E) Schematic of in vivo experiments using AAV vectors. $n=9$ per group. (F) Mouse hearts transduced with AAV vectors. Scale bar, 1 mm. (G) Ratio between heart and body weight. (H) CM cross-sectional area. (I) Percentage of cells positive for H3S10ph. (J) Confocal microscopy of H3S10ph-stained mouse hearts transduced with AAV. Scale bar, 10 μm. All panels, mean ± SEM; $^{**}p<.01$, $^{***}p<.001$ relative to control.

Reprinted from Eulalio A, Mano M, Dal Ferro M, Zentilin L, Sinagra G, Zacchigna S, et al. Functional screening identifies miRNAs inducing cardiac regeneration. Nature 2012;492:376–81.

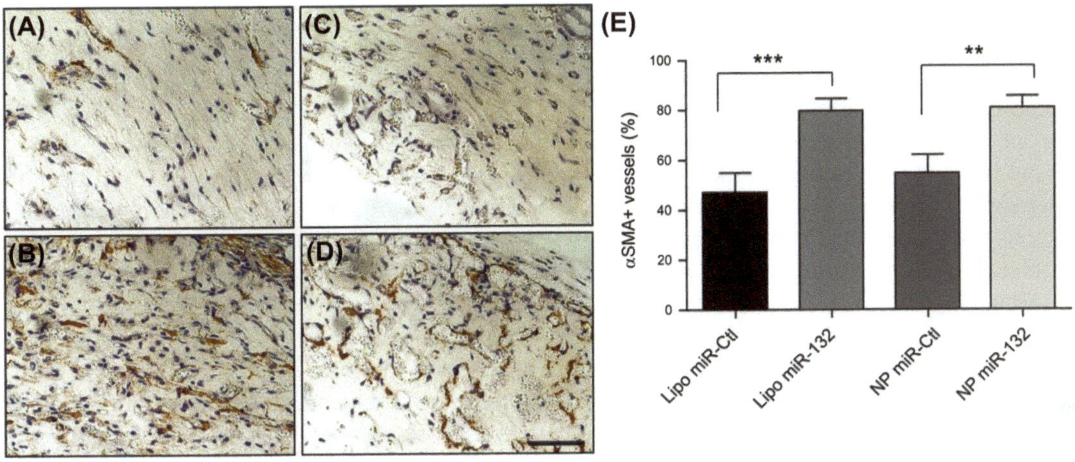

FIGURE 7.7

MiR-132 delivery results in increased number of SMA-invested vessels. HUVECs were transfected, suspended in gel, and implanted into abdominal wall of C.B-17 SCID/beige mice. Implants were retrieved after 2 weeks, and sections were stained with mouse-specific smooth muscle α-actin (SMA) antibody. (A–D) Lipofectamine miR-Ctl (A), Lipofectamine miR-132 (B), NP miR-Ctl (C), and NP miR-132 (D). Scale bar = 100 μm. (E) Quantitation of positive SMA vessels (percentage of total vessel number; means ± SEM); $n=5$. *$p<.05$, **$p<.01$, ***$p<.0005$.

Reprinted from Devalliere J, Chang WG, Andrejecsk JW, Abrahimi P, Cheng CJ, Jane-wit D, et al. Sustained delivery of proangiogenic microRNA-132 by nanoparticle transfection improves endothelial cell transplantation. FASEB J 2014;28:908–22.

coupling [124]. The results showed enhanced bone formation coordinated with vascularization in both mouse subcutaneous implantation and calvarial bone defect models.

OTHER APPLICATIONS

Type 1 diabetes results from the autoimmune destruction of the insulin-producing pancreatic β-cells. Poy et al. found that overexpression of miR-375 suppressed glucose-induced insulin secretion [125]. Hence, they suggested that inhibition of endogenous miR-375 function enhanced insulin secretion. The mechanism by which secretion is modified by miR-375 is independent of changes in glucose metabolism or intracellular Ca21-signaling but correlated with a direct effect on insulin exocytosis. Myotrophin was predicted to be and validated as a target of miR-375. Inhibition of myotrophin by siRNA mimicked the effects of miR-375 on glucose-stimulated insulin secretion and exocytosis. This indicates that miR-375 is a regulator of insulin secretion and may thereby constitute a novel pharmacological target for the treatment of diabetes.

In renal regeneration, adult renal progenitor cells have been recently identified in the cortex of the renal parenchyma, and it has been demonstrated that they expressed PAX-2, CD133, and CD24 and exhibited renal regeneration capacity. Recent studies on stem cells indicated that miRNAs may play a key role in stem cell self-renewal and differentiation. Sallustio et al. investigated that miR-1915 and miR-1225-5p regulated the expression of important markers of renal progenitor cells, such as CD133 and PAX-2, and important genes involved in the repair mechanisms of renal progenitor cells, such as toll-like receptor 2 [126].

SUMMARY AND FUTURE DIRECTIONS

The function of small RNAs in selectively controlling target gene expression has been increasingly studied for basic and clinical researches due to its immense therapeutic potential. Many researches focus on genetic diseases and their cures, while other researches have been devoted to regenerative therapy for traumatic injury. Unlike growth factors, small RNAs, both siRNA and miRNA, have the target-specific nature that can modulate target-specific genes. Current progress on small RNA delivery has applied the RNAi strategy for tissue engineering and regenerative medicine as a robust treatment method for in situ tissue regeneration. This strategy has a synergistic effect on regeneration with immunogenic advantages compared to DNA treatment, and it can be used for transient or long-term treatment, since it is an easily reversible process. For this reason, small RNAs make more pharmaceutical sense as therapeutic drugs. Moreover, incorporating small RNAs into a tissue-specific scaffolding system can be easily achieved because many synthetic materials used in small RNA delivery have also been applied in tissue engineering purposes. Choosing appropriate small RNAs and biomaterials for the target and purpose is required to maximize the regeneration capacity of the tissue. For a more efficient therapeutic outcome, an improved understanding of the complex interactions and pathways of the molecules that are involved in the target-specific tissue regeneration will be necessary.

LIST OF ACRONYMS AND ABBREVIATIONS

ALS Amyotrophic lateral sclerosis
ATF3 Activating transcription factor 3
BM Basal membrane
BMP-2 Bone morphogenic protein 2
CNS Central nerve system
COMP Cartilage oligomeric matrix protein
CPP Cell-penetrating peptide
dsRNA Double-stranded RNA
E2F3 E2F transcription factor 3
ECM Extracellular matrix
ESCs Embryonic stem cells
GAPDH Glyceraldehyde-3-phosphate dehydrogenase
GATA2 Globin transcription factor binding protein 2
HDAC4 Histone deacetylase 4
HIF-1α Hypoxia-inducible factor 1α
HNF-3β Hepatocyte nuclear factor 3 beta
HNF-4α Hepatocyte nuclear factor 4 alpha
HSP47 Heat shock protein 47
IFN Interferon
IGFBP Insulin-like growth factor binding protein
IL-1β Interleukin 1β
iPSCs Induced pluripotent stem cells
Klf4 Kruppel-like factor 4
MEF2 Myocyte enhancer factor 2

MHC class II Major histocompatibility complex class II
miRNA MicroRNA
MMP Matrix metallopeptidase
MSCs Mesenchymal stem cells
NPCs Neural progenitor cells
NSCs Neural stem cells
PCL Poly(ε-caprolactone)
PD Polydopamine
pDNA Plasmid DNA
PEG Poly(ethylene glycol)
PEI Polyethylenimine
PLGA Poly(lactide-*co*-glycolide)
PU Polyurethane
REST RE-1 silencing transcription factor
RISC RNA-induced silencing complex
RNAi RNA interference
RNase Ribonuclease
ROS Reactive oxygen species
Runx2 Runt-related transcription factor 2
SCs Satellite cells
shRNA Short-hairpin RNA
siRNA Small interfering RNA
SIRPα Signal-regulatory protein α
SRF Serum response factor
TA Tibialis anterior
Tet-GA Dipeptide Gly–Ala linked with biphenyl-substituted tetrazole
TGF Transforming growth factor
TLR2 Toll-like receptor 2
TNF-α Tumor necrosis factor α

ACKNOWLEDGMENT

This study is supported by the Musculoskeletal Transplant Foundation (MTF).

REFERENCES

[1] Behlke MA. Progress towards in vivo use of siRNAs. Mol Ther 2006;13:644–70.
[2] Fire A, Xu S, Montgomery MK, Kostas SA, Driver SE, Mello CC. Potent and specific genetic interference by double-stranded RNA in *Caenorhabditis elegans*. Nature 1998;391:806–11.
[3] Romano G, Pacilio C, Giordano A. Gene transfer technology in therapy: current applications and future goals. Stem Cells 1999;17:191–202.
[4] Carthew RW, Sontheimer EJ. Origins and Mechanisms of miRNAs and siRNAs. Cell 2009;136:642–55.
[5] Peng B, Chen Y, Leong KW. MicroRNA delivery for regenerative medicine. Adv Drug Deliv Rev 2015;88:108–22.
[6] Langer R. Tissue engineering. Mol Ther 2000;1:12–5.

[7] Atala A. Tissue engineering and regenerative medicine: concepts for clinical application. Rejuvenation Res 2004;7:15–31.
[8] Lee SJ, Van Dyke M, Atala A, Yoo JJ. Host cell mobilization for in situ tissue regeneration. Rejuvenation Res 2008;11:747–56.
[9] Ko IK, Ju YM, Chen T, Atala A, Yoo JJ, Lee SJ. Combined systemic and local delivery of stem cell inducing/recruiting factors for in situ tissue regeneration. FASEB J 2011;26(1):158–68.
[10] Ju YM, Atala A, Yoo JJ, Lee SJ. In situ regeneration of skeletal muscle tissue through host cell recruitment. Acta Biomater 2014;10:4332–9.
[11] Launay T, Armand A-S, Charbonnier F, Mira J-C, Donsez E, Gallien CL, et al. Expression and neural control of myogenic regulatory factor genes during regeneration of mouse soleus. J Histochem Cytochem 2001;49:887–99.
[12] Nakasa T, Ishikawa M, Shi M, Shibuya H, Adachi N, Ochi M. Acceleration of muscle regeneration by local injection of muscle-specific microRNAs in rat skeletal muscle injury model. J Cell Mol Med 2010;14:2495–505.
[13] Ten Broek RW, Grefte S, Von den Hoff JW. Regulatory factors and cell populations involved in skeletal muscle regeneration. J Cell Physiol 2010;224:7–16.
[14] Aigner A. Applications of RNA interference: current state and prospects for siRNA-based strategies in vivo. Appl Microbiol Biotechnol 2007;76:9–21.
[15] Akhtar S, Benter IF. Nonviral delivery of synthetic siRNAs in vivo. J Clin Invest 2007;117:3623–32.
[16] Caplen NJ, Fleenor J, Fire A, Morgan RA. dsRNA-mediated gene silencing in cultured *Drosophila* cells: a tissue culture model for the analysis of RNA interference. Gene 2000;252:95–105.
[17] Gan L, Anton KE, Masterson BA, Vincent VAM, Ye S, Gonzalez-Zulueta M. Specific interference with gene expression and gene function mediated by long dsRNA in neural cells. J Neurosci Methods 2002;121:151–7.
[18] Cheng JC, Sakamoto KM. The emerging role of RNA interference in the design of novel therapeutics in oncology. Cell Cycle 2004;3:1398–401.
[19] Salem AK, Behlke MA. siRNA delivery vehicles. RNA interference: application to drug discovery and challenges to pharmaceutical development. John Wiley & Sons Inc.; 2010.
[20] Karpala AJ, Doran TJ, Bean AG. Immune responses to dsRNA: implications for gene silencing technologies. Immunol Cell Biol 2005;83:211–6.
[21] Nieth C. Modulation of the classical multidrug resistance (MDR) phenotype by RNA interference (RNAi). FEBS Lett 2003;545:144–50.
[22] Bernstein E, Caudy AA, Hammond SM, Hannon GJ. Role for a bidentate ribonuclease in the initiation step of RNA interference. Nature 2001;409:363–6.
[23] Dang LT, Kondo H, Aoki T, Hirono I. Engineered virus-encoded pre-microRNA (pre-miRNA) induces sequence-specific antiviral response in addition to nonspecific immunity in a fish cell line: convergence of RNAi-related pathways and IFN-related pathways in antiviral response. Antivir Res 2008;80:316–23.
[24] Elbashir SM, Harborth J, Lendeckel W, Yalcin A, Weber K, Tuschl T. Duplexes of 21-nucleotide RNAs mediate RNA interference in cultured mammalian cells. Nature 2001;411:494–8.
[25] John M, Constien R, Akinc A, Goldberg M, Moon Y-A, Spranger M, et al. Effective RNAi-mediated gene silencing without interruption of the endogenous microRNA pathway. Nature 2007;449:745–7.
[26] Olejniczak M, Galka P, Krzyzosiak WJ. Sequence-non-specific effects of RNA interference triggers and microRNA regulators. Nucleic Acids Res 2010;38:1–16.
[27] Zamore PD, Tuschl T, Sharp PA, Bartel DP. RNAi: double-stranded RNA directs the ATP-dependent cleavage of mRNA at 21 to 23 nucleotide intervals. Cell 2000;101:25–33.
[28] Elbashir SM, Lendeckel W, Tuschl T. RNA interference is mediated by 21- and 22-nucleotide RNAs. Genes Dev 2001;15:188–200.
[29] Grimm D, Streetz KL, Jopling CL, Storm TA, Pandey K, Davis CR, et al. Fatality in mice due to oversaturation of cellular microRNA/short hairpin RNA pathways. Nature 2006;441:537–41.

[30] Lewis BP, Shih I-h, Jones-Rhoades MW, Bartel DP, Burge CB. Prediction of mammalian microRNA targets. Cell 2003;115:787–98.

[31] Caplen NJ, Parrish S, Imani F, Fire A, Morgan RA. Specific inhibition of gene expression by small double-stranded RNAs in invertebrate and vertebrate systems. Proc Natl Acad Sci USA 2001;98:9742–7.

[32] Elbashir SM, Martinez J, Patkaniowska A, Lendeckel W, Tuschl T. Functional anatomy of siRNAs for mediating efficient RNAi in *Drosophila melanogaster* embryo lysate. EMBO J 2001;20:6877–88.

[33] Ambros V. The functions of animal microRNAs. Nature 2004;431:350–5.

[34] Bartel DP. MicroRNAs: genomics, biogenesis, mechanism, and function. Cell 2004;116:281–97.

[35] Lee Y, Ahn C, Han J, Choi H, Kim J, Yim J, et al. The nuclear RNase III Drosha initiates microRNA processing. Nature 2003;425:415–9.

[36] Lee Y, Jeon K, Lee J-T, Kim S, Kim VN. MicroRNA maturation: stepwise processing and subcellular localization. EMBO J 2002;21:4663–70.

[37] Yi R, Qin Y, Macara IG, Cullen BR. Exportin-5 mediates the nuclear export of pre-microRNAs and short hairpin RNAs. Genes Dev 2003;17:3011–6.

[38] Zeng Y, Yi R, Cullen BR. MicroRNAs and small interfering RNAs can inhibit mRNA expression by similar mechanisms. Proc Natl Acad Sci USA 2003;100:9779–84.

[39] Lund E, Güttinger S, Calado A, Dahlberg JE, Kutay U. Nuclear export of microRNA precursors. Science 2004;303:95–8.

[40] Valencia-Sanchez MA, Liu J, Hannon GJ, Parker R. Control of translation and mRNA degradation by miRNAs and siRNAs. Genes Dev 2006;20:515–24.

[41] Collins R, Cheng X. Structural domains in RNAi. FEBS Lett 2005;579:5841–9.

[42] Matranga C, Tomari Y, Shin C, Bartel DP, Zamore PD. Passenger-strand cleavage facilitates assembly of siRNA into Ago2-containing RNAi enzyme complexes. Cell 2005;123:607–20.

[43] Nykänen A, Haley B, Zamore PD. Atp requirements and small interfering RNA structure in the RNA interference pathway. Cell 2001;107:309–21.

[44] Hammond SM, Boettcher S, Caudy AA, Kobayashi R, Hannon GJ. Argonaute2, a link between genetic and biochemical analyses of RNAi. Science 2001;293:1146–50.

[45] Liu J, Carmell MA, Rivas FV, Marsden CG, Thomson JM, Song J-J, et al. Argonaute2 is the catalytic engine of mammalian RNAi. Science 2004;305:1437–41.

[46] Rand TA, Ginalski K, Grishin NV, Wang X. Biochemical identification of Argonaute 2 as the sole protein required for RNA-induced silencing complex activity. Proc Natl Acad Sci USA 2004;101:14385–9.

[47] Martinez J, Patkaniowska A, Urlaub H, Lührmann R, Tuschl T. Single-stranded antisense siRNAs guide target RNA cleavage in RNAi. Cell 2002;110:563–74.

[48] Pillai RS, Artus CG, Filipowicz W. Tethering of human Ago proteins to mRNA mimics the miRNA-mediated repression of protein synthesis. RNA 2004;10:1518–25.

[49] Lim LP, Lau NC, Garrett-Engele P, Grimson A, Schelter JM, Castle J, et al. Microarray analysis shows that some microRNAs downregulate large numbers of target mRNAs. Nature 2005;433:769–73.

[50] Baek D, Villen J, Shin C, Camargo FD, Gygi SP, Bartel DP. The impact of microRNAs on protein output. Nature 2008;455:64–71.

[51] Selbach M, Schwanhausser B, Thierfelder N, Fang Z, Khanin R, Rajewsky N. Widespread changes in protein synthesis induced by microRNAs. Nature 2008;455:58–63.

[52] Banan M, Puri N. The ins and outs of RNAi in mammalian cells. Curr Pharm Biotechnol 2004;5:441–50.

[53] Zhang X, Godbey WT. Viral vectors for gene delivery in tissue engineering. Adv Drug Deliv Rev 2006;58:515–34.

[54] Goff SP, Berg P. Construction of hybrid viruses containing SV40 and lambda phage DNA segments and their propagation in cultured monkey cells. Cell 1976;9:695–705.

[55] Martin SE, Caplen NJ. Applications of RNA interference in mammalian systems. Annu Rev Genom Hum Genet 2007;8:81–108.

[56] Kim WJ, Kim SW. Efficient siRNA delivery with non-viral polymeric vehicles. Pharm Res 2009;26:657–66.

[57] Ruponen M, Honkakoski P, Ronkko S, Pelkonen J, Tammi M, Urtti A. Extracellular and intracellular barriers in non-viral gene delivery. J Control Release 2003;93:213–7.

[58] Kim N, Jiang D, Jacobi AM, Lennox KA, Rose SD, Behlke MA, et al. Synthesis and characterization of mannosylated pegylated polyethylenimine as a carrier for siRNA. Int J Pharm 2011;427(1):123–33.

[59] Hobel S, Aigner A. Polyethylenimines for siRNA and miRNA delivery in vivo. Wiley Interdiscip Rev Nanomed Nanobiotechnol 2013;5:484–501.

[60] Liang GF, Zhu YL, Sun B, Hu FH, Tian T, Li SC, et al. PLGA-based gene delivering nanoparticle enhance suppression effect of miRNA in HePG2 cells. Nanoscale Res Lett 2011;6:447.

[61] Chien Y, Chang YL, Li HY, Larsson M, Wu WW, Chien CS, et al. Synergistic effects of carboxymethyl-hexanoyl chitosan, cationic polyurethane-short branch PEI in miR122 gene delivery: accelerated differentiation of iPSCs into mature hepatocyte-like cells and improved stem cell therapy in a hepatic failure model. Acta Biomater 2015;13:228–44.

[62] Louw AM, Kolar MK, Novikova LN, Kingham PJ, Wiberg M, Kjems J, et al. Chitosan polyplex mediated delivery of miRNA-124 reduces activation of microglial cells in vitro and in rat models of spinal cord injury. Nanomedicine 2015;12(3):643–53.

[63] Suh JS, Lee JY, Choi YS, Chung CP, Park YJ. Peptide-mediated intracellular delivery of miRNA-29b for osteogenic stem cell differentiation. Biomaterials 2013;34:4347–59.

[64] Crombez L, Aldrian-Herrada G, Konate K, Nguyen QN, McMaster GK, Brasseur R, et al. A new potent secondary amphipathic cell-penetrating peptide for siRNA delivery into mammalian cells. Mol Ther 2009;17:95–103.

[65] Morris MC, Deshayes S, Heitz F, Divita G. Cell-penetrating peptides: from molecular mechanisms to therapeutics. Biol Cell 2008;100:201–17.

[66] Li H, Zheng X, Koren V, Vashist YK, Tsui TY. Highly efficient delivery of siRNA to a heart transplant model by a novel cell penetrating peptide-dsRNA binding domain. Int J Pharm 2014;469:206–13.

[67] Nguyen MK, Jeon O, Krebs MD, Schapira D, Alsberg E. Sustained localized presentation of RNA interfering molecules from in situ forming hydrogels to guide stem cell osteogenic differentiation. Biomaterials 2014;35:6278–86.

[68] Li J, Kooger R, He M, Xiao X, Zheng L, Zhang Y. A supramolecular hydrogel as a carrier to deliver microRNA into the encapsulated cells. Chem Commun (Camb) 2014;50:3722–4.

[69] Cao H, Jiang X, Chai C, Chew SY. RNA interference by nanofiber-based siRNA delivery system. J Control Release 2010;144:203–12.

[70] Ji W, Sun Y, Yang F, van den Beucken JJ, Fan M, Chen Z, et al. Bioactive electrospun scaffolds delivering growth factors and genes for tissue engineering applications. Pharm Res 2011;28:1259–72.

[71] Low WC, Rujitanaroj PO, Lee DK, Messersmith PB, Stanton LW, Goh E, et al. Nanofibrous scaffold-mediated REST knockdown to enhance neuronal differentiation of stem cells. Biomaterials 2013;34:3581–90.

[72] Kanellopoulou C, Muljo SA, Kung AL, Ganesan S, Drapkin R, Jenuwein T, et al. Dicer-deficient mouse embryonic stem cells are defective in differentiation and centromeric silencing. Genes Dev 2005;19:489–501.

[73] Murchison EP, Partridge JF, Tam OH, Cheloufi S, Hannon GJ. Characterization of Dicer-deficient murine embryonic stem cells. Proc Natl Acad Sci USA 2005;102:12135–40.

[74] Wang Y, Medvid R, Melton C, Jaenisch R, Blelloch R. DGCR8 is essential for microRNA biogenesis and silencing of embryonic stem cell self-renewal. Nat Genet 2007;39:380–5.

[75] Judson RL, Babiarz JE, Venere M, Blelloch R. Embryonic stem cell-specific microRNAs promote induced pluripotency. Nat Biotechnol 2009;27:459–61.

[76] Anokye-Danso F, Trivedi CM, Juhr D, Gupta M, Cui Z, Tian Y, et al. Highly efficient miRNA-mediated reprogramming of mouse and human somatic cells to pluripotency. Cell Stem Cell 2011;8:376–88.

[77] Luningschror P, Hauser S, Kaltschmidt B, Kaltschmidt C. MicroRNAs in pluripotency, reprogramming and cell fate induction. Biochim Biophys Acta 2013;1833:1894–903.

[78] Frith JE, Porrello ER, Cooper-White JJ. Concise review: new frontiers in microRNA-based tissue regeneration. Stem Cells Transl Med 2014;3:969–76.
[79] Zhang Y, Xie RL, Croce CM, Stein JL, Lian JB, van Wijnen AJ, et al. A program of microRNAs controls osteogenic lineage progression by targeting transcription factor Runx2. Proc Natl Acad Sci USA 2011;108:9863–8.
[80] Eskildsen T, Taipaleenmaki H, Stenvang J, Abdallah BM, Ditzel N, Nossent AY, et al. MicroRNA-138 regulates osteogenic differentiation of human stromal (mesenchymal) stem cells in vivo. Proc Natl Acad Sci USA 2011;108:6139–44.
[81] Tardif G, Hum D, Pelletier JP, Duval N, Martel-Pelletier J. Regulation of the IGFBP-5 and MMP-13 genes by the microRNAs miR-140 and miR-27a in human osteoarthritic chondrocytes. BMC Musculoskelet Disord 2009;10:148.
[82] Tuddenham L, Wheeler G, Ntounia-Fousara S, Waters J, Hajihosseini MK, Clark I, et al. The cartilage specific microRNA-140 targets histone deacetylase 4 in mouse cells. FEBS Lett 2006;580:4214–7.
[83] Pais H, Nicolas FE, Soond SM, Swingler TE, Clark IM, Chantry A, et al. Analyzing mRNA expression identifies Smad3 as a microRNA-140 target regulated only at protein level. RNA 2010;16:489–94.
[84] Lin EA, Kong L, Bai XH, Luan Y, Liu CJ. miR-199a, a bone morphogenic protein 2-responsive microRNA, regulates chondrogenesis via direct targeting to Smad1. J Biol Chem 2009;284:11326–35.
[85] Akhtar N, Rasheed Z, Ramamurthy S, Anbazhagan AN, Voss FR, Haqqi TM. MicroRNA-27b regulates the expression of matrix metalloproteinase 13 in human osteoarthritis chondrocytes. Arthritis Rheum 2010;62:1361–71.
[86] Ohgawara T, Kubota S, Kawaki H, Kondo S, Eguchi T, Kurio N, et al. Regulation of chondrocytic phenotype by micro RNA 18a: involvement of Ccn2/Ctgf as a major target gene. FEBS Lett 2009;583:1006–10.
[87] Kim D, Song J, Jin EJ. MicroRNA-221 regulates chondrogenic differentiation through promoting proteosomal degradation of slug by targeting Mdm2. J Biol Chem 2010;285:26900–7.
[88] Dudek KA, Lafont JE, Martinez-Sanchez A, Murphy CL. Type II collagen expression is regulated by tissue-specific miR-675 in human articular chondrocytes. J Biol Chem 2010;285:24381–7.
[89] Yan C, Wang Y, Shen XY, Yang G, Jian J, Wang HS, et al. MicroRNA regulation associated chondrogenesis of mouse MSCs grown on polyhydroxyalkanoates. Biomaterials 2011;32:6435–44.
[90] Rao PK, Kumar RM, Farkhondeh M, Baskerville S, Lodish HF. Myogenic factors that regulate expression of muscle-specific microRNAs. Proc Natl Acad Sci USA 2006;103:8721–6.
[91] Rosenberg MI, Georges SA, Asawachaicharn A, Analau E, Tapscott SJ. MyoD inhibits Fstl1 and Utrn expression by inducing transcription of miR-206. J Cell Biol 2006;175:77–85.
[92] Sokol NS, Ambros V. Mesodermally expressed *Drosophila* microRNA-1 is regulated by Twist and is required in muscles during larval growth. Genes Dev 2005;19:2343–54.
[93] Zhao Y, Samal E, Srivastava D. Serum response factor regulates a muscle-specific microRNA that targets Hand2 during cardiogenesis. Nature 2005;436:214–20.
[94] Chen C-Z, Li L, Lodish HF, Bartel DP. MicroRNAs modulate hematopoietic lineage differentiation. Science 2004;303:83–6.
[95] Liu N, Williams AH, Kim Y, McAnally J, Bezprozvannaya S, Sutherland LB, et al. An intragenic MEF2-dependent enhancer directs muscle-specific expression of microRNAs 1 and 133. Proc Natl Acad Sci USA 2007;104:20844–9.
[96] Crist CG, Montarras D, Pallafacchina G, Rocancourt D, Cumano A, Conway SJ, et al. Muscle stem cell behavior is modified by microRNA-27 regulation of Pax3 expression. Proc Natl Acad Sci USA 2009;106(32):13383–7.
[97] Yuasa K, Hagiwara Y, Ando M, Nakamura A, Takeda S, Hijikata T. MicroRNA-206 is highly expressed in newly formed muscle fibers: implications regarding potential for muscle regeneration and maturation in muscular dystrophy. Cell Struct Funct 2008;33:163–9.

[98] Gordon KJ, Blobe GC. Role of transforming growth factor-β superfamily signaling pathways in human disease. Biochim Biophys Acta 2008;1782:197–228.
[99] Kollias HD, McDermott JC. Transforming growth factor-β and myostatin signaling in skeletal muscle. J Appl Physiol 1985;2008(104):579–87.
[100] Allen RE, Boxhorn LK. Regulation of skeletal muscle satellite cell proliferation and differentiation by transforming growth factor-beta, insulin-like growth factor I, and fibroblast growth factor. J Cell Physiol 1989;138:311–5.
[101] Haugk KL, Roeder RA, Garber MJ, Schelling GT. Regulation of muscle cell proliferation by extracts from crushed muscle. J Anim Sci 1995;73:1972–81.
[102] Robertson TA, Maley MAL, Grounds MD, Papadimitriou JM. The role of macrophages in skeletal muscle regeneration with particular reference to chemotaxis. Exp Cell Res 1993;207:321–31.
[103] Amthor H, Huang R, McKinnell I, Christ B, Kambadur R, Sharma M, et al. The regulation and action of myostatin as a negative regulator of muscle development during avian embryogenesis. Dev Biol 2002;251:241–57.
[104] McCroskery S, Thomas M, Maxwell L, Sharma M, Kambadur R. Myostatin negatively regulates satellite cell activation and self-renewal. J Cell Biol 2003;162:1135–47.
[105] McPherron AC, Lee S-J. Double muscling in cattle due to mutations in the myostatin gene. Proc Natl Acad Sci USA 1997;94:12457–61.
[106] Massagué J, Cheifetz S, Endo T, Nadal-Ginard B. Type beta transforming growth factor is an inhibitor of myogenic differentiation. Proc Natl Acad Sci USA 1986;83:8206–10.
[107] Sato K, Li Y, Foster W, Fukushima K, Badlani N, Adachi N, et al. Improvement of muscle healing through enhancement of muscle regeneration and prevention of fibrosis. Muscle Nerve 2003;28:365–72.
[108] Kim N, Yoo JJ, Atala A, Lee SJ. Combination of small RNAs for skeletal muscle regeneration. FASEB J 2015;30(3):1198–206.
[109] Hutchison ER, Okun E, Mattson MP. The therapeutic potential of microRNAs in nervous system damage, degeneration, and repair. Neuromol Med 2009;11:153–61.
[110] Cui Y, Xiao Z, Chen T, Wei J, Chen L, Liu L, et al. The miR-7 identified from collagen biomaterial-based three-dimensional cultured cells regulates neural stem cell differentiation. Stem Cells Dev 2014;23:393–405.
[111] Yu YM, Gibbs KM, Davila J, Campbell N, Sung S, Todorova TI, et al. MicroRNA miR-133b is essential for functional recovery after spinal cord injury in adult zebrafish. Eur J Neurosci 2011;33:1587–97.
[112] Jeng S-F, Rau C-S, Liliang P-C, Wu C-J, Lu T-H, Chen Y-C, et al. Profiling muscle-specific microRNA expression after peripheral denervation and reinnervation in a rat model. J Neurotrauma 2009;26:2345–53.
[113] Williams AH, Valdez G, Moresi V, Qi X, McAnally J, Elliott JL, et al. MicroRNA-206 delays ALS progression and promotes regeneration of neuromuscular synapses in mice. Science 2009;326:1549–54.
[114] Jankowski MP, McIlwrath SL, Jing X, Cornuet PK, Salerno KM, Koerber HR, et al. Sox11 transcription factor modulates peripheral nerve regeneration in adult mice. Brain Res 2009;1256:43–54.
[115] Cannon 3rd RO. Mechanisms, management and future directions for reperfusion injury after acute myocardial infarction. Nat Clin Pract Cardiovasc Med 2005;2:88–94.
[116] Hullinger TG, Montgomery RL, Seto AG, Dickinson BA, Semus HM, Lynch JM, et al. Inhibition of miR-15 protects against cardiac ischemic injury. Circ Res 2012;110:71–81.
[117] Eulalio A, Mano M, Dal Ferro M, Zentilin L, Sinagra G, Zacchigna S, et al. Functional screening identifies miRNAs inducing cardiac regeneration. Nature 2012;492:376–81.
[118] Wang Z, Li L. Adenovirus-mediated RNA interference against collagen-specific molecular chaperone 47-KDa heat shock protein suppresses scar formation on mouse wounds. Cell Biol Int 2008;32:484–93.
[119] Monaghan M, Browne S, Schenke-Layland K, Pandit A. A collagen-based scaffold delivering exogenous microRNA-29B to modulate extracellular matrix remodeling. Mol Ther 2014;22:786–96.
[120] Biswas S, Roy S, Banerjee J, Hussain SR, Khanna S, Meenakshisundaram G, et al. Hypoxia inducible microRNA 210 attenuates keratinocyte proliferation and impairs closure in a murine model of ischemic wounds. Proc Natl Acad Sci USA 2010;107:6976–81.

[121] Anand S, Majeti BK, Acevedo LM, Murphy EA, Mukthavaram R, Scheppke L, et al. MicroRNA-132-mediated loss of p120RasGAP activates the endothelium to facilitate pathological angiogenesis. Nat Med 2010;16:909–14.
[122] Devalliere J, Chang WG, Andrejecsk JW, Abrahimi P, Cheng CJ, Jane-wit D, et al. Sustained delivery of proangiogenic microRNA-132 by nanoparticle transfection improves endothelial cell transplantation. FASEB J 2014;28:908–22.
[123] Collin-Osdoby P. Role of vascular endothelial cells in bone biology. J Cell Biochem 1994;55:304–9.
[124] Li Y, Fan L, Liu S, Liu W, Zhang H, Zhou T, et al. The promotion of bone regeneration through positive regulation of angiogenic-osteogenic coupling using microRNA-26a. Biomaterials 2013;34:5048–58.
[125] Poy MN, Eliasson L, Krutzfeldt J, Kuwajima S, Ma X, Macdonald PE, et al. A pancreatic islet-specific microRNA regulates insulin secretion. Nature 2004;432:226–30.
[126] Sallustio F, Serino G, Costantino V, Curci C, Cox SN, De Palma G, et al. miR-1915 and miR-1225-5p regulate the expression of CD133, PAX2 and TLR2 in adult renal progenitor cells. PLoS One 2013;8:e68296.
[127] Zhu D, Pan C, Li L, Bian Z, Lv Z, Shi L, et al. MicroRNA-17/20a/106a modulate macrophage inflammatory responses through targeting signal-regulatory protein alpha. J Allergy Clin Immunol 2013;132:426–36.e8.
[128] Zhou J, Ju W, Wang D, Wu L, Zhu X, Guo Z, et al. Down-regulation of microRNA-26a promotes mouse hepatocyte proliferation during liver regeneration. PLoS One 2012;7:e33577.
[129] Gao J, Yang T, Han J, Yan K, Qiu X, Zhou Y, et al. MicroRNA expression during osteogenic differentiation of human multipotent mesenchymal stromal cells from bone marrow. J Cell Biochem 2011;112:1844–56.
[130] Xu W, Li P, Qin K, Wang X, Jiang X. miR-124 regulates neural stem cells in the treatment of spinal cord injury. Neurosci Lett 2012;529:12–7.
[131] Motohashi N, Alexander MS, Shimizu-Motohashi Y, Myers JA, Kawahara G, Kunkel LM. Regulation of IRS1/Akt insulin signaling by microRNA-128a during myogenesis. J Cell Sci 2013;126:2678–91.
[132] Barter MJ, Tselepi M, Gomez R, Woods S, Hui W, Smith GR, et al. Genome-wide microRNA and gene analysis of mesenchymal stem cell chondrogenesis identifies an essential role and multiple targets for miR-140-5p. Stem Cells 2015;33:3266–80.
[133] Wang YS, Li SH, Guo J, Mihic A, Wu J, Sun L, et al. Role of miR-145 in cardiac myofibroblast differentiation. J Mol Cell Cardiol 2014;66:94–105.
[134] Liu J, van Mil A, Aguor EN, Siddiqi S, Vrijsen K, Jaksani S, et al. MiR-155 inhibits cell migration of human cardiomyocyte progenitor cells (hCMPCs) via targeting of MMP-16. J Cell Mol Med 2012;16:2379–86.
[135] Chan YC, Roy S, Khanna S, Sen CK. Downregulation of endothelial microRNA-200b supports cutaneous wound angiogenesis by desilencing GATA binding protein 2 and vascular endothelial growth factor receptor 2. Arterioscler Thromb Vasc Biol 2012;32:1372–82.
[136] Liu N, Williams AH, Maxeiner JM, Bezprozvannaya S, Shelton JM, Richardson JA, et al. microRNA-206 promotes skeletal muscle regeneration and delays progression of Duchenne muscular dystrophy in mice. J Clin Invest 2012;122:2054–65.
[137] Bork S, Horn P, Castoldi M, Hellwig I, Ho AD, Wagner W. Adipogenic differentiation of human mesenchymal stromal cells is down-regulated by microRNA-369-5p and up-regulated by microRNA-371. J Cell Physiol 2011;226:2226–34.
[138] Wang Y, Huang C, Reddy Chintagari N, Bhaskaran M, Weng T, Guo Y, et al. miR-375 regulates rat alveolar epithelial cell trans-differentiation by inhibiting Wnt/beta-catenin pathway. Nucleic Acids Res 2013;41:3833–44.

CHAPTER

MICRO- AND NANOTOPOGRAPHICAL CUES GUIDING BIOMATERIAL HOST RESPONSE

8

D.M. Kalaskar, F. Alshomer

University College London, London, United Kingdom

CHAPTER OUTLINE

In Situ Tissue Regeneration. http://dx.doi.org/10.1016/B978-0-12-802225-2.00008-8

INTRODUCTION

Cells in their native niche interact with various cues guiding their future behavior. This niche comprises of various chemical, mechanical, and topographical clues. The presence of such features also ranges in different sizes and spatial distribution. Niche topography in particular poses a remarkable variation in such matter involving macro- to micro- and finally nanotopographic features [1].

Meticulous work in the field of tissue engineering and cell–material interactions proved the importance of topographical mimicry for successful integration, both in vitro and in vivo [2]. Work of Harrison, 1911, has established the concept of physical guidance (stereotropism) after directing the cell growth along spider web fibers [3]. This work later evolved with the advancements in different fabrication techniques creating topographically smart surfaces with an essential impact on cell adhesion and subsequent spreading and differentiation [4]. Since then, there has been a surge in the number of scientific publications investigating the different manufacturing techniques and their effect on various cellular and host responses, as shown in Fig. 8.1. In this chapter, the importance of topographic features of the native extracellular matrix (ECM) (cell niche) is explored. Further understating of the effect of surface topography on cells of various lines, which are modulating the cellular cytoskeleton, is elaborated. Such surface features dictate and guide certain physiologic phenomena like cell morphology, proliferation, and migration, together with stem cell differentiation and commitment. The effect of manipulating the niche surrounding cells with the production of different synthetic substrates having variable micro- and nanotopographic features creating smart material for better tissue engineering approaches are presented. The chapter is concluded by providing case studies highlighting in vivo response to topographically modified scaffolds for various applications in orthopedic implants and the host inflammatory response.

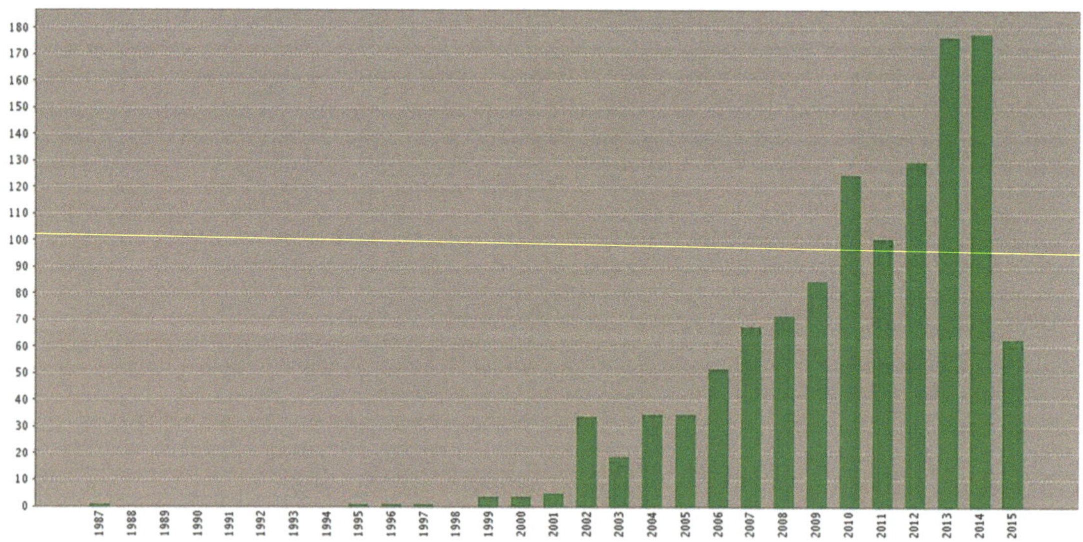

FIGURE 8.1

This figure reflects the incremental increase in the rate of published articles under the topic "Nanotopography."

Adapted from www.webofknowledge.com.

EXTRACELLULAR MATRIX TOPOGRAPHY AND ITS EFFECT ON CELLULAR RESPONSE

The ECM-surrounding cells (cell niche) possess complex topographical features involving fibers, pores, or crystals from nano- to microlevels. Their interaction determines certain cellular behavior that is mediated through intrinsic and/or extrinsic cell signaling pathways [4].

Different investigative efforts have evaluated the topographical nature of the basement membrane. It has been shown that the corneal epithelial basement membrane has different nanotopographic features, including an average fiber width of 77 nm and an average height of 147 and 191 nm with shared features between primate and human basement membrane [2,5]. Assessment of the glomerular and tubular basement membrane of different species has shown a distinctive topographical architecture. Different fibrils range in thickness from 5 to 9 nm and 6 to 11 nm in both lamina rare interna and lamina rare externa, respectively, of rat's kidney, forming a mesh-like structure [6]. Yamasaki et al. have reported fibrous strands with width ranging from 3 to 15 nm and pores having a diameter approximately 10 and 12 nm in both glomerular and tubular membranes, respectively, of bovine origin [7].

Cells sense and respond to surface and niche topography via different pathways that involve direct mechanical and indirect mechanochemical signaling pathways, as shown in Fig. 8.2. This topographic effect is mediated through various rearrangements of the actin cytoskeleton and integrin receptors, forcing cells to different fates [8]. The integrin superfamily is a group of *trans*membrane receptors that act as reciprocal signaling pathways between the cell and the ECM [9]. The direct mechanical pathway is mediated through the attachment of the extracellular domain of integrin to certain ECM ligands. Integrins also are linked to the cytoskeletal actin on the cytoplasmic domain that is mediated through different integrin-associated proteins such as Paxillin, focal adhesion kinase, and vinculin, forming the cell adhesion complex [10–13]. The actin cytoskeleton then transmits the signaling pathway through its connection to the nucleus inner membrane through its attachment to different membrane-bound proteins like Nesprins. This results in different alteration in the nuclear morphology with subsequent effect on gene transcription [14]. The cell adhesion complex also mediates the signal transduction in an indirect fashion through an alternative chemical signaling cascade that transmits the mechanical input to the nucleus. Such signaling pathways were shown to involve different pathways like YAP (yes-associated protein)/TAZ (transcriptional coactivator with PDZ-binding motif) signaling, Ras (part of GTPase superfamily)/mitogen-activated protein kinases [Ras–Raf–MEK–extracellular signal-regulated kinase (ERK)] signaling, and Ras/PI3K (phosphoinositide 3-kinase)/Akt (serine/threonine kinase and known as protein kinase B) signaling pathways with different physiologic effects like cell differentiation, proliferation, and self-renewal, respectively [8].

CONTROLLED SUBSTRATE TOPOGRAPHY GUIDING IN VIVO HOST RESPONSE

Following the implantation of different substrates within the body, serial physiologic cascades occur, defining the host response mechanism. This phenomena is clear when different substrates behave differently following in vitro versus in vivo assessment. Biomaterial surface is considered an important interface dictating this interaction. These physiologic events involve the first contact with bodily fluids, namely water, with subsequent interaction with host proteins and lately cells, as summarized in Fig. 8.3. Each of those events involves a series of complex interactions with significant overall effect [15].

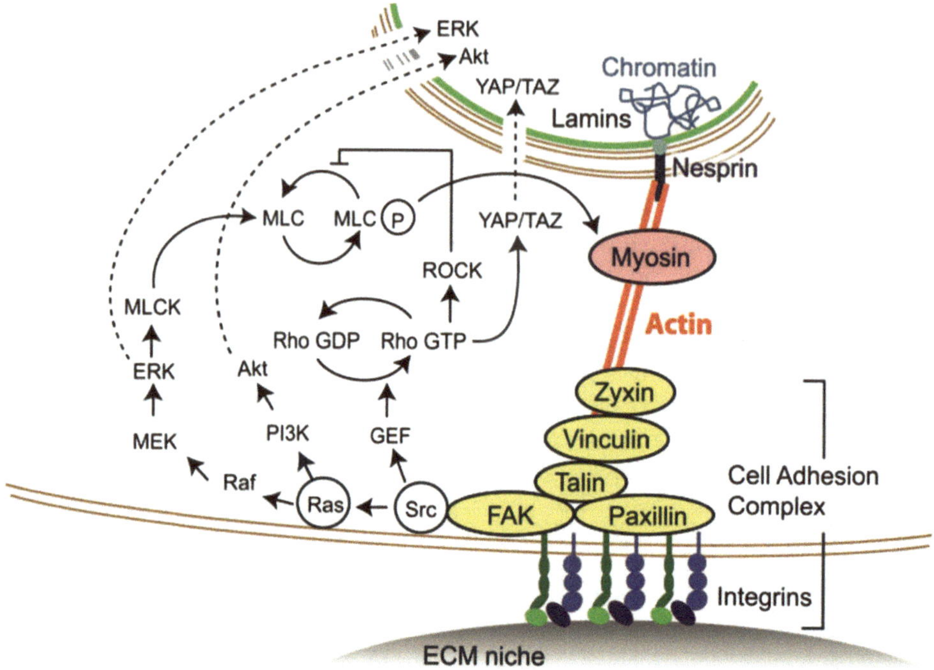

FIGURE 8.2

Schematic representation of intracellular cellular signaling affected by ECM interaction. Cells interact with ECM via two different pathways, namely the mechanical and topographical signaling from the ECM through the actin cytoskeleton or indirect signaling pathway, which involves a different chemical pathway that is initiated at the cell adhesion complex.

Adapted from Miyoshi H, Adachi T. Topography design concept of a tissue engineering scaffold for controlling cell function and fate through actin cytoskeletal modulation. Tissue Eng Part B Rev 2014;20(6):609–27.

MICRO- AND NANOTOPOGRAPHY AND ITS EFFECT ON WATER INTERACTION

Biomaterial surface wettability is an essential concept related to its subsequent contact with water. This leads to a material surface that is either water loving (ie, hydrophilic) or water repealing (ie, hydrophobic). Surface roughness residing in its micro- and nanoscale topographic features was investigated for its effect on modulating such surface property. Different theories were postulated accounting for the effect of surface topography (ie, roughness) on its subsequent wettability, like Wenzel's and Cassie's theories. In Wenzel's theory, it states that for a hydrophilic surface (contact angle reading <90), its associated roughness will enhance its hydrophilicity, whereas for hydrophobic surfaces, their hydrophobicity will predominate. It is also important to mention that in cases of certain hydrophobic surfaces, air pockets can form between the surface and the water molecules, creating what is a so-called "lotus effect" with a higher degree of hydrophobicity [16]. All of this clearly delineates the clear effect that substrate topography has on its subsequent wettability with an essential effect on the subsequent physiologic phenomena.

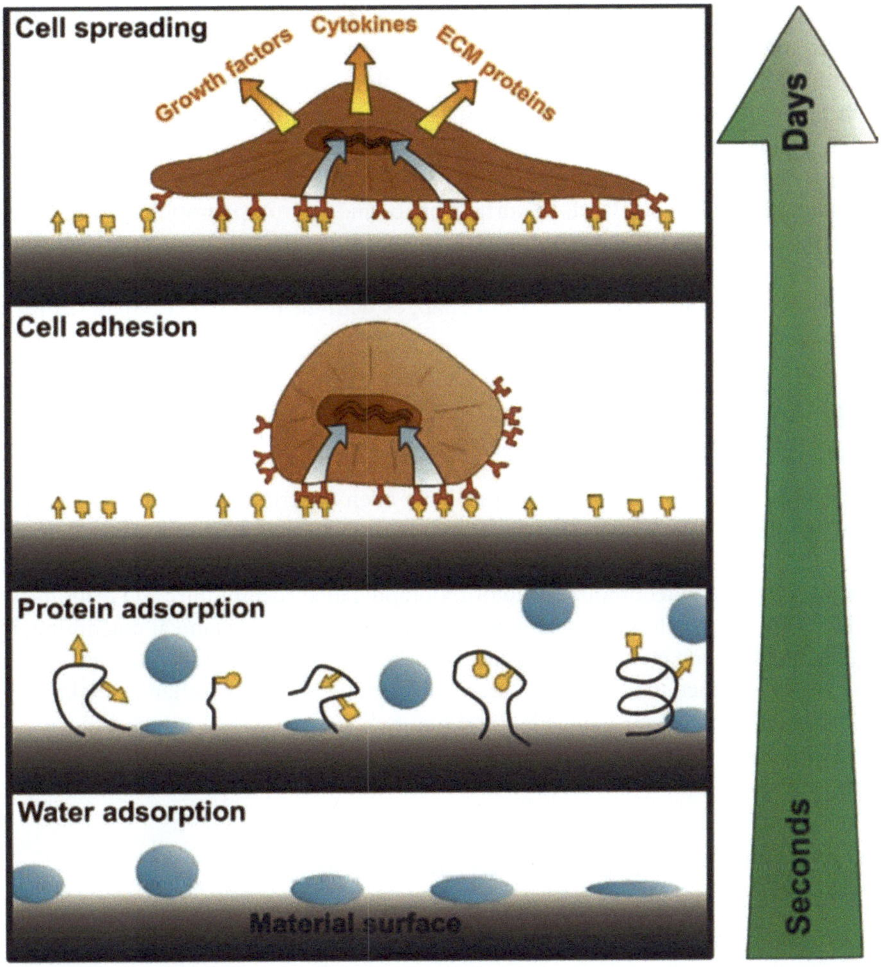

FIGURE 8.3

A time-lapse schematic diagram that shows the cascade of events occurring on the biomaterial surface after implantation into the host body. Water molecules will encounter the surface that is followed by protein adsorption. This will enable the later attachment and recognition of host cells.

Adapted from Jell G, Minelli C, Stevens MM. Biomaterial-related approaches: surface structuring. Fundamentals of tissue engineering and regenerative medicine. Springer; 2009. p. 469–84.

MICRO- AND NANOTOPOGRAPHY AND ITS EFFECT ON PROTEIN ADSORPTION

Similarly, substrate topography was shown to have an essential effect of the subsequent protein adsorption that is mediated directly or indirectly through its effects on water attachment. Among the additional effects substrate topography postulated to modulate protein attachment is by its increased surface area, allowing more proteins to adsorb together with providing clues for subsequent structural changes in the attached proteins [16]. This, however, was challenged by showing an increased amount of attached globulins on nanostructured tantalum oxide substrate with only 7% increase in their surface area [17]. Additionally, the characteristic size and geometry of the substrate surface topographic features all affect the way proteins are interacting with the biomaterial of interest. As an example, work of the Dolatshahi-Pirouz et al. group has shown an increased rate of fibronectin protein attachment on surfaces having nanotopographic deep pit features on a scale of 14 nm compared to other surfaces with similar nanotopographic features but with different scales [16].

This eventually delineates the effects of surface nano- and microtopographic modulation on the cellular process associated. Cell adhesion, relying on the specific structural and conformational changes of the surface-bounded proteins, will follow. This will be associated with the latter on focal adhesion formations, cellular morphologic, and structural changes with the eventual cellular host response [15].

DIFFERENT FABRICATION TECHNIQUES USED TO CREATE MICRO-/NANOSURFACE TOPOGRAPHY

Different micro- and nanofabrication techniques have been described to produce a synthetic surface topography, which mimics the ECM. These methods are usually tailored toward applying the desired effect based on the material of interest that might range from polymers to ceramics and metallic substrates. Different lithography techniques, photolithography, electrospinning, 3-D printing, embossing, microfluidic layer-by-layer patterning, self-assembled monolayers, mechanical machining, ion milling, sandblasting, and reactive ion etching have been described [18,19]. These techniques have aided in the production of various surface topographic features like grooves, ridges, pillars, or islands at different scales and orientations, as shown in Table 8.1 and Fig. 8.4.

Among the techniques described earlier, few key techniques that are widely explored for production of defined topographical features are discussed as follows:

PHOTOLITHOGRAPHY AND ELECTRON BEAM LITHOGRAPHY

In this method, a light is used to modulate surface topography. UV light is used to treat a light-sensitive polymer using a photoresist. Exposure to UV light causes cross-linking of a photosensitive polymer. Based on features of the photoresist, various 2-D topographical morphologies are produced, whereas in case of electron beam lithography (EBL), instead of UV light, high-energy electrons are exposed over an electron-sensitive material to produce desired topographic features.

SOFT LITHOGRAPHY

Soft lithography, on the other hand, is a technique that utilizes elastomeric polymers that are embossed, molded, or printed to develop the required pattern. This technique has three main processes that involve microstamping, stencil patterning, and microfluidic patterning. This technique is relatively easy to use with low cost [20].

ELECTROSPINNING

Electrospinning is another technique in which nanofibrous structures are formed. The uses of electrically-charged mobilization of polymer melt or solution droplets mediate such processes with both

Table 8.1 Examples of Different Approaches to Fabricate Surface Topography With Varying Features

Fabrication Technique	Topographic Feature	Studied Material	Cellular Effect
Photolithography in combination with other techniques, like ion etching [24,25]	Grooves	Quartz	Cellular spread and elongation along wider grooves in a depth-dependent fashion.
Diamond cutting [26]		Glass	Cells were highly likely to migrate along the grooves.
Electron-beam lithography in combination with other techniques, like wet etching and glow discharge [27]		Poly(dimethyl siloxane) cast	Cellular alignment along the direction of the grooves together proved orientation of vinculin and focal adhesion complex.
Electrospinning [28]	Fibers	Polymer blend of poly(ε-caprolactone) (PCL) and poly(3-hydroxybutyrate-co-3-hydroxyvalerate) (PHBV) of varying concentrations	Increased cell attachment, proliferation, and differentiation on smoother fibrous substrate.
Rapid prototyping and electrospinning [29]		Patterned resin formers and poly(D, L-lactide-co-glycolide)	Cellular adhesion and proliferation over the guided 3-D microtopography.
Microporous filter [30]	Pores	Silicon filters (coated and uncoated)	Increased inflammatory cellular infiltrated with scaffolds having larger pores (in this case, it was 3.3 μm).
Rapid prototyping [31]		Polylactic acid (PLA), PLA/calcium phosphate glass or chitosan	Increased proinflammatory marker from microphages with increased scaffold pore size with filopodia-like and podosome-like cellular morphology.
Evaporative coating [32]	Ridges	Polystyrene with silicon oxide	Seeded mouse neuroblastoma cells were shown to have increased cellular alignment along the silicon line ridges produced.
UV lithographic technique [33]	Pillars and pits	Polystyrene	Cellular migration on pillar substrate toward the sidewall, whereas on pits, substrate cells tended to move toward the sidewalls and bottom.
Lithography, electroplating, and forming/molding (LIGA) [34]	Grooves, pillars, and wells	HAPEX and AWPEX high-density polyethylene composites	Increased cell alignment along grooves, pillars, and wells were seen.
Ultrafast laser surface texturing [35]	Laser-induced periodic surface structures, nanopillars, and micro-columns	Titanium alloy Ti 6Al-4V	Seeded hMSCs showed enhanced matrix mineralization and bone-like nodule formation on surfaces having laser-induced periodic surface structures and nanopillars.

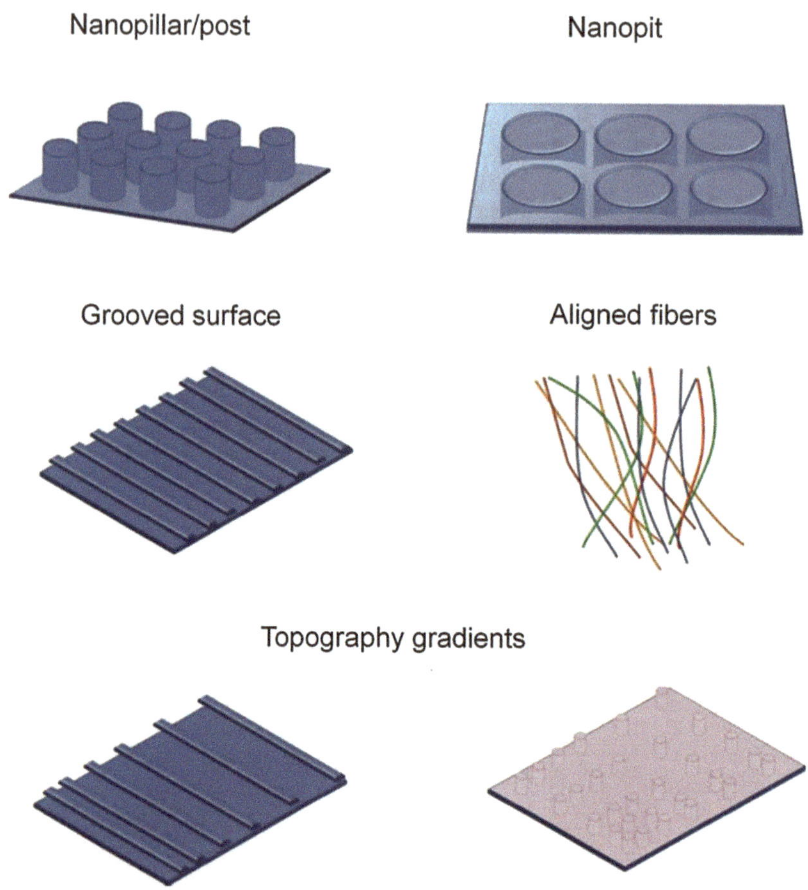

FIGURE 8.4

Different types of topographic features produced at the micro- and nanoscale level.

Adapted from Park S, Im GI. Stem cell responses to nanotopography. J Biomed Mater Res Part A 2014;103(3):1238–45.

ordered and unordered morphologies [20,21]. Different modifications can be applied in order to control the morphology, diameter, and chemical composition of the produced nanostructures [22].

MICROSTEREOLITHOGRAPHY

Other techniques like microstereolithography were also utilized to fabricate a delicate 3-D construct with precise topography. This technique usually involves the use of layer-by-layer fabrication with the use of a UV light source, combined with a digital micromirror masking device and a conventional computer projector. This combination allows the fabrication of complex internal structures, together with precise spatial distribution inside a scaffold of interest [23].

Methods described above can be used alone or in combination to produce such controlled physical surface topographies. An example of such a combination in order to gain a combination of micro- and

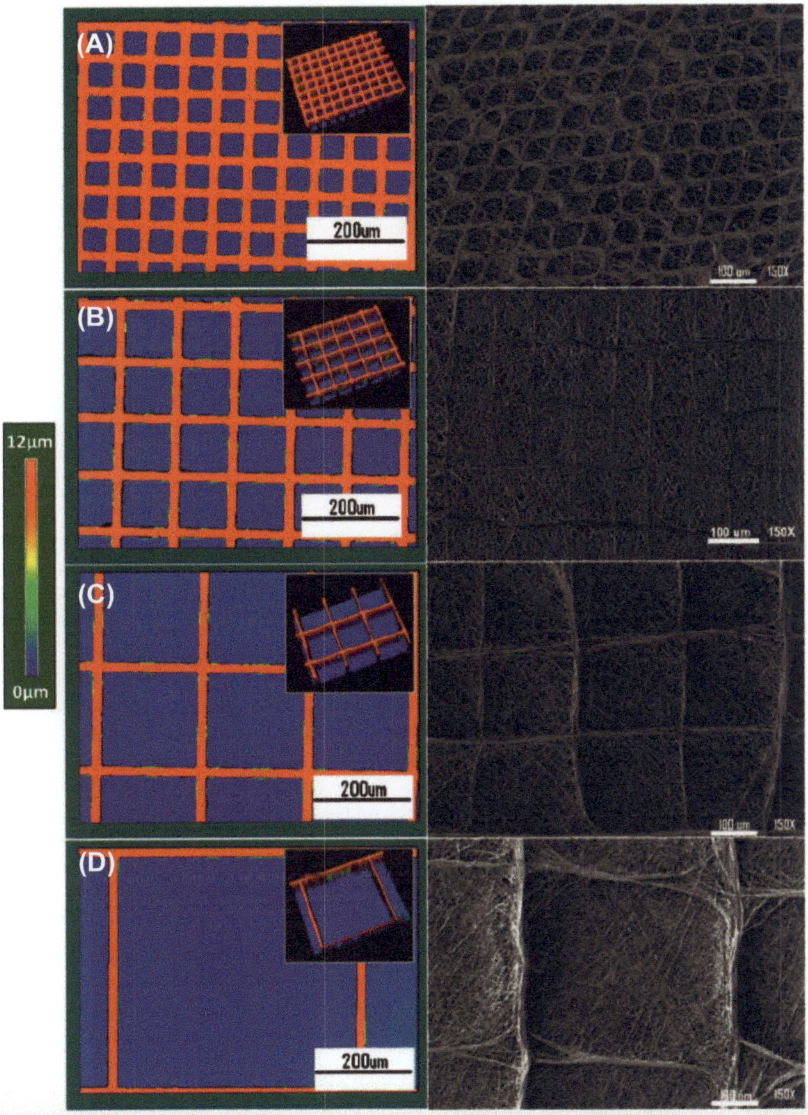

FIGURE 8.5

Example of combination of soft lithography and electrospinning to produce micro- and nanotopographies. Serial fabrication steps that involve the use of patterned silicon-based poly(dimethylsiloxane) (PDMS) collector are shown on the left side. This is followed by electrospinning of polyurethane fibers with variable spacing from 50 (A), 100 (B), 200 (C), and 500 (D) micrometers as shown on the right side SEM images.

Adapted from Dempsey DK, Schwartz CJ, Ward RS, Iyer AV, Parakka JP, Cosgriff-Hernandez EM. Micropatterning of electrospun polyurethane fibers through control of surface topography. Macromol Mater Eng 2010;295(11):990–4.

Table 8.2 Different Classification Methods of Other Nanotopographic Fabrication Techniques Applied

Energy Source	Technique	Characteristics	Advantages and Disadvantages
Thermal	Thermal nanoimprint lithography	Depends on the physical deformation of the thermo-plastic polymer above glass transition temperature.	Gives high resolution with high throughput and low cost, but associated with the use of high temperature, high pressure (50–100 bar), mechanical tension.
	Reverse nanoimprint lithography	Depends on the thermal cure to the liquid resist and then is formed on the mold and finally to substrate.	Associated with short process with no external pressure, but challenging pattern transfer.
Optical	UV nanoimprint lithography	Depends on curable polymer resist that is dispensed and coated on substrate.	Associated with the use of low pressure, short process, and with low cost, but with hard reproducibility of patterns with high density.
	Reverse UV nanoimprint lithography	Depends on the use of curable liquid resist. Pattern is formed on the mold then transferred to the substrate.	Associated with reduced temperature, reduced pressure, and 3-D patterning, but challenging pattern transfer.
Chemical	Microcontact printing	Pattern is transferred to a substrate that is based on relative difference between the surface energies of both stamp and substrate.	Associated with simple and low-cost process with versatile technique, but with lower resolution of patterning and decreased reproducibility of the required pattern.
Electrical	Electrochemical deposition	Depends on the oxidation/reduction between conductive and ionic interfaces.	Associated with high accuracy but limited material choice.

Adapted from Elsayed M, Merkel OM. Nanoimprinting of topographical and 3D cell culture scaffolds. Nanomedicine 2014;9(2):349–66.

nanotopographic features is shown in Fig. 8.5. Dempsey et al. [21] have utilized soft lithography creating micropattern on a silicon collector substrate. This was followed by electrospinning of controlled deposition of polyurethane fibers with different dimensions that range from 50 to 500 μm.

The resolution of topographical modifications achieved by each technique is variable and it depends on the type of energy sources (thermal, optical, chemical, and electrical) used as a part of instrumentation. Table 8.2 provides classification of the most common techniques based on energy sources with their advantages and disadvantages.

IN VITRO ASSESSMENT OF MICRO- AND NANOTOPOGRAPHIC FEATURES

In this section, various effects of controlled topography on cellular behavior are presented. We would like to mention early on that most investigative work done so far suggests cell type-specific response to topography, ie, different cell types can respond differently to the same substrate topography. In response to topographical modification, various changes occur to cell adhesion, morphology, proliferation, and their differentiation. In the following sections, we will look at the effect that topography has on each of these essential cell functions.

THE EFFECTS OF MICRO-/NANOSURFACE TOPOGRAPHY ON CELL MORPHOLOGY AND MIGRATION

Surface topography can alter subsequent cell attachment, morphology, and migration. Different synthetic topographic features like grooves, pillars, and ridges were shown to influence the migration behavior of various cell lines. This control is guided by the actin cytoskeleton modulation. It has been shown that cells of different origins, like fibroblasts, osteoblasts, and glial cells, align and migrate along the longitudinal axis of such surface features [8]. A gradient density of topographic features was also shown to affect cell migration on a surface having a variable rectangular lattice array with noticeable effect on single cells, as well as the larger cell population [38]. Miyoshi et al. have categorized the various extracellular topographic features acting as a cell constrainer at different scale levels. For features that are at a scale of tens of micrometers, they were said to act primarily on single cells or on cells on cluster. For features that are on a scale of 10 μm to submicrometer levels, they were said to modulate primarily the actin cytoskeleton, whereas for features on a lower scale (nanometer level), they were said to act primarily on the integrin clustered. This classification aimed to better understand the different topographic levels modulating the actin cytoskeleton and eventually the cellular behavior [8].

The effect of topography on cellular migration is elegantly shown by Mahmud et al. in their study [1]. They demonstrated a directional migration and directed cellular extension of cells seeded on a microchanneled device with ratchets, as shown in Fig. 8.6. Different efforts to further analyze this phenomenon were made with the use of nanogratings demonstrating an altered cellular polarization with changed orientation of the microtubule organization center on an unpatterned surface toward the needed direction and along the longitudinal axis of the cell on patterned surface [39]. To further understand the importance of surface topography guiding the cellular attachment, morphology, and migration, chemical surface treatment was challenged with the presence of such physical cues. Seeded preosteoblasts were assessed on a microscopic gratings polymeric scaffold with gold and titanium (Ti) coating. This was later microcontact printed with a different orientation of fibronectin lines. It was shown that cells are preferably aligned along the underlying physical microtopography, regardless of the fibronectin orientation present [40].

All of the earlier mentioned examples represent the importance of controlling the surface topography for better tissue engineering approaches.

THE EFFECTS OF MICRO-/NANOSURFACE TOPOGRAPHY ON CELL PROLIFERATION

Controlled nano- and microsurface topography was also investigated for its effect on cellular proliferation. It is observed that challenged cells with altered adhesion and spreading rates possess increased rates of cellular growth and DNA synthesis [42]. This phenomena is linked to the activation of Rho-ROCK (Rho-associated protein kinase) pathway through actin cytoskeleton tension formed after cell spreading, forming mature focal adhesions. Subsequent activation of ERK follows that leads to the promotion of cellular growth with the induction of cyclin D1 [8]. Several studies have shown variable levels of success in such matters. It has been shown that nanostructured silicon substrate with densely packed sharp peaks of fractals promote fibroblast proliferation when compared to other surfaces with regular ridges [43]. Wood et al. have investigated the role surfaces with

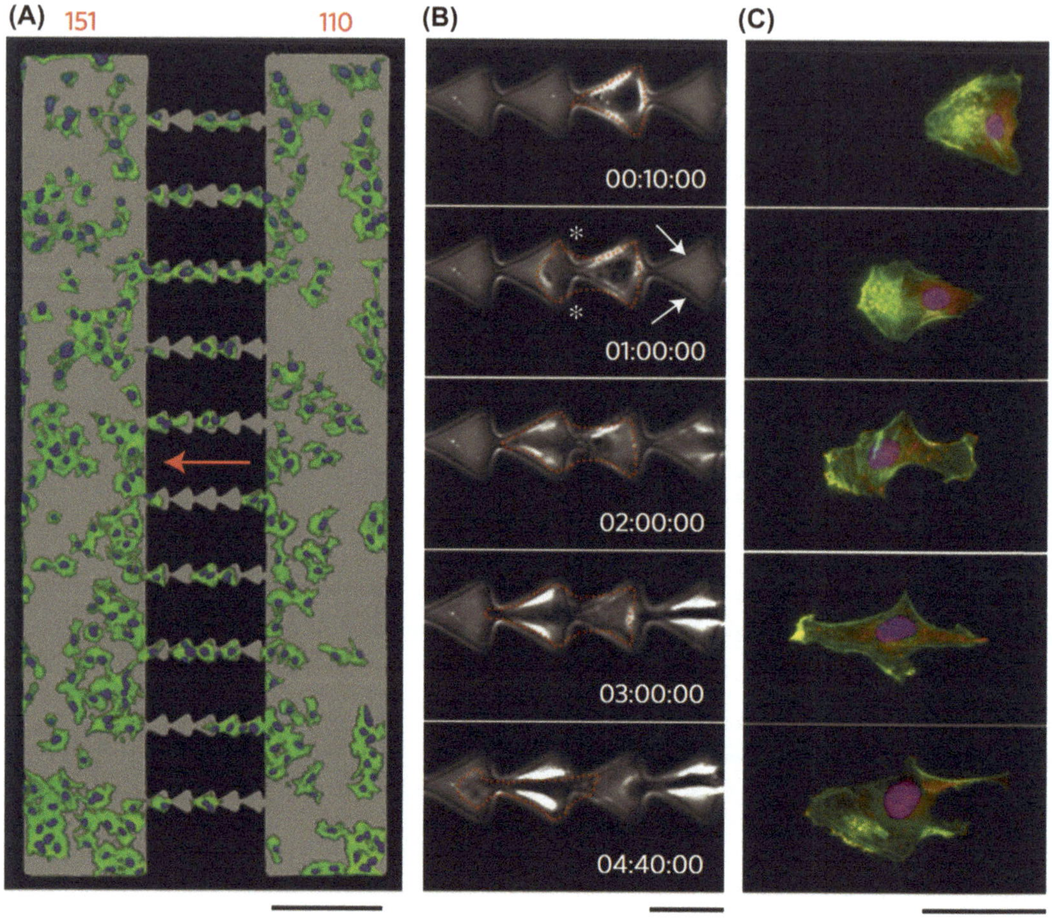

FIGURE 8.6

(A) Different distribution of B16F1 mouse melanoma cells between two reservoirs having a distribution bias with 151 cells on the left and 110 on the right, creating 57.8% directional bias toward the left connected by 10 ratchets. The scale bar represents 250 μm. (B) Phase contrast live images taken at 10-min intervals with cell migration across the ratchets. The dotted line surrounding cells indicates the cellular edge. The scale bar represents 50 **μm. (C)** Structural deformation of the cell as it passes through the guiding channels is delineated. Actin cytoskeleton (*green*) deformation is shown constraining the migration of cell and retracting its rare end. Arp2/3 complex (*yellow*), which is a polarity marker localized at the leading edge of the migrating cell indicating the direction of migration. The scale bar represents 50 μm.

Adapted from Mahmud G, Campbell CJ, Bishop KJ, Komarova YA, Chaga O, Soh S, et al. Directing cell motions on micropatterned ratchets. Nat Phys 2009;5(8):606–12.

anisotropically ordered nanoridges and isotropically ordered holes and showed increased alignment, elongation, migration, and proliferation rates of canine mesenchymal stem cells (MSCs) [44]. Interestingly, submicron nanogratings of polyurethane creating topographically patterned ridges and grooves did not affect the proliferation rates of human MSCs. Although it was demonstrated that cells grown on surfaces with 1400- or 4000-nm pitches showed greater elongation and alignment, others grown on 400-nm pitch demonstrated significant increases in protein expression and extracellular calcium deposition [45].

Nanostructured titanium oxide (TiO_2) nanotubes were also tested with various cell lines and with various topographies. In one study, vascular smooth muscle cells were grown on tubes with an average pore size of 30 nm and were shown to disrupt actin stress fibers with an overall decrease in cellular proliferation compared to flat control [46]. In another effort, rat MSCs were grown on self-assembled Ti nanotubes with vertical orientation. These cells were shown to have higher proliferation rates together integrin clustering and focal adhesion formation when grown over tubes with 15-nm diameter in comparison to others with 100-nm diameter [47]. Nanorough Ti films with surface roughness ranging between 2 and 21 nm were also investigated in which human osteoblast proliferation on such surface was the same as smooth surface controls [48]. Khang et al. investigated different levels of surface roughness of similar Ti films and concluded that only nanoscale to submicron hybrid surfaces were able to show an effect on integrin activation with subsequent proliferation and differentiation of MSCs [49].

This concept was utilized to create nanogratings with various depth and width on poly(methyl methacrylate) as promoters of osteogenic differentiation of MSCs. It was shown that the osteogenic phenotype was minimally affected by such surface topography with reduced early effect on the proliferation potential of the seeded cells. However, later increased proliferation (day 14) was noticed that is different from control [50]. Such discrepancy in the desired effect of controlled surface topography over cellular proliferation might indicate cell type-specific and material-specific responses that all play a role influencing such behavior.

THE EFFECTS OF MICRO-/NANOSURFACE TOPOGRAPHY ON STEM CELL DIFFERENTIATION

Along with chemical signals, topographic modification has a profound effect on cellular differentiation [51]. The use of topographical modification is especially an easy way forward to direct stem cell differentiation, both in presence or absence of chemical clues. Table 8.3 provides an overview of some of the key studies where directed differentiation of various stem cells is achieved by providing them with various topographical clues.

The effect of topographic modulation on mesenchymal stem cell differentiation

The modulation of actin cytoskeleton was shown to have an effect on stem cell commitment and differentiation, especially toward osteogenic lineage [52]. Such modulation and commitment was investigated in MSCs of different species and showed to be mediated again through RhoA and ROCK [8]. Dalby et al. have investigated the effect of growing human MSCs on surfaces having different grooves and pits that are 300–500 nm deep and 5–50 mm wide and showed an increased focal adhesions formation and osteoblastic activity [53]. EBL was utilized to create nanopits with different morphologies, including a hexagonal pattern, disordered square, or random morphology on a poly(methyl methacrylate) surface. Such topographical features were then tested to induce osteogenic differentiation of osteoprogenitor cells and human MSCs. It was shown that surfaces with disordered squares were associated with the highest bone differentiation whereas surfaces with high symmetry were associated with the lowest results [54]. Others have investigated the response of similar human MSCs (hMSCs) on polyethylene terephthalate (PET) having nanotopographic features with varying sizes and showed that osteogenic differentiation was highest on surfaces with 100-nm features compared to the ones with 10-nm features [52].

Table 8.3 Various Examples From the Literature Were How Stem Cells' Fate and Differentiation Potential is Affected by the Substrate Topography

Cell Type	Scaffold	Topographic Features	Cellular Effect
Human MSCs	Polymethylmethacrylate [53]	• Grooves and pits scaled to 300–500 nm deep and 5–50 mm wide.	• Increased focal adhesion formation and osteoblastic activity.
	Polymethylmethacrylate [54]	• Nanopits with different morphologies including hexagonal pattern, disordered square, or random.	• Increased bone differentiation on surfaces with disordered squares compared to others.
	Polyethylene terephthalate [52]	• Islands with microtopographic features and different nanotopographic depth sizes.	• Small (10 nm) depth surface features promoted cell adhesion without noticeable differentiation. • Larger depth patterns (100 nm) induced differentiation into osteoblast-like cells.
	Polydimethylsiloxane [60]	• Grooves with 10 μm width, 3 μm depth, and 10 μm spacing.	• Alignment of cells within the grooves aided in their response to parallel mechanical tension applied and helped in smooth muscle cell differentiation in vascular tissue engineering.
Human ESCs	Polydimethylsiloxane [56]	• Microsize grooves with different scales.	• Surfaces with 2-μm grooves associated with 1.7-fold increase in neuronal growth. • As the groove pitch size decreases, neuronal differentiation increases.
	Polydimethylsiloxane [61]	• Islands of micropattern with different surface areas (100 × 100 μm and 32 × 32 μm) with fibronectin and pluronic F127 treatment.	• With cells spreading, TGFβ3 activates Rac1, which increases N-cadherin expression, leading to the upregulation of smooth muscle cell markers. • If cell spreading is restricted, TGFβ3 fails to activate Rac1, and cells instead will induce chondrogenic markers.

	Polystyrene [62]	• Nanotopographic surface treatment with well-defined hexagonal and honeycomb configurations having various spacing.	• High stem cell survival rates with retaining of cell stemness.
	Polyurethane acrylate [63]	• Nanoscale ridges and grooves with 350 nm width, 500 nm height, and 350 nm spacing.	• Neuronal lineage differentiated after 5 days in the absence of any other differentiation agents.
Human ADSCs	Quartz [58]	• Nanograting with alternating ridges and grooves that are 250 and 500 nm.	• Increase of vWF, PECAM-1, and VE-cadherin on the nanograting substrates.
	Polycaprolactone [59]	• Nanotopographic modification having nanowire surfaces.	• Increased adipogenic differentiation of cell seeded on nanowire surfaces.
IPS cells	Polyethersulfone [64]	• Electrospun nanofibers.	• Increased capacity for differentiation into osteoblast-like cells with flattened and spread morphology aided with differentiation media.
Human neuronal stem cells	Polyurethane acrylate [65]	• Nanotopographic groove and pillar with different dimensions, ranging from 300 to 1500 nm for both groove width and pillar gap.	• Smaller scale features (300–300 nm groove ridges and 300–300 nm pillar diameter gaps) were associated with increased formation of focal adhesion. • This was associated with increased differentiation toward neurons and astrocytes.
	Polydimethylsiloxane [66]	• Micron-size grooves with different scales (5, 10, 20, and 60 μm). Followed by O_2 plasma treatment and coating with polylysine and laminin.	• Increased neurite growth on grooved surfaces where the groove width had a high impact on the development and differentiation.

Different dispersion tendencies of actin cytoskeleton stress fibers and integrin clusters were shown to be associated with a different commitment profile of MSCs. It was shown that when MSCs are committed toward neurogenic lineage, actin and integrin complexes were more likely to be dispersed inside the cell. In contrast, adipogenic and myogenic commitment were associated with more bundled structures [55].

The effect of topographic modulation on embryonic stem cells

Embryonic stem cells (ESCs) also showed different responses to various surface topographies. Microfabrication techniques were utilized, for example, to commit ESCs toward neurogenic lineage. Lu et al. showed polydimethylsiloxane surfaces with microsize grooves having different pitches to be associated with size-dependent cellular growth and differentiation responses. It was shown that as the groove pitch size decreases, neuronal differentiation increases. Interestingly, surfaces having 2-μm grooves were shown to be associated with a 1.7-fold increase in neuronal growth [56]. Nanotopographic surface grating was also investigated for its role in ESCs commitment. It was shown that an increase in osteogenic differentiation is noticed when the cells are grown over a poly-L-lactide (PLLA) scaffold having fibrous nanoarchitecture with diameters of 50–500 nm in comparison with other techniques utilized [57].

The effect of topographic modulation on adipose-derived stem cells

Adipose-derived stem cells (ADSCs) were also investigated for their differentiation in response to the topographic features. Surface nanograting on quartz with alternating ridges and grooves that are 250 and 500 nm was utilized to investigate the endothelial differentiation of ADSCs. It was shown that upregulation of von Willebrand factor (vWF), platelet endothelial cell adhesion molecule (PECAM-1), and vascular endothelial cadherin at the gene level on the nanograting substrates. Nanograting Matrigel also showed enhanced capillary tube formation during in vitro angiogenesis assay [58]. In another report, fabrication of polycaprolactone (PCL) nanowire surfaces was investigated to guide the differentiation potential of ADSCs. It was shown that such surfaces supported cell adhesion and proliferation with induced elongated morphologies of grown cells, as shown in Fig. 8.7. Also, surfaces with nanowires supported the adipogenic differentiation of ADSCs rather than chondrogenic differentiation compared to surfaces without such features [59].

All of this delineates clearly the essential effect of substrate micro- and nanotopography in guiding the desired stem cell fate. Further understanding of such essential cues might help in improving the overall outcome of different tissue engineering protocols.

USE OF TOPOGRAPHICAL MODIFICATIONS TO ENGINEER FUNCTIONAL TISSUE-ENGINEERED CONSTRUCTS

Different tissue engineering approaches have incorporated the fundamental concepts of manipulating substrate topography to improve the intended tissue engineering approaches. A few examples will be discussed in the following section that delineate such implications in tissue-specific approaches, such as tendon, vascular, and cardiac tissue engineering.

Tendon tissue engineering

Tendons tissue possesses an interesting structural hierarchy in which highly organized engineered matrices are required for successful integration. Several investigative works have incorporated the concept of engineered contact guidance to promote organization of cells and their matrix. Bagnaninchi et al.

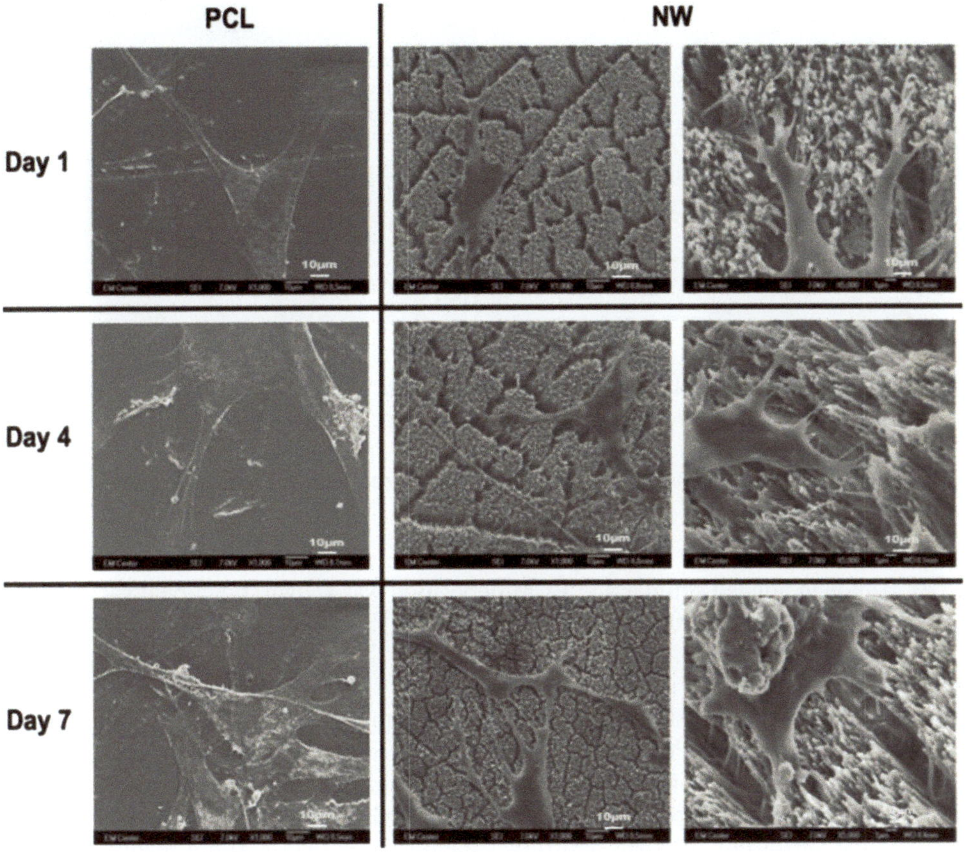

FIGURE 8.7

Different SEM images of ADSCs seeded on PCL at different time periods (day 1, day 4, and day 7), either with surface nanowires or without. Adhesions, cellular extensions, and change in morphology of ADSCs are clearly delineated on surfaces with nanowires at higher magnification level.

Adapted from Trujillo NA, Popat KC. Increased adipogenic and decreased chondrogenic differentiation of adipose derived stem cells on nanowire surfaces. Materials 2014;7(4):2605–30.

have utilized porous microchannels with diameters close to 250 μm in a chitosan scaffold. The scaffold was then seeded with porcine tenocytes in which they were shown to proliferate in bundle-like structures within these channels [67]. In another effort, capillary channels with open grooves were utilized to create a scaffold that is made of either poly (L-lactic acid) and PET. Seeded fibroblasts were shown to align and proliferate along the long axis of these grooves, as shown in Fig. 8.8. The ECM produced was shown to be deposited on and parallel to the direction of the grooves [68]. In a similar fashion, collagen membranes were produced with grooved surfaces as a potential scaffold for tendon tissue engineering. It was shown that seeded human dermal fibroblasts align themselves in the direction of the grooved surface, as shown by scanning electron microscope (SEM) imaging and F-actin staining [69]. Despite this, several limitations and variable levels of success were obtained from those

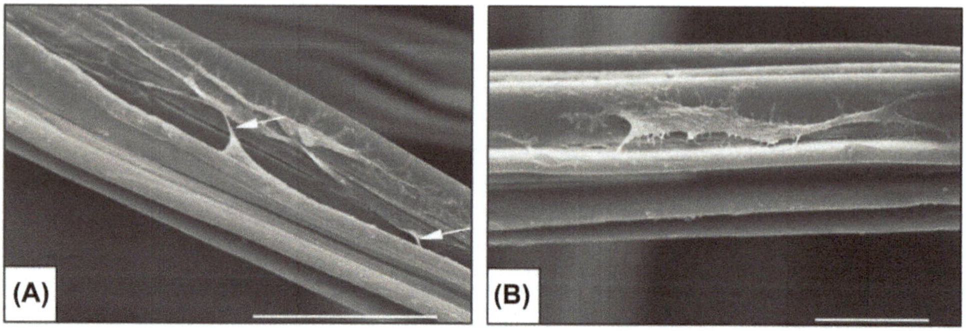

FIGURE 8.8

(A) SEM images of seeded fibroblast on PLA microchanneled fiber. Cellular spreading and parallel alignment of the cell is seen together with an evidence of cytoplasmic connection between the cells (*arrows*). (B) Shows SEM images of seeded fibroblast on PET fiber with similar alignment profile to (A).

Adapted from Lu Q, Simionescu A, Vyavahare N. Novel capillary channel fiber scaffolds for guided tissue engineering. Acta Biomater 2005;1(6):607–14.

approaches. Although aligned cellular and ECM deposition was shown, functional success needs further biomechanical evaluation [70].

Vascular tissue engineering

Endothelial cells were also investigated for their response to various topographic stimuli in vascular tissue engineering approaches. Polyurethane with a modified topographic surface having ridges and grooves that range in pitch from 400 to 4000 nm was investigated. Human endothelial cells from different origins (aortic and umbilical vein) seeded on modified surfaces showed parallel alignment and orientation on the anisotropic grooves and ridges having more than 800-nm features in size. Cells also exhibited migratory potential along the longitudinal axis of these grooves [71]. Biela et al. investigated human coronary artery endothelial cells and smooth muscle cells for their response to topographic features. Topographic modification of polydimethylsiloxane substrate having surface grooves with different depth and width were used in their assessment. The groove depth ranges from 50 to 200 nm, and the width was variable from 2, 3, 5, and 10 μm. It was shown that surfaces with grooves of smaller width or greater depth induced significant directed migration of the seeded cells [72]. Human microvascular endothelial cells were seeded on surface-modified collagen films. The collagen films were modified creating channels with different groove and ridge depth and width. They investigated grooves with widths of 650 nm and depth of 300 nm, widths of 500 nm with 250 nm in depth, and 332.5 nm in width with 200 nm in depth. Seeded constructs were also subjected to shear flow conditions. It was shown that seeded cells were not affected by the modified topography in terms of cellular proliferation. However, increased cell retention was seen on cells seeded over modified surfaces under shear flow conditions [73]. Polydimethylsiloxane was also modified to include ridges and grooves with pitches from 400 to 4000 nm and groove depth that is at least 300 nm. The cells were also subjected to shear flow conditions. It was shown that seeded human aortic endothelial cells showed greater cellular alignment when exposed to both topographic and flow condition stimuli, as shown in Fig. 8.9 [74].

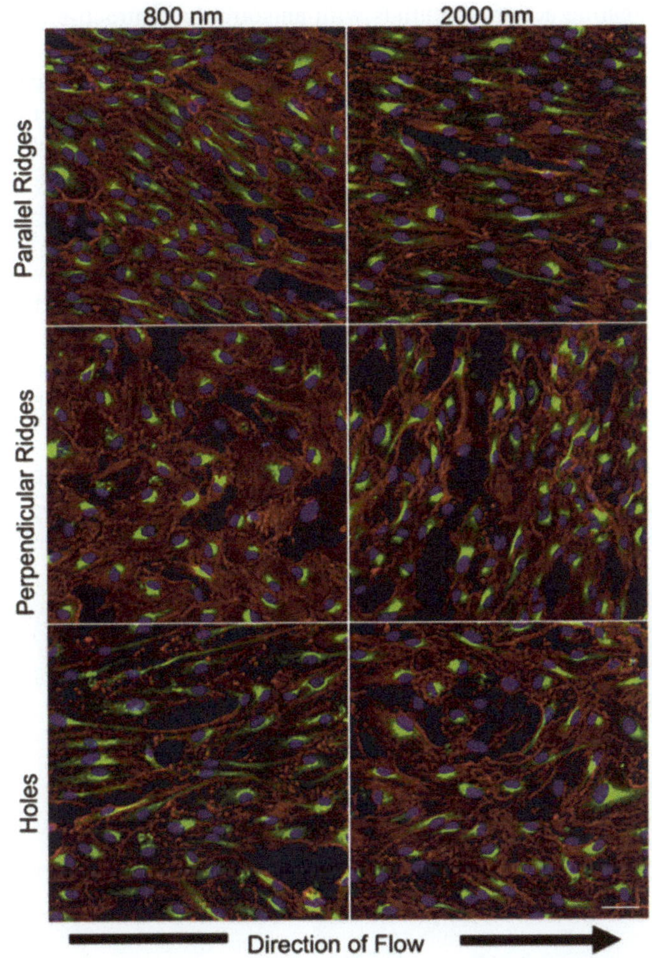

FIGURE 8.9

The combined effect of surface topography and shear flow conditions on seeded human aortic endothelial cells is delineated. Synergistic effect of grooves parallel to the flow direction over cellular alignment was noticed as antagonistic effect was seen when the grooves were perpendicular to the flow direction.

Adapted from Morgan JT, Wood JA, Shah NM, Hughbanks ML, Russell P, Barakat AI, et al. Integration of basal topographic cues and apical shear stress in vascular endothelial cells. Biomaterials 2012;33(16):4126–35.

Cardiac tissue engineering

Cardiac myocytes were also evaluated for their response when seeded on a synthetic topographically modified surface. PEG hydrogel was surface modified creating nanotopographic features with the use of UV-assisted lithography and later chemically modified with fibronectin attachment. Seeded myocytes showed parallel alignment to that topography with higher cell-to-cell and cell-to-surface adhesion and connexin 43 expression than the unmodified surfaces. It was also shown that cells were able to produce propagating action potentials with anisotropic contractile forces than control [75]. Wang et al. have investigated the use of EBL and dry etching-creating polydimethylsiloxane molds that were later used to fabricate nanogrooved polystyrene and polyurethane with variable levels (450 nm in groove/ridge width; 100 or 350 nm in depth). It was shown that cultured myocytes assumed a spindled shape with appropriate response to the surface topography applied, as shown in Fig. 8.10. Cell contractility was shown also to be anisotropic and parallel to the direction of the grooves in comparison to flat controls. The beating rate, however, was shown to be variable (50 beats per minute on day 1, postseeding decreasing to 15 beats per minute on day 7) with more sustained and efficient contraction on polyurethane substrates [76]. Electrospinning was also investigated to fabricate various substrates for cardiac engineering approaches. In one study, knitting of cotton or polyester yarns was applied as a template prior to the electrospinning process in which poly(lactic-co-glycolic) acid and thermoplastic polycarbonate–urethane were later spun with anisotropic morphology. Cardiac myoblast cells were shown to be successfully guided into the same anisotropic

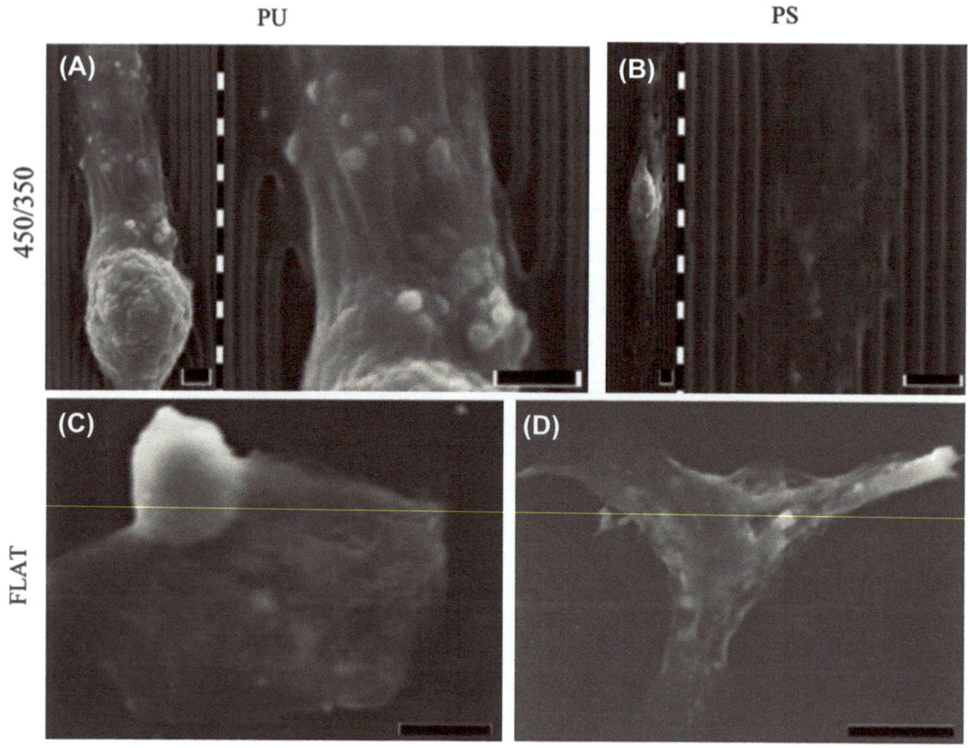

FIGURE 8.10

SEM images of cardiac myocytes seeded on different substrates (PU = polyurethane, PS = polystyrene) having surface nanogrooves (450 nm in width and 350 nm in depth) and flat control. Cells as shown have responded to the morphology of the substrate as compared to the flat controls.

Adapted from Wang P-Y, Yu J, Lin J-H, Tsai W-B. Modulation of alignment, elongation and contraction of cardiomyocytes through a combination of nanotopography and rigidity of substrates. Acta Biomater 2011;7(9):3285–93.

orientation. Spontaneous contractility was demonstrated for 10 days with frequency of ~120 beats per minutes on such constructs [77].

Knowing this, one understands the importance of modulating surface topography to aid in the needed engineering approaches. Directed alignment of cells and subsequently the produced ECM were shown to be fundamental for specific types of tissues as was shown here for both tendon and cardiac tissue engineering.

MODULATION OF SURFACE TOPOGRAPHY AND ITS EFFECT ON ASSOCIATED IN VIVO RESPONSE

One of the most important factors to discuss in this section is the associated inflammatory response and subsequent capsular formation and/or integration with the implanted substrate. Surface micro- and nanotopographic features were investigated for their role in modulating these outcomes. It has been shown that TiO_2 nanotube-modified implants were associated with significant reduction in the thickness of associated capsules after 6 weeks of implantation. This effect was thought to be mediated by the increased surface area of the modified implants, although other factors also play a role, such as surface chemistry and wettability [78]. Capsular formation was also shown to be affected at the micron-scale level where silicone and PLLA implants, having either parallel microgrooves (depth of 1.0 μm and width of 10.0 μm) or random roughness on a micrometer scale were evaluated. It was shown that capsules formed around the microgrooved substrates were thicker, whereas the ones surrounding the roughened implants were thinner. This, however, was associated with a stronger and prolonged inflammatory response surrounding the randomly roughened implants [79]. Rosengren et al. have utilized low-density polyethylene with smooth to coarse surfaces. They have shown that substrates with smoother surfaces were associated with a thicker capsule than the ones having rougher surfaces [80]. They also showed that mechanical shear surrounding the implants with thicker capsules (smooth surfaces) were associated with increased rates of cellular necrosis with subsequent increase in the inflammatory cells and later, thicker capsule formation [81].

EFFECTS ON THE BONE IMPLANTS TISSUE INTEGRATION

Topographic modification of implants creating micro- and nanofeatures were extensively investigated to improve their intended integration. The introduction of surface microroughness was shown to be beneficial at different in vitro, in vivo, and clinically applied investigations [82]. Ti alloy (Ti6Al4V) screws were produced, having either relatively smoothed surfaces obtained through machining or with microtopographic features applied with grit-blasted techniques. It has been shown that higher bone-to-implant contact was obtained with the grit-blasted screws compared to the machined ones. This was also associated with higher force to pull the implant from the surrounding bone [83]. It also appears that surfaces with complex microtopographic geometry are more osteointegrated than others with solo types of surface features. Szmukler-Moncler et al. have compared the dual surface treatment of Ti implants utilizing both sandblasting and acid etching to the single treatment with acid etching techniques. They reported an increased microtopographic roughness obtained with the combined treatments than the solo acid etching modification. Significantly higher force to pull the implant from the implanted bone was also obtained with combined surface treatment than the single acid etching technique [84].

Aided with the preference of complex geometry for better integration, efforts were made to evaluate a topographic size-specific preference for improved response. It has been shown that Ti implants blasted with 25- and 75-μm particles were associated with increased removal force and bone-to-implant contact compared to machined ones [85]. This, however, was inversely related when the particle size was increased to 250 μm. It was shown that implants blasted with particles of the size range of 250 μm were associated with decreased bone-to-implant contact when compared to the ones blasted with 25-μm particles [86].

Nonotopographic features were also investigated for their effects, either alone or in combination with microtopography, creating more biomimetic implants. This, however, was associated with a degree of limitation in which most of the modifications introduced at the nanoscale level are associated with other changes in the implant characteristics, like surface chemistry with its eventual effect on the cellular response [82]. Mendonça, Gustavo, et al. have compared sol–gel nanosurface-modified Ti implants to machined smooth controls and showed certain crystal structural changes in the former ones. This was also associated with higher bone-to-implant contact together with higher expression of osteoblastic markers surrounding nanomodified implants compared to machined smooth ones [87]. Feature size on the nanoscale level seems also to play a role in dictating the host response. It has been shown that Ti implants with colloidal lithographic surface treatment creating nanobumps have a size-dependent preference. Ballo et al. have showed an increased bone-to-implant contact with surfaces having 60-nm sized bumps compared to ones having 120-nm features or machined control [88].

Tsukimura et al. have evaluated the combined effect of micro- and nanotopographic modifications on the overall bone implant integration. The effect of sandblasting and chemical nanomodification using alkali (NaOH) and heat (600°C) treatments of Ti alloy (Ti–15Mo–5Zr–3Al) to sandblasting alone was compared. The results showed increased bone-to-implant contact with higher push-in forces for the combined modification than the solo sandblasting treatment [89].

Different efforts have tried to evaluate and compare microtopographic modification to the nanotopographic modalities for their in vivo tissue response. Bjursten et al. have assessed grit-blasted implants in comparison to anatase nanotube surface-modified implants through electrochemical anodization and annealing. Higher bone-to-implant contact with the nanomodified surfaces compared to micromodified ones was shown. Higher pullout force and bone retention on the nanotube-containing surfaces were seen in comparison to the microtreated ones [90].

SUMMARY

Success and failure of artificial implant largely depends on how it interacts with site of implantation. Successful implantation is achieved when there is a minimum or no long-term immune response from host. Especially with use of synthetic materials, their interaction with the surrounding cellular environment depends on how closely it mimics the host tissue and helps minimize immune reaction. In order to design such smart biomaterials, huge efforts have been put forward in understanding the native cellular environment called "niche environment." By closely mimicking this environment, it is possible to design successful biomaterials for various applications. Topography at macro-, micro-, and nanoscale has a definitive role in biomimetic process to enhance biomaterial integration. It can direct cell response to specific tissue type. With the advent of new technologies to process material at micro- and nanoscale level, our understanding of cellular interaction with these materials has increased significantly. There is a large body of literature with in vitro work, but in vivo work is limited to very specific areas, such as orthopedic implants, where tissue integration has been a priority area. More work is thus required, focusing on in vivo assessment of various topographical features for better understanding of long-term effects and benefits of topographical modifications.

REFERENCES

[1] Abrams GA, Goodman SL, Nealey PF, Franco M, Murphy CJ. Nanoscale topography of the basement membrane underlying the corneal epithelium of the rhesus macaque. Cell Tissue Res 2000;299(1):39–46.

[2] Flemming RG, Murphy CJ, Abrams GA, Goodman SL, Nealey PF. Effects of synthetic micro- and nano-structured surfaces on cell behavior. Biomaterials 1999;20(6):573–88.

[3] Harrison RG. On the stereotropism of embryonic cells. Science 1911;34(870):279–81.

[4] Martinez E, Engel E, Planell JA, Samitier J. Effects of artificial micro- and nano-structured surfaces on cell behaviour. Ann Anat 2009;191(1):126–35.

[5] Abrams G, Schaus S, Goodman S, Nealey P, Murphy C. Nanoscale topography of the corneal epithelial basement membrane and Descemet's membrane of the human. Cornea 2000;19(1):57–64.

[6] Shirato I, Tomino Y, Koide H, Sakai T. Fine structure of the glomerular basement membrane of the rat kidney visualized by high-resolution scanning electron microscopy. Cell Tissue Res 1991;266(1):1–10.

[7] Yamasaki Y, Makino H, Ota Z. Meshwork structures in bovine glomerular and tubular basement membrane as revealed by ultra-high resolution scanning electron microscopy. Nephron 1994;66(2):189–99.

[8] Miyoshi H, Adachi T. Topography design concept of a tissue engineering scaffold for controlling cell function and fate through actin cytoskeletal modulation. Tissue Eng Part B Rev 2014;20(6):609–27.

[9] Salsmann A, Schaffner-Reckinger E, Kieffer NRGD. The Rho'd to cell spreading. Eur J Cell Biol 2006;85(3):249–54.

[10] Berrier AL, Yamada KM. Cell–matrix adhesion. J Cell Physiol 2007;213(3):565–73.

[11] Wehrle-Haller B. Structure and function of focal adhesions. Curr Opin Cell Biol 2012;24(1):116–24.

[12] Dumbauld DW, Lee TT, Singh A, Scrimgeour J, Gersbach CA, Zamir EA, et al. How vinculin regulates force transmission. Proc Natl Acad Sci 2013;110(24):9788–93.

[13] Roca-Cusachs P, Del Rio A, Puklin-Faucher E, Gauthier NC, Biais N, Sheetz MP. Integrin-dependent force transmission to the extracellular matrix by α-actinin triggers adhesion maturation. Proc Natl Acad Sci 2013;110(15):E1361–70.

[14] Wang N, Tytell JD, Ingber DE. Mechanotransduction at a distance: mechanically coupling the extracellular matrix with the nucleus. Nat Rev Mol Cell Biol 2009;10(1):75–82.

[15] Jell G, Minelli C, Stevens MM. Biomaterial-related approaches: surface structuring. Fundamentals of tissue engineering and regenerative medicine. Springer; 2009. p. 469–84.

[16] Wang G, Moya S, Lu Z, Gregurec D, Zreiqat H. Enhancing orthopedic implant bioactivity: refining the nanotopography. Nanomedicine 2015;10(8):1327–41.

[17] Müller B, Riedel M, Michel R, De Paul SM, Hofer R, Heger D, et al. Impact of nanometer-scale roughness on contact-angle hysteresis and globulin adsorption. J Vac Sci Technol B 2001;19(5):1715–20.

[18] Griffin MF, Butler PE, Seifalian AM, Kalaskar DM. Control of stem cell fate by engineering their micro and nanoenvironment. World J Stem Cells 2015;7(1):37–50.

[19] Janson IA, Putnam AJ. Extracellular matrix elasticity and topography: material-based cues that affect cell function via conserved mechanisms. J Biomed Mater Res Part A 2014;103(3):1246–58.

[20] Chong D, Lindsey B, Dalby M, Gadegaard N, Seifalian A, Hamilton G. Luminal surface Engineering,'Micro and Nanopatterning': potential for self endothelialising vascular grafts? Eur J Vasc Endovascular Surg 2014;47(5):566–76.

[21] Dempsey DK, Schwartz CJ, Ward RS, Iyer AV, Parakka JP, Cosgriff-Hernandez EM. Micropatterning of electrospun polyurethane fibers through control of surface topography. Macromol Mater Eng 2010;295(11):990–4.
[22] Li D, Xia Y. Electrospinning of nanofibers: reinventing the wheel? Adv Mater 2004;16(14):1151–70.
[23] Lu Y, Mapili G, Suhali G, Chen S, Roy K. A digital micro-mirror device-based system for the microfabrication of complex, spatially patterned tissue engineering scaffolds. J Biomed Mater Res Part A 2006;77(2):396–405.
[24] Wood A. Contact guidance on microfabricated substrata: the response of teleost fin mesenchyme cells to repeating topographical patterns. J Cell Sci 1988;90(4):667–81.
[25] Wójciak-Stothard B, Madeja Z, Korohoda W, Curtis A, Wilkinson C. Activation of macrophage-like cells by multiple grooved substrata. Topographical control of cell behaviour. Cell Biol Int 1995;19(6):485–90.
[26] Wilkinson P, Shields J, Haston WS. Contact guidance of human neutrophil leukocytes. Exp Cell Res 1982;140(1):55–62.
[27] Meyle J, Gültig K, Brich M, Hämmerle H, Nisch W. Contact guidance of fibroblasts on biomaterial surfaces. J Mater Sci Mater Med 1994;5(6–7):463–6.
[28] Kh PR, Pavasant P, Supaphol P. Effect of the surface topography of electrospun poly(epsilon-caprolactone)/poly(3-hydroxybuterate-co-3-hydroxyvalerate) fibrous substrates on cultured bone cell behavior. Langmuir 2011;27(17):10938–46.
[29] Rogers CM, Morris GE, Gould TW, Bail R, Toumpaniari S, Harrington H, et al. A novel technique for the production of electrospun scaffolds with tailored three-dimensional micro-patterns employing additive manufacturing. Biofabrication 2014;6(3):035003.
[30] Campbell CE, Von Recum AF. Microtopography and soft tissue response. Investig Surg 1989;2(1):51–74.
[31] Almeida CR, Serra T, Oliveira MI, Planell JA, Barbosa MA, Navarro M. Impact of 3-D printed PLA-and chitosan-based scaffolds on human monocyte/macrophage responses: unraveling the effect of 3-D structures on inflammation. Acta Biomater 2014;10(2):613–22.
[32] Cooper A, Munden H, Brown G. The growth of mouse neuroblastoma cells in controlled orientations on thin films of silicon monoxide. Exp Cell Res 1976;103(2):435–9.
[33] Kim M-H, Sawada Y, Taya M, Kino-oka M. Influence of surface topography on the human epithelial cell response to micropatterned substrates with convex and concave architectures. J Biol Eng 2014;8(1):13.
[34] Rea SM, Brooks RA, Schneider A, Best SM, Bonfield W. Osteoblast-like cell response to bioactive composites—Surface-topography and composition effects. J Biomed Mater Res Part B Appl Biomaterials 2004;70(2):250–61.
[35] Cunha A, Zouani OF, Plawinski L, Botelho do Rego AM, Almeida A, Vilar R, et al. Human mesenchymal stem cell behavior on femtosecond laser-textured Ti-6Al-4V surfaces. Nanomedicine 2015;10(5):725–39.
[36] Elsayed M, Merkel OM. Nanoimprinting of topographical and 3D cell culture scaffolds. Nanomedicine 2014;9(2):349–66.
[37] Park S, Im GI. Stem cell responses to nanotopography. J Biomed Mater Res Part A 2014;103(3):1238–45.
[38] Kim DH, Seo CH, Han K, Kwon KW, Levchenko A, Suh KY. Guided cell migration on microtextured substrates with variable local density and anisotropy. Adv Funct Mater 2009;19(10):1579–86.
[39] Yim EK, Reano RM, Pang SW, Yee AF, Chen CS, Leong KW. Nanopattern-induced changes in morphology and motility of smooth muscle cells. Biomaterials 2005;26(26):5405–13.
[40] Charest JL, Eliason MT, García AJ, King WP. Combined microscale mechanical topography and chemical patterns on polymer cell culture substrates. Biomaterials 2006;27(11):2487–94.
[41] Mahmud G, Campbell CJ, Bishop KJ, Komarova YA, Chaga O, Soh S, et al. Directing cell motions on micropatterned ratchets. Nat Phys 2009;5(8):606–12.
[42] Folkman J, Moscona A. Role of cell shape in growth control. Nature 1978;273.
[43] Gentile F, Medda R, Cheng L, Battista E, Scopelliti PE, Milani P, et al. Selective modulation of cell response on engineered fractal silicon substrates. Sci Rep 2013;3.

[44] Wood JA, Ly I, Borjesson DL, Nealey PF, Russell P, Murphy CJ. The modulation of canine mesenchymal stem cells by nano-topographic cues. Exp Cell Res 2012;318(19):2438–45.
[45] Watari S, Hayashi K, Wood JA, Russell P, Nealey PF, Murphy CJ, et al. Modulation of osteogenic differentiation in hMSCs cells by submicron topographically-patterned ridges and grooves. Biomaterials 2012;33(1):128–36.
[46] Peng L, Eltgroth ML, LaTempa TJ, Grimes CA, Desai TA. The effect of TiO_2 nanotubes on endothelial function and smooth muscle proliferation. Biomaterials 2009;30(7):1268–72.
[47] Park J, Bauer S, von der Mark K, Schmuki P. Nanosize and vitality: TiO_2 nanotube diameter directs cell fate. Nano Lett 2007;7(6):1686–91.
[48] Cai K, Bossert J, Jandt KD. Does the nanometre scale topography of titanium influence protein adsorption and cell proliferation? Colloids Surf B Biointerfaces 2006;49(2):136–44.
[49] Khang D, Choi J, Im YM, Kim YJ, Jang JH, Kang SS, et al. Role of subnano-, nano- and submicron-surface features on osteoblast differentiation of bone marrow mesenchymal stem cells. Biomaterials 2012;33(26):5997–6007.
[50] Janson IA, Kong YP, Putnam AJ. Nanotopographic substrates of poly (methyl methacrylate) do not strongly influence the osteogenic phenotype of mesenchymal stem cells in vitro. PLoS One 2014;9(3):e90719.
[51] Seidlits SK, Lee JY, Schmidt CE. Nanostructured scaffolds for neural applications. Nanomedicine 2008;3.
[52] Zouani OF, Chanseau C, Brouillaud B, Bareille R, Deliane F, Foulc M-P, et al. Altered nanofeature size dictates stem cell differentiation. J Cell Sci 2012;125(5):1217–24.
[53] Dalby MJ, McCloy D, Robertson M, Wilkinson CD, Oreffo RO. Osteoprogenitor response to defined topographies with nanoscale depths. Biomaterials 2006;27(8):1306–15.
[54] Dalby MJ, Gadegaard N, Tare R, Andar A, Riehle MO, Herzyk P, et al. The control of human mesenchymal cell differentiation using nanoscale symmetry and disorder. Nat Mater 2007;6(12):997–1003.
[55] Yim EK, Pang SW, Leong KW. Synthetic nanostructures inducing differentiation of human mesenchymal stem cells into neuronal lineage. Exp Cell Res 2007;313(9):1820–9.
[56] Lu D, Chen CS, Lai CS, Soni S, Lam T, Le C, et al. Microgrooved surface modulates neuron differentiation in human embryonic stem cells. Methods Mol Biol 2014;1307:281–7.
[57] Smith LA, Liu X, Hu J, Wang P, Ma PX. Enhancing osteogenic differentiation of mouse embryonic stem cells by nanofibers. Tissue Eng Part A 2009;15(7):1855–64.
[58] Shi Z, Neoh KG, Kang ET, Poh CK, Wang W. Enhanced endothelial differentiation of adipose-derived stem cells by substrate nanotopography. J Tissue Eng Regen Med 2014;8(1):50–8.
[59] Trujillo NA, Popat KC. Increased adipogenic and decreased chondrogenic differentiation of adipose derived stem cells on nanowire surfaces. Materials 2014;7(4):2605–30.
[60] Kurpinski K, Chu J, Hashi C, Li S. Anisotropic mechanosensing by mesenchymal stem cells. Proc Natl Acad Sci USA 2006;103(44):16095–100.
[61] Gao L, McBeath R, Chen CS. Stem cell shape regulates a chondrogenic versus myogenic fate through Rac1 and N-cadherin. Stem Cells 2010;28(3):564–72.
[62] Kong YP, Tu CH, Donovan PJ, Yee AF. Expression of Oct4 in human embryonic stem cells is dependent on nanotopographical configuration. Acta Biomater 2013;9(5):6369–80.
[63] Lee MR, Kwon KW, Jung H, Kim HN, Suh KY, Kim K, et al. Direct differentiation of human embryonic stem cells into selective neurons on nanoscale ridge/groove pattern arrays. Biomaterials 2010;31(15):4360–6.
[64] Ardeshirylajimi A, Hosseinkhani S, Parivar K, Yaghmaie P, Soleimani M. Nanofiber-based polyethersulfone scaffold and efficient differentiation of human induced pluripotent stem cells into osteoblastic lineage. Mol Biol Rep 2013;40(7):4287–94.
[65] Yang K, Jung K, Ko E, Kim J, Park KI, Kim J, et al. Nanotopographical manipulation of focal adhesion formation for enhanced differentiation of human neural stem cells. ACS Appl Mater Interfaces 2013;5(21):10529–40.

[66] Beduer A, Vieu C, Arnauduc F, Sol JC, Loubinoux I, Vaysse L. Engineering of adult human neural stem cells differentiation through surface micropatterning. Biomaterials 2012;33(2):504–14.
[67] Bagnaninchi P, Yang Y, Zghoul N, Maffulli N, Wang R, Haj AE. Chitosan microchannel scaffolds for tendon tissue engineering characterized using optical coherence tomography. Tissue Eng 2007;13(2):323–31.
[68] Lu Q, Simionescu A, Vyavahare N. Novel capillary channel fiber scaffolds for guided tissue engineering. Acta Biomater 2005;1(6):607–14.
[69] Vernon RB, Gooden MD, Lara SL, Wight TN. Microgrooved fibrillar collagen membranes as scaffolds for cell support and alignment. Biomaterials 2005;26(16):3131–40.
[70] Liu Y, Ramanath H, Wang D-A. Tendon tissue engineering using scaffold enhancing strategies. Trends Biotechnol 2008;26(4):201–9.
[71] Liliensiek SJ, Wood JA, Yong J, Auerbach R, Nealey PF, Murphy CJ. Modulation of human vascular endothelial cell behaviors by nanotopographic cues. Biomaterials 2010;31(20):5418–26.
[72] Biela SA, Su Y, Spatz JP, Kemkemer R. Different sensitivity of human endothelial cells, smooth muscle cells and fibroblasts to topography in the nano–micro range. Acta Biomater 2009;5(7):2460–6.
[73] Zorlutuna P, Rong Z, Vadgama P, Hasirci V. Influence of nanopatterns on endothelial cell adhesion: enhanced cell retention under shear stress. Acta Biomater 2009;5(7):2451–9.
[74] Morgan JT, Wood JA, Shah NM, Hughbanks ML, Russell P, Barakat AI, et al. Integration of basal topographic cues and apical shear stress in vascular endothelial cells. Biomaterials 2012;33(16):4126–35.
[75] Kim D-H, Lipke EA, Kim P, Cheong R, Thompson S, Delannoy M, et al. Nanoscale cues regulate the structure and function of macroscopic cardiac tissue constructs. Proc Natl Acad Sci USA 2010;107(2):565–70.
[76] Wang P-Y, Yu J, Lin J-H, Tsai W-B. Modulation of alignment, elongation and contraction of cardiomyocytes through a combination of nanotopography and rigidity of substrates. Acta Biomater 2011;7(9):3285–93.
[77] Ayaz HGŞ, Perets A, Ayaz H, Gilroy KD, Govindaraj M, Brookstein D, et al. Textile-templated electrospun anisotropic scaffolds for regenerative cardiac tissue engineering. Biomaterials 2014;35(30):8540–52.
[78] Svensson S. Molecular and cellular interactions on noble metal nanopatterned surfaces– applications towards bone, soft tissue and infection control. 2014.
[79] Parker JA, Walboomers XF, Von den Hoff JW, Maltha JC, Jansen JA. Soft-tissue response to silicone and poly-L-lactic acid implants with a periodic or random surface micropattern. J Biomed Mater Res 2002;61(1):91–8.
[80] Rosengren A, Bjursten LM, Danielsen N, Persson H, Kober M. Tissue reactions to polyethylene implants with different surface topography. J Mater Sci Mater Med 1999;10(2):75–82.
[81] Rosengren A, Danielsen N, Bjursten LM. Reactive capsule formation around soft-tissue implants is related to cell necrosis. J Biomed Mater Res 1999;46(4):458–64.
[82] Gittens RA, Olivares-Navarrete R, Schwartz Z, Boyan BD. Implant osseointegration and the role of microroughness and nanostructures: lessons for spine implants. Acta Biomater 2014;10(8):3363–71.
[83] Schwartz Z, Raz P, Zhao G, Barak Y, Tauber M, Yao H, et al. Effect of micrometer-scale roughness of the surface of Ti6Al4V pedicle screws in vitro and in vivo. J Bone & Jt Surg 2008;90(11):2485–98.
[84] Szmukler-Moncler S, Perrin D, Ahossi V, Magnin G, Bernard J. Biological properties of acid etched titanium implants: effect of sandblasting on bone anchorage. J Biomed Mater Res Part B Appl Biomaterials 2004;68(2):149–59.
[85] Wennerberg A, Albrektsson T, Andersson B, Krol J. A histomorghometric study of screw-shaped and removal torque titanium implants with three different surface topographies. Clin Oral Implants Res 1995;6(1):24–30.
[86] Wennerberg A, Albrektsson T, Andersson B. Bone tissue response to commercially pure titanium implants blasted with fine and coarse particles of aluminum oxide. Int J Oral Maxillofac Implants 1995;11(1):38–45.
[87] Mendonça G, Mendonça DBS, Simões LGP, Araújo AL, Leite ER, Golin AL, et al. Nanostructured implant surface effect on osteoblast gene expression and bone-to-implant contact in vivo. Mater Sci Eng C 2011;31(8):1809–18.

[88] Ballo A, Agheli H, Lausmaa J, Thomsen P, Petronis S. Nanostructured model implants for in vivo studies: influence of well-defined nanotopography on de novo bone formation on titanium implants. Int J Nanomedicine 2011;6:3415.
[89] Tsukimura N, Ueno T, Iwasa F, Minamikawa H, Sugita Y, Ishizaki K, et al. Bone integration capability of alkali-and heat-treated nanobimorphic Ti–15Mo–5Zr–3Al. Acta Biomater 2011;7(12):4267–77.
[90] Bjursten LM, Rasmusson L, Oh S, Smith GC, Brammer KS, Jin S. Titanium dioxide nanotubes enhance bone bonding in vivo. J Biomed Mater Res Part A 2010;92(3):1218–24.

CHAPTER

9 MECHANOBIOLOGY AND MECHANOTHERAPY IN TISSUE ENGINEERING

R. Ogawa
Nippon Medical School, Tokyo, Japan

CHAPTER OUTLINE

INTRODUCTION

The 3-D structure of living organisms is influenced by various physical factors, including gravity, atmospheric pressure, and water pressure. These constant, seemingly unremarkable mechanical forces are in fact essential for forming, maintaining, and changing the dynamic structures and functions of our cells, tissues, and organs. “Mechanobiology” is the study of the molecular cascades and cellular responses that are triggered by mechanical forces. A more comprehensive and improved understanding of mechanobiology may greatly facilitate the development of new therapies that act by controlling mechanical forces and thereby specifically induce desired molecular, cellular, tissue, and/or organ formation, changes, or repair. We have denoted these therapies as “mechanotherapies.” In this chapter, we review the concepts of mechanobiology and mechanotherapy and discuss the future of tissue engineering mechanotherapies.

In Situ Tissue Regeneration. http://dx.doi.org/10.1016/B978-0-12-802225-2.00009-X

CELLS AND THE PHYSICAL ENVIRONMENT

The 3-D structure of living organisms is influenced by various physical factors, including gravity, atmospheric pressure, and water pressure (Fig. 9.1) [1,2]. This physical environment certainly also played a crucial role in the beginnings of life on Earth. For example, the evolution of multicellular organisms from unicellular organisms was probably facilitated by the fact that unicellular organisms had already evolved certain mechanosensory, molecular signaling, and genetic regulatory mechanisms that allowed them to respond and adapt to mechanical stimuli from their environment [3]. These preexisting mechanosensitive pathways were then adapted in multicellular organisms to mediate the communal functions of their cells. For example, when individual cells are moved and stretched via the cell adhesion molecules (CAMs) that connect them to other cells, they all undergo cellular changes that ultimately lead to physiological adaptation to the mechanical force in question.

In the human body, the musculoskeletal system (which includes the bones, cartilage, tendons, and muscles) supports our body weight, implements movement, and grows or develops in response to changing physical demands. At the same time, the skin stretches to accommodate musculoskeletal growth. The heart beats constantly, blood flows through vessels, and the lungs expand and contract as we breathe. Thus every part of our body is stretching, shrinking, and/or moving as we perform our daily activities. These constant, seemingly unremarkable mechanical forces are in fact essential for forming, maintaining, and changing the dynamic structures and functions of our cells, tissues, and organs [1]. An illuminating example of this is the fact that when astronauts return to Earth after being in outer space, they are less capable of standing and working compared to before their space flight; they exhibit cardiovascular deconditioning, muscle atrophy, immune dysfunction, and bone loss [4,5]. This suggests

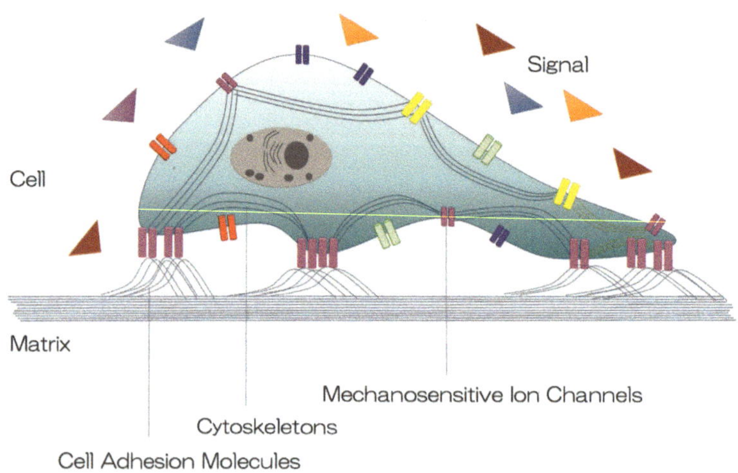

FIGURE 9.1 Types of mechanical forces.

The microenvironment around cells imposes many types of mechanical force. In general, cell shape is changed by stretch and shear forces but not by hydrostatic pressure. The change in cell shape affects the cytoskeleton, thereby transducing the mechanical force into the cell. Hydrostatic pressure acts more directly by opening ion channels in the plasma membrane of the cells.

that if life evolved on another planet with a different surface gravity compared to Earth, the 3-D form of the living organisms would probably be completely different to those on Earth; perhaps they would be flatter/thicker and softer/harder.

Thus when devising methods to induce tissue repair and regeneration, we must focus as much on the physical environment (including body weight, gravity, and atmospheric pressure) as on the cells themselves. This notion is supported by another example: when we walk on Earth, the articular cartilage of our knee joint is subjected to 30 atm of water pressure (ie, equal to the pressure experienced at a depth of 300 m in the sea) [6]. In space, the pressure on the knee is hugely reduced, and it is likely that over time, the articular cartilage of the knee will begin to weaken. However, even if, in an effort to preserve astronaut knee function, we injected the knees of astronauts under zero gravity with the "ultimate" multipotent stem cells (such as embryonic stem cells [7] or induced pluripotent stem cells [8]) and chondrocytes indeed formed, the absence of pressure on the cartilage would mean that functional cartilage tissue would probably not develop.

MECHANOSENSITIVITY OF CELLS

Each cell type seems to respond differently to the various mechanical forces. Fibroblasts seem to respond particularly strongly to stretching force, as shown by several in vitro models. Thus lung fibroblasts that are subjected to stretching force exhibit Ca^{2+} influx and adenosine triphosphate (ATP) release [9]. Stretched dermal fibroblasts migrate faster and for a longer distance than unstretched cells, and the increased migration results in the reorientation of the cells perpendicular to the direction of stretching [10]. This associates with reduced cellular apoptosis but unchanged proliferation [10]. By contrast, coronary artery fibroblasts do proliferate more strongly when stretched than when unstretched [11]. They also secrete more hydroxyproline and express higher mRNA levels of matrix metalloproteinase-9/tissue inhibitor metalloproteinase, alpha-smooth muscle actin, interleukin-6 (IL-6), heat shock transcription factor-1, and heat shock protein-70. Thus mechanical stretch increases the ability of coronary artery fibroblasts to form collagen and secrete inflammatory factors. Similarly, stretching of patellar tendon fibroblasts [12] and anterior cruciate ligament fibroblasts [13] increases their collagen type I gene expression/synthesis. These studies indicate that fibroblasts are sensitive to mechanical stretch and that it increases their secretion of collagen and inflammatory mediators, migration, and cell proliferation. These observations are entirely consistent with the clinical symptoms of our bodies when they are exposed to stretching force. For example, when cutaneous scars are persistently stretched by the daily movements of our body, they can become inflamed, accumulate collagen, and become thicker [14,15]. Similarly, although tendons are metabolically active structures that readily adapt their biochemical, biomechanical, and structural properties to chronic exercise, abnormal adaptations due to inappropriate mechanical force can lead to tendinopathy and pain [16]. Thus although an appropriately strong mechanical force can make fibroblasts produce the correct response, forces that are too strong yield inflammation and pathological fibrosis.

Osteocytes, which are the most abundant cells in the bone, appear to be the most mechanosensitive cells in bone; they play key roles in the transduction of mechanical stress on the skeletal system into a biological response [17]. Osteocytes respond differently to various mechanical stimuli. When subjected to pulsating fluid flow, they respond with the sustained release of prostaglandin E2 [18] and increased expression of nitric oxide (NO) [19]. However, if they experience cyclic strain, they release NO but not prostaglandin E2. Similarly, whereas substrate strain enhances their production of bone matrix protein collagen I, fluid shear reduces their collagen I production. Thus these mechanical forces and their strengths may strongly affect bone growth and remodeling. We also found that hydrostatic pressure affects the viability, distribution, and osteogenic differentiation and maturation of bone marrow mesenchymal stem cells that have been seeded in 3-D hydroxyapatite scaffolds and cultured in osteogenic medium; the cells under hydrostatic pressure expressed significantly more osteocalcin, osteopontin, osteonectin, and collagen type 1 than the cells without this pressure [17]. These observations also cast a new light on mechanobiology in general: although the main physiological mechanical forces on osteocytes are the compression force that is produced by body weight and the tension from retracting/extending tendons/muscles, the studies described above [17–19] indicate that osteocytes are also sensitive to fluid flow and water pressure. Thus many kinds of cells may be highly sensitive to different types of mechanical forces even when they are not forces to which the cells are regularly exposed in normal daily life.

The mechanobiology of chondrocytes has also been well studied. The chondrocytes in cartilage tissue are affected by various intrinsic and extrinsic mechanical stimuli, including the shear forces, compression pressure, hydrostatic pressure, and osmotic pressure that are produced by joint movement. When tissue-engineered articular cartilage is subjected to fluid flow, its type II collagen production increases [20]. Hydrostatic pressure also seems to enhance the matrix synthesis of chondrocytes [21] by increasing intracellular Ca^{2+} levels via mechanosensitive ion channels [22]. Moreover, when we subjected chondrocytes from articular cartilage to repeated changes in hydrostatic and osmotic pressure, we found this affected not only their proliferation and differentiation but also their anabolic and catabolic gene expression profiles [23]. In particular, we found that osmotic and hydrostatic pressure changes had similar effects on metabolic gene expression. We speculated that chondrocyte phenotypes can be maintained by finely orchestrating hydrostatic and osmotic pressure [23]. Two studies also showed that chondrocytes are sensitive to stretch force; stretched chondrocytes exhibit potassium channel activation and mechanosignaling pathway changes [24,25].

It is easy to imagine that mechanical force increases the volume of muscle, as this is the principle underlying exercise and rehabilitation. Muscle can grow in three ways, namely, by increasing muscle cell numbers, muscle fiber diameter, and fiber length [26]. Skeletal muscle exhibits hypertrophy when it is subjected to a sustained increase of mechanical loading via exercise or rehabilitation. By contrast, when the mechanical loading is weak, the muscle atrophies. A key molecule in these responses to mechanical load is myostatin: when it is inactivated, it induces skeletal muscle hypertrophy, whereas its overexpression or systemic administration causes muscle atrophy [27]. Myostatin negatively regulates the activity of the Akt pathway, which promotes protein synthesis and increases ubiquitin–proteasome system activity, which in turn mediates atrophy [27]. Notably, cardiac muscle cells also have an intrinsic ability to sense and respond to mechanical load [28]. It has been proposed that the Z-disc muscle LIM protein– a Tcap gene–titin complex in these cells functions as a stretch sensor and that defects in this complex can lead to cardiomyopathy and heart failure [28,29].

Keratinocytes exhibit various changes after mechanical force loading. Stretching accelerates their migration in the in vitro wound closure model [30] and increases their ATP release and intracellular Ca^{2+} levels. Since this reaction is impaired in knockout mice that lack terminal porphyrin (TPPC6) (a mechanosensitive calcium channel on the cell membrane), it may be that TPPC6 is an important mechanosensor of keratinocytes. Moreover, keratinocytes subjected to stretching force in vitro exhibit endotheline-1 upregulation. It was also suggested that keratinocyte-derived endotheline-1 upregulation may play a significant role in the pathogenesis of pigmented disorders that are caused by mechanical stress (eg, friction melanosis) [31]. To further examine the effects of stretching on epidermal cells, we developed a servo-controlled skin stretching device for mice. When we subjected the skin of mice to static and cyclical stretching forces, we found that cyclic stretching was superior to static stretching in terms of increasing the skin expression of epidermal growth factor, transforming growth factor beta1, and nerve growth factor [32]. Both types of stretching also induced epidermal proliferation and skin angiogenesis. However, the cyclically stretched skin exhibited significant upregulation of hypoxia-induced factor 1alpha, *unlike the statically stretched skin*: nevertheless, poststretch analysis revealed that the skin was well oxygenated. This suggests that waveform-specific mechanical loads, not static stretching, induce transient hypoxia that accelerates the growth of skin in response to mechanical stretching [32].

The endothelium is constantly subjected to the fluid shear stress that is produced by blood flow, and numerous in vitro and in vivo studies have shown that shear stress greatly influences the endothelial cell phenotype [33]. Moreover, fluid flow markedly increases the secretion by both endothelial cells and vascular smooth muscle cells of cytokines and vasoactive mediators such as growth factors, NO, prostaglandin, and other molecules [34]. Fluid flow also opens mechanosensitive transmembrane K^+ and Ca^{2+} channels in endothelial cells [35], upregulates their heterotrimeric G-proteins [36], and activates many of their intracellular signaling cascades, including the calcium-dependent phosphorylation and activation of endothelial nitric oxide synthase: this results in increased NO production, phosphoinositide 3-kinase activation, and integrin-mediated signaling [33,36,37].

Whereas the musculoskeletal system and fibrous tissues tend to increase their volume when mechanical forces are loaded, adipose tissues tend to decrease their volume. Several studies have investigated the effects of mechanical forces on adipogenesis in vitro because it is increasingly being understood that various adipose tissue cells, including adipocytes and preadipocytes, are both mechanosensitive and mechanoresponsive. It has been shown that the *same* mechanical force has totally different effects on stem cells, preadipocytes, and adipocytes in terms of their adipogenic ability. A recent study showed that when mature adipocytes undergo prolonged uniaxial static stretching, the MAPK/ERK kinase/mitogen-activated protein kinase (MAPK) signaling pathway is activated and adipocyte hypertrophy ensues [38]. However, when preadipocytes undergo the same mechanical stretching procedure, adipogenic differentiation is inhibited [39]. Moreover, different mechanical forces seem to have different effects in terms of adipogenesis overall, possibly because different signaling pathways are evoked; static stretching seems to promote adipogenesis, whereas dynamic mechanical forces, such as cyclic stretching or vibration and static compression, inhibit it. This pattern may also explain why subcutaneous fat tends to localize in the abdominal and gluteofemoral regions, especially in obesity [40]; the abdominal and gluteofemoral regions are under less tension than other regions of our body. This could also explain why the crunch exercise, which places cyclic stretching force on the abdominal fat, is an efficient way to lose abdominal fat. This notion is supported by the study of Findlay et al. [41], who subcutaneously implanted the groins of pigs with a polycarbonate tissue engineering chamber that surrounded a pedicled fat flap. This approach increased the volume of the fat flaps by more than fivefold, whereas fat flaps that were not supplied with a chamber exhibited little growth [41]. We speculated that the chamber not only provided a space for adipose tissue regeneration, but it also decreased the tension on the flap [42]. It is possible that the decreased tension on the flap allowed the cells to maintain a round morphology and that this promoted adipogenesis. This notion is supported by the fact that cell shape strongly regulates the commitment of mesenchymal stem cells to a particular adipocyte fate via several signaling pathways, including the RhoA/Rho-associated protein kinase (ROCK) signaling pathway [43].

MECHANOSENSORS, MECHANORECEPTORS, AND MECHANOSENSITIVE NOCICEPTORS

Mechanical forces, including stretching tension, shear force, scratch, compression, and hydrostatic and osmotic pressure, are perceived by both cellular mechanosensors (Fig. 9.2) and the nerve fiber receptors (including mechanosensitive nociceptors) that produce the somatic sensation of mechanical force [44]. Cellular mechanosensors include the mechanosensitive ion channels (eg, Ca^{2+}, K^{+}, Na^{2+}, and Mg^{2+}), the cytoskeleton (eg, actin filaments), and CAMs (eg, integrins) [45]. These three sensor structures/molecules operate together with the extracellular matrix (ECM) to transduce a mechanical force into tissue-resident cells; the CAMs are attached to both the ECM and the cytoskeleton, and the cytoskeleton is also connected to mechanosensitive ion channels. Thus when the ECM is distorted by mechanical forces such as tension, the cytoskeleton is altered, and this activates the mechanosensitive ion channels. Notably, not all mechanical forces activate mechanosensitive ion channels via cytoskeletal alteration; extracellular fluid-based hydrostatic pressure impacts ion inflow but not cell shape [21,22,46]. The mechanical stimuli that are received by the mechanosensors are then passed down various mechanotransduction pathways (mechanosignaling pathways) [1,45,47] and converted into electrical and biochemical signals that ultimately change cell proliferation and activity.

At the tissue level, sensory fibers act as mechanosensitive nociceptors in various tissues and organs [48,49]. When these nociceptors receive a mechanical stimulus, the signals are transmitted to dorsal root ganglia that contain neuronal cell bodies in the afferent spinal nerves. This results in neuropeptide release from the peripheral terminals of primary afferent sensory neurons, which innervate the tissue and are often in contact with tissue-resident cells. These neuropeptides can directly modulate the functions of tissue-resident cells such as keratinocytes, fibroblasts, and mast,

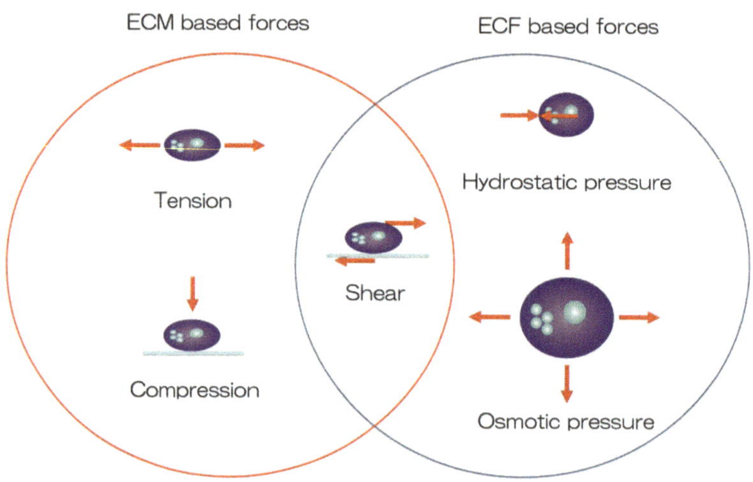

FIGURE 9.2 Mechanosensors of cells.

Cellular mechanosensors include the mechanosensitive ion channels, the cytoskeleton, and CAMs. In recent years, many other sensors have also been discovered.

microvascular endothelial, and infiltrating immune cells. These neuropeptides include substance P, calcitonin gene-based peptide (CGRP), neurokinin A, vasoactive intestinal peptide, and somatostatin, and they each may activate specific nociceptors; for example, substance P and CGRP act through the neurokinin 1 receptor and CGRP1 receptor, respectively. The neuropeptides that are generated under physiological and pathophysiological conditions ultimately modulate tissue and immune cell functions, including cell proliferation, cytokine production, antigen presentation, sensory neurotransmission, mast cell degradation, vasodilation, and vascular permeability. When proinflammatory responses arise from mechanical stimuli that are transmitted by neuropeptides, they are termed neurogenic inflammation.

The relationship between cellular mechanosensors and mechanosensitive nociceptors is interesting. Of particular interest is the question, which of these mechanosensitive structures/molecules is the primary mechanical force sensor of tissues? In the case of skin, it may be cellular mechanosensors of the epithelium, such as transient receptor potential channel V4 (TRPV4) [50]. This mechanosensitive ion channel occurs in keratinocytes and is activated by mechanical stimuli applied on the skin. Thereafter, TRPV4 converts the mechanical stimuli into electrical signals, and these signals are conveyed to nociceptors. Thus in skin at least, mechanosensitive nociceptors may simply serve as electric wires that transmit signals rather than being the primary mechanical sensors.

MECHANOSIGNALING PATHWAYS

Mechanotransduction is the process by which physical forces are sensed and converted into biochemical and electrical signals that then result in cellular responses. The discovery and elucidation of the various molecular pathways involved in this process have revolutionized the fundamental and clinical understanding of the formation and subsequent development of tissues and organs. The mechanosignaling pathways that participate in the formation and growth of tissues include thetransforming growth factor (TGF)-β/Smad, integrin, calcium ion pathways, MAPK and G protein, Wnt/β-catenin, tumor necrosis factor (TNF)-α/NF-κB, and interleukin pathways (Fig. 9.3) [47,51]. During tissue development, these cellular mechanosignaling pathways interact actively with the ECM. A better understanding of these interactions will be useful for the tissue engineering field [6,17,51] and may facilitate the development of pharmacological interventions that could ultimately induce the formation and development of tissues and organs.

MECHANOBIOLOGY AND MECHANOTHERAPY

At the cellular level, mechanical forces can induce cells to change shape and cause molecules to be transferred into and out of the cell through the cell membrane. These changes activate molecular cascades within the cells that alter gene expression and thereby play an important role in the life cycle of the cell. "Mechanobiology" is the study of how cells sense the mechanical forces of the physical microenvironment and what molecular cascades and cellular responses ensue when they are sensed [1,2]. A more comprehensive and improved understanding of mechanobiology may greatly facilitate the development of new therapies that control mechanical forces and thereby specifically induce desired molecular, cellular, tissue, and/or organ formation, changes, or repair. Recently, we denoted these therapies

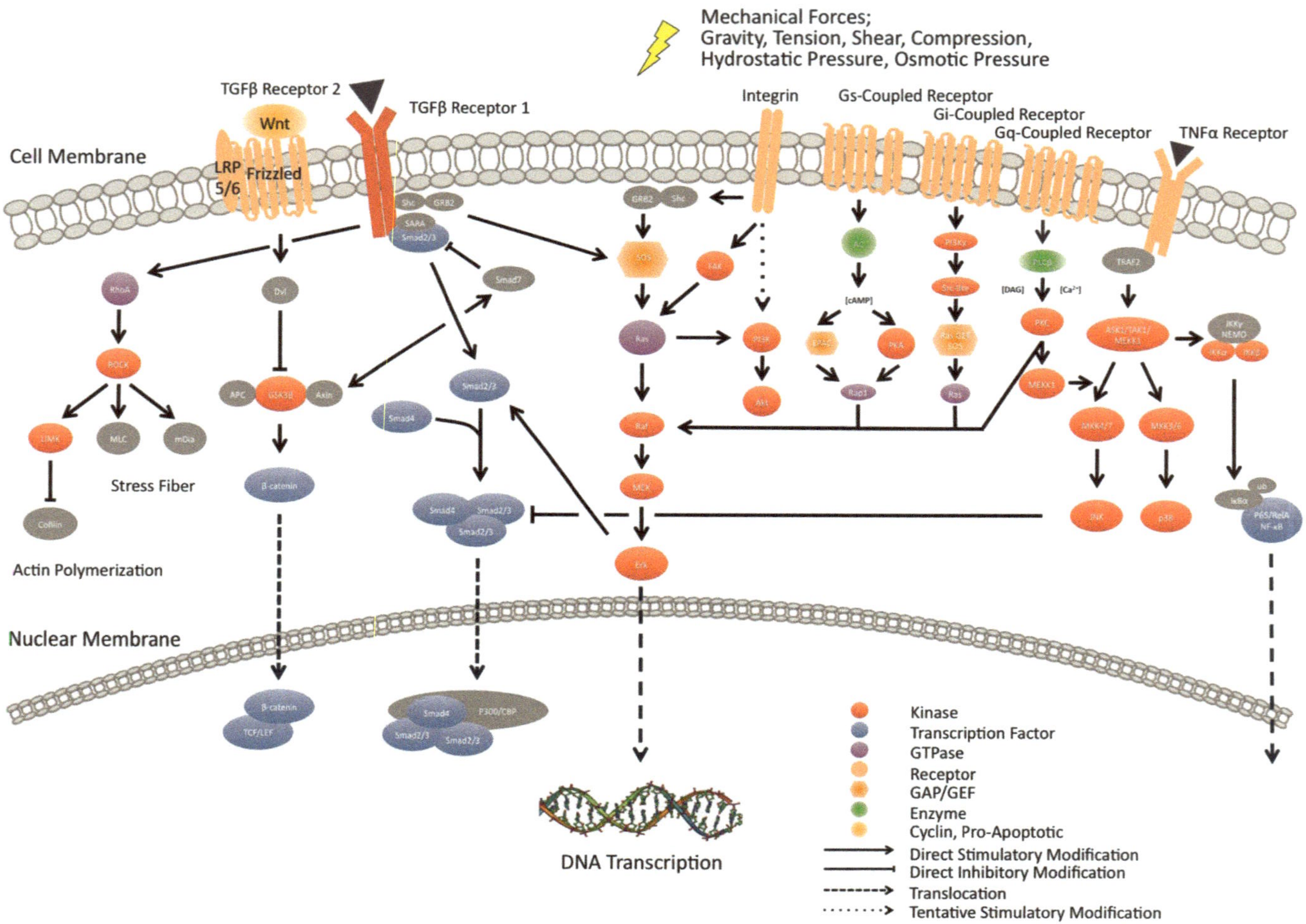

FIGURE 9.3 Mechanosignaling pathways.

Physical forces are sensed by cellular mechanosensors and converted into biochemical and electrical signals that result in cellular responses. These signaling pathways are called mechanosignaling pathways. For example, while the TGFβ signaling pathway can be activated by applying a TGFβ ligand, it can also be activated by cellular stretch alone.

Reproduced with permission from Huang C, Akaishi S, Ogawa R. Mechanosignaling pathways in cutaneous scarring. Arch Dermatol Res October 2012;304(8):589–597.

as "mechanotherapies" [1]. While the term mechanotherapy was originally synonymous with physical therapy, massotherapy, and the rehabilitation of the musculoskeletal system, our new definition reflects the multidimensional medical possibilities of the field that now exist. We recently proposed several potential mechanotherapies for various skin disorders, including keloids, namely, the use of sutures, surgical procedures, and dressings that eliminate the tension on the disordered skin [14,52,53]. Mechanobiology-mediated medicine could also be used to analyze and/or treat many disorders/diseases, accelerate wound healing, reduce scarring during wound healing, and repair and regenerate injured/aged tissues and organs. There has been a significant increase in the basic and clinical research into mechanobiology and mechanotherapy recently. This has caused expansion of the target tissues/organs to the nail [54] and hair [55] and has attracted considerable attention from the aesthetics and antiaging fields.

The observations above indicate that the ultimate target of future tissue engineering mechanotherapies is the direct and specific control of mechanosignaling pathways [1]. These pathways could be activated in vivo by various devices that produce actual mechanical forces and electrical stimuli. Moreover, methodologies such as massage that involve hand manipulation should be revisited in light of the new definition of mechanotherapy and further optimized. In addition, it would be of interest to identify pharmacological approaches that can activate or block mechanosignaling pathways and lead to the same cellular responses that are induced by the actual mechanical stimulation.

MECHANOTHERAPY AT THE MOLECULAR LEVEL

Since mechanosignaling pathways are activated by mechanical force loading, the same responses may be obtained by pharmacological intervention that targets one or more mechanosignaling pathways. Candidate pathways that are involved in musculoskeletal system responses to mechanical forces are intracellular calcium ion signaling, prostaglandin and NO signaling, and Wingless-type (Wnt)/β-catenin signaling [51], while good candidates for preventing or treating benign or malignant fibroproliferative disorders may be the integrin signaling, TGF-β/Smad, MAPK signaling, RhoA/ROCK signaling, TNF-α/NF-κB signaling, and Wnt/β-Catenin pathways [52].

The pharmacological interventions could be mediated by small interfering RNA (siRNA), neutralizing antibodies, or competitive inhibitor proteins [1]. Naturally, because many molecules play multiple roles in various pathways and the different pathways crosstalk, such molecular therapies will have to be sufficiently specific to avoid uncontrollable and unwanted effects [56].

Mechanotherapies that target mechanotransduction signaling pathways can mainly aim to modulate one of their four phases [57]: (1) the mechanocoupling phase, where the external mechanical signal is converted into a mechanical signal in the vicinity of the cell; (2) the biochemical coupling phase, where the local mechanical signal is transduced into a biochemical signal, resulting ultimately in genetic or protein changes; (3) signal transmission, where the biochemical signal is then passed from the sensor cells to the effector cells; and (4) the effector cell response [1]. For example, inhibiting focal adhesion kinase (FAK) effectively prevents mechanical forces from inducing pathological scarring [58]. Moreover, siRNA-induced FAK knockdown impairs the proliferation, differentiation, and collagen synthesis of cardiac fibroblasts in response to cyclic stretch, which indicates that it has the potential to reduce myocardial fibrosis [59].

MECHANOTHERAPY AT A CELLULAR LEVEL

The well-defined integrin-mediated mechanisms that alter various cellular functions, including cytoskeleton-related tensegrity, cell–matrix interactions, and cell shape-dependent functions, are particularly interesting for mechanotherapy research [1,2]. Tensile forces received by the cytoskeleton of a cell from the ECM not only change the cell that receives the signals, but they are also transferred to neighboring cells through cadherin-containing cell–cell adhesion complexes [60]. Thus cells are connected to each other and to the ECM, thereby forming a dynamic system that can be manipulated by potential mechanotherapeutic interventions at the cellular level.

A relatively simple mechanotherapeutic strategy would be to manipulate the elasticity/rigidity of the ECM microenvironment, which profoundly shapes cell migration and differentiation. Several lines of evidence suggest that manipulating this mechanical equilibrium could promote tissue regeneration [61–63]. In particular, fibroblasts have a preference for stiff substrates; thus when they are placed on flexible polyacrylamide sheets, they will migrate from the soft to the stiff side [63]. In the case of breast surgery, this observation could be useful when combined with the observation of Findlay et al. [41], who found that surrounding a pedicled fat flap in a pig groin with a polycarbonate chamber caused the flap to expand to the exact chamber shape. Thus instead of using breast implants, hollow polycarbonate chambers could be implanted subcutaneously around small pedicled fat flaps. Fibrous tissue would eventually cover the inside and outside surfaces of the chamber, while the adipose tissue inside the chamber would expand until stopped by the tension of the stiff fibrotic capsule. Thus simply by manipulating ECM elasticity/rigidity, one could obtain the desired cellular behavior and tissue reactions.

The fact that integrin acts as a mechanosensor and could participate in mechanotherapy has heightened interest in the relationship between integrins and several other cellular mechanosensors, namely, gap junctions, hemichannels, primary cilia, and transient receptor potential channels [1]. Gap junctions are transmembane-spanning channels that are composed of two juxtaposed hemichannels formed by connexins [64]. Primary cilia are the microtubule-based organelles that project from the cell surface. In chondrocytes and endothelial cells, they can serve as mechanosensory organelles that sense compression [65] and compression fluid shear [66], respectively. The transient receptor potential channels are a group of ion channels that are mostly located on plasma membranes. It has been suggested that these channels are important in relaying mechanical stimuli, although they may participate in mechanosensitivity indirectly rather than via their direct activation [67,68].

MECHANOTHERAPY AT THE TISSUE LEVEL

In the clinic, many devices that are based on mechanobiology theory have been developed and used. They include the devices used to rehabilitate and straighten teeth, the scalp massage devices that promote hair growth, the shape memory alloys that straighten curved nails, distraction osteogenesis, the use of shockwaves to destroy kidney stones or accelerate wound healing (extracorporeal shockwave therapy), the negative pressure wound treatment device that accelerates wound healing, tissue expanders that serve to enlarge normal skin, and silicone gel sheets that reduce tension around cutaneous scars. Other procedures that shape mechanobiology at the tissue level include hyperbaric oxygen and lung protective and cardiac offloading strategies.

Negative pressure wound therapy involves applying a porous polyurethane sponge onto a cutaneous wound, sealing it, and applying a vacuum. The vacuum pressure distorts the granulation tissues, thereby causing various cell types to sense the mechanical force and change their behavior [69,70]. As a result, angiogenesis [71], nerve fiber numbers [49], and matrix (granulation tissue) volume increases [49]. This associates with not only a change in gene expression profile and cell morphology [72] but also the accumulation of neuropeptides [49]. This supports the notion that nerve systems relate closely to mechanobiology. It may also explain why negative pressure wound therapy is effective for denervated wounds such as diabetic ulcers.

The shockwaves that are commonly used in extracorporeal shockwave therapy [73] are biphasic high-energy acoustic waves that can be generated by electrohydraulic, electromagnetic, or piezoelectric technologies [1]. Clinical trials have shown that it reduces wound size [74], accelerates reepithelialization after wounding [75], improves the blood flow in wounded skin in a diabetes model [76], decreases the pain associated with chronic ulcers [77], and reduces ischemic necrosis [78]. Tissues that are treated with this technology exhibit increased neovascularization [79], revascularization [80], and collagen synthesis [81]. At the molecular level, it upregulates TGF-β1 and suppresses the production of the proinflammatory cytokines IL-1β, IL-6, and tumor necrosis factor-α [82].

Tissue expanders are widely used for burn and breast reconstruction. They are implanted subcutaneously, and saline solution is gradually injected into the expander over the following weeks. This skin stretching generates new skin that is highly vascular. It has been proposed that this increased vascularity reflects the elaboration of hypoxia-induced factor alpha1, which elevates vascular endothelial growth factor production [83,84]. However, our study with a skin stretching model suggests that the mechanical force that is loaded onto cells can also directly increase angiogenesis [31].

A noninvasive form of soft tissue expansion therapy is the traction-assisted dermatogenesis technique [85]. This technique involves the application of serial intermittent strips of skin tape to the normal skin around defects. The aim is to stretch the normal skin as much as possible so that the resulting lax skin can later be used to cover the defects. Similarly, external volume expansion devices apply force to enhance cell and tissue engraftment and to directly augment tissue volume, mainly for breast augmentation [86]. It is suggested that angiogenesis is increased by mechanical force loading, but fat tissue grows in the results of edema induced by EVE-like adipose tissue deposition in lower limb edema [87].

A widely applied distraction osteogenesis method is the Ilizarov technique. It can effectively correct limb deformities caused by congenital defects, mal- or nonunion open fractures, osteomyelitis, and tumor resection. This method involves the use of the Ilizarov external fixator, which is composed of metal rings, threaded rods, and Kirschner wires. Direct membranous ossification across the distraction gap is induced by turning the nuts on the rods. This eventually results in the bridging of the large bony defect [88]. In a mouse model, distraction osteogenesis was found to activate bone morphogenic protein signaling molecules [89]. In craniofacial complex reconstruction, distraction osteogenesis effectively induces mandibular distraction and widening, ridge augmentation, and midface distraction [90]. Interestingly, high strain was found to induce the formation of fibrous or cartilaginous tissue, whereas low strain induced bone formation [91].

All of the above devices are just a few examples of the many mechanotherapy devices that exist at present. This suggests that many devices that are based on mechanobiology theory could be developed in the near future.

MECHANOTHERAPY FOR DISEASES

Mechanotherapies for specific diseases have already been developed. For example, keloids and hypertrophic scars are fibroproliferative disorders of the skin that are characterized by red, elevated, and chronically inflamed scars. There is increasing evidence that the local microenvironment, especially mechanical force distribution, plays a significant role in the development of these scars [15,92]. First, keloids show a marked preference for sites of the body that are constantly or frequently subjected to mechanical forces (such as the anterior chest and scapular regions); however, they seldom occur in areas where stretching/contraction of the skin is rare (such as the parietal region or anterior lower leg), even in patients with multiple keloids. Second, keloids commonly adopt distinct site-specific shapes (eg, butterfly, crab's claw, or dumbbell shapes) that appear to be largely determined by the direction of the mechanical forces on and around the wound site [92]. Thus it has been suggested that the formation of keloids and hypertrophic scars is driven by mechanosignaling pathway deficiencies [47]. Since these lesions develop in the dermis, it is likely that a better understanding of dermal mechanobiology will help to elucidate their pathogenic mechanisms. The fact that local skin tension plays an important role in these mechanisms explains why tension-reducing flap surgery (eg, z-plasty) and sutures effectively decrease the development and recurrence of these scars [93]. Silicone gel sheeting and taping fixation, which also reduce mechanical force on wounds, are also effective [94].

Mechanobiology also explains the pathogenesis of several nail deformities, namely, koilonychia (characterized by spooning of the nails) and pincer nail (characterized by transverse overcurvature of the nail plate that increases along the longitudinal axis). Our recent studies show that when toenails and fingernails undergo extensive physical stimulation, they tend to have a flat/concave shape; by contrast, toenails and fingernails that receive little stimulation tend to curve inward [95–97]. Our mechanobiology-based hypothesis is that therapies that limit (or increase) the degree of mechanical stimulus on the nail will improve the balance between the automatic curvature force of each nail and the upward mechanical forces, thereby correcting the nail deformity. Such therapies include several current treatments, namely, those that use an elastic wire or plastic device to reinforce the daily upward mechanical force on the nail.

DEVELOPMENT OF NEW MECHANOTHERAPIES FOR TISSUE ENGINEERING

Our increasing understanding of mechanobiology and the development of techniques in mechanobiology research open the door to many potential novel mechanotherapies. This is particularly true for tissue engineering that aims to generate tissue and organs. The appropriate application of mechanical stimuli will help to optimize the stem cell niche and enhance nutrient transport and waste removal (which will improve cell viability); it can also be used to customize scaffold compliance and substrate stiffness and facilitate the synergistic effects of biochemical and mechanical factors. Physical interventions can also be used to directly regulate cell fates and functions into the desired direction.

The field of mechanobiology-based mechanotherapy is expanding. To best exploit it for medical gain, it is necessary to consider our body structure from the perspective of the environment on Earth. The fact that human bodies cannot survive in outer space without spacesuits suggests that the environment has played, and is still playing, an absolutely essential (yet at present, still rather overlooked) role in the evolution of life and multicellular organisms on Earth. We believe that mechanobiology theory promises many viable and novel medical therapies in the near future.

CONCLUSION

We reviewed the concepts of mechanobiology and mechanotherapy and discussed the future of tissue engineering mechanotherapies. The appropriate application of mechanical stimuli will help to optimize the stem cell niche and enhance nutrient transport and waste removal; it can also be used to customize scaffold compliance and substrate stiffness and facilitate the synergistic effects of biochemical and mechanical factors. Physical interventions can also be used to directly regulate cell fates and functions into the desired direction. We believe that mechanobiology theory promises many viable and novel medical therapies in the near future.

REFERENCES

[1] Huang C, Holfeld J, Schaden W, Orgill D, Ogawa R. Mechanotherapy: revisiting physical therapy and recruiting mechanobiology for a new era in medicine. Trends Mol Med September 2013;19(9):555–64.

[2] Ingber DE. Mechanobiology and diseases of mechanotransduction. Ann Med 2003;35(8):564–77.

[3] Martinac B, Kloda A. Evolutionary origins of mechanosensitive ion channels. Prog Biophys Mol Biol May–July 2003;82(1–3):11–24.

[4] Payne MW, Williams DR, Trudel G. Space flight rehabilitation. Am J Phys Med Rehabil July 2007;86(7):583–91.

[5] Guéguinou N, Huin-Schohn C, Bascove M, Bueb JL, Tschirhart E, Legrand-Frossi C, et al. Could spaceflight-associated immune system weakening preclude the expansion of human presence beyond Earth's orbit? J Leukoc Biol November 2009;86(5):1027–38.

[6] Ogawa R, Mizuno S, Murphy GF, Orgill DP. The effect of hydrostatic pressure on three-dimensional chondroinduction of human adipose-derived stem cells. Tissue Eng Part A October 2009;15(10):2937–45.

[7] Strelchenko N, Verlinsky O, Kukharenko V, Verlinsky Y. Morula-derived human embryonic stem cells. Reprod Biomed Online December 2004;9(6):623–9.

[8] Takahashi K, Tanabe K, Ohnuki M, Narita M, Ichisaka T, Tomoda K, et al. Induction of pluripotent stem cells from adult human fibroblasts by defined factors. Cell November 30, 2007;131(5):861–72.

[9] Murata N, Ito S, Furuya K, Takahara N, Naruse K, Aso H, et al. Ca^{2+} influx and ATP release mediated by mechanical stretch in human lung fibroblasts. Biochem Biophys Res Commun October 10, 2014;453(1):101–5.

[10] Huang C, Miyazaki K, Akaishi S, Watanabe A, Hyakusoku H, Ogawa R. Biological effects of cellular stretch on human dermal fibroblasts. J Plast Reconstr Aesthet Surg December 2013;66(12):e351–61.

[11] Li J, Zhang Y, Cui L, Wang J, Pang X, Lai Y, et al. Mechanical stretch changes coronary artery fibroblasts function by upregulating HSF1 protein expression. Int J Biol Macromol August 2013;59:105–10.

[12] Jiang C, Shao L, Wang Q, Dong Y. Repetitive mechanical stretching modulates transforming growth factor-β induced collagen synthesis and apoptosis in human patellar tendon fibroblasts. Biochem Cell Biol October 2012;90(5):667–74.

[13] Tetsunaga T, Furumatsu T, Abe N, Nishida K, Naruse K, Ozaki T. Mechanical stretch stimulates integrin alphaVbeta3-mediated collagen expression in human anterior cruciate ligament cells. J Biomech September 18, 2009;42(13):2097–103.

[14] Ogawa R, Hsu CK. Mechanobiological dysregulation of the epidermis and dermis in skin disorders and in degeneration. J Cell Mol Med July 2013;17(7):817–22.

[15] Ogawa R, Okai K, Tokumura F, Mori K, Ohmori Y, Huang C, et al. The relationship between skin stretching/contraction and pathologic scarring: the important role of mechanical forces in keloid generation. Wound Repair Regen March–April 2012;20(2):149–57.

[16] Tardioli A, Malliaras P, Maffulli N. Immediate and short-term effects of exercise on tendon structure: biochemical, biomechanical and imaging responses. Br Med Bull September 2012;103(1):169–202.

[17] Huang C, Ogawa R. Effect of hydrostatic pressure on bone regeneration using human mesenchymal stem cells. Tissue Eng Part A October 2012;18(19–20):2106–13.
[18] Klein-Nulend J, van der Plas A, Semeins CM, Ajubi NE, Frangos JA, Nijweide PJ, et al. Sensitivity of osteocytes to biomechanical stress in vitro. FASEB J 1995;9:441–5.
[19] Mullender M, El Haj AJ, Yang Y, van Duin MA, Burger EH, Klein-Nulend J. Mechanotransduction of bone cells in vitro: mechanobiology of bone tissue. Med Biol Eng Comput January 2004;42(1):14–21.
[20] Gemmiti CV, Guldberg RE. Fluid flow increases type II collagen deposition and tensile mechanical properties in bioreactor-grown tissue-engineered cartilage. Tissue Eng March 2006;12(3):469–79.
[21] Mizuno S, Tateishi T, Ushida T, Glowacki J. Hydrostatic fluid pressure enhances matrix synthesis and accumulation by bovine chondrocytes in three-dimensional culture. J Cell Physiol December 2002;193(3):319–27.
[22] Mizuno S. A novel method for assessing effects of hydrostatic fluid pressure on intracellular calcium: a study with bovine articular chondrocytes. Am J Physiol Cell Physiol February 2005;288(2):C329–37.
[23] Mizuno S, Ogawa R. Using changes in hydrostatic and osmotic pressure to manipulate metabolic function in chondrocytes. Am J Physiol Cell Physiol June 2011;300(6):C1234–45.
[24] Hdud IM, Mobasheri A, Loughna PT. Effects of cyclic equibiaxial mechanical stretch on α-BK and TRPV4 expression in equine chondrocytes. Springerplus January 29, 2014;3:59.
[25] Mobasheri A, Lewis R, Maxwell JE, Hill C, Womack M, Barrett-Jolley R. Characterization of a stretch-activated potassium channel in chondrocytes. J Cell Physiol May 2010;223(2):511–8.
[26] Pearson AM. Muscle growth and exercise. Crit Rev Food Sci Nutr 1990;29(3):167–96.
[27] Rodriguez J, Vernus B, Chelh I, Cassar-Malek I, Gabillard JC, Hadj Sassi A, et al. Myostatin and the skeletal muscle atrophy and hypertrophy signaling pathways. Cell Mol Life Sci November 2014;71(22):4361–71.
[28] Lyon RC, Zanella F, Omens JH, Sheikh F. Mechanotransduction in cardiac hypertrophy and failure. Circ Res April 10, 2015;116(8):1462–76.
[29] Knöll R, Hoshijima M, Hoffman HM, et al. The cardiac mechanical stretch sensor machinery involves a Z disc complex that is defective in a subset of human dilated cardiomyopathy. Cell 2002;111:943–55.
[30] Takada H, Furuya K, Sokabe M. Mechanosensitive ATP release from hemichannels and Ca^{2+} influx through TRPC6 accelerate wound closure in keratinocytes. J Cell Sci October 01, 2014;127(Pt. 19):4159–71.
[31] Kurita M, Okazaki M, Fujino T, Takushima A, Harii K. Cyclic stretch induces upregulation of endothelin-1 with keratinocytes in vitro: possible role in mechanical stress-induced hyperpigmentation. Biochem Biophys Res Commun May 27, 2011;409(1):103–7.
[32] Chin MS, Ogawa R, Lancerotto L, Pietramaggiori G, Schomacker KT, Mathews JC, et al. In vivo acceleration of skin growth using a servo-controlled stretching device. Tissue Eng Part C Methods June 2010;16(3):397–405.
[33] Collins C, Tzima E. Hemodynamic forces in endothelial dysfunction and vascular aging. Exp Gerontol February–March 2011;46(2–3):185–8.
[34] Shi ZD, Tarbell JM. Fluid flow mechanotransduction in vascular smooth muscle cells and fibroblasts. Ann Biomed Eng June 2011;39(6):1608–19.
[35] Naruse K, Sokabe M. Involvement of stretch-activated ion channels in Ca^{2+} mobilization to mechanical stretch in endothelial cells. Am J Physiol April 1993;264(4 Pt. 1):C1037–44.
[36] Gudi S, Nolan JP, Frangos JA. Modulation of GTPase activity of G proteins by fluid shear stress and phospholipid composition. Proc Natl Acad Sci USA March 03, 1998;95(5):2515–9.
[37] Tzima E, del Pozo MA, Shattil SJ, Chien S, Schwartz MA. Activation of integrins in endothelial cells by fluid shear stress mediates Rho-dependent cytoskeletal alignment. EMBO J September 03, 2001;20(17):4639–47.
[38] Shoham N, Gottlieb R, Sharabani O, Zaretsky U, Benayahu D, Gefen A. Static mechanical stretching accelerates lipid production in 3T3-L1 adipocytes by activating the MEK signaling pathway. Am J Physiol Cell Physiol 2012;302:429–41.
[39] Tanabe Y, Koga M, Saito M, Matsunaga Y, Nakayama K. Inhibition of adipocyte differentiation by mechanical stretching through ERK-mediated downregulation of PPARγ2. J Cell Sci 2004;117:3605–14.

[40] Arner P. Obesity and the adipocyte. Regional adipocity in man. J Endocrinol 1997;155:191–2.
[41] Findlay MW, Dolderer JH, Trost N, et al. Tissue-engineered breast reconstruction: bridging the gap toward large-volume tissue engineering in humans. Plast Reconstr Surg 2011;128:1206–15.
[42] Yuan Y, Ogawa R. Tissue-engineered breast reconstruction: bridging the gap toward large-volume tissue engineering in humans. Plast Reconstr Surg January 2015;135(1):236e–7e.
[43] Xu B, Ju Y, Song G. Role of p38, ERK1/2, focal adhesion kinase, RhoA/ROCK and cytoskeleton in the adipogenesis of human mesenchymal stem cells. J Biosci Bioeng May 2014;117(5):624–31.
[44] Akaishi S, Ogawa R, Hyakusoku H. Keloid and hypertrophic scar: neurogenic inflammation hypotheses. Med Hypotheses 2008;71(1):32–8.
[45] Hayakawa K, Tatsumi H, Sokabe M. Mechano-sensing by actin filaments and focal adhesion proteins. Commun Integr Biol November 01, 2012;5(6):572–7.
[46] Watanabe S, Inagaki S, Kinouchi I, Takai H, Masuda Y, Mizuno S. Hydrostatic pressure/perfusion culture system designed and validated for engineering tissue. J Biosci Bioeng July 2005;100(1):105–11.
[47] Huang C, Akaishi S, Ogawa R. Mechanosignaling pathways in cutaneous scarring. Arch Dermatol Res October 2012;304(8):589–97.
[48] Chin MS, Lancerotto L, Helm DL, Dastouri P, Prsa MJ, Ottensmeyer M, et al. Analysis of neuropeptides in stretched skin. Plast Reconstr Surg July 2009;124(1):102–13.
[49] Younan G, Ogawa R, Ramirez M, Helm D, Dastouri P, Orgill DP. Analysis of nerve and neuropeptide patterns in vacuum-assisted closure-treated diabetic murine wounds. Plast Reconstr Surg July 2010;126(1): 87–96.
[50] Denda M, Sokabe T, Fukumi-Tominaga T, Tominaga M. Effects of skin surface temperature on epidermal permeability barrier homeostasis. J Invest Dermatol March 2007;127(3):654–9.
[51] Huang C, Ogawa R. Mechanotransduction in bone repair and regeneration. FASEB J October 2010;24(10):3625–32.
[52] Huang C, Ogawa R. Fibroproliferative disorders and their mechanobiology. Connect Tissue Res 2012;53(3):187–96.
[53] Ogawa R. Mechanobiology of scarring. Wound Repair Regen September 2011;19(Suppl. 1):s2–9.
[54] Sano H, Ogawa R. Role of mechanical forces in hand nail configuration asymmetry in hemiplegia: an analysis of four hundred thumb nails. Dermatology 2013;226(4):315–8.
[55] Koyama T, Ogawa R, Kobayashi K, Hama T, Hyakusoku H. Effect of stretching force on human hair dermal papilla cells: possibility of manipulating mechanobiology to induce hair regeneration. In: The 7th World Congress for Hair Research (Edinburgh), May 2013.
[56] Varga J, Pasche B. Antitransforming growth factor-beta therapy in fibrosis: recent progress and implications for systemic sclerosis. Curr Opin Rheumatol 2008;20:720–8.
[57] Turner CH, Pavalko FM. Mechanotransduction and functional response of the skeleton to physical stress: the mechanisms and mechanics of bone adaptation. J Orthop Sci 1998;3:346–55.
[58] Wong VW, et al. Focal adhesion kinase links mechanical force to skin fibrosis via inflammatory signaling. Nat Med 2011;18:148–52.
[59] Dalla Costa AP, Clemente CF, Carvalho HF, Carvalheira JB, Nadruz Jr W, Franchini KG. FAK mediates the activation of cardiac fibroblasts induced by mechanical stress through regulation of the mTOR complex. Cardiovasc Res 2010;86:421–31.
[60] Stamenovic D, Ingber DE. Tensegrity-guided self assembly: from molecules to living cells. Soft Matter 2009;5:1137–45.
[61] Paszek MJ, Weaver VM. The tension mounts: mechanics meets morphogenesis and malignancy. J Mammary Gland Biol Neoplasia 2004;9:325–42.
[62] Engler AJ, et al. Matrix elasticity directs stem cell lineage specification. Cell 2006;126:677–89.
[63] Lo CM, et al. Cell movement is guided by the rigidity of the substrate. Biophys J 2006;79:144–52.
[64] Donahue HJ. Gap junctions and biophysical regulation of bone cell differentiation. Bone 2000;26:417–22.

[65] Wann AK, et al. Primary cilia mediate mechanotransduction through control of ATP-induced Ca^{2+} signaling in compressed chondrocytes. FASEB J 2012;26:1663–71.

[66] Nauli SM, et al. Endothelial cilia are fluid shear sensors that regulate calcium signaling and nitric oxide production through polycystin-1. Circulation 2008;117:1161–71.

[67] Patel A, et al. Canonical TRP channels and mechanotransduction: from physiology to disease states. Pflugers Arch 2010;460:571–81.

[68] Christensen AP, Corey DP. TRP channels in mechanosensation: direct or indirect activation? Nat Rev Neurosci 2007;8:510–21.

[69] Saxena V, et al. A set of genes previously implicated in the hypoxia response might be an important modulator in the rat ear tissue response to mechanical stretch. BMC Genomics 2007;8:430.

[70] Orgill DP, Bayer LR. Update on negative-pressure wound therapy. Plast Reconstr Surg 2011;127:105S–15S.

[71] Erba P, Ogawa R, Ackermann M, Adini A, Miele LF, Dastouri P, et al. Angiogenesis in wounds treated by microdeformational wound therapy. Ann Surg 2011;253:402–9.

[72] Lu F, Ogawa R, Nguyen DT, Chen B, Guo D, Helm DL, et al. Microdeformation of three-dimensional cultured fibroblasts induces gene expression and morphological changes. Ann Plast Surg 2011;66:296–300.

[73] Qureshi AA, Ross KM, Ogawa R, Orgill DP. Shock wave therapy in wound healing. Plast Reconstr Surg 2011;128:721e–7e.

[74] Schaden W, et al. Shock wave therapy for acute and chronic soft tissue wounds: a feasibility study. J Surg Res 2007;143:1–12.

[75] Ottomann C, et al. Prospective randomized phase II trial of accelerated reepithelialization of superficial second-degree burn wounds using extracorporeal shock wave therapy. Ann Surg 2012;255:23–9.

[76] Kuo YR, et al. Extracorporeal shock-wave therapy enhanced wound healing via increasing topical blood perfusion and tissue regeneration in a rat model of STZ-induced diabetes. Wound Repair Regen 2009;17:522–30.

[77] Saggini R, et al. Extracorporeal shock wave therapy for management of chronic ulcers in the lower extremities. Ultrasound Med Biol 2008;34:1261–71.

[78] Reichenberger MA, et al. Preoperative shock wave therapy reduces ischemic necrosis in an epigastric skin flap model. Ann Plast Surg 2009;63:682–4.

[79] Wang CJ, et al. Shock wave therapy induces neovascularization at the tendon-bone junction. A study in rabbits. J Orthop Res 2003;21:984–9.

[80] Mittermayr R, et al. Extracorporeal shock wave therapy (ESWT) minimizes ischemic tissue necrosis irrespective of application time and promotes tissue revascularization by stimulating angiogenesis. Ann Surg 2011;253:1024–32.

[81] Yang G, et al. Extracorporeal shock wave treatment improves incisional wound healing in diabetic rats. Tohoku J Exp Med 2011;225:285–92.

[82] Davis TA, et al. Extracorporeal shock wave therapy suppresses the early proinflammatory immune response to a severe cutaneous burn injury. Int Wound J 2009;6:11–21.

[83] Bennett RG, Hirt M. A history of tissue expansion. Concepts, controversies, and complications. J Dermatol Surg Oncol 1993;19:1066–73.

[84] Johnson TM, et al. Histology and physiology of tissue expansion. J Dermatol Surg Oncol 1993;19:1074–8.

[85] Daya M, Nair V. Traction-assisted dermatogenesis by serial intermittent skin tape application. Plast Reconstr Surg 2008;122:1047–54.

[86] Del Vecchio DA, Bucky LP. Breast augmentation using preexpansion and autologous fat transplantation: a clinical radiographic study. Plast Reconstr Surg 2011;127:2441–50.

[87] Heit YI, Lancerotto L, Mesteri I, et al. External volume expansion increases subcutaneous thickness, cell proliferation, and vascular remodeling in a murine model. Plast Reconstr Surg 2012;130:541–7.

[88] Simard S, Marchant M, Mencio G. The Ilizarov procedure: limb lengthening and its implications. Phys Ther January 1992;72(1):25–34.

[89] Haque T, Hamade F, Alam N, Kotsiopriftis M, Lauzier D, St-Arnaud R, et al. Characterizing the BMP pathway in a wild type mouse model of distraction osteogenesis. Bone June 2008;42(6):1144–53.
[90] Maull DJ. Review of devices for distraction osteogenesis of the craniofacial complex. Semin Orthod March 1999;5(1):64–73.
[91] Meyer U, Kruse-Lösler B, Wiesmann HP. Principles of bone formation driven by biophysical forces in craniofacial surgery. Br J Oral Maxillofac Surg August 2006;44(4):289–95.
[92] Akaishi S, Akimoto M, Ogawa R, et al. The relationship between keloid growth pattern and stretching tension: visual analysis using the finite element method. Ann Plast Surg 2008;60:445–51.
[93] Ogawa R, Akaishi S, Huang C, et al. Clinical applications of basic research that shows reducing skin tension could prevent and treat abnormal scarring: the importance of fascial/subcutaneous tensile reduction sutures and flap surgery for keloid and hypertrophic scar reconstruction. J Nippon Med Sch 2011;78:68–76.
[94] Akaishi S, Akimoto M, Hyakusoku H, Ogawa R. The tensile reduction effects of silicone gel sheeting. Plast Reconstr Surg 2010;126:109e–11e.
[95] Sano H, Ichioka S. Influence of mechanical forces as a part of nail configuration. Dermatology 2012;225:210–4.
[96] Sano H, Ogawa R. Role of mechanical forces in hand nail configuration asymmetry in hemiplegia: an analysis of 400 thumb nails. Dermatology 2013;226:315–8.
[97] Sano H, Shionoya K, Ogawa R. Impact of mechanical forces on finger nail curvature: an analysis of the impact of different occupations on 332 finger nails. Dermatol Surg 2014;40:441–5.

PART

4

SMART BIOMATERIALS DEVELOPMENT

CHAPTER

A BIOMIMETIC STRATEGY TO DESIGN BIOMATERIALS FOR IN SITU TISSUE REGENERATION

10

J.H. Kim, S.J. Lee

Wake Forest School of Medicine, Winston-Salem, NC, United States

CHAPTER OUTLINE

INTRODUCTION

Restoration and maintenance of normal function of injured or damaged tissues and organs with biological substitutes is the primary objective of tissue engineering, a major component of regenerative medicine that adheres to standards established in the areas of cell transplantation, materials science, and engineering [1,2]. Engineered tissue constructs that are composed of biomaterial scaffolds preseeded with tissue-specific cells are among the most promising approaches to generate biologically and/or mechanically functional tissue replacements. Clinical applications of tissue engineering and regenerative medicine technologies, however, have been relatively restricted due to the limitation in clinically approved biomaterials [2]. Most of biomaterials that has been developed to date has

In Situ Tissue Regeneration. http://dx.doi.org/10.1016/B978-0-12-802225-2.00010-6

encountered delays in translation to clinical practice, because tissue morphogenesis is greatly influenced by the interactions between cells and the extracellular matrix (ECM) proteins. The conventional simple polymers as a artificial ECM, which have been used historically to provide architectural support for neo-tissue development, poorly mimic the complex interactions between cells and ECM that can promote tissue formation and maturation. Consequently, tissue engineering and regenerative medicine strategies will advance as biomimetic materials that can provide proper microenvironment for tissue regeneration are developed [2–4].

Indeed, nature provides numerous systems that possess exceptional properties and performance that might be replicated for many biomedical applications. Thus scientists have observed phenomena of nature, learned the principles, and incorporated various characteristics to mimic biological systems. For example, the fabric hook-and-loop fastener was inspired by the seeds of the burdock plant [5]. And, adhesive biomaterials have been fabricated by using microfabrication techniques inspired by the feet of the gecko, which have extraordinary climbing ability [5]. Multifunctional biomaterials that mimic the chemical composition, physical structure, and biologically functional moieties of natural living systems could contribute to the development of new biomimetic materials for tissue engineering applications. Accordingly, advanced progresses in tissue engineering and regenerative medicine strategies have led to a paradigm shift in biomaterials research, whereby the concepts of bioinspiration and biomimetics play a more active role in small-scale structures and their time-dependent biological interactions with the host.

This chapter will review the biomimetic materials that contribute to tissue engineering and regenerative medicine strategies to achieve multifunctional and integrated tissues or organs that incorporate biological, chemical, mechanical, topographical, and electrical cues derived from nature, as well as offer space as a scaffold (Fig. 10.1). By reproducing principles or structures of biological systems,

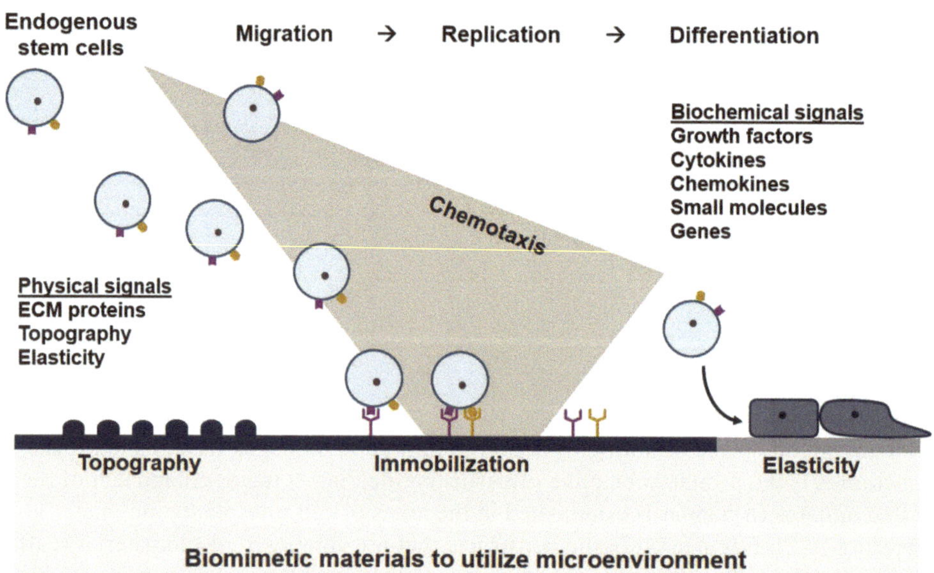

FIGURE 10.1

Schematic illustration of interactions between endogenous stem cells and biomimetic materials. Stem cell fate in a particular microenvironment is regulated by intricate reciprocal molecular interactions with its surroundings.

biomimetic materials offer several aspects of higher-level integration in biological systems: sophistication, miniaturization, hierarchical organizations, hybridization, resistance, and adaptability [6]; moreover, these materials could participate in functional in situ tissue regeneration. The present chapter will describe the current state and trend of biomimetic materials that are being used for tissue engineering and regenerative medicine research.

BIOMIMETIC MATERIALS

This section classifies the biomimetic materials used in tissue engineering and regenerative medicine strategies. Three major approaches of biomimetics are introduced: (1) ECM-mimetic bioactive materials; (2) physicochemical signals for controlling cell fates; and (3) designed structure of peptide-based molecules.

EXTRACELLULAR MATRIX-MIMETIC BIOACTIVE MATERIALS

A variety of synthetic biodegradable polymers have been used as tissue-engineered scaffolds because they possess adjustable mechanical properties, biodegradability, and functionality [3,7]. Synthetic polymers, however, often lack biological recognition. Naturally derived hydrogels, such as fibrin and collagen, have biological functions that enhance cell adhesion, proliferation, and differentiation, which are lacking in synthetic polymers. Therefore synthetic polymers have been modified to mimic ECM functions using short peptide sequences derived from the bioactive domains of ECM components, including adhesive peptides, enzyme-sensitive peptides, and growth factors.

Cell-adhesive or enzyme-sensitive peptides

In the tissue regeneration process, the interactions between cells and tissue-specific ECM are critical, since cell attachment to the ECM regulates various cellular functions such as proliferation, migration, and differentiation [8,9]. Also, the proteolytic degradation of the ECM is an essential feature of cell migration, tissue regeneration, and remodeling [10,11]. Most synthetic biomaterials have inferior cell adhesion ability, and their degradation rates are much slower than naturally derived materials. Therefore synthetic biomaterials have been modified by introducing cell adhesive molecules or enzyme-sensitive peptides to mimic the functions of the ECM.

Several cell-adhesive peptides, such as Arg-Gly-Asp (RGD) derived from fibronectin, Tyr-Ile-Gly-Ser-Arg (YIGSR) and Ile-Lys-Val-Ala-Val (IKVAV) from laminin, Asp-Gly-Glu-Ala (DGEA) and Gly-Phe-Hyp-Gly-Glu-Arg (GFOGER) from collagen, and Val-Ala-Pro-Gli (VAPG) from elastin, have been introduced to the synthetic polymeric biomaterials to improve the cell adhesion capability [12]. Yamada et al. have identified a number of cell-adhesive peptides from laminin, which is a major component of basement membranes [13], and these peptides are potential sources for incorporating cell-binding activities into biomaterial scaffolds for tissue engineering applications. This research group conjugated laminin-derived cell-adhesive peptides, a mixture of A99 (AGTFALRGDNPQG, binds to integrin $\alpha v\beta 3$), AG73 (RKRLQVQLSIRT, binds to syndecans) (A99/AG73), to hyaluronic acid (HA) scaffolds. The A99/AG73-HA scaffolds showed improvement in biological properties, such as cell attachment, cell spreading, and cell viability. In order to accelerate the biodegradability of synthetic polymeric scaffolds, various enzymatic-sensitive peptides, including matrix metalloproteinases

[MMPs, eg, Gly-Pro-Gln-Gly-Ile-Ala-Gly-Gln (GPQGIAGQ), Gly-Pro-Gln-Gly-Ile-Trp-Gly-Gln (GPQGIWGQ), Ala-Pro-Gly-Leu (APGL), and Leu-Gly-Pro-Ala (LGPA)], plasmin [eg, Tyr-Lys-Asn-Arg-Asp (YKNRD) and Val-Arg-Asn (VRN)], and elastase [eg, Ala-Ala-Pro-Val-Arg-Gly-Gly-Gly (AAPVRGGG) and Ala-Ala-Ala-Ala-Ala-Ala-Ala (AAAAAAA)], have been utilized. For instance, Sokic et al. developed cell-adhesive and protease-sensitive peptides with Tyr-Arg-Gly-Asp-Ser (YRGDS) with multiple proteolytic cleavage sites that can be covalently incorporated into the backbone of poly(ethylene glycol) (PEG) that forms hydrogels with enhanced degradation properties and vascularization [14]. In addition, Miller et al. have developed a synthetic approach to mediate degradation rates of cell-adhesive peptide-immobilized PEG using three different types of MMP-sensitive peptides, which, when modified, can support rapid vascular invasion [15].

Growth factor bearing or binding biomaterials

Growth factors, which are naturally occurring substances, are capable of stimulating cell growth, proliferation, and differentiation [16]. For this regard, many researchers have incorporated various growth factors into tissue-engineered scaffolding systems using protein delivery strategies, including direct loading, carrier-encapsulating, and covalent bonding. The simplest approach incorporates growth factors into hydrogels during hydrogel formation. Growth factors are entrapped within the cross-linked hydrogel network and, subsequently, released from the hydrogel network by diffusion [17]. While numerous studies endeavor to deliver growth factors using hydrogels in vivo, the main drawback to the direct loading method is burst release [17,18]. Therefore a variety of protein delivery systems for growth factors have been designed and fabricated, such as micro- or nanoencapsulation. This method of encapsulation allows for sustainable release of growth factors and prevents rapid degradation within tissues [19]. Wei et al. have reported that platelet-derived growth factor-BB (PDGF-BB) incorporated in poly(lactide-*co*-glycolide) (PLGA) nanoparticles could be released in a controlled fashion poly(lactide-*co*-glycolide [20]. Xie et al. have shown that glycidyl methacrylate dextran and gelatin-based nanoparticles could provide sustained release of vascular endothelial growth factor (VEGF) to induce angiogenesis in vivo [21]. Growth factors can also be covalently attached to the hydrogel network. Various functional groups, such as thiol, acrylate, and azide, have been used for covalent binding of growth factors. Moon et al. developed synthetic, biomimetic PEG hydrogels conjugated with VEGF, MMP-sensitive peptides, and cell-adhesive peptides [22]. Their study showed that the rapid formation of a stable and mature vascular network was promoted by the provision of an angiogenic environment.

In the body, spatial localization and activity of growth factors can be controlled by glycosaminoglycans (GAGs), such as heparin, chondroitin sulfate, and HA [23]. One of the representative methods to mimic the growth factor binding mechanism of GAGs includes utilization of heparin or heparin-binding peptides (HBPs). Because their application is limited to certain growth factors that have an affinity for GAGs, this method effectively maintains stability of growth factors and provides their controlled release. Our group developed heparin-conjugated electrospun poly(ε-caprolactone) (PCL)/gelatin scaffolds to provide controlled release and prolonged bioactivity of PDGF-BB to enhance interactions between smooth muscle cells (SMCs) and the scaffold material [24]. The heparin-conjugated scaffolds allow the immobilization of PDGF-BB via electrostatic interactions. A combination of the large pore structure in the scaffolds and the heparin-mediated delivery of PDGF-BB provides controlled release of PDGF-BB and promotes effective cellular infiltration. In addition, Rajangam et al. have developed heparin-binding hydrogels that contain a heparin-binding domain to bind heparin (HBPA) as well as other growth factors of interest (Fig. 10.1A) [25]. The results suggested that the conformation of heparin on nanostructures exhibiting the consensus sequence of the HBPA molecules is optimal for bioactivity and that heparin binding to synthetic peptides and the consequent interaction with proteins are highly specific.

Advanced studies indicate that the delivery of a single growth factor may be insufficient to recapitulate natural complex processes, so attention has turned to novel delivery approaches that allow the release of multiple growth factors at different doses and release rates [26,27]. Richardson et al. suggested a multiple protein delivery system for accelerating vascularization and tissue formation because the development of tissues and organs is typically driven by the action of a number of growth factors [28]. They reported a novel polymeric system that allows for the tissue-specific delivery of two or more growth factors with controlled dose and rate of delivery. Controlling sustained release of multiple growth factors with different release kinetics enables effective tissue regeneration. Likewise, Chen et al. have shown various methods of sustained release of bioactive molecules [29]. The sustained release of multiple growth factors mimics in vivo tissue regeneration and contributes to effective and rapid tissue regeneration. Another study in skeletal muscle regeneration has shown effective and functional skeletal muscle regeneration using alginate that simultaneously released insulin-like growth factor-1 and VEGF [30]. In addition to increased angiogenesis, a functional skeletal muscle tissue with activation of muscle satellite cells was created; furthermore, this delivery system of combined multiple growth factors displays potential for enhanced tissue regeneration in vivo.

PHYSICOCHEMICAL SIGNALS FOR CONTROLLING CELL FATES

Cells are exposed to a tissue-specific microenvironment in vivo, and they respond to numerous chemical and physical stimuli. As a result, cellular functions like cell adhesion and proliferation, protein synthesis, and cytoskeletal architecture are critically influenced by the microenvironment of the cells. To maintain the phenotype expression and differentiation of tissue-specific cells, numerous cues have been applied to biomaterial scaffolds to mimic natural ECM microenvironments. Especially, the growth and specific differentiation of stem cells (embryonic or adult) are significantly affected by their microenvironments, including chemical, topographical, mechanical, and electrical cues. The following section will introduce these cues that are addressed in in situ tissue regeneration.

Bioactive molecules for controlling stem cell fates

Bioactive molecules (or signaling molecules), including proteins and small molecules, involved in tissue regeneration play an important role in controlling the microenvironment in vivo. Chemotactic signals from bioactive molecules are responsible for inducing host cell mobilization; moreover, an anatomic destination is identified according to certain concentration gradients of chemicals produced at injured sites within the microenvironment. Bioactive molecules are able to regulate host cell migration, proliferation, and differentiation and allow cells to interact via specific receptors for chemical recognition with their surrounding microenvironment. Thus incorporation of a suitable bioactive molecule through the design of a tissue-engineered scaffold can promote tissue regeneration by stimulating the transplanted cells or adjacent host cells.

Bioactive signals can directly stimulate stem cells and control tissue-specific differentiation in vitro. Additionally, these signals can be integrated with scaffolding materials to induce differentiation of specific cell types in vivo. Specific differentiation of stem cells from bioactive signals is being investigated actively. Chemical agents, including dexamethasone, ascorbic acid, and β-glycerophosphate, have been used for osteogenic differentiation [31]. For chondrogenic differentiation, a pelleted cell aggregate has been treated with transforming growth factor-β or bone morphogenic protein (BMP) families [32,33]. Neural differentiation of stem cells has been achieved using insulin, retinoic acid, nerve growth factor (NGF), basic fibroblast growth factor (bFGF), or brain-derived neurotrophic factor [34]. Amniotic fluid-derived stem cells (AFSCs) have been used as a stem cell source for tissue engineering applications [35,36]. Our group has demonstrated that AFSCs have important and unique features that may lead to novel and successful applications toward the regeneration of a composite tissue (bone and cartilage) in a single scaffolding system that incorporates biochemical signals [37]. We have developed a bilayered scaffolding system that includes a starch/PCL scaffold for osteogenesis and an agarose hydrogel for chondrogenesis, and we studied the influence of medium supplements in the osteogenic and chondrogenic differentiations of AFSCs [38]. Additionally, we investigated the induction of pancreatic development in AFSCs following combination of adenoviral-delivered Pdx1transduction and biochemical signals from activin A, bFGF, and nicotinamide [39].

Another approach to recruit host stem cells into the targeted sites in vivo is through chemotactic signals. The body has an endogenous healing mechanism involving several recruiting factors to mobilize host stem cells or progenitor cells to the injured site for tissue regeneration. Thus many researchers have been inspired by in situ tissue regeneration, which induces mobilization of host stem cells and controls cell differentiation into tissue-specific cell types [40]. Unlike cell-based tissue engineering, this strategy eliminates donor cell procurement and ex vivo cell manipulation. Stem cell recruiting or inducing factors that have been applied to mobilize host stem cells include stromal cell-derived factor-1, substance P, granulocyte colony-stimulating factor, and granulocyte-macrophage colony-stimulating factor [41,42]. For successful tissue regeneration by host stem cell recruitment, it is essential to direct stem cells to the site of interest and to provide the recruited stem cells with a local microenvironment that mimics the ECM to promote proliferation and differentiation.

Substrates with controlled topographical cues

The interactions of cells with biomaterials are critically important for the successful outcome of tissue engineering applications. Thus the behavior of cells grown on a biomaterial surface, including adhesion to the material, development of appropriate cellular structures, and maintenance of proper cell phenotype and function, must be investigated to identify the characteristics of the biomaterial. Cells encounter topographical cues in the form of the physical features of their surrounding microenvironment. The topography of the surface of a biomaterial can directly influence cell adhesion and proliferation, which further affects cellular functions. It has been determined that natural ECM has a nano-scaled fibrous protein structure that supports cellular interactions and stimulates cellular functions. This substrate nanoscale topography provides a tool for investigating complex cell functions such as adhesion, migration, cytoskeleton reorganization, and cell polarization [43,44]. Thus researchers have attempted to develop nano-scaled fibrous scaffolds that mimic the structure of the natural ECM using a variety of fabrication methods, including self-assembly, phase separation, and electrospinning.

Among the fabrication methods used, electrospinning technology offers many advantages that include the production of nano-scaled fibers with spatial orientation, high aspect ratio, high surface area, and controlled pore geometry, depending on target configurations. This electrospinning process allows for fabrication of tissue-engineered scaffolds with a nano-scaled topography, high porosity, and interconnectivity similar to natural ECM. In addition, many parameters can be optimized to enhance cellular growth and function in vitro and in vivo, leading to improved cell adhesion, cellular expression, and diffusion of oxygen and nutrients [45]. A variety of natural materials and synthetic polymers have been intricately fabricated with aligned, multilayered, core-shelled, hybrid, and protein-loaded nanofibers [46]. We have demonstrated that aligned nanofibers assist muscle cell organization and enhance myotube formation [47]. The myotubes formed on aligned nanofibrous scaffolds are highly organized and are significantly longer than myotubes formed on randomly oriented scaffolds (Fig. 10.2A). The diameter of the myotubes was comparable between the aligned and randomly oriented nanofiber scaffolds; however, the myotubes on the aligned nanofibrous scaffolds are double the length of the myotubes on the randomly oriented scaffolds [47]. These findings indicate that electrospun aligned nanofibrous scaffolds are better able to guide and orient skeletal muscle cells into organized structures that closely mimic native tissues. To enhance infiltration of SMCs into the vascular scaffold, we have developed an electrospun bilayered scaffolding system that provides a variety of pore sizes to facilitate adequate cellular interactions [48]. This bilayered scaffolding system permits endothelial cell (EC) adhesion on the lumen and SMC infiltration into the outer layer and mimics the native vessel structure.

Substrate elasticity/stiffness and mechanical cues

Physical contact of cells on substrates is essential to anchorage dependence and function. While stem cell differentiation induced by soluble biochemical signals has been well established, current findings reveal that stem cell fates can be significantly influenced by the substrate elasticity/stiffness from the surrounding microenvironment. For example, neural cell differentiation can be induced on soft matrices, which mimic brain tissue, while myogenic and osteogenic differentiation require stiffer matrices that mimic muscle and collagenous bone, respectively. Soft matrices that mimic brain are neurogenic, stiffer matrices that mimic muscle are myogenic, and comparatively rigid matrices that mimic collagenous bone prove osteogenic [49]. Several studies have demonstrated specific stem cell differentiation can be achieved using substrates or matrices with particular surface elasticity/stiffness. Modification of the cross-linking degree of polymeric hydrogels is the basis of substrate-controlled elasticity. To mimic the matrix elasticity, Engler et al. used polyacrylamide gels in which the concentration of bis-acrylamide cross-linking determines elasticity [49]. The substrate stiffness increases cell adhesion and cytoskeletal organization (Fig. 10.2B). They observed the effect of the substrate elasticity using cultures of bone marrow-derived mesenchymal stem cells (MSCs), which can be differentiated into neurons, myoblasts, and osteoblasts. Identification of the substrate elasticity/stiffness of a target tissue was found to be important for efficient regeneration in tissue engineering applications. We have studied the interaction of AFSCs with substrates of varying elasticity [50]. AFSCs cultured on substrates of varying elasticity exhibited significant changes in cell proliferation, morphology, and increased MSC surface marker (CD44, CD90, CD105, and N-cadherin) expression [50]. Therefore we strongly suggest that mimicking the physical characteristics of biomaterials and culture microenvironments to specific physiological values will improve efficacy of stem cell therapy applications.

External mechanical stimuli are also important for maintaining phenotype, controlling stem cell differentiation, and establishing functional tissues [51]. Tissues can experience compressive forces, or tensile forces such as mechanical loading or stretch, and fluid-applied forces such as shear flow. Chemical cues, including growth factors and cytokines, are well-known regulators of cell behavior and stem cell differentiation. Interestingly, these chemical cues are strongly modified by mechanical cues, which modify cell morphology, function, and differentiation [51]. Therefore to provide mechanical forces to cells in vivo or in vitro, external mechanical stimuli have been artificially applied for stem cell differentiation and functional tissue regeneration. In response to compression, native cartilage responds through altered matrix synthesis, cell metabolism, and chondrogenesis [52]. Thus mechanical compression could be an effective method of enhancing the development of tissue-engineered cartilage both

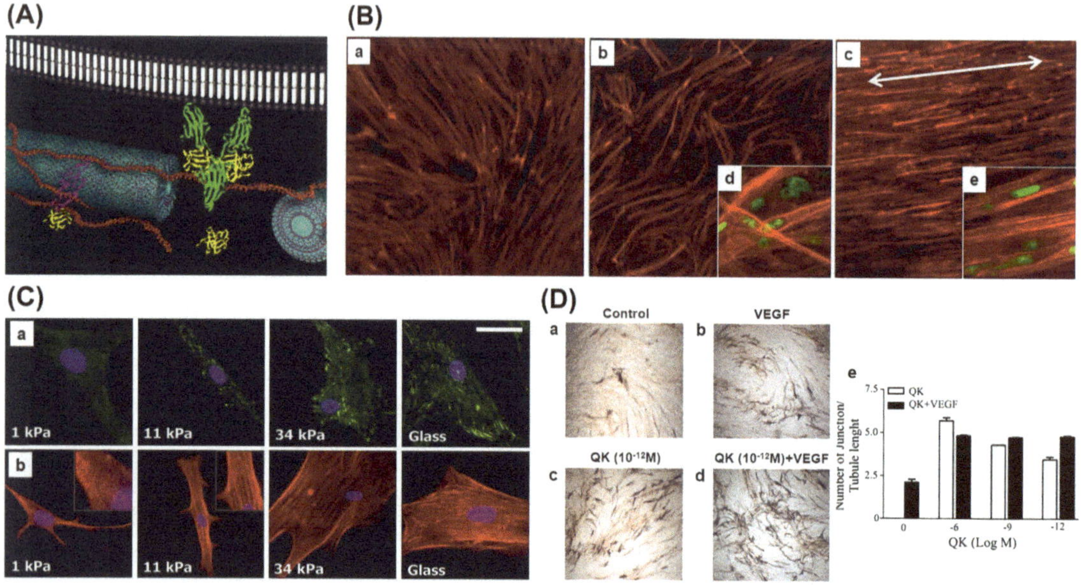

FIGURE 10.2

(A) Schematic illustration of heparin-nucleated HBPA nanofibers interacting with growth factors and receptors. The HBPA nanofibers (blue) are shown with adsorbed heparin chains on them (red). Heparin is known to bind and activate VEGF (purple), FGF-2 (yellow), and FGF receptor (green). The schematic proposes that the heparin–FGF-2–FGF receptor complex is further stabilized by their anchoring on HBPA nanofibers. *(Reprinted from Rajangam K, Arnold MS, Rocco MA, Stupp SI. Peptide amphiphile nanostructure-heparin interactions and their relationship to bioactivity. Biomaterials 2008;29:3298–305.)* (B) Immunofluorescent images of F-actin of skeletal muscle cells on electrospun PCL/collagen nanofibers: (a) culture dish, (b) randomly oriented, and (c) aligned electrospun nanofibers (×40 magnification). Laser confocal microscopy images of F-actin of skeletal muscle cells seeded on the (d) randomly oriented and (e) aligned electrospun nanofibers (×600 magnification). *(Reprinted from Choi JS, Lee SJ, Christ GJ, Atala A, Yoo JJ. The influence of electrospun aligned poly(epsilon-caprolactone)/collagen nanofiber meshes on the formation of self-aligned skeletal muscle myotubes. Biomaterials 2008;29:2899–906.)* (C) Adhesions grow and cytoskeletal organization increases with substrate stiffness: (a) Paxillin-labeled adhesions grow from undetectable diffuse "contacts" on neurogenic, soft gels (1 kPa) to punctate adhesions on stiffer, myogenic gels (11 kPa). On the stiffest, osteogenic gels (34 kPa), the adhesions are long, thin, and slightly more peripheral than they appear on glass. (b) F-actin organization shows a similar trend, from diffuse on soft gels to progressively organized on stiffer substrates (as stress fibers). *(Reprinted from Engler AJ, Sen S, Sweeney HL, Discher DE. Matrix elasticity directs stem cell lineage specification. Cell 2006;126:677–89.)* Scale bar is 20 μm. (D) In vitro angiogenic properties of QK. Human ECs were cocultured with other human cells in a specially designed medium in a 24-well plate. Every 3 days, QK alone (c) or a combination of QK and VEGF165 (100 ng/mL) (d) was added. On the 11th day, cells were fixed with ice cold 70% ethanol, and tubule formation was visualized by staining for antihuman CD31 [Platelet endothelial cell adhesion molecule (PECAM-1)]. (a–d) Sample images are reported. Suramine (20 μM) (a) and VEGF165 (b) were used as negative and positive controls, respectively. (e) The number of cellular connections and the total tubule length were determined by using software that analyzes the images after digitalization. *(Reprinted from D'Andrea LD, Iaccarino G, Fattorusso R, Sorriento D, Carannante C, Capasso D, et al. Targeting angiogenesis: structural characterization and biological properties of a de novo engineered VEGF mimicking peptide. Proc Natl Acad Sci USA 2005;102:14215–20.)*

in vitro and in vivo. Many studies have employed compressive forces in the development of artificial cartilage, and short-term (>24 h) compression has been shown to stimulate the accumulation of cartilage-like ECM and increase chondrocyte-like gene expression [53]. In addition, specifically designed bioreactor devices have been developed to influence in vivo adaptive physical stimulation that include compression as well as shear, hydrostatic pressure, and combinations thereof to generate artificial cartilage [52].

In the musculoskeletal system, tensional forces, which arise from movement of articulated tissues, are critical to cell differentiation. Powell et al. developed mechanical cell stimulator hardware to apply in vivo-like forces directly to the engineered muscle tissue fabricated by a suspension of muscle cells in collagen/Matrigel [54]. Following eight days of repetitive stretch/relaxation, the elasticity, myofiber diameter, and myofiber area of the engineered muscle tissue were increased [54]. To improve the contractility of engineered skeletal muscle, we have developed an in vitro preconditioning protocol that uses a cyclic strain in a computer-controlled bioreactor system [55]. The in vitro bioreactor preconditioning of the engineered skeletal muscle caused acceleration of tissue maturation and improved contractility of subsequently implanted muscle constructs in vivo.

Fluid shear stress is another important mechanical force, which is frequently applied in cardiovascular tissue engineering [56]. Shear flow reportedly promotes endothelial differentiation of MSCs or endothelial progenitor cells, as well as cardiac differentiation of embryonic stem cells [57]. To mimic shear flow, bioreactors have been applied to engineered heart and blood vessels. In cardiac tissue engineering, for example, researchers have constructed a perfusion bioreactor that provides pulsatile fluid flow resulting in physiologically relevant shear stresses and flow rates [56]. Lee et al. have designed a perfusion system that allows direct investigation of the effects of shear stress on the development of microvasculature [58]. Coculture of ECs and MSCs in a porous collagen gel and in the presence of a bulk fluid flow field has resulted in the formation of microvasculature in a biomimetic environment [58].

Electrical stimuli

A biomimetic system has been designed to deliver electrical signals similar to those of native tissue. The results observed include progressive development of conductive and contractile properties of tissue such as cardiac, neural, and muscular tissues. In cardiac tissue engineering, electrical stimulation has been frequently applied to stimulate tissue contractility. The Vunjak-Novakovic group has a well-designed protocol for tissue engineering of synchronously contractile cardiac constructs where cultured cardiac cells with pulsatile electrical fields mimic the native heart [59].

Additionally, electrical stimulation can promote nerve regeneration when applied to the proximal nerve stump and has become a promising guiding cue to promote axonal regeneration in nerve injury repair. A microenvironment with electrical stimulation localized at the conductive scaffold has been shown to accelerate nerve regeneration and promote functional recovery in a 15-mm nerve defect in rats [60]. The Schmidt group has also developed an electrospun PLGA nanofiber scaffold with a nanometer-thick coating of electrically conducting polypyrrole for applications in neural engineering applications [61]. NGF was chemically conjugated to the scaffolds, and electrical stimulation of neural cells on the NGF-conjugated scaffolds was shown to improve neurite development when compared to unstimulated cells on the NGF-conjugated scaffolds [61]. The combination of a neurotrophic factor and electrical stimulation appears to be a promising approach for neural tissue engineering applications.

DESIGNED STRUCTURE OF PEPTIDE-BASED MOLECULES

Biomimetic materials are desirable as tissue engineered scaffolds because they mimic the native microenvironment of the ECM. Successfully designed scaffold materials should include synthetic peptide-based molecules (short peptide sequences and peptide amphiphiles) to develop biomaterial scaffolding systems. Peptide sequences could provide biological, chemical, mechanical, and structural functions that are inspired from nature [62]. Supramolecular self-assembly of specific designed peptide sequences to fabricate biomimetic materials has shown promise in in situ tissue regeneration.

Growth factor-mimicking peptides

Biomimetic materials have been developed by conjugating synthetic peptide sequences to biomaterials. Growth factor-derived peptides can be directly applied to the polymeric biomaterials. While the covalent bonding strategy may cause structural damages to the biomaterial due to modifications of growth factors, this method prevents the initial burst release of growth factors from the scaffold. The development of VEGF-mimicking peptides, named QK peptides, has been favored to promote angiogenesis and has replaced recombinant VEGF proteins [63,64]. Another growth factor, the BMP-derived peptide (KIPKASSVPTELSAISTLYL), has been used to induce osteogenic differentiation of MSCs. He et al. have developed a poly(lactide-*co*-ethylene oxide fumarate) (PLEOF) hydrogel combined with RGD, BMP, and osteopontin (OPN, SVVYGLR) peptides that provides a favorable microenvironment for osteogenic and vasculogenic differentiation of MSCs [65].

Peptide amphiphiles

A feature of protein self-assembly is the ability to form nanoscale structures with remarkable structural specificity [66], which has inspired the field of self-assembled scaffolding systems and the potential to provide unique therapeutic strategies for tissue regeneration. Chemical cross-linking, which can result in toxicity, shrinkage, or limited degradation rates, remains a drawback to using traditional hydrogels [67]. An alternative approach includes the design of self-assembled peptides or proteins using fully degradable small molecules [68,69]. Supramolecular chemistry, which encompasses self-assembling peptide-based molecules held together by noncovalent intermolecular forces, favors larger and more complicated assemblies [70,71].

Peptide amphiphiles, or peptide-based molecules, have dual hydrophobic and hydrophilic characteristics with the functionality of delivering bioactive molecules to the site of interest. The chemical composition of peptide amphiphiles includes four structural features: (1) the hydrophobic domain for self-assembly and typically consists of a long alkyl tail; (2) a short peptide sequence that is capable of forming intermolecular hydrogen bonding; (3) charged amino acids for enhanced solubility and specific pH and salt responsive nanostructures; and (4) the presentation of bioactive signals, usually through epitopes that can interact with cells or proteins. The self-assembling peptides are composed of 8–16 amino acids and are characterized by periodic repeats of alternating ionic hydrophilic and hydrophobic amino acids [66]. Once assembled, reversible and stable β-sheet structures composed of fibers (5–10 nm) are formed in water. Hydrophobic van der Waals interactions, which combine with an array of ionic and peptide backbone hydrogen bonds, serve as the driving force behind self-assembling peptides. Under physiological conditions, the peptides form fibers that gel and self-assemble into 3-D microenvironments, which closely mimic the porosity and ECM-like structure with elevated hydration. These structures are made less immunogenic and less toxic due to the use of synthetic amino acids [68,72]; therefore, self-assembling peptides are promising candidates for scaffold materials in tissue engineering and regenerative medicine.

Self-assembling peptides have been applied to a variety of tissue repairs and establish a suitable microenvironment for normal cellular functions. Ellis-Behnke et al. and Guo et al. have shown that self-assembling peptides provide a 3-D microenvironment similar to ECM and enable the regeneration of axons by preventing scar tissue formation in the damaged brain [73,74]. Self-assembling peptides have also been shown to enhance angiogenesis through recruitment of vascular ECs and promotion of capillary-like formation [75,76]. Along with angiogenic potential, self-assembling peptides aid local sustained delivery of various angiogenic factors into myocardium [77]. Lin et al. have reported that injection of RADA16-II along with MSCs can increase retention and differentiation of transplanted cells as well as increase angiogenesis after infarction [78]. Active and functional motifs from the ECM have been employed to significantly enhance the interactions of self-assembling peptides with cells and tissues. Kim et al. have reported that the sustained delivery of a specific combination of growth factors, bFGF and PDGF-BB, with hydrogels composed of self-assembling peptides resulted in improved cardiac function and formation of mature vessels in infarcted hearts [77]. Furthermore, Kim et al. have developed bioactive peptides by immobilizing substance P into self-assembling peptides; consequently, these bioactive peptides are becoming valuable tools for treatment of ischemia-induced tissue damage due to recruitment of autologous MSCs and promotion of angiogenesis without cell transplantation [41]. Designer self-assembling peptides, which are directly coupled with biologically active and functional peptide motifs, are actively being studied [72,79].

The Stupp group has designed peptide amphiphiles that form cylindrical nanofibers under physiological conditions [69,80]. The incorporation of peptide epitopes into networks of peptide amphiphile assemblies allows for both structural and functional mimicry of native ECM. The use of cell-binding epitopes, including RGDS and IKVAV, as bioactive sequences on peptide amphiphiles has been investigated for a variety of regenerative medicine applications [81–83]. The IKVAV epitope has been incorporated into peptide amphiphiles as a bioactive sequence for neural applications [82].

SUMMARY AND FUTURE PERSPECTIVES

Development of in situ tissue regeneration strategies continues to be a critical component of the research pursuits in the field of tissue engineering and regenerative medicine [2]. Future advances in these strategies rely on the development of the biomimetic materials that can utilize microenvironment for efficient tissue regeneration and better integration with host tissue. Desirable biomimetic materials could be designed as a smart scaffolding system that mimics the natural biological system and integrates the necessary structural and biological properties (Table 10.1). Thorough understanding of materials science, combined with extensive knowledge of the clinical challenges and cell biology, is vital for development of clinically applicable biomaterials to be used for in situ tissue regeneration. Therefore interdisciplinary collaboration between materials scientists, engineers, cell biologists, physiologists, and clinicians should be encouraged to develop novel biomimetic materials for in situ tissue regeneration that might enhance or improve regenerative medicine therapies.

Table 10.1 Biomimetic Materials for Tissue Engineering Applications

	Scaffold Design	Biomimetic	Outcomes	References
Nervous tissue	Electrospun PCL fibers and multichannel nerve guides	Fascicular architecture and fibrous ECM found in native nerve	A greater number of defined paths Schwann cells infiltration into channels	[84]
	Conductive PPy/chitosan scaffold	Local electrical environments	Acceleration of nerve regeneration and functional recovery	[60]
Epithelial tissue	Microwell patterned PDMS scaffolds coated with fibronectin	Small intestinal crypt-villus surface topography	Protrusions extending to microwell side walls of small intestinal epithelial cells	[85]
Cartilage	PEG containing the pendant photo-cleavable peptide sequence	The physical and chemical properties of native tissue	Chondrogenic differentiation of encapsulated MSCs, temporal and spatial regulation of the 3-D culture	[86]
	Agarose hydrogel with dynamic compression	Compression circumstances of native cartilage	Accumulation of proteoglycan and chondrocyte-like gene expression	[53]
Bone	Adhesive PLEOF hydrogel grafted with osteopontin and BMP-derived peptides	ECM-mimic geometry with bioactive molecules	Osteogenic and vasculogenic differentiation of MSCs, high extent of mineralization	[65]
	Polyacrylamide hydrogels coated with type I collagen	Matrix stiffness	Osteogenic differentiation of MSCs	[87]
Musculoskeletal tissues	Water-responsible dynamic PEE-rigid PPy composite film	Rigid and elastic network structure of animal dermis	Rapid and continuous locomotion, expansion, and contraction driven by water gradients	[88]
	Electrospun aligned fibrous scaffolds/microgrooved methacrylated gelatin hydrogels	Native muscle fiber architecture	Aligned myoblasts and muscle-like fibrous structure formation	[47,89]
Cardiovascular tissues	Bilayered electrospun PCL/collagen vascular scaffolds	Blood vessel structure	EC adhesion on the lumen and SMC infiltration into the outer layer	[48]
	Heparin-biding peptides amphiphiles	Protein self-assembly and molecular-scale matrix–heparin microstructure	Binding of growth factors mediated by heparin induces new blood vessel formation in vivo	[90]
Immune system	Nanoporous silicon particles coated with cellular membranes from leukocytes	Leukocyte-based biomimetic camouflage	Avoided opsonization and improved accumulation in a tumor	[91]
	Substance P-immobilized self-assembling peptides	Wound healing process in nature with chemical factors	Recruiting MSCs and promoting angiogenesis	[41]

BMP, *bone morphogenetic protein-2;* ECM, *extracellular matrix;* MSC, *mesenchymal stem cells;* PCL, *poly(ε-carprolactone);* PDMS, *poly(dimethylsiloxane);* PEE, *pentaerythritol ethoxylate;* PEG, *polyethylene glycol;* PLEOF, *poly(lactide-co-ethylene oxide fumarate);* PPy, *polypyrrole.*

LIST OF ACRONYMS AND ABBREVIATIONS

AFSCs Amniotic fluid-derived stem cells
BDGF Brain-derived neurotrophic factor
bFGF Basic fibroblast growth factor
BMP Bone morphogenic protein
ECM Extracellular matrix
ECs Endothelial cells
EPCs Endothelial progenitor cells
ESCs Embryonic stem cells
GAGs Glycosaminoglycans
G-CSF Granulocyte colony-stimulating factor
GM-CSF Granulocyte-macrophage colony-stimulating factor
HA Hyaluronic acid
HBPs Heparin-binding peptides
IGF-1 Insulin-like growth factor-1
MMPs Matrix metalloproteinases
MSCs Bone marrow-derived mesenchymal stem cells
NGF Nerve growth factor
PCL Poly(ε-caprolactone)
PDGF-BB Platelet-derived growth factor-BB
PDMS Poly(dimethylsiloxane)
PECAM-1 Platelet endothelial cell adhesion molecule
PEE Pentaerythritol ethoxylate
PEG Poly(ethylene glycol)
PLEOF Poly(lactide-*co*-ethylene oxide fumarate)
PLGA Poly(lactide-*co*-glycolide)
PPy Polypyrrole
SDF-1α Stromal cell-derived factor-1α
SMCs Smooth muscle cells
TGF-β Transforming growth factor-β
VEGF Vascular endothelial growth factor

ACKNOWLEDGMENTS

The authors thank Dr. Heather Hatcher for editorial assistance. This study was supported by the Basic Science Research Program through the National Research Foundation of Korea (NRF) funded by the Ministry of Education, Science and Technology (NRF-2012R1A6A3A03040684).

REFERENCES

[1] Atala A. Tissue engineering of reproductive tissues and organs. Fertil Steril 2012;98:21–9.
[2] Atala A, Kasper FK, Mikos AG. Engineering complex tissues. Sci Transl Med 2012;4:160rv12.
[3] Pashuck ET, Stevens MM. Designing regenerative biomaterial therapies for the clinic. Sci Transl Med 2012;4:160sr4.
[4] Furth ME, Atala A, Van Dyke ME. Smart biomaterials design for tissue engineering and regenerative medicine. Biomaterials 2007;28:5068–73.

[5] Geim AK, Dubonos SV, Grigorieva IV, Novoselov KS, Zhukov AA, Shapoval SY. Microfabricated adhesive mimicking gecko foot-hair. Nat Mater 2003;2:461–3.
[6] Sanchez C, Arribart H, Guille MM. Biomimetism and bioinspiration as tools for the design of innovative materials and systems. Nat Mater 2005;4:277–88.
[7] Nair LS, Laurencin CT. Polymers as biomaterials for tissue engineering and controlled drug delivery. Adv Biochem Eng Biotechnol 2006;102:47–90.
[8] Rhodes JM, Simons M. The extracellular matrix and blood vessel formation: not just a scaffold. J Cell Mol Med 2007;11:176–205.
[9] Scott JE. Extracellular matrix, supramolecular organisation and shape. J Anat 1995;187(Pt 2):259–69.
[10] Shin H, Jo S, Mikos AG. Biomimetic materials for tissue engineering. Biomaterials 2003;24:4353–64.
[11] Lutolf MP, Hubbell JA. Synthetic biomaterials as instructive extracellular microenvironments for morphogenesis in tissue engineering. Nat Biotechnol 2005;23:47–55.
[12] Rahmany MB, Van Dyke M. Biomimetic approaches to modulate cellular adhesion in biomaterials: a review. Acta Biomater 2013;9:5431–7.
[13] Yamada Y, Hozumi K, Katagiri F, Kikkawa Y, Nomizu M. Laminin-111-derived peptide-hyaluronate hydrogels as a synthetic basement membrane. Biomaterials 2013;34:6539–47.
[14] Sokic S, Papavasiliou G. Controlled proteolytic cleavage site presentation in biomimetic PEGDA hydrogels enhances neovascularization in vitro. Tissue Eng Part A 2012;18:2477–86.
[15] Miller JS, Shen CJ, Legant WR, Baranski JD, Blakely BL, Chen CS. Bioactive hydrogels made from step-growth derived PEG-peptide macromers. Biomaterials 2010;31:3736–43.
[16] Chen RR, Mooney DJ. Polymeric growth factor delivery strategies for tissue engineering. Pharm Res 2003;20:1103–12.
[17] Hiemstra C, Zhong Z, van Steenbergen MJ, Hennink WE, Feijen J. Release of model proteins and basic fibroblast growth factor from in situ forming degradable dextran hydrogels. J Control Release 2007;122:71–8.
[18] Lin CC, Anseth KS. PEG hydrogels for the controlled release of biomolecules in regenerative medicine. Pharm Res 2009;26:631–43.
[19] Lee K, Silva EA, Mooney DJ. Growth factor delivery-based tissue engineering: general approaches and a review of recent developments. J R Soc Interface 2011;8:153–70.
[20] Wei G, Jin Q, Giannobile WV, Ma PX. Nano-fibrous scaffold for controlled delivery of recombinant human PDGF-BB. J Control Release 2006;112:103–10.
[21] Xie J, Wang H, Wang Y, Ren F, Yi W, Zhao K, et al. Induction of angiogenesis by controlled delivery of VEGF using nanoparticles. Cardiovasc Ther 2013;31:e12–8.
[22] Moon JJ, Saik JE, Poche RA, Leslie-Barbick JE, Lee SH, Smith AA, et al. Biomimetic hydrogels with pro-angiogenic properties. Biomaterials 2010;31:3840–7.
[23] Schultz GS, Wysocki A. Interactions between extracellular matrix and growth factors in wound healing. Wound Repair Regen 2009;17:153–62.
[24] Lee J, Yoo JJ, Atala A, Lee SJ. The effect of controlled release of PDGF-BB from heparin-conjugated electrospun PCL/gelatin scaffolds on cellular bioactivity and infiltration. Biomaterials 2012;33:6709–20.
[25] Rajangam K, Arnold MS, Rocco MA, Stupp SI. Peptide amphiphile nanostructure-heparin interactions and their relationship to bioactivity. Biomaterials 2008;29:3298–305.
[26] Xu W, Atala A, Yoo JJ, Lee SJ. Controllable dual protein delivery through electrospun fibrous scaffolds with different hydrophilicities. Biomed Mater 2013;8:014104.
[27] Chen FM, Zhang M, Wu ZF. Toward delivery of multiple growth factors in tissue engineering. Biomaterials 2010;31:6279–308.
[28] Richardson TP, Peters MC, Ennett AB, Mooney DJ. Polymeric system for dual growth factor delivery. Nat Biotechnol 2001;19:1029–34.
[29] Chen FM, An Y, Zhang R, Zhang M. New insights into and novel applications of release technology for periodontal reconstructive therapies. J Control Release 2011;149:92–110.

[30] Borselli C, Storrie H, Benesch-Lee F, Shvartsman D, Cezar C, Lichtman JW, et al. Functional muscle regeneration with combined delivery of angiogenesis and myogenesis factors. Proc Natl Acad Sci USA 2010;107:3287–92.
[31] Jaiswal N, Haynesworth SE, Caplan AI, Bruder SP. Osteogenic differentiation of purified, culture-expanded human mesenchymal stem cells in vitro. J Cell Biochem 1997;64:295–312.
[32] Bosnakovski D, Mizuno M, Kim G, Ishiguro T, Okumura M, Iwanaga T, et al. Chondrogenic differentiation of bovine bone marrow mesenchymal stem cells in pellet cultural system. Exp Hematol 2004;32:502–9.
[33] Shen B, Wei A, Whittaker S, Williams LA, Tao H, Ma DD, et al. The role of BMP-7 in chondrogenic and osteogenic differentiation of human bone marrow multipotent mesenchymal stromal cells in vitro. J Cell Biochem 2010;109:406–16.
[34] Krabbe C, Zimmer J, Meyer M. Neural transdifferentiation of mesenchymal stem cells – a critical review. Apmis 2005;113:831–44.
[35] De Coppi P, Bartsch Jr G, Siddiqui MM, Xu T, Santos CC, Perin L, et al. Isolation of amniotic stem cell lines with potential for therapy. Nat Biotechnol 2007;25:100–6.
[36] Joo S, Ko IK, Atala A, Yoo JJ, Lee SJ. Amniotic fluid-derived stem cells in regenerative medicine research. Arch Pharm Res 2012;35:271–80.
[37] Rodrigues MT, Lee BK, Lee SJ, Gomes ME, Reis RL, Atala A, et al. The effect of differentiation stage of amniotic fluid stem cells on bone regeneration. Biomaterials 2012;33:6069–78.
[38] Rodrigues MT, Lee SJ, Gomes ME, Reis RL, Atala A, Yoo JJ. Bilayered constructs aimed at osteochondral strategies: the influence of medium supplements in the osteogenic and chondrogenic differentiation of amniotic fluid-derived stem cells. Acta Biomater 2012;8:2795–806.
[39] Chun SY, Mack DL, Moorefield E, Oh SH, Kwon TG, Pettenati MJ, et al. Pdx1 and controlled culture conditions induced differentiation of human amniotic fluid-derived stem cells to insulin-producing clusters. J Tissue Eng Regen Med 2015;9:540–9.
[40] Lee SJ, Van Dyke M, Atala A, Yoo JJ. Host cell mobilization for in situ tissue regeneration. Rejuvenation Res 2008;11:747–56.
[41] Kim JH, Jung Y, Kim BS, Kim SH. Stem cell recruitment and angiogenesis of neuropeptide substance P coupled with self-assembling peptide nanofiber in a mouse hind limb ischemia model. Biomaterials 2013;34:1657–68.
[42] Ko IK, Ju YM, Chen T, Atala A, Yoo JJ, Lee SJ. Combined systemic and local delivery of stem cell inducing/recruiting factors for in situ tissue regeneration. FASEB J 2012;26:158–68.
[43] Bettinger CJ, Langer R, Borenstein JT. Engineering substrate topography at the micro- and nanoscale to control cell function. Angew Chem Int Ed Engl 2009;48:5406–15.
[44] Ross AM, Jiang Z, Bastmeyer M, Lahann J. Physical aspects of cell culture substrates: topography, roughness, and elasticity. Small 2012;8:336–55.
[45] Li WJ, Laurencin CT, Caterson EJ, Tuan RS, Ko FK. Electrospun nanofibrous structure: a novel scaffold for tissue engineering. J Biomed Mater Res 2002;60:613–21.
[46] Norman JJ, Desai TA. Methods for fabrication of nanoscale topography for tissue engineering scaffolds. Ann Biomed Eng 2006;34:89–101.
[47] Choi JS, Lee SJ, Christ GJ, Atala A, Yoo JJ. The influence of electrospun aligned poly(epsilon-caprolactone)/collagen nanofiber meshes on the formation of self-aligned skeletal muscle myotubes. Biomaterials 2008;29:2899–906.
[48] Ju YM, Choi JS, Atala A, Yoo JJ, Lee SJ. Bilayered scaffold for engineering cellularized blood vessels. Biomaterials 2010;31:4313–21.
[49] Engler AJ, Sen S, Sweeney HL, Discher DE. Matrix elasticity directs stem cell lineage specification. Cell 2006;126:677–89.
[50] Skardal A, Mack D, Atala A, Soker S. Substrate elasticity controls cell proliferation, surface marker expression and motile phenotype in amniotic fluid-derived stem cells. J Mech Behav Biomed Mater 2013;17:307–16.

[51] Maul TM, Chew DW, Nieponice A, Vorp DA. Mechanical stimuli differentially control stem cell behavior: morphology, proliferation, and differentiation. Biomech Model Mechanobiol 2011;10:939–53.
[52] Schulz RM, Bader A. Cartilage tissue engineering and bioreactor systems for the cultivation and stimulation of chondrocytes. Eur Biophys J 2007;36:539–68.
[53] Kisiday JD, Frisbie DD, McIlwraith CW, Grodzinsky AJ. Dynamic compression stimulates proteoglycan synthesis by mesenchymal stem cells in the absence of chondrogenic cytokines. Tissue Eng Part A 2009;15:2817–24.
[54] Powell CA, Smiley BL, Mills J, Vandenburgh HH. Mechanical stimulation improves tissue-engineered human skeletal muscle. Am J Physiol Cell Physiol 2002;283:C1557–65.
[55] Moon du G, Christ G, Stitzel JD, Atala A, Yoo JJ. Cyclic mechanical preconditioning improves engineered muscle contraction. Tissue Eng Part A 2008;14:473–82.
[56] Brown MA, Iyer RK, Radisic M. Pulsatile perfusion bioreactor for cardiac tissue engineering. Biotechnol Prog 2008;24:907–20.
[57] Krawiec JT, Vorp DA. Adult stem cell-based tissue engineered blood vessels: a review. Biomaterials 2012;33:3388–400.
[58] Lee EJ, Niklason LE. A novel flow bioreactor for in vitro microvascularization. Tissue Eng Part C Methods 2010;16:1191–200.
[59] Tandon N, Cannizzaro C, Chao PH, Maidhof R, Marsano A, Au HT, et al. Electrical stimulation systems for cardiac tissue engineering. Nat Protoc 2009;4:155–73.
[60] Huang J, Lu L, Zhang J, Hu X, Zhang Y, Liang W, et al. Electrical stimulation to conductive scaffold promotes axonal regeneration and remyelination in a rat model of large nerve defect. PLoS One 2012;7:e39526.
[61] Lee JY, Bashur CA, Milroy CA, Forciniti L, Goldstein AS, Schmidt CE. Nerve growth factor-immobilized electrically conducting fibrous scaffolds for potential use in neural engineering applications. IEEE Trans Nanobioscience 2012;11:15–21.
[62] Altunbas A, Pochan DJ. Peptide-based and polypeptide-based hydrogels for drug delivery and tissue engineering. Top Curr Chem 2012;310:135–67.
[63] Webber MJ, Tongers J, Newcomb CJ, Marquardt KT, Bauersachs J, Losordo DW, et al. Supramolecular nanostructures that mimic VEGF as a strategy for ischemic tissue repair. Proc Natl Acad Sci USA 2011;108:13438–43.
[64] D'Andrea LD, Iaccarino G, Fattorusso R, Sorriento D, Carannante C, Capasso D, et al. Targeting angiogenesis: structural characterization and biological properties of a de novo engineered VEGF mimicking peptide. Proc Natl Acad Sci USA 2005;102:14215–20.
[65] He X, Yang X, Jabbari E. Combined effect of osteopontin and BMP-2 derived peptides grafted to an adhesive hydrogel on osteogenic and vasculogenic differentiation of marrow stromal cells. Langmuir 2012;28:5387–97.
[66] Loo Y, Zhang S, Hauser CA. From short peptides to nanofibers to macromolecular assemblies in biomedicine. Biotechnol Adv 2012;30:593–603.
[67] Billiet T, Vandenhaute M, Schelfhout J, Van Vlierberghe S, Dubruel P. A review of trends and limitations in hydrogel-rapid prototyping for tissue engineering. Biomaterials 2012;33:6020–41.
[68] Zhang S, Gelain F, Zhao X. Designer self-assembling peptide nanofiber scaffolds for 3D tissue cell cultures. Semin Cancer Biol 2005;15:413–20.
[69] Cui H, Webber MJ, Stupp SI. Self-assembly of peptide amphiphiles: from molecules to nanostructures to biomaterials. Biopolymers 2010;94:1–18.
[70] Menger FM, Azov VA. Synthesis and properties of water-soluble asterisk molecules. J Am Chem Soc 2002;124:11159–66.
[71] Estroff LA, Hamilton AD. Water gelation by small organic molecules. Chem Rev 2004;104:1201–18.
[72] Horii A, Wang X, Gelain F, Zhang S. Biological designer self-assembling peptide nanofiber scaffolds significantly enhance osteoblast proliferation, differentiation and 3-D migration. PLoS One 2007;2:e190.

[73] Ellis-Behnke RG, Liang YX, You SW, Tay DK, Zhang S, So KF, et al. Nano neuro knitting: peptide nanofiber scaffold for brain repair and axon regeneration with functional return of vision. Proc Natl Acad Sci USA 2006;103:5054–9.
[74] Guo J, Leung KK, Su H, Yuan Q, Wang L, Chu TH, et al. Self-assembling peptide nanofiber scaffold promotes the reconstruction of acutely injured brain. Nanomedicine 2009;5:345–51.
[75] Davis ME, Motion JP, Narmoneva DA, Takahashi T, Hakuno D, Kamm RD, et al. Injectable self-assembling peptide nanofibers create intramyocardial microenvironments for endothelial cells. Circulation 2005;111:442–50.
[76] Narmoneva DA, Oni O, Sieminski AL, Zhang S, Gertler JP, Kamm RD, et al. Self-assembling short oligopeptides and the promotion of angiogenesis. Biomaterials 2005;26:4837–46.
[77] Kim JH, Jung Y, Kim SH, Sun K, Choi J, Kim HC, et al. The enhancement of mature vessel formation and cardiac function in infarcted hearts using dual growth factor delivery with self-assembling peptides. Biomaterials 2011;32:6080–8.
[78] Lin YD, Yeh ML, Yang YJ, Tsai DC, Chu TY, Shih YY, et al. Intramyocardial peptide nanofiber injection improves postinfarction ventricular remodeling and efficacy of bone marrow cell therapy in pigs. Circulation 2010;122:S132–41.
[79] Gelain F, Horii A, Zhang S. Designer self-assembling peptide scaffolds for 3-D tissue cell cultures and regenerative medicine. Macromol Biosci 2007;7:544–51.
[80] Stupp SI. Self-assembly and biomaterials. Nano Lett 2010;10:4783–86.
[81] Webber MJ, Tongers J, Renault MA, Roncalli JG, Losordo DW, Stupp SI. Development of bioactive peptide amphiphiles for therapeutic cell delivery. Acta Biomater 2010;6:3–11.
[82] Silva GA, Czeisler C, Niece KL, Beniash E, Harrington DA, Kessler JA, et al. Selective differentiation of neural progenitor cells by high-epitope density nanofibers. Science 2004;303:1352–5.
[83] Tysseling VM, Sahni V, Pashuck ET, Birch D, Hebert A, Czeisler C, et al. Self-assembling peptide amphiphile promotes plasticity of serotonergic fibers following spinal cord injury. J Neurosci Res 2010;88:3161–70.
[84] Jeffries EM, Wang Y. Biomimetic micropatterned multi-channel nerve guides by templated electrospinning. Biotechnol Bioeng 2012;109:1571–82.
[85] Wang L, Murthy SK, Fowle WH, Barabino GA, Carrier RL. Influence of micro-well biomimetic topography on intestinal epithelial Caco-2 cell phenotype. Biomaterials 2009;30:6825–34.
[86] Kloxin AM, Kasko AM, Salinas CN, Anseth KS. Photodegradable hydrogels for dynamic tuning of physical and chemical properties. Science 2009;324:59–63.
[87] Shih YR, Tseng KF, Lai HY, Lin CH, Lee OK. Matrix stiffness regulation of integrin-mediated mechanotransduction during osteogenic differentiation of human mesenchymal stem cells. J Bone Miner Res 2011;26:730–8.
[88] Ma M, Guo L, Anderson DG, Langer R. Bio-inspired polymer composite actuator and generator driven by water gradients. Science 2013;339:186–9.
[89] Hosseini V, Ahadian S, Ostrovidov S, Camci-Unal G, Chen S, Kaji H, et al. Engineered contractile skeletal muscle tissue on a microgrooved methacrylated gelatin substrate. Tissue Eng Part A 2012;18:2453–65.
[90] Rajangam K, Behanna HA, Hui MJ, Han X, Hulvat JF, Lomasney JW, et al. Heparin binding nanostructures to promote growth of blood vessels. Nano Lett 2006;6:2086–90.
[91] Parodi A, Quattrocchi N, van de Ven AL, Chiappini C, Evangelopoulos M, Martinez JO, et al. Synthetic nanoparticles functionalized with biomimetic leukocyte membranes possess cell-like functions. Nat Nanotechnol 2013;8:61–8.

CHAPTER

IMPACT OF MATRIX DYNAMIC PROPERTIES ON STEM CELL VIABILITY

11

M.B. Taraban, Y. Li, K.A. Joyner, J.P. Stains, Y.B. Yu
University of Maryland, Baltimore, MD, United States

CHAPTER OUTLINE

INTRODUCTION

Modern regenerative medicine focuses on tissue replacement and/or repair via transplantation of the stem cell to a patient in need [1]. It is the most challenging task to find a cue, physical or chemical, which allows to efficiently direct the differentiation of the stem cells and to promote their proliferation. Since early 2000s [2], stiffness became a major consideration in the design of artificial extracellular matrices (ECMs) for stem cells in prospective tissue repair/regeneration applications. Indeed, among all other properties, physical factors of the stem cell's environment, its viscoelastic properties, such as stiffness, contribute significantly to stem cell survival and targeted transformation into desired tissue cells. For example, tuning the elasticity of the supportive scaffold could serve as an effective tool to regulate the expansion of hematopoietic [3] and skeletal muscle stem cells [4]. Proper selection of scaffold stiffness stimulates chondrocytes to develop true cartilage-like ECMs, with the properties very close to mechanically functional tissues [5].

The sensitivity of stem cells toward the physical parameters of ECMs provides a tool to control cell biology by using the scaffold material with preprogrammed physical characteristics [6]. Of these, stiffness is widely believed to be the most important regulator of stem cell growth, differentiation [7], and even malignization [8]. But it is difficult to isolate stiffness from other ECM parameters for investigation. For example, the chemical composition of ECM could affect the adhesion of stem cells to the matrix. Another factor is porosity, which is, of course, related to stiffness, and defines the space

In Situ Tissue Regeneration. http://dx.doi.org/10.1016/B978-0-12-802225-2.00011-8

available for stem cells. Numerous attempts have been made to isolate stiffness from other ECM attributes in order to assess its impact on stem cells. When the stiffness of acrylamide-based hydrogels was varied without changing the porosity and ligand tethering, it was concluded that stiffness alone could control the adipogenic and osteogenic differentiation of stem cells [7]. However, in this case, the hydrogel stiffness was changed by varying the ratio between acrylamide and *bis*-acrylamide [7]. This, of course, resulted in other structural and chemical differences in addition to difference in stiffness. In another study, Ca^{2+} was used to tune the stiffness of alginate-based hydrogels. It was shown that changes in the stiffness alone without variation of basement membrane ligands could trigger the proliferation of malignant phenotypes of epithelial cells [8]. However, the introduction of Ca^{2+}, especially in the form of the low soluble $CaSO_4$, does more than changing the stiffness of alginate hydrogels. It is also capable of eliciting significant structural changes in the 3-D organization of the alginate chain network, such as correlation length, fiber thickness, entanglement points of the network, etc. Even though it was not possible to fully separate the influence stiffness from other factors, such as porosity [7] or ECM composition [8], it was nonetheless concluded that it is the scaffolds stiffness rather than any other ECM attributes that controls stem cell biology.

The stiffness of a viscoelastic material is often represented by its shear modulus G, which has both elastic (G') and viscous (G'') components with $G=(G'^2+G''^2)^{1/2}$. In solid-like viscoelastic hydrogels, $G' >> G''$, thus the stiffness is determined largely by the elastic modulus G'. On the other hand, the viscous modulus G'' reflects the capability of a biomaterial to dissipate the energy of ECM deformation. Indeed, it has been demonstrated [9] that the increase in the viscous modulus of polyacrylamide hydrogels promotes the proliferation and differentiation of human mesenchymal stem cells (hMSCs).

While G (or G') captures the static aspect of the viscoelasticity of a soft material, it misses its dynamic aspect, which reflects the capacity of such a material to release stress—its stress relaxation capability. This is because shear modulus data are usually collected at a single oscillatory angular frequency and thereby contain little dynamic information. However, one might expect that the ability of a matrix to release mechanical stress should have a significant impact on stem cell behavior. The dynamic properties of ECMs could mediate the interaction between stem cells and ECMs over the course of cell proliferation and/or differentiation by reducing the mechanical tension generated during cell growth. Hence, properly designed ECMs should be responsive to the stress generated by cells, similar to native biological tissues. Indeed, in 2013 it has been shown [10] that hydrogel networks capable to adapt to stress exerted by myoblasts better stimulate cell proliferation as opposed to more rigid ECMs. Comparison of covalently cross-linked elastic (almost zero stress relaxation) and ionically cross-linked viscoelastic (significant stress relaxation) alginate hydrogels [11] shows that the latter promote much greater spreading of cells on such substrates. These observations lead to the conclusion that stress relaxation capability of ECMs might have significant influence on stem cells.

Mechanical properties of ECMs could be also altered due to posttranslational modifications (PTMs) of ECM proteins in a number of pathologies. For example, cancer cells are known to remodel ECMs by introducing PTMs, which increase stiffness, thus enhancing tumor cell migration or metastasis [12]. Among a wide range of different PTMs, N-terminal acetylation and C-terminal amidation are two very common modifications of a protein [13]. Posttranslational acetylation of N-terminal is known to occur in more than 80% of human proteins [14]. Amidation of C-terminal might promote the stability and activity of a protein and provides for better binding of a protein to cell receptor [13]. One might reasonably expect that PTMs could also change the dynamic properties of ECMs, as a result, modulating cells' behavior.

In this chapter, we explore the impact of ECM dynamic properties on stem cells. Specifically, we assess how the dynamic properties of engineered ECM affect the viability of hMSCs. Such an assessment requires the isolation of the impact dynamic properties from that of stiffness and chemical composition. To this end, we prepared a pair of hydrogels of the identical stiffness and nearly identical chemical composition. They are assembled from oligopeptides with identical amino acid sequences, the only difference being acetylation and amidation of N- and C-terminals, respectively, mimicking two very common PTMs. This subtle difference nonetheless produced hydrogels with very different dynamic properties, as revealed by the relaxation spectral analysis of the shear modulus of the two hydrogels. Cell culture data show that this difference in the relaxation spectra of the two hydrogels leads to significant difference in hMSC viability. Specifically, greater relaxation capability at shorter relaxation times, a result of higher fiber flexibility, better supports stem cell growth.

Understanding the effects of relaxation characteristics of ECM will allow one to use PTMs to tune the material properties to provide ECMs, which will be highly beneficial for stem cell proliferation and will widen the range of tools to regulate their differentiation and survival.

VIABILITY OF HUMAN MESENCHYMAL STEM CELLS IN TWO HYDROGELS

In an attempt to single out the influence of the dynamic properties of the matrix on the viability of hMSCs, we compared two hydrogels with nearly identical chemical composition. One hydrogel was constructed from a pair of oppositely charged undecapeptides with the sequences *acetyl-KW(KA)$_3$KWK-amide* (***K***$^{6+}$, carrying six positive charges at neutral pH) and *acetyl-EW(EA)$_3$-EWE-amide* (***E***$^{6-}$, carrying six negative charges at neutral pH). To construct another hydrogel, the *N*-terminal acetyl group in ***K***$^{6+}$ was removed, leading to a peptide carrying seven positive charges at neutral pH (*H$_3$N$^+$-KW(KA)$_3$KWK-amide*, ***K***$^{7+}$), while the *C*-terminal amide group in ***E***$^{6-}$ was removed, leading to a peptide carrying seven negative charges at neutral pH (*acetyl-EW(EA)$_3$EWE-COO$^-$*, ***E***$^{7-}$). Four undecapeptides, ***K***$^{6+}$ and ***E***$^{6-}$ (6-charged), and ***K***$^{7+}$ and ***E***$^{7-}$ (7-charged) were synthesized (Table 11.1), as described in details in our earlier work [15].

These peptide sequences were based on the design principle of self-repulsion but mutual attraction [16]. Gelation is initiated by mixing oppositely charged peptides. The advantage of mixing-induced gelation (coassembly) over other modes of gelation initiation (eg, pH, salt, heat, etc., in self-assembling

Table 11.1 Sequence, Molecular Weight, and Charges of Undecapeptides

Peptide Module Sequences	Charges	M.W. (Da)
acetyl-KW(KA)$_3$KWK-*amide* (***K***$^{6+}$)	+6	1413
H$_3$N$^+$-KW(KA)$_3$KWK-*amide* (***K***$^{7+}$)	+7	1372
acetyl-EW(EA)$_3$EWE-*amide* (***E***$^{6-}$)	−6	1419
acetyl-EW(EA)$_3$EWE-COO$^-$ (***E***$^{7-}$)	−7	1420

A, alanine; E, glutamic acid; K, lysine; W, tryptophan. Terminal charges are controlled by blocking N- *or* C-*terminals by the acetyl or amide groups, respectively.*

peptide hydrogels) is that it preserves the physiological pH, ionic strength, and temperature of the original peptide solutions. As a result, the hydrogels are highly biocompatible. For example, the resulting hydrogels preserve the native conformation of encapsulated protein molecules [17]. Also, the hydrogels can support stem cell growth [18].

These hydrogels have been extensively characterized. Here is a brief summary of their properties most relevant to stem cell growth. These hydrogels are shear responsive [16], a feature that makes them injectable. From the standpoint of mechanical stiffness, the optimal chain length of the peptides is 8–12 amino acid residues [19,20]. The hydrogels slow down the diffusion of small molecules to a modest 10–15%, and the exact extent of slowing down increases linearly with the $\log P_{oct}$ value (the 1-octanol/water partition coefficient) of the diffusant [21]. The relative free diffusion of small molecules (nutrients, wastes, etc.) inside the hydrogels is important for using these hydrogels to grow stem cells. Structurally, the hydrogels comprise of peptide nanofibers, as revealed by small-angle X-ray and neutron scattering studies [19,22]. Such nanofibers provide anchoring points for stem cells. Additional properties of these hydrogels, including their interaction with polysaccharide, dependence of their properties on chirality, temperature, ionic strength, and charge distribution, as well as the prospect of their applications in contrast agents for MRI, can be found in our published works [15,23–33]. The potential of these hydrogels in drug delivery and tissue repair applications was also reviewed in a previous publication [34].

The synthesis was performed using an automated peptide synthesizer based on standard solid phase fluorenylmethyloxycarbonyl chemistry [35]. After cleavage and purification, 16mM stock solutions of each peptide in phosphate buffered saline (PBS) buffer (pH 7.4) were used for hydrogel assembly. One hydrogel, made by mixing $\boldsymbol{K^{6+}}$ and $\boldsymbol{E^{6-}}$ at 1:1 M ratio, is denoted as $\boldsymbol{K^{6+}E^{6-}}$. Another hydrogel, denoted as $\boldsymbol{K^{7+}E^{7-}}$, was made by mixing $\boldsymbol{K^{7+}}$ and $\boldsymbol{E^{7-}}$ at 1:1 M ratio. This approach minimizes the chemical difference between the two hydrogels. Also, the peptide sequences were designed to avoid any motifs known to promote specific binding of the peptides to cell membranes.

hMSCs were grown in these two hydrogels in both 3-D (in the scaffolds volume) and 2-D (on the scaffolds surface) fashions, with collagen as the control. For 3-D culture, hMSCs (50,000 cells/well) were mixed with an equal volume of the respective peptide solution ($\boldsymbol{K^{7+}E^{7-}}$ or $\boldsymbol{K^{6+}E^{6-}}$) or rat-tail collagen (control). Cell-containing peptide solutions were then added to a 96-well plate and allowed to set at 37°C in a 5% CO_2 incubator. The following day, fresh media were added to the cultures. For the 2-D cell culture, the respective peptide solutions or rat-tail collagen were coated onto the wells of a 96-well plate and allowed to dry overnight. Subsequently, hMSCs (50,000 cells/well) were seeded onto the coated wells. At day 7 of culture, cell proliferation and viability were assessed using a Cell Counting Kit-8 (CCK-8) colorimetric assay according to the manufacturer's (Dojindo Molecular Technologies) directions. Experiments were repeated a minimum of three times with triplicate wells; the resulting cell counts were averaged and standard deviations calculated. Statistical comparison was conducted using ANOVA for unpaired samples with a Tukey's *post hoc* test, using the *Prism 6* software. A p-value $<.05$ was used as the threshold for statistical significance.

In both 3-D and 2-D cultures, $\boldsymbol{K^{7+}E^{7-}}$ support hMSCs proliferation better than $\boldsymbol{K^{6+}E^{6-}}$ (Fig. 11.1). Since $\boldsymbol{K^{7+}E^{7-}}$ and $\boldsymbol{K^{6+}E^{6-}}$ have almost identical chemical composition, one might have attributed their difference in supporting hMSCs growth to a difference in stiffness. However, comparison of the mechanical properties of $\boldsymbol{K^{7+}E^{7-}}$ and $\boldsymbol{K^{6+}E^{6-}}$ hydrogels revealed a quite unexpected result.

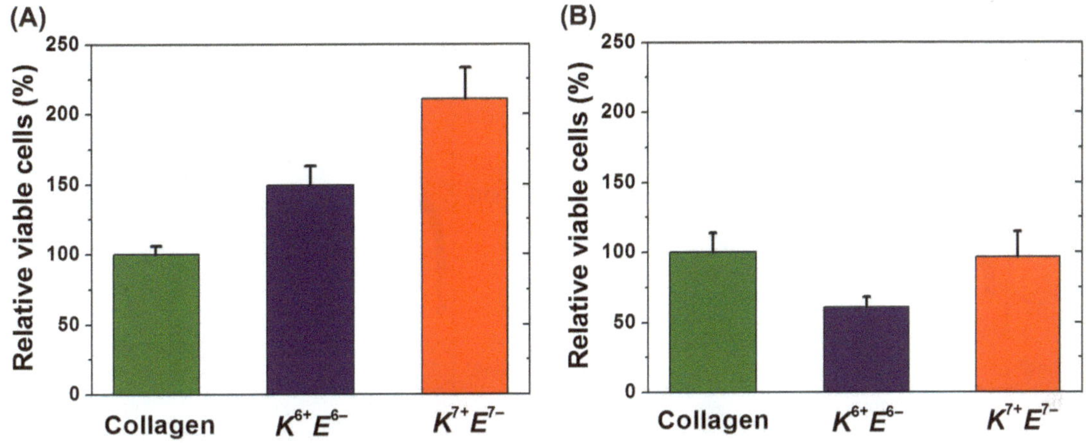

FIGURE 11.1 Viability of hMSCs examined by the CCK-8 assay after 7 days.

(A) 3-D culture; (B) 2-D culture. Cell count in the collagen control (■) is set to 100%. Data are represented as means ± standard deviations, which confirm the statistical significance of the observed differences. Data for the $K^{7+}E^{7-}$ hydrogel (■) show that it is more beneficial for cell growth than the $K^{6+}E^{6-}$ hydrogel (■) in both 3-D and 2-D cell cultures.

STIFFNESS AND RELAXATION SPECTRA OF TWO HYDROGELS

Hydrogels for oscillatory rheological experiments were prepared by mixing the solutions of two oppositely charged peptides (16 mM each) through a Y-shaped connector in the humidified sealed cell of the rheometer, followed by time sweep monitoring of the hydrogelation process at 25°C. The sequence of rheological experiments and the experimental setup for longtime monitoring of gelation has been described in details in our earlier work [25]. The formation of hydrogels was monitored in time sweep measurements; strain amplitude $\gamma = 0.2\%$ and angular frequency $\omega = 1$ rad/s. Frequency sweep measurements at identical normal force (~3.0 N) were done at $\gamma = 0.2\%$ within the ω range from 0.01 to 100 rad/s with 18 data points per frequency decade.

As it is seen from the rheological measurements, $K^{7+}E^{7-}$ and $K^{6+}E^{6-}$ have very similar stiffness, as judged by the plateau shear modulus $G \sim 80$ kPa (Fig. 11.2A). Both gels form dynamic viscoelastic networks with $G' >> G''$. At the same time, despite the identical G values observed at fixed angular frequency ($\omega = 1$ rad/s), noticeable differences in the frequency spectra of $K^{7+}E^{7-}$ and $K^{6+}E^{6-}$ in the higher frequency range are detected (Fig. 11.2B). These observations point to possible distinctive features of the dynamic network behavior of the two hydrogels. The differences in dynamic properties of two equally stiff hydrogels could be revealed through the analysis of relaxation spectra.

The relaxation spectra of $K^{7+}E^{7-}$ and $K^{6+}E^{6-}$ hydrogels were derived from their corresponding frequency sweep data (Fig. 11.2B) using the computer program for Bayesian analysis, *BayesRelax* [36]. Theory and applications of the advanced Bayesian analysis approach to derive the relaxation spectra from the frequency sweep data were discussed in detail and illustrated using the frequency

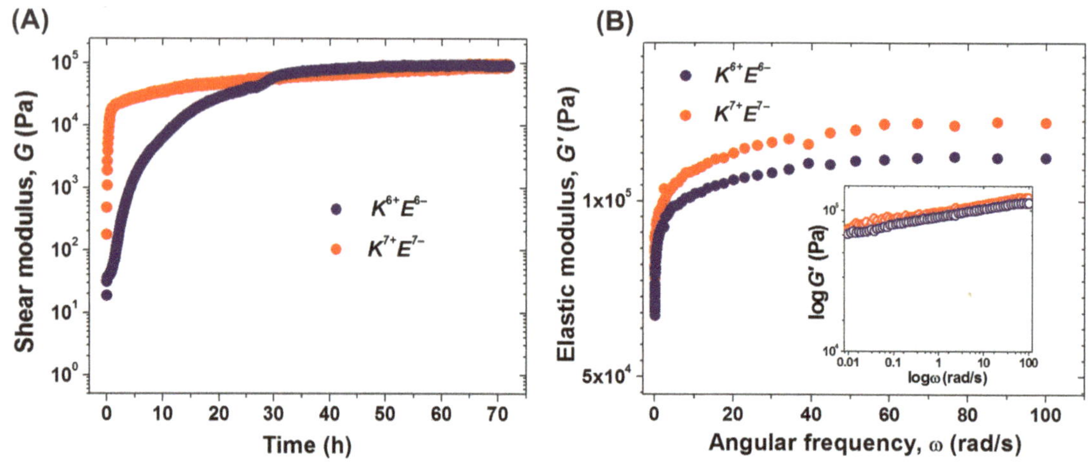

FIGURE 11.2 Viscoelastic properties of hydrogel fibrous networks.

(A) Rheological time sweep monitoring of the assembly of $K^{7+}E^{7-}$ (•) and $K^{6+}E^{6-}$ (•) hydrogels. (B) Frequency sweep of $K^{7+}E^{7-}$ (•) and $K^{6+}E^{6-}$ (•). Inset in B shows the linearity of frequency spectra in log$G'(\omega)$ versus logω coordinates, which point to the viscoelastic nature of both hydrogels under study.

sweep data of plant cell walls [36,37]. Briefly [38], the derivation procedure is based on two Fredholm integral equations (11.1) and (11.2)

$$G'(\omega) = G_0 + \int_0^{\infty} H(\tau)\frac{\omega^2\tau^2}{1+\omega^2\tau^2}\frac{d\tau}{\tau} \tag{11.1}$$

$$G''(\omega) = \int_0^{\infty} H(\tau)\frac{\omega\tau}{1+\omega^2\tau^2}\frac{d\tau}{\tau} \tag{11.2}$$

where G_0 is the residual modulus, which is $\neq 0$ for the viscoelastic solid-like hydrogels studied in the present work. The *BayesRelax* computer program [36] calculates the relaxation spectrum, $H(\tau)$, and compares the model $G'(\omega)$ and $G''(\omega)$ values obtained by substituting $H(\tau)$ to the Fredholm equations (11.1) and (11.2) with the experimental $G'(\omega)$ and $G''(\omega)$ values. A best fit is selected based on minimum χ^2 depicting the deviation of model $G'(\omega)$ and $G''(\omega)$ from the corresponding frequency spectrum. In this work, $\chi^2 \leq 0.2$ for both hydrogels, indicating excellent fit.

To describe the relaxation process, the generalized Maxwell model of viscoelastic material [39] is approximated by a set of 100 discrete elements with the relaxation time, τ, spanning 5 decades from 10^{-2} to 10^3 s, the range where reliable predictions could be made. The relaxation time, τ, of any such discrete element is the time necessary to observe $(1-1/e)$ or 63.2% of stress decline under constant strain; hence, shorter τ means faster stress release.

Stress relaxation in a fibrous hydrogel network reflects the time-dependent changes in a position of the entangled hydrogel fibers where different portions/segments of the fibers move to relax the applied stress. Shorter τ is characteristic of local fiber mobility, whereas longer τ is attributed to movements of

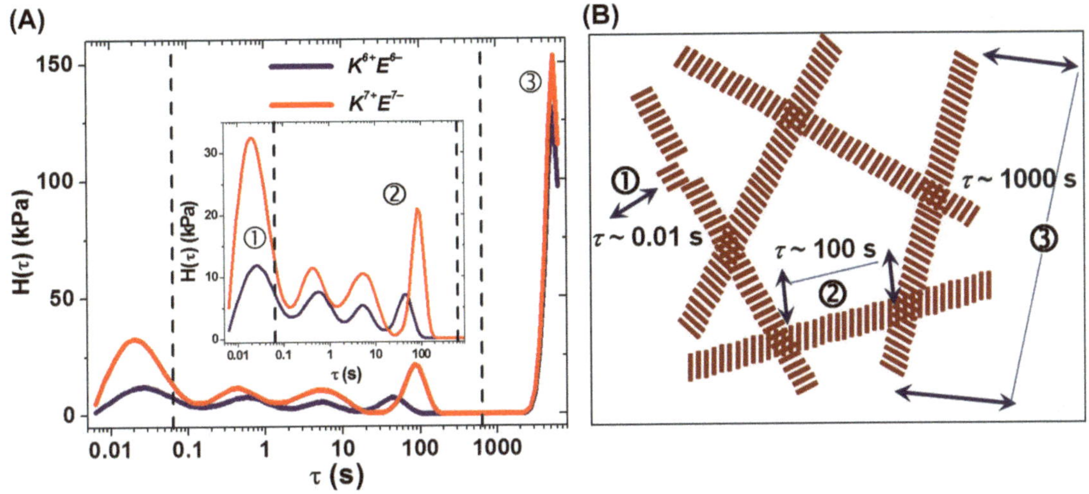

FIGURE 11.3 Relaxation spectra and network mobility.

(A) Relaxation spectra $H(\tau)$ versus $\log\tau$ derived from the frequency sweep data based on Bayesian analysis of the frequency sweep data presented in Fig. 11.2B for $\boldsymbol{K^{7+}E^{7-}}$ (—) and $\boldsymbol{K^{6+}E^{6-}}$ (—). Inset in A shows enlarged region for $\tau \sim 0–700$ s. Fitted range of τ from 10^{-3} to 10^4 s is the most reliable range from the viewpoint of maximum Bayesian likelihood, and the range of τ from 0.0628 to 628 s (denoted by two *vertical dashed lines*) corresponds to the timescale of our frequency sweep experiments (from 100 to 0.01 rad/s). (B) Pictorial presentation of different motions present in the entangled fibrous hydrogel network with their characteristic ranges of the relaxation time τ: ① local displacements of the individual peptide modules within the fiber structure; ② movements of fiber portions between the points of contact; ③ slow movements of the entire fiber.

large network segments. The relaxation time distribution function $H(\tau)$ reflects the presence of different discrete elements, corresponding to different relaxation mechanisms, in a material. The larger is the value of $H(\tau)$ at certain τ, higher relaxation capability, the more stress the scaffold can release via the relaxation mechanism characterized by this τ value. For fibrous hydrogels networks, higher relaxation capability within the short and intermediate τ ranges result from higher flexibility of local fibers and segments between entangled fibers. One might reasonably expect that the material with higher relaxation capabilities in the short to intermediate τ range would be less restrictive for cell movement and thereby more beneficial for their growth.

Indeed, such differences are evident from the relaxation spectra $H(\tau)$ versus $\log\tau$ (Fig. 11.3A) derived from the corresponding frequency sweep data of the two hydrogels ($G'(\omega)$ and $G''(\omega)$) using the *BayesRelax* program [36]. The best fitted range of τ stretches from 10^{-3} to 10^4 s and is the most reliable range from the viewpoint of maximum Bayesian likelihood. Multipeak relaxation spectra in Fig. 11.3A are characteristic of the formation of fibrous hydrogels where the fibers are long enough for kinking and entanglement and creating "the points of contact," thus resulting in a complex hydrogel network [39]. Simplified pictorial presentation of a hydrogel network in Fig. 11.3B could be helpful to illustrate the observed peaks in the relaxation spectra (Fig. 11.3A) to different movements of the elements of the fibrous network. Specifically, peaks observed at the lowest τ decade ~0.01 s (①, Fig. 11.3A), are assigned to fast movement of local fiber segments. Based on the earlier revealed fiber structure of the $\boldsymbol{K^{6+}E^{6-}}$ hydrogel [15], such movements are consistent with fast local displacements of the individual peptide units stacked within the fiber structure (①, Fig. 11.3B). The interpretation of the smaller peaks in the τ decades of ~1 and ~10 s is less obvious, but one might attribute their appearance to the movement of larger stacked segments of the individual peptide fiber. Whereas, peaks in the intermediate τ decade ~100 s (②, Fig. 11.3A) result from the movement of fiber portions/segments between the points of contact (②, Fig. 11.3B), while peaks at the longest τ decade ~1000 s (③, Fig. 11.3A) arise from very slow movements of the entire fiber network (③, Fig. 11.3B).

Comparison of the relaxation spectra of $\boldsymbol{K^{7+}E^{7-}}$ and $\boldsymbol{K^{6+}E^{6-}}$ hydrogels (Fig. 11.3A) shows that the $\boldsymbol{K^{7+}E^{7-}}$ hydrogel has much greater relaxation capability [higher $H(\tau)$ values] attributed to local fiber displacements (τ ~0.01 s) and fiber movements between the points of contact (τ ~100 s) as opposed to the $\boldsymbol{K^{6+}E^{6-}}$ hydrogel. This distinction suggests that better mobility of the fiber portions, which define the boundaries of the niche available for cells, is more beneficial (since it is less restrictive) for cell survival and proliferation. In contrast, the $\boldsymbol{K^{6+}E^{6-}}$ hydrogel has less contribution from these relaxation components and is comparatively more rigid, which makes it less beneficial as a cell growth matrix. Indeed, this is in agreement with our observations in both 2-D and 3-D cell culture studies, demonstrating that the $\boldsymbol{K^{7+}E^{7-}}$ hydrogel is more beneficial for the hMSCs than the $\boldsymbol{K^{6+}E^{6-}}$ hydrogel (Fig. 11.1).

NANOSCALE STRUCTURAL DIFFERENCES DEFINING FIBER DYNAMICS

What structural differences of $\boldsymbol{K^{7+}E^{7-}}$ and $\boldsymbol{K^{6+}E^{6-}}$ hydrogels can result in their different dynamic behaviors? Small-angle neutron scattering (SANS) is a versatile tool, which allows one to unravel these structural distinctions at the nanoscale level of individual fiber and the fibrous network as a whole. The advantage of SANS as a tool for biomaterial structure analysis is that it permits the biomaterial to be investigated under the fully hydrated state. Indeed, significant insight on hydrogel structures can be gleaned from SANS analysis [22].

For SANS experiments, $\boldsymbol{K^{7+}E^{7-}}$ and $\boldsymbol{K^{6+}E^{6-}}$ hydrogels were prepared by mixing respective oppositely charged peptides in deuterated PBS buffer (pH 7.4, no pD correction). The peptides were mixed in a titanium cell with 1-mm path length between a pair of quartz windows, each of 30 mm in diameter. SANS data were collected 72 h after mixing (the gelation was completed, see Fig. 11.2A) using the 30-m SANS instrument (NG-7) at National Institute of Standards and Technology (NIST) [40]. Monochromatic neutrons at $\lambda = 6$ Å with a wavelength spread ($\Delta\lambda/\lambda$) of 0.14 were detected on a 64 cm × 64 cm 2-D detector. Data on SANS intensity were collected with a Q-range from 0.001 to 0.4 Å^{-1}. Scattering intensities were normalized using direct beam transmission measurements and were reduced according to published protocols [41]. ATSAS software [42] has been used to estimate the radius of gyration of the fiber cross-section R_c and the zero-angle scattering intensity of the fiber cross-section $I_c(0)$ in both hydrogels, which is based on the Guinier analysis of $\ln Q \times I(Q)$ versus Q^2 plots for rod-like particles. This software suite was also instrumental to produce the Guinier plots for flat elements in hydrogels, $\ln Q^2 \times I(Q)$ versus Q^2.

SANS profiles shown in Fig. 11.4A suggest that both hydrogels assemble into fibrous network. Sharp increase in the scattering intensity at low Q-values (Fig. 11.4A) is consistent with the formation of large molecular assemblies. The presence of elongated asymmetrical rod-like particles (such as hydrogel fibers) is evident from the linearity of Guinier plots for rod-like particles (inset, Fig. 11.4A). Also, these linear Guinier plots for rod-like particles, $\ln Q \times I(Q)$ versus Q^2, allow one to derive the

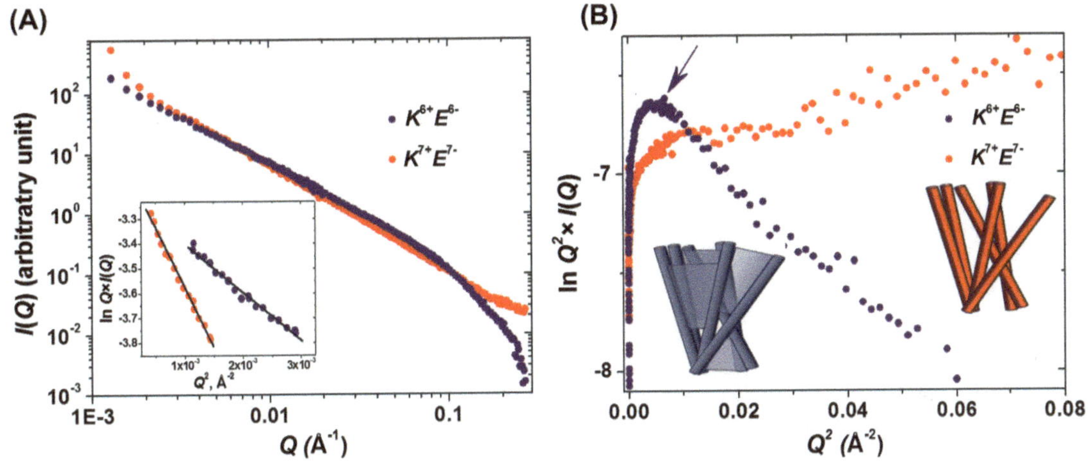

FIGURE 11.4 Organization of hydrogel fibrous networks reconstructed from SANS data.

(A) SANS scattering profiles *I(Q)* versus *Q* of $K^{7+}E^{7-}$ (●) and $K^{6+}E^{6-}$ (●) hydrogels. Inset shows Guinier plots for rod-like particles, ln*Q*× *I(Q)* versus Q^2, and the linearity in this region indicates the formation of elongated fibers in all hydrogels. (B) Guinier plots for flat particles, lnQ^2× *I(Q)* versus Q^2, show the characteristic upturn marked by the *blue arrow,* which indicates the formation of flat, lappet-like webs interconnecting the peptide fibers in the $K^{6+}E^{6-}$ hydrogel (●), while such webs are absent in the $K^{7+}E^{7-}$ (●) hydrogel (also shown by two pictorial inset cartoons in corresponding colors).

Table 11.2 Structural Parameters of the Hydrogel Fibrous Networks From SANS Data

Hydrogel	R_c (Å)	$I_c(0) \times 10^2$ (aU/Å)	S_c (Å^2)	$\rho \times 10^5$ (aU/Å^3)
$K^{6+}E^{6-}$	19.2±0.6	3.9±0.01	2316.2	1.7
$K^{7+}E^{7-}$	29.0±0.6	4.2±0.07	5284.2	0.8

R_c, *the radius of gyration of the fiber cross-section; for cylindrical rods, the radius of the cylinder* $R = R_c\sqrt{2}$; $I_c(0)$, *mass per unit length of the fiber in arbitrary unit per Å;* S_c, *area of the fiber cross-section in* Å^2, $S_c = \pi R^2 = 2\pi R_c^2$; ρ $(= I_c(0)/S_c)$, *fiber density in arbitrary unit per* Å^3 *(aU/Å^3).*

cross-sectional radius of gyration R_c of the fibers (from the slope) and their zero-angle scattering intensity $I_c(0)$ of cross-section (from the intercept), which is proportional to the mass per unit length of the fiber. For simplicity, under the assumption of cylindrical fibers, one could estimate the cross-sectional area S_c and, using the above values of mass per unit length, $I_c(0)$, to derive the mass density ϱ of the fibers (Table 11.2).

SANS data analysis (Table 11.2) shows that the $K^{7+}E^{7-}$ hydrogel is assembled from much thicker fibers (larger cross-section area) as compared to the $K^{6+}E^{6-}$ hydrogel. However, $K^{7+}E^{7-}$ fibers are more than two times less dense than $K^{6+}E^{6-}$ fibers (smaller ϱ value) and, therefore, have more mobile local fiber segments, consistent with the relaxation spectra (①, Fig. 11.3A and B). In addition, the characteristic upturn observed for the $K^{6+}E^{6-}$ hydrogel in the Guinier plot for flat structural elements (*arrow* in

Fig. 11.4B) suggests that fibers in this hydrogel network are interconnected by lappet-like webs that are not observed for the $K^{7+}E^{7-}$ hydrogel (cf. Fig. 11.4B). The formation and 3-D organization of such webs in the $K^{6+}E^{6-}$ hydrogel has been explored in detail in our earlier work [15]. On the other hand, the absence of web connections between the fibers in the $K^{7+}E^{7-}$ gel could explain its greater relaxation capabilities due to the more pronounced mobility of the fiber portion between the network entanglements consistent with the relaxation spectra (②, Fig. 11.3A and B).

CONCLUSIONS

In summary, the observed differences in two hydrogels with very similar chemical composition and stiffness in supporting stem cell growth suggest that stiffness is not the only viscoelastic property important for scaffold performance. Aside from stiffness, the relaxation capacity of the scaffold should also be taken into account when designing artificial ECMs. Greater relaxation capability of the fibrous scaffold network is generally a result of better flexibility and mobility of different fiber segments. This leads to a scaffold that is more beneficial for cell growth, proliferation, and survival. The relaxation spectra extracted from the frequency sweep of hydrogels allow one to delineate the contribution to stress release by the various fiber elements. We have found that commonly encountered PTMs of acetylation and amidation of a protein could be used to modulate the dynamic properties of a peptide-based ECM without changing its stiffness. It is our belief that successful design of supportive scaffolds should consider not only matrix stiffness but also matrix dynamics. This chapter also suggests PTMs could be an effective strategy in tuning the mechanical characteristics of peptide- or protein-based ECMs.

GLOSSARY

***G* (shear modulus)** A measure of the material stiffness, described as the ratio of shear stress to shear strain when the material is deformed by a force parallel to its surface.

***G′* (elastic or storage modulus)** Estimate of the energy stored in the material, elastic portion of the shear modulus.

***G″* (viscous or loss modulus)** Estimate of the energy dissipated in the material, viscous portion of the shear modulus.

τ (relaxation time) The time necessary to observe $(1-1/e)$ or 63.2% of stress decline under constant strain.

$H(_\tau)$ (relaxation spectrum) The relaxation time distribution function reflecting the contributions from differently relaxing elements in a material corresponding to distinctive relaxation processes (mechanisms).

$I_c(0)$ (zero-angle scattering intensity of the cross-section) Intensity of the neutron scattering of the fiber cross-section when scattering angle tends to zero, reflects the mass of the unit length of the fiber.

R_c (the radius of gyration of the fiber cross-section; for cylindrical rods) The contrast-weighted root–mean–square distance of all area elements from the center of scattering density of the fiber cross-section.

LIST OF ACRONYMS AND ABBREVIATIONS

ECM extracellular matrix
hMSC human mesenchymal stem cell
PTM posttranslational modification
SANS small-angle neutron scattering

ACKNOWLEDGMENTS

Financial support provided by the NIH (EB004416) is gratefully acknowledged. We also thank Dr. B. Hammouda (NIST, NCNR) for help with SANS experiments. This work has been done in the frames of NIST NCNR Proposal No. S31-50 and is based upon activities supported in part by the National Science Foundation under Agreement No. DMR-0944772.

REFERENCES

[1] Lane SW, Williams DA, Watt FM. Modulating the stem cell niche for tissue regeneration. Nat Biotechnol 2014;32:795–803.

[2] Engler AJ, Sen S, Sweeney HL, Disher DE. Matrix elasticity directs stem cells lineage specifications. Cell 2006;126:677–89.

[3] Holst J, Watson S, Lord MS, Eamegdool SS, Bax DV, Nivison-Smith LB, et al. Substrate elasticity provides mechanical signals for the expansion of hemopoietic stem and progenitor cells. Nat Biotechnol 2010;28:1123–8.

[4] Gibbert PM, Havenstrite KL, Magnusson KEG, Sacco A, Leonardi NA, Kraft P, et al. Substrate elasticity regulates skeletal muscle stem cell self-renewal in culture. Science 2010;329:1078–81.

[5] Kisiday J, Jin M, Kurz B, Hung H, Semino C, Zhang S, et al. Self-assembling peptide hydrogel fosters chondrocyte extracellular matrix production and cell division: implications for cartilage tissue repair. Proc Natl Acad Sci USA 2002;99:9996–10001.

[6] Kumar S. Stiffness does matter. Nat Mater 2014;13:918–20.

[7] Wen JH, Vincent LG, Fuhrmann A, Choi YS, Hribar KC, Taylor-Weiner H, et al. Interplay of matrix stiffness and protein tethering in stem cell differentiation. Nat Mater 2014;13:979–87.

[8] Chaudhouri O, Koshy ST, da Cunha CB, Shin J-W, Verbeke CS, Allison KH, et al. Extracellular matrix stiffness and composition jointly regulates the induction of malignant phenotypes in mammary epithelium. Nat Mater 2014;13:970–8.

[9] Cameron AR, Frith JE, Cooper-White JJ. The influence of substrate creep on mesenchymal stem cell behaviour. Biomaterials 2011;32:5979–93.

[10] McKinnon DD, Domaille DW, Cha JN, Anseth KS. Biophysically defined and cytocompatible covalently adaptable networks as viscoelastic 3D cell culture systems. Adv Mater 2013;26:865–72.

[11] Chaudhuri O, Gu L, Darnell M, Klumpers D, Bencherif SA, Weaver JC, et al. Substrate stress relaxation regulates cell spreading. Nat Commun 2015;6:6365.

[12] Leeming DJ, Bay-Jensen AC, Vassiliadis E, Larsen MR, Henriksen K, Karsdal MA. Post-translational modifications of the extracellular matrix are key events in cancer progression: opportunities for biochemical marker development. Biomarkers 2011;16:193–205.

[13] Walsh G, Jefferis R. Post-translational modifications in the context of therapeutic proteins. Nat Biotechnol 2006;24:1241–52.

[14] Mogk A, Bukau B. When beginning marks the end. Science 2010;327:966–7.

[15] Taraban MB, Feng Y, Hammouda B, Hyland LL, Yu YB. Chirality-mediated mechanical and structural properties of oligopeptide hydrogels. Chem Mater 2012;24:2299–310.

[16] Ramachandran S, Tseng Y, Yu YB. Repeated shear-responsiveness of peptide hydrogels with tunable shear-modulus. Biomacromolecules 2005;6:1316–21.

[17] Ramachandran S, Flynn P, Tseng Y, Yu YB. Electrostatically controlled hydrogelation of oligopeptides and protein entrapment. Chem Mater 2005;17:6583–8.

[18] Hyland LL, Twomey JD, Vogel S, Hsieh AH, Yu YB. Enhancing of biocompatibility of *D*-oligopeptide hydrogels by negative charges. Biomacromolecules 2013;14:406–12.

[19] Ramachandran S, Trewhella J, Tseng Y, Yu YB. Co-assembling peptide-based biomaterials: effect of pairing equal and unequal chain-length oligopeptides. Chem Mater 2006;18:6157–62.

[20] Taraban MB, Ramachandran S, Gryczynski I, Gryczynski Z, Trewhella J, Yu YB. Effects of chain length on oligopeptide hydrogelation. Soft Matter 2011;7:2624–31.

[21] Feng Y, Lee M, Taraban M, Yu YB. Diffusion of small molecules inside a peptide hydrogel. Chem Commun 2011;47:10455–7.

[22] Hyland LL, Taraban MB, Yu YB. Using small-angle scattering techniques to understand mechanical properties of biopolymer-based biomaterials. Soft Matter 2013;9:10218–28.

[23] Ramachandran S, Taraban MB, Trewhella J, Gryczynski I, Gryczanski Z, Yu YB. Effect of temperature during assembly on the structure and mechanical properties of peptide-based materials. Biomacromolecules 2010;11:1502–6.

[24] Hyland LL, Taraban MB, Hammouda B, Yu YB. Mutually reinforced multicomponent polysaccharide network. Biopolymers 2011;95:840–51.

[25] Hyland LL, Taraban MB, Feng Y, Hammouda B, Yu YB. Viscoelastic properties and nanoscale structures of composite oligopeptide-polysaccharide hydrogels. Biopolymers 2012;97:177–88.

[26] Weerasekare M, Taraban MB, Shi X, Jeong E-K, Trewhella J, Yu YB. Sol and gel states visualized by Gd(III)-enhanced magnetic resonance imaging. Biopolymers 2011;96:734–43.

[27] Taraban MB, Weerasekare M, Trewhella J, Shi X, Jeong E-K, Yu YB. Effects of gadolinium chelate on the evolution of nanoscale structure in peptide hydrogels. Biopolymers 2012;98:50–8.

[28] Joyner K, Taraban MB, Feng Y, Yu YB. An interplay between electrostatic and polar interactions in peptide hydrogels. Biopolymers 2013;100:174–83.

[29] Feng Y, Taraban MB, Yu YB. Linear dependency of NMR relaxation rates on shear modulus in hydrogels. Soft Matter 2011;7:9890–3.

[30] Feng Y, Taraban MB, Yu YB. The effect of ionic strength on the mechanical, structural and transport properties of peptide hydrogels. Soft Matter 2012;8:11723–31.

[31] Feng Y, Taraban MB, Yu YB. Linear dependence of the water proton transverse relaxation rate on the shear modulus of hydrogels. Chem Commun 2012;50:12120–2.

[32] Hyland LL, Taraban M, Vogel S, Lai L-C, Feng Y, Chiou W-A, et al. Cryo-TEM characterization of chiral peptide hydrogel networks. Microsc Microanal 2012;18(Suppl. 2):278–9.

[33] Taraban MB, Hyland LL, Yu YB. Split of chiral degeneracy in mechanical and structural properties of oligopeptide-polysaccharide biomaterials. Biomacromolecules 2013;14:3192–201.

[34] Ramachandran S, Yu YB. Peptide-based viscoelastic matrices for drug-delivery and tissue repair. BioDrugs 2006;20:263–9.

[35] Chan WC, White PD. Fmoc solid phase peptide synthesis: a practical approach. New York: Oxford University Press; 2000.

[36] Hansen SL. Estimation of the relaxation spectrum from dynamic experiments using Bayesian analysis and a new regularization constraint. Rheol Acta 2008;47:169–78.

[37] Hansen SL, Ray RP, Karlsson AO, Jørgensen B, Borkhardt B, Petersen BL, et al. Mechanical properties of plant cell walls probed by relaxation spectra. Plant Physiol 2011;155:246–58.

[38] Tschoegl NW. The phenomenological theory of linear viscoelastic behaviour. Berlin: Springer; 1989.

[39] Ferry JD. Viscoelastic properties of polymers. New York: Wiley; 1980.

[40] Glinka CJ, Barker JG, Hammouda B, Krueger S, Moyer JJ, Orts WJ. The 30 m small-angle neutron scattering instruments at the National Institute of Standards and Technology. J Appl Crystallogr 1998;31:430–45.

[41] Kline SR. Reduction and analysis of SANS and USANS data using IGOR Pro. J Appl Crystallogr 2006;39:895–900.

[42] Konarev PV, Volkov VV, Sokolova AV, Koch MHJ, Svergun DI. PRIMUS: a Windows PC-based system for small-angle scattering data analysis. J Appl Crystallogr 2003;36:1277–82.

CHAPTER

FUNCTIONALIZED POLYMERIC BIOMATERIALS FOR IN SITU TISSUE REGENERATION

12

S.H. Park, B.K. Lee, M.S. Kim
Ajou University, Suwon, Korea

CHAPTER OUTLINE

INTRODUCTION

Annually, millions of patients experience the functional loss of, or damage to, organs, tissues, or other body parts. Although several clinical trials have attempted to regenerate the function of damaged tissue or organs by using donor organs, many of these patients experienced various limitations, such as donor organ or tissue unavailability and procedure-related complications. Regenerative medicine has received considerable attention as a clinical solution for the regeneration of damaged tissue or organs [1]. Regenerative medicine is defined as the regeneration of lost or damaged organs through the transplantation of ex vivo-fabricated body parts or as the restoration of some level of function of damaged tissues or organs. Thus regenerative medicine has huge potential to solve the problem of the shortage of organs available for donation.

The goals of regenerative medicine can be ultimately achieved by research contributions from a number of fields, such as stem cell engineering, tissue engineering, gene and drug delivery engineering, artificial and biological organ engineering, etc. Particularly, stem cell engineering is generating a great deal of interest in the treatment of various diseases [2]. The various types of stem/progenitor cells can act as potential therapeutic cells for a wide variety of tissue damage and diseases. Numerous transplantation studies using stem/progenitor cells showed tissue repair or regeneration, either by the

In Situ Tissue Regeneration. http://dx.doi.org/10.1016/B978-0-12-802225-2.00012-X

differentiation of the cells into many different cell types or by their trophic effects. Stem/progenitor cells are well characterized, easily available, and they can meet the cellular demand for tissue regeneration. The use of stem/progenitor cells typically necessitates a donor tissue biopsy, and sometimes donor cells are unavailable because of extensive tissue damage. The biopsy of primary cells, including stem/progenitor cells, is sequentially followed by cell isolation and ex vivo expansion procedures, which require extensive cell manipulation before in vivo transplantation.

Unfortunately, the in vitro expansion of primary cells has several disadvantages [3]. For example, in vitro expansion to obtain adequate cell numbers can result in the dedifferentiation of cells into the original source cell type and differentiation into undesirable cell types. In some cases, the use of stem/progenitor cells requires differentiation technology to produce specific cell lineages for transplantation. However, upon repeated subculture in vitro, primary stem/progenitor cells can lose their multipotency and self-renewal capacity, leading to senescence. Furthermore, in vivo stem cell transplantation often causes problems such as low cell survival rates and tumorigenesis.

Tissue engineering offers various advances and new opportunities for the treatment of tissue and organ deficits, and thus, it has received considerable attention as a promising strategy in regenerative medicine [4]. Tissue engineering has great potential and is likely to have a profound impact in the future. Regeneration or reconstruction of damaged or diseased tissues and organs by tissue engineering requires three components: (1) cells harvested from various donor tissues, including adult stem or progenitor cells derived from bone, nerve, liver, cartilage, or embryonic and induced pluripotent stem cells; (2) scaffolds, on which cells are able to attach during proliferation and/or differentiation; and (3) biologic molecules, such as cytokines and growth factors, which promote growth and/or differentiation in the desired tissue or organ.

A scaffold-based approach is one of the major challenges in tissue engineering research fields, as well as in regenerative medicine. Scaffold-based approaches play a critical role in tissue engineering strategies because scaffolds provide an architectural context in which cells and growth factors can interact, literally and figuratively serving as the framework for regenerative medicine. Various scaffold-based approaches have allowed for the development of biological molecules that are designed to regenerate and maintain normal tissue and organ function. Thus cell and/or growth factor-loaded scaffolds have been applied to damaged tissue. The cell and/or growth factor-loaded scaffolds represent a fascinating treatment option for tissue regeneration, providing a structural basis for the regeneration of damaged tissue or organs, and stimulating the healing processes of damaged tissue or organs.

The challenges associated with classic scaffold-based approaches have been overcome by implementing scaffolds that are preseeded with desirable cells and/or growth factors to generate functional tissues that progressively mature when introduced in vivo. The cell and/or growth factor-loaded scaffolds have been demonstrated in various preclinical and clinical studies. However, despite good and promising results, cell and/or growth factor-loaded scaffold research is still in its infancy, especially in the clinical setting, and many controversial aspects have yet to be clarified, such as the best stem/progenitor cell source, dosage, the use of concentrated or expanded stem/progenitor cells, the use of growth factors, etc.

STRATEGIES FOR THE FUNCTIONALIZED POLYMERIC SCAFFOLD

BIOMATERIALS FOR FUNCTIONALIZED POLYMERIC SCAFFOLD

The functionalized polymeric scaffolds can be fabricated using a variety of biomaterials.There is an impetus to develop and design functional groups-modified biomaterials with optimized physical properties and desirable performance for use in practical in vivo applications. There are two commonly used functionalization strategies: (1) functional groups are introduced to the biomaterials, sometimes in a protected form, to be deprotected before or after the preparation of polymeric scaffolds; and (2) functional groups are introduced by direct modification of the as-prepared polymeric scaffolds. Regardless of any functionalization strategies, functional groups are needed to prepare the functionalized polymeric scaffolds. Biomaterials can be divided into two main categories of natural and synthetic biomaterials.

Natural biomaterials have a number of advantages such as remarkable biocompatibility, relative abundance, and ease of processing, even though natural biomaterials exhibit different mechanical properties due to different composition for batch-to-batch variations and have the potential immunogenic properties. There is a large number of natural biomaterials, including collagens, gelatin, sodium carboxymethylcellulose, small intestine submucosa, alginate, chitosan, hyaluronic acid, fibrins, etc. [5], which exhibit only mild inflammatory responses in vivo. In theory, natural biomaterials are eventually broken down into CO_2 and water under microorganisms. In addition, they can be adjusted into the targeted in vivo microenvironment. In addition, most natural biomaterials are good candidate materials for functionalization of various biologic factors because they possess functionalizable side and/or end chains (carboxyl, amino, hydroxyl, thiol, etc.) that can easily meet the need for functionalization of biomaterials.

In contrast to natural biomaterials, synthetic biomaterials can be prepared as materials with uniform composition even on a large scale without batch-to-batch variation and can elicit the reduced immune responses or none at all. Meanwhile, synthetic biomaterials or their degraded product can induce inflammatory responses. Functionalization of synthetic biomaterials can be performed before or after the preparation of synthetic biomaterials. In particular, synthetic biomaterials can be tailored by functional groups, such as carboxyl, amino, hydroxyl, thiol, aldehyde, azide, halogen, carbon–carbon double or triple bonds, etc., in side and/or end chains [6–8]. The functional groups of synthetic biomaterials can be further modified by biologic factors before or after fabrication of polymeric scaffolds. In addition, they can allow precise design of geometric scaffold structure and can be tailored to produce a scaffold with more tunable and predictable properties such as hydrophilicity, biodegradation rates, bioadhesion, etc.

Thus various biomaterials can be used to modify the physical and mechanical properties of polymeric scaffolds because functionalization is possible to prepare properly designed biomaterials or polymeric scaffolds without altering the bulk properties. Various natural and synthetic biomaterials are in use and have been adapted for the manufacture of functionalized polymeric scaffolds that create a more natural in vivo microenvironment for tissue regeneration through supporting of biological signals.

SCAFFOLDING SYSTEM

Generally, functionalized polymeric scaffolds have been developed to support targeted tissue regeneration and are characterized by their biological and physical features. Several promising results have been shown in the clinical setting, as well as for the treatment of complex cases otherwise doomed to a poorer prognosis with other treatment procedures. Advances in cell-seeded and/or growth factor-loaded polymeric scaffolds are not surprising because in past years, huge steps have been made in regards to cell-based approaches for tissue engineering applications. A new generation of polymeric scaffolds has been developed, which are able to mimic the characteristics of healthy tissues and exploit the intrinsic tissue regeneration capability and to avoid the risk linked to in vitro cell management (such as bacterial contamination and phenotype loss during extensive cell manipulation), reducing costs and simplifying the procedure. Although the fundamental principles of cell-seeded and/or growth factor-loaded scaffolding systems have been successfully applied in various preclinical and clinical studies, it is essential to obtain the appropriate cell sources for conventional tissue engineering applications. Clinical studies have focused on cell-seeded scaffolds [9], even though the actual role of cells in the cell-based approaches remains a controversial issue. A more technical aspect could also be an important confounding factor when trying to address the problem of understanding the contribution of cells in tissue regeneration. However, the quality of the implanted cells is not implied in most of the cell-seeded scaffolds, or their results regarding the clinical outcomes through the studies are not documented.

It is well known that during in vitro cultivation of cells, several stem/progenitor cells can undergo dedifferentiation, losing their phenotype and thus the ability to regenerate the damaged tissue. Even after being cultured in the 3-D structure of the scaffolds, stem/progenitor cells may not be completely recovered, and concerns could be raised regarding their distribution and vitality after being cultured, as well as after surgical manipulation and implantation of the scaffold. Some clinical studies have also directly focused on scaffolds without cells, but almost no successful clinical results have been reported using these scaffolds without cells [10]. In situ tissue regeneration using a cell-free scaffolding system has high potential to overcome these limitations. Ideally, cell-free scaffold-based regeneration would be achieved by using an off-the-shelf product capable of recruiting host cells and stimulating tissue development. Hence, the functionalized polymeric scaffolding system seems eligible for in situ tissue regeneration through the migration and adhesion of host cells from around the damaged tissue or circulating cells from the blood stream into the region of interest.

In situ tissue regeneration using the functionalized polymeric scaffold presents formidable challenges, such as how to immediately attract and recruit cells upon implantation of the scaffold, how to achieve in situ tissue regeneration upon implantation, how to avoid adverse developments, such as hyperplasia, how to modulate the foreign body response, and how to maintain functionality throughout the patient's lifespan. Thus this cell-free scaffold with a specific cell recruiting motif can address in vivo endogenous tissue regeneration mechanisms, where the recruited cells' capability of aiding the production and remodeling of new tissue plays an important role.

CHEMOKINE SIGNALING

Tissue damage may occur because of several reasons, resulting in a complex inflammatory environment in response to hypoxia of the damaged tissue site. The hypoxic environment causes damaged cells to locally release intracellular content and chemokines such as hypoxia-inducible factor 1α, followed by the release of first signaling factors, such as vascular endothelial growth factor (VEGF), stromal cell-derived factor-1 (SDF-1), monocyte chemoattractant protein 1 (MCP-1), platelet-derived growth factor β (PDGF-β), macrophage chemotactic factor (MCF), and so on. The chemokine signaling factors spread in a gradient pattern, with the highest concentration being in the vicinity of the damaged area (Fig. 12.1) [11,12]. The chemokine signaling factors can stimulate the expression of cellular adhesion molecules, like integrins. The extracellular matrix (ECM) and endothelium may be adhered in the area surrounding the damaged area. This process allows circulating cells to reach the ECM and endothelium. Neovascularization is then initiated at the damaged area. Cells exposed to hypoxic conditions for prolonged periods undergo lysis by autodigestive enzymes, and intracellular materials are then released into the surrounding area.

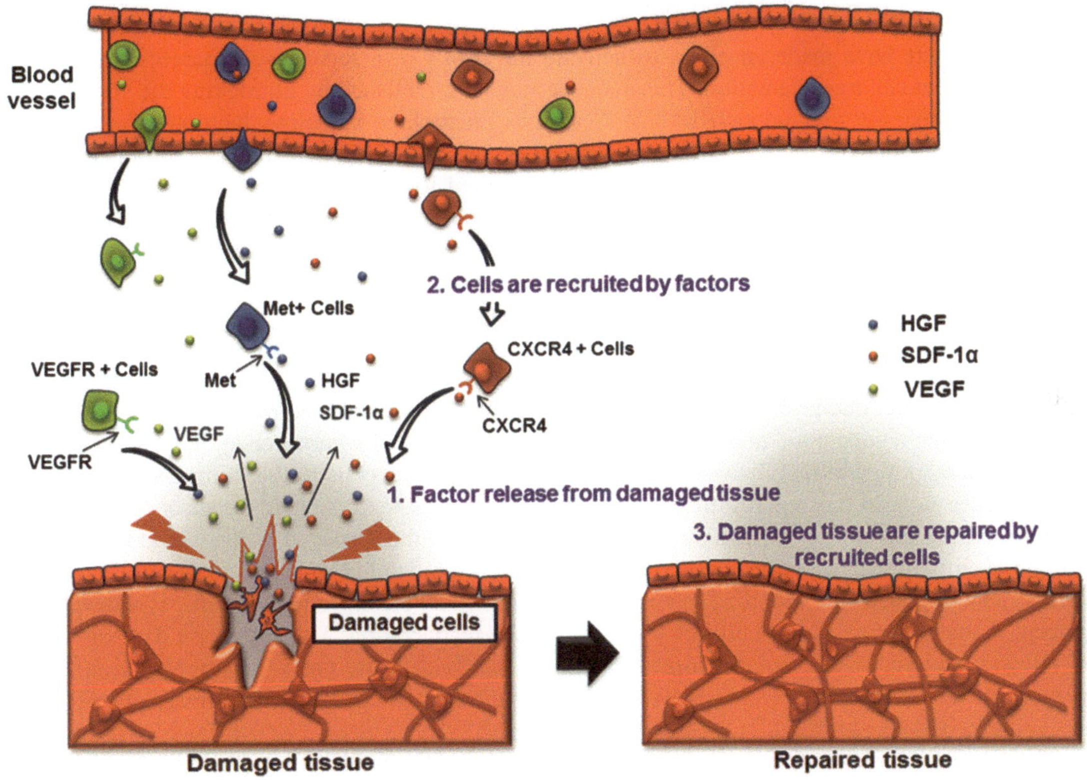

FIGURE 12.1

Schematic image for repairing of damaged tissue via cellular attraction. Damaged tissue (cells) locally release chemokine signaling factors in a gradient pattern toward the vicinity of the damaged area. The chemokine signaling factors mobilize or recruit host stem/progenitor cells toward damaged tissue for in situ tissue regeneration.

The images were drawn by SHP and BKL using software of Adobe Photoshop 7.0.

The immune system is activated by priming resident macrophages, as well as the complement and coagulation systems. Additional chemokine signaling factors, as well as free radicals, are released into this environment, stimulating adjacent endothelial cells and fibroblasts, as well as mast cells, neutrophils, and monocytes, which participate in the inflammatory response. Macrophages, pericytes, and mesenchymal stem cells (MSCs) are attracted along this gradient toward the highest concentration in the vicinity of the damaged area. The attracted macrophages, pericytes, and MSCs produce a complex secondary signaling environment of interleukins (ILs) and chemokines that further influences the inflammatory and endogenous tissue regeneration processes. Collectively, the dynamics of the initial signaling and subsequent secondary chemokine signaling factors play a crucial role in cellular attraction toward damaged tissue. In this process, the chemokine signaling factors may provide clues as to which signaling proteins might be used to trigger a beneficial cellular response for spontaneous regenerative capacity. Thus the understanding of signaling factors may serve as a good starting point for the development of a functionalized scaffolding system.

STEM CELL RECRUITING FACTORS

Many researchers have made an effort to activate the host's own reparative capability, rather than attempting direct cell transplantation. This concept may be established by mimicking the spontaneous regeneration processes. As previously stated, various chemokine signaling factors are secreted in response to tissue damage in order to initiate the processes of stem cell recruitment. In this regard, if the host stem/progenitor cells' potential could be recruited to the sites of interest, without ex vivo expansion, the in situ tissue regeneration of damaged tissue may be possible. This strategy does not include donor cell procurement and in vitro cell manipulation, unlike the use of cell-seeded tissue constructs.

For efficient and successful in situ tissue regeneration, appropriate numbers of host stem/progenitor cells must be recruited by host cell recruitment factors. However, the populations of host stem/progenitor cells are transient and too small to have a significant effect on endogenous tissue regeneration. To overcome this issue, one promising approach may be the recruitment of circulating host cells to the target site so that regeneration may be enhanced in vivo. Several exogenous chemokine signaling factors have been applied to mobilize or recruit host stem/progenitor cells to the injured sites for in situ tissue regeneration. In this regard, if exogenous cell recruitment factors could be attached to the scaffold surface, the recruitment of host stem/progenitor cells into the damaged tissue would be mediated through chemokine signaling on the scaffold. Thus the mobilization of exogenous cell recruitment factors, which induces the mobilization or recruitment of host stem/progenitor cells, is a developing concept in the use of cell-free scaffolds for in situ tissue regeneration. The key to the development of an efficient and successful functionalized polymeric scaffold is the proficient mobilization of cell recruitment factors to the scaffold, as well as the recruitment of appropriate numbers of host stem/progenitor cells to the scaffold.

The recruitment of stem/progenitor cells into the damaged tissue is mediated by cell recruiting factors that could be incorporated into a polymeric scaffold. Several types of exogenous cell recruiting factors have been applied to mobilize or recruit host stem/progenitor cells to the injured sites for in situ tissue regeneration (Table 12.1) [13–19]. Thus such factors are candidates for use in the preparation of the polymeric scaffolds for in situ tissue regeneration.

SDF-1α has been shown to provide the main chemotactic signals to stem cells, especially MSCs [19]. SDF-1α plays a major role in the mobilization, integration, homing, survival, proliferation, and differentiation of stem cells. In addition, SDF-1α has been shown to enhance MSC recruitment to the damaged site via CXCR4 receptor signaling. MPC-1 is another likely signaling pathway for the recruitment of MSCs from systemic circulation. As a member of the cysteine–cysteine chemokine family,

Table 12.1 Recruitment Factors to Mobilize or Recruit Host Stem/Progenitor Cells

Recruitment Factors	Recruited Cell	References
Stromal cell derived factor-1 (SDF-1)	Bone-marrow derived stem cells, haematopoietic stem cells, mesenchymal stem cells, monocytes, lymphocytes	[14,15]
Hepatocyte growth factor (HGF)	Mesenchymal stem cells, neural stem cells	[16]
Monocyte chemoattractant protein 1 (MCP-1)	Monocytes, bone-marrow stromal cells, mesenchymal stem cells, macrophages, dendritic cells	[17,18]
Substance P	Mesenchymal stem cells, angiogenic cells	[19]

MPC-1 is a key mediator of proinflammatory pathways, activating leukocytes by binding to several chemokine receptors. MPC-1 recruits monocytes, memory T cells, and dendritic cells to the sites of inflammation produced by damaged tissue. Thus MPC-1 is believed to be effective in in situ tissue regeneration by promoting the recruitment of MSCs to damaged tissues [17,20,21]. Substance P (SP) is a highly conserved, 11-amino acid neuropeptide that mediates pain perception. SP is known to be involved in many processes, such as the regulation of inflammation, wound healing, and angiogenesis. SP elicits the mobilization and recruitment of stromal-like CD291 cells, hematopoietic stem cells, and MSCs [22]. SP has been reported to be effective in tissue regeneration by promoting the recruitment of MSCs to damaged tissues, making it an ideal candidate for the recruitment of endogenous stem cells, which are able to participate in the regeneration process at the damaged site. Transforming growth factor (TGF) plays a crucial role in tissue regeneration, cell differentiation, embryonic development, and regulation of the immune system [23]. Three isoforms of TGF-β are expressed in mammals (TGF-β1, -β2, and -β3). Latent TGF-β is abundant in the bone matrix. A gradient of active TGF-β then signals to transiently recruit perivascular MSCs to damaged bone sites for osteoblast differentiation and new bone formation. Hepatocyte growth factor (HGF) regulates and stimulates cell growth, cell motility, and morphogenesis and plays a central role in angiogenesis, tumorigenesis, adult organ regeneration, and wound healing [24]. In addition, HGF has been shown to be a chemoattractant that recruits human MSCs.

Besides the cell recruitment factors outlined above, several exogenous chemokine signaling factors, such as the granulocyte colony-stimulating factor, granulocyte-macrophage colony-stimulating factor, IL-3, IL-7, IL-8, IL-12, VEGF, insulin-like growth factor, PDGF-β, etc., can recruit host stem/progenitor cells to the injured sites for endogenous tissue regeneration. Additionally, more than two recruitment factors can effectively recruit stem cells.

DESIGN CONSIDERATIONS OF FUNCTIONALIZED POLYMERIC SCAFFOLDS

The optimal polymeric scaffold for in situ tissue regeneration should promote cell recruitment from the tissue surrounding the implanted scaffold and/or from the bloodstream, control the fate and differentiation of recruited cells, and stimulate tissue formation and remodeling from recruited cells (Fig. 12.2). In addition, it should be mechanically robust to avoid failure once introduced into the hemodynamic environment. The scaffold's properties are strictly reliant on the chosen design and the biomaterial used. The polymeric biomaterials used for scaffolding system (1) should have suitable mechanical properties for the regeneration of damaged tissues and organs; (2) must not cause excessive immune responses, properties collectively referred to as biocompatibility; (3) must be nontoxic, according to degradation over the appropriate experimental time frame, such that the ECM secreted by the recruited cells may compromise the mechanical integrity; (4) should act as a support for adhesion and proliferation of the recruited cells; (5) must be capable of facilitating cell–cell contact and cell migration through providing an optimal protective and nurturing environment over a prolonged period of time; and (6) must be adaptable to manufacturing techniques of the scaffold. Therefore the choice of the scaffold material is focused on the fulfillment of several requirements.

Efficacy of the prepared polymeric scaffold depends on two main properties, namely macroscopic and microscopic properties. Macroscopic properties refer to the mechanical properties regarding the scaffold architecture, while microscopic properties involve surface chemistry, bioactivity, local

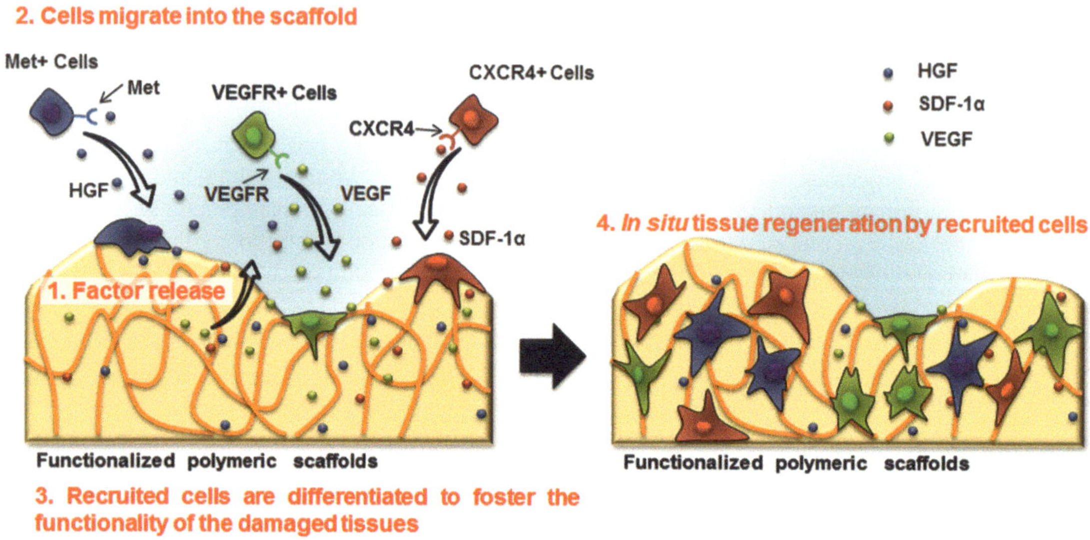

FIGURE 12.2

Schematic image for in situ tissue regeneration by functionalized polymeric scaffolds. The recruitment factors-immobilized scaffolds facilitate cell recruitment from the host tissue and/or blood to stimulate in situ tissue regeneration of damaged tissues.

The images were drawn by SHP and BKL using software of Adobe Photoshop 7.0.

stiffness, porosity, and topography. The macroscopic properties of the scaffolds are key to achieve optimal geometry and the overall mechanical properties of the scaffold. The microscopic properties of the scaffold are important to control the recruited cell fate through cell–scaffold interactions. Thus both the microscopic and macroscopic features can provide guidelines for the design of the scaffold.

One critical aspect of the scaffold design for in situ tissue regeneration is that it should have 3-D porous structures, since the cells from the surrounding tissue and/or bloodstream should be able to recruit onto the scaffold, and then homogeneously colonize the whole scaffold to regenerate the damaged tissue. Thus the first parameter of concern for the scaffold design is the pore size of the scaffold. The macroscopic architecture of a scaffold should provide the optimal geometry for tissue development and functionality. 3-D porous scaffolds are ideal for in situ tissue regeneration because they allow cell infiltration into the graft. The size of the recruited stem cells should be taken into consideration for the design of the pores in order to avoid the recruitment of cells in only some parts of the scaffold. Various scaffold fabrication methods can accurately control the pore structures to match the size of the recruited stem cells. Meanwhile, the pore is particularly relevant for both the scaffold's mechanical properties and cell recruitment. The scaffold design must take into consideration the relationship between being able to withstand the physiological mechanical environment and providing enough void volume for cell recruitment.

The scaffold's mechanical properties have often been designed and adapted to avoid mismatch at the time of in vivo implantation. It should be noted in this respect that the biodegradable properties of the scaffolds most often fail to mimic newly formed tissues or organs, almost inevitably leading to changes in the mechanical properties over time. However, it is difficult to predict the changes of the scaffold's mechanical properties over time after implantation. Therefore the scaffold should be designed as close as possible to that of the native tissue or organ in which it is implanted. Thus it is relevant to control the scaffold mechanical properties and tissue formation in time, as well as their combined effects on tissue mechanical properties. Despite significant advances in scaffold design, the ability of the scaffold to create an appropriate microenvironment in vivo during tissue regeneration remains an important and unresolved issue.

The cell recruiting factors can be immobilized onto the scaffold to mobilize stem cells from the tissue and/or bloodstream and to keep recruited cells adhered onto the scaffold surface. The concept of the immobilization of bioactive molecules onto the scaffold surface is well known. The immobilization is carried out either by the noncovalent bonding approach (physical adsorption) or by the covalent bonding approach (chemical adsorption). Both of these approaches allow for the introduction of recruitment factors onto the scaffold. Covalent bonding allows the stable immobilization of the cell recruitment factors by using several cross-linkers. This method usually requires surface modification to create a functional group that can be used for the immobilization of the recruitment factors. Thus the cell recruitment factors can be anchored directly onto the surface of the scaffold material. However, during this reaction, the scaffolds may result in side reactions, such as scaffold breakdown. In addition, the covalent bonding efficiency with sequential reaction of the recruitment factors is generally low. In contrast, physical adsorption utilizes noncovalent bonding through hydrogen bonding, van der Waals forces, and hydrophobic bonding. Thus the preparation of the scaffold with recruitment factors is simple when using intermolecular interactions between the scaffold surface and the recruiting factors. However, the strength of these interactions is mainly dependent on the surface chemistry of the scaffold material. Therefore physical adsorption may not provide enough stability of the recruitment factors. Moreover, the content of the recruitment factors and the conformation upon physical adsorption cannot be precisely controlled.

A drug delivery system can be used in the introducing of recruiting factors by physical adsorption. The concept of loading recruitment factors into a drug carrier is well known. The recruiting factors are loaded into a delivery drug carrier by several methods used in drug delivery systems. The recruiting factor-loaded scaffold allows for a timed release via a mainly passive release. Sustained release from the recruiting factor-loaded scaffold can create a gradient of recruitment factors capable of attracting cells at a distance of hundreds of microns. The recruiting factor-loaded scaffold influences local cellular processes by its slow release [13,25]. A scaffold prepared by two approaches may be used to induce selective cell recruitment in the scaffold. Various strategies on how to modify the local concentration of recruiting factors in the polymeric scaffold must be considered. It is apparent that the recruiting factors in the scaffold are maintained with stable and efficient activity at the initially immobilized concentration. An appealing mechanism by which scaffolds recruit host cells is by the action of the recruiting factors, which then induce the response of the surrounding endogenous cells.

IN SITU TISSUE REGENERATION USING THE FUNCTIONALIZED POLYMERIC SCAFFOLDS

The scaffold-based research represents a fascinating treatment option for in situ tissue engineering, the recruitment of cells from host tissue and/or blood, and stimulating the self-healing processes of damaged tissues. Various functionalized scaffolds, with or without cell recruiting factors, have been designed to support the attachment, proliferation, and differentiation of the recruited cells and to foster the mechanical functionality of the damaged tissues or organs. Lee SJ et al., as well as other researchers, have used conventional polyglycolic acid (PGA)/poly-L-lactic acid (PLLA) scaffolds without cell recruiting factors to investigate whether the host biologic resources and environmental conditions could be used for in situ tissue regeneration. Their study demonstrated that the host endogenous stem cells or tissue-specific progenitor cells could be mobilized into an implanted scaffold and that the infiltrated cells were capable of differentiating into multiple cells or target cell lineages if appropriate conditions were provided [26–30]. Meanwhile, the potential in vitro and in vivo results showed that the scaffolds with cell recruiting factors could induce in situ tissue regeneration, even though there is still much to learn about the design and clinical applications of the scaffolds with cell recruiting factors. Nevertheless, implantation of the scaffolds with cell recruiting factors, performed by several research groups, showed that these strategies are feasible for in situ tissue regeneration (Table 12.2) [31–57].

As discussed, SDF-1α, MCP, SP, and TGF were shown to be useful cell recruiting factors. Various cell recruiting factors have been reported to be useful in the in situ tissue regeneration of various organs, such as the brain, vasculature, heart, kidney, bone, cartilage, and liver. Superior results were reported by the functionalized polymeric scaffolds with cell recruiting factors compared with using a scaffold alone. Preclinical research regarding different scaffold materials, dosages of recruitment factors, recruited cells, animal models, and defect types attempt to understand the clinical need for the scaffolds. The cell recruiting factors can be introduced into various natural polymers (eg, collagen, fibrin, gelatin, alginate, and hyaluronic acids), synthetic polymers [eg, poly(lactic-*co*-glycolic acid) (PLGA), PLLA, polycaprolactone (PCL), polyethylene glycol (PEG), and their derivatives], and mixtures of natural and synthetic polymers (Table 12.2) [31–57].

SDF-1α was the most investigated cell recruiting factor. The scaffold with SDF-1α was shown to be useful in the in situ tissue regeneration of vasculature, heart, kidney, bone, cartilage, and liver tissue. The polymeric scaffold with SDF-1α showed great potential for in situ vascular regeneration [57–59].

Table 12.2 Functionalized Polymeric Scaffolds With Cell Recruitment Factors

Factors Involved	Scaffold Material	References
Stromal cell derived factor-1 (SDF-1)	Synthesis polymer: PLGA, PCL, PU, PLEOF, PGA, PLLA, PNIPAM	[32–36]
	Natural polymer: heparin, gelatin, chitosan, hyaluronic acid, collagen	[37–44]
	Synthesis polymer/natural polymer: PLLA/gelatin, PLGA/fibrin	[45–47]
Monocyte chemoattractant protein (MCP)	Synthesis polymer: PDO, PCL	[48,49]
	Natural polymer: gelatin, fibirin	[50,51]
Substance P (SP)	Synthesis polymer: PCLA, PCL	[52,53]
	Natural polymer: gelatin, peptide	[14,54]
Transforming growth factor (TGF)	Synthesis polymer: PCL	[55]
	Natural polymer: chitosan, collagen	[56]
Hepatocyte growth factor (HGF)	Natural polymer: hyaluronic acid, gelatin	[57]

PCL, *(polycaprolactone);* PCLA, *poly(caprolactone-*co*-L-lactic acid);* PDO, *polydioxanone;* PGA, *polyglycolic acid;* PLEOF, *poly(lactide ethylene oxide fumarate);* PLGA, *poly(lactic-*co*-glycolic acid);* PLLA, *poly-L-lactic acid;* PNIPAM, *poly(*N*-isopropylacrylamide);* PU, *polyurethane.*

Several groups have reported that using the polymeric scaffolds with SDF-1α could be a promising strategy for tissue regeneration, such as cartilage and subchondral bone regeneration [33,41,47,60–64]. Kim et al. examined whether the scaffolds with SP would significantly enhance the recruitment of stem cells and promote the regeneration of bone, cartilage, limb ischemia, and fat cells [51–53,65]. For decades, many polymeric scaffolds, with and without cell recruiting factors, have been developed and have received considerable attention for their potential to induce in situ tissue regeneration. Specifically, in the field of cardiology, the scaffolds have already been used in the clinical practice of cardiac surgery [66]. The functionalized polymeric scaffolds can lead to the manipulation of cellular responses, are available off-the-shelf, have minimal batch-to-batch variation, and most importantly, result in fully autologous, living in situ tissue regeneration.

CONCLUSION AND FUTURE TECHNOLOGICAL CHALLENGES

Research on developing the functionalized polymeric scaffolds has increasingly become a subject of investigation due to its potential for in situ tissue regeneration via host stem cell mobilization. The number of developments of the polymeric scaffolds will certainly continue to grow. Although many advances have been rapidly made, there are still many important hurdles to overcome before researchers can ensure the safety and efficacy of the polymeric scaffolds. The polymeric scaffolds could incorporate the cell recruiting factors that are necessary to induce the desired cells from the adjacent tissue and/or blood circulation. The polymeric scaffold with cell recruiting factors must induce an appropriate cell source from the surrounding damaged tissue, then attach and grow the recruited cells, and allow successful in situ tissue regeneration at the target site. Following further research, in which cell recruitment factors yield the best results in cell recruitment, it is important to investigate the in vivo performance of implanted polymeric scaffolds.

Further consideration of the polymeric scaffolds is the prediction of the in vivo responses to novel materials. Ideally, polymeric materials selected for the scaffolds will both minimize the immune response through thoughtful material selection and design and contain a sufficient comprehension of the immune response to enable effective antirejection strategies with minimal side effects. In addition, to support these various functions in the tissue regeneration process, the polymeric scaffolds must possess appropriate mechanical properties and 3-D structures that mimic the ECM. The polymeric scaffold must function in the same environment as the original tissue, or during the desired period, and suppress malfunctioning. A great challenge lies in the precise control of the mechanical properties of the scaffold. Combining the precise in vivo target cell recruitment using the polymeric scaffolds, the development of biocompatible materials, the maintenance of appropriate mechanical properties, and the complete understanding of the complex in situ tissue regeneration processes, the polymeric scaffolds should be available off-the-shelf, have minimal batch-to-batch variation, and most importantly, result in fully autologous, living in situ tissue regeneration.

Although considerable research focused on increasing the number of clinically successful polymeric scaffold lies ahead, recent developments in science and technology have ushered in a new era of regenerative medicine. There will no doubt be significant crossover in the functionalized polymeric scaffold research that leads to better, safer, and more integrated in situ tissue engineering in order to regenerate human tissue or organs. The present scaffold materials have been successfully applied in animal models, and thus new challenges will arise when those strategies are translated to human applications. The key advances in research for human applications must address the efficiency of host cell recruitment, immunological issues of the scaffold materials, and understanding the in situ tissue regeneration process and the changeability of the polymeric scaffolds in clinical environments regarding surrounding damaged tissue, age, and physical activity.

At this time, a united effort including researchers in various fields is urgently needed to develop and apply original technologies that might help to realize the tremendous potential of the polymeric scaffold, which can undoubtedly perform the specific requirements for regenerative medicine in human health in the near future. The emerging clinically relevant knowledge and technology regarding the polymeric scaffolds is growing exponentially. Realizing the potential of in situ tissue regeneration through the functionalized polymeric scaffolds will require substantial and continuing collaborative research among material, pharmaceutical, biological, and clinical scientists.

REFERENCES

[1] Atala A, et al. Principles of regenerative medicine. Academic Press; 2007.

[2] Bianco P, et al. Stem cells in tissue engineering. Nature 2001;414:118–21.

[3] Kirkpatrick CJ, et al. Theoretical and practical aspects of testing potential biomaterilas in vitro. J Mater Sci 1990;1:9–13.

[4] Griffith LG, et al. Tissue engineering–current challenges and expanding opportunities. Science 2002;295:1009–14.

[5] Kim MS, et al. Polymeric scaffolds for regenerative medicine. Polym Rev 2011;51:1–30.

[6] Kim JI, et al. An injectable biodegradable temperature-responsive gel with an adjustable persistence window. Biomaterials 2012;33:2823–34.

[7] Shim SW, et al. Preparation of zwitterionic sulfobetaine end-functionalized poly(ethylene glycol)-*b*-poly(caprolactone) diblock copolymers and examination of their thermogelling properties. J Polym Sci Part A Polym Chem 2014;52:2185–91.

[8] Kim JI, et al. Examination of phase transition behavior of ion group functionalized MPEG-b-PCL diblock copolymers. Soft Matter 2011;7:8650–6.

[9] Cancedda R, et al. Tissue engineering and cell theraphy of cartilage and bone. Matrix Biol 2003;22:81–91.

[10] Kon E, et al. Scaffold-based cartilage treatments: with or without cells? A systematic review of preclinical and clinical evidence. Arthroscopy 2015;31:767–75.

[11] Kollet O, et al. HGF, SDF-1, and MMP-9 are involved in stress-induced human CD34+ stem cell recruitment to the liver. J Clin Invest 2003;112:160–9.

[12] Muylaert DEP, et al. Combining tissue repair and tissue engineering; bioactivating implantable cell-free vascular scaffolds. Heart 2014;100:1825–30.

[13] Askari AT, et al. Effect of stromal-cell-derived factor 1 on stem-cell homing and tissue regeneration in ischaemic cardiomyopathy. Lancet 2003;362:697–703.

[14] Kitoari T, et al. Stromal cell-derived factor1/CXCR4 signaling is critical for the recruitment of mesenchymal stem cells to the fracture site during skeletal repair in a mouse model. Athritis Rheum 2009;60:813–23.

[15] van de Kamp J, et al. Hepatocyte growth factor-loaded biomaterials for mesenchymal stem cell recruitment. Stem Cells Int 2013;2013:892065.

[16] Schenk S, et al. Monocyte chemotactic protein-3 is a myocardial mesenchymal stem cell homing factor. Stem Cells 2007;25:245–51.

[17] Ishikawa M, et al. MCP/CCR2 signaling is essential for recruitment of mesenchymal progenitor cells during the early phase of fracture healing. PLoS One 2014;9:e105954.

[18] Kim JH, et al. Stem cell recruitment and angiogenesis of neuropeptide substance P coupled with self-assembling peptide nanofiber in a mouse hind limb ischemia model. Biomaterials 2013;34:1657–68.

[19] Liu X, et al. SDF-1/CXCR4 axis modulates bone marrow mesenchymal stem cell apoptosis, migration and cytokine secretion. Protein Cell 2011;2:845–54.
[20] Monika K, et al. Monocyte chemoattractant protein 1-mediated migration of mesenchymal stem cells is a source of intimal hyperplasia. Arterioscler Thromb Vasc Biol 2013;33:1271–9.
[21] Andreas S. Chemokines in vascular dysfunction and remodeling the chemokine network to enable therapeutic intervention. Arterioscler Thromb Vasc Biol 2008;28:1950–9.
[22] Bowden JJ, et al. Direct observation of substance P-induced internalization of neurokinin 1 (NK1) receptors at sites of inflammation. Proc Natl Acad Sci USA 1994;91:8964–8.
[23] Moustakas A, et al. Mechanism of TGF-β signaling in regulation of cell growth and differentiation. Immunol Lett 2002;82:85–91.
[24] Neuss S. Functional expression of HGF and HGF receptor/c-met in adult human mesenchymal stem cells suggests a role in cell mobilization, tissue repair, and wound healing. Stem Cells 2004;22:405–14.
[25] Zhang F. Surface-engineering of glycidyl methacrylated dextran/gelatin microcapsules with thermos-responsive poly(*N*-isopropylacrylamide) gates for controlled delivery of stromal cell-derived factor-1α. Biomaterials 2013;34:6515–27.
[26] Ju YM, et al. In situ regeneration of skeletal muscle tissue through host cell recruitment. Acta Biomater 2014;10:4332–9.
[27] Lee SJ, et al. Host cell mobilization for in situ tissue regeneration. Rejuvenation Res 2008;11:747–56.
[28] Ko IK, et al. In situ tissue regeneration through host stem cell recruitment. Exp Mol Med 2013;15:45–57.
[29] Lyons FG, et al. The healing of bony defects by cell-free collagen-based scaffolds compared to stem cell-seeded tissue engineered constructs. Biomaterials 2010;31:9323–43.
[30] Sandeep T, et al. Injectable, porous, and cell-responsive gelatin cryogels. Biomaterials 2014;35:2477–87.
[31] Reyes R, et al. Cartilage repair by local delivery of transforming growth factor-beta1 or bone morphogenetic protein-2 from a novel, segmented polyurethane/polylactic-co-glycolic bilayered scaffold. J Biomed Mater Res A 2014;102:1110–20.
[32] Thevenot PT, et al. The effect of incorporation of SDF-1alpha into PLGA scaffolds on stem cell recruitment and the inflammatory response. Biomaterials 2010;31:3997–4008.
[33] Schantz JT, et al. Cell guidance in tissue engineering: SDF-1 mediates site-directed homing of mesenchymal stem cells within three-dimensional polycaprolactone scaffolds. Tissue Eng 2007;13:2615–24.
[34] He X, et al. Migration of marrow stromal cells, in response to sustained release of stromal-derived factor-1alpha from poly(lactide ethylene oxide fumarate) hydrogels. Int J Pharm 2010;390:107–16.
[35] Torikai K, et al. A self-renewing, tissue-engineered vascular graft arterial reconstruction. J Thorac Cardiovasc Surg 2008;136:37–45.
[36] Yu J, et al. The effect of stromal cell-derived factor-1alpha/heparin coating of biodegradable vascular grafts on the recruitment of both endothelial and smooth muscle progenitor cells for accelerated regeneration. Biomaterials 2012;33:8062–74.
[37] Kimura Y, et al. Controlled release of stromal-cell-derived factor-1 from gelatin hydrogels enhances angiogenesis. J Biomater Sci Polym Ed 2010;21:37–51.
[38] Prokoph S, et al. Sustained delivery of SDF-1alpha from heparin-based hydrogels to attract circulating pro-angiogenic cells. Biomaterials 2012;33:4792–800.
[39] Purcell BP, et al. Synergistic effects of SDF-1alpha chemokine and hyaluronic acid release from degradable hydrogels on directing bone marrow derived cell homing to the myocardium. Biomaterials 2012;33:7849–57.
[40] Huang YC, et al. Mobilization of mesenchymal stem cells by stromal cell derived factor-1 released from chitosan/tripolyphosphate/fucoidan nanoparticles. Acta Biomater 2012;8:1048–56.
[41] Zhang W, et al. The use of type 1 collagen scaffold containing stromal cell-derived factor-1 to create a matrix environment conducive to partial-thickness cartilage defects repair. Biomaterials 2013;34:713–23.
[42] Segal MS, et al. Nitric oxide cytoskeletal-induced alterations reverse the endothelial progenitor cell migratory defect associated with diabetes. Diabetes 2006;55:102–9.

[43] Yin Y, et al. SDF-1α involved in mobilization and recruitment of endothelial progenitor cells after arterial injury in mice. Cardiovasc Pathol 2010;19:218–27.
[44] Ko IK, et al. Combined systemic and local delivery of stem cell inducing/recruiting factors for in situ tissue regeneration. FASEB J 2012;26:158–68.
[45] Wang W, et al. The restoration of full-thickness cartilage defects with BMSCs and TGF-beta 1 loaded PLGA/fibrin gel constructs. Biomaterials 2010;31:8964–73.
[46] Ertan AB, et al. Effect of double growth factor release on cartilage tissue engineering. J Tissue Eng Regen Med 2013;7:149–60.
[47] Shinohara K, et al. Stromal cell-derived factor-1 and monocyte chemotactic protein-3 improve recruitment of osteogenic cells into sites of musculoskeletal repair. J Orthop Res 2011;29:1064–9.
[48] Smith MJ, et al. Feasibility of electrospun polydioxanone monocyte chemotactic protein-1 (MCP-1) hybrid scaffold as potential cellular homing devices. J Eng Fibers Fabr 2010;5:1–9.
[49] Garcia Cruz DM, et al. Gelatin microparticles aggregates as three-dimensional scaffolding system in cartilage engineering. J Mater Sci Mater Med 2013;24:503–13.
[50] Smits AIPM, et al. Shear flow affects selective monocyte recruitment into MCP-1-loaded scaffolds. J Cell Mol Med 2014;18:2176–88.
[51] Kim SH, et al. Self-assembling peptide nanofibers coupled with neuropeptide substance P for bone tissue engineering. Tissue Eng Part A 2015;21:1237–46.
[52] Shafiq M, et al. Stem cell recruitment, angiogenesis, and tissue regeneration in substance P-conjugated poly(l-lactide-co-ε-caprolactone) nonwoven meshes. J Biomed Mater Res Part A 2015;103:2673–88.
[53] Kohara H, et al. Angiogenesis induced by controlled release of neuropeptide substance P. Biomaterials 2010;31:8617–25.
[54] Huang Q, et al. In vivo mesenchymal cell recruitment by a scaffold loaded with transforming growth factor beta1 and the potential for in situ chondrogenesis. Tissue Eng 2002;8:469–82.
[55] Zhang Y, et al. Novel chitosan/collagen scaffold containing transforming growth factor-β1 DNA for periodontal tissue engineering. Biochem Biophys Res Commun 2006;344:362–9.
[56] Jing Z, et al. Recruitment of endogenous stem cells for tissue repair. Macromol Biosci 2008;8:836–42.
[57] Blumenthal B, et al. Functional regeneration of ischemic myocardium by transplanted cells overexpressing stromal cell-derived factor-1 (SDF-1): intramyocardial injection versus scaffold-based application. Eur J Cardiothorac Surg 2011;40:134–41.
[58] Lee KW, et al. Human progenitor cell recruitment via SDF-1α coacervate-laden PGS vascular grafts. Biomaterials 2013;34:9877–86.
[59] Blumenthal B, et al. Polyurethane scaffolds seeded with genetically engineered skeletal myoblasts: a promising tool to regenerate myocardial function. Artif Organs 2010;34:46–54.
[60] Chen P, et al. Radially oriented collagen scaffold with SDF-1 promotes osteochondral repair by facilitating cell homing. Biomaterials 2015;39:114–23.
[61] Liu Y, et al. Mineralised collagen scaffolds loaded with stromal cell-derived factor-1 improve mandibular bone regeneration. Chin J Dent Res 2014;17:23–9.
[62] Liu YS, et al. The effect of simvastatin on chemotactic capability of SDF-1α and the promotion of bone regeneration. Biomaterials 2014;34:4489–98.
[63] Zhang F, et al. A transduced living hyaline cartilage graft releasing transgenic stromal cell-derived factor-1 inducing endogenous stem cell homing in vivo. Tissue Eng Part A 2013;19:1091–9.
[64] Shen W, et al. The effect of incorporation of exogenous stromal cell-derived factor-1 alpha within a knitted silk-collagen sponge scaffold on tendon regeneration. Biomaterials 2010;31:7239–49.
[65] Song M, et al. Regeneration of chronic myocardial infarction by injectable hydrogels containing stem cell homing factor SDF-1 and angiogenic peptide Ac-SDKP. Biomaterials 2014;34:2436–45.
[66] Kurobe H, et al. Concise review: tissue-engineered vascular grafts for cardiac surgery: past, present, and future. Stem Cells Transl Med 2012;1:566–71.

CHAPTER

TISSUE-DERIVED MATRICES

13

H.C. Ott, T.K. Rajab

Harvard Medical School, Boston, MA, United States

CHAPTER OUTLINE

In Situ Tissue Regeneration. http://dx.doi.org/10.1016/B978-0-12-802225-2.00013-1

INTRODUCTION

The etymology of *matrix* derives from Latin *mater* (mother) and refers to a supporting or enclosing structure. Tissue-derived matrices are biomaterials that are generated from the extracellular matrix (ECM) of specific tissues. The ECM refers to the material in which cells of metazoan organisms are embedded [1]. This material forms a dynamic 3-D structure and fulfills important functions that depend on the respective tissue type. The ECM functions as a structural foundation by providing a scaffold that supports the embedded cells. In addition, the ECM has biological functions that allow it to regulate the activity of extracellular molecules and affect cellular processes such as gene expression and migration [2]. The specialized properties of the ECM make tissue-derived matrices a promising substrate for use in tissue engineering and biomaterial design [3].

COMPOSITION OF THE EXTRACELLULAR MATRIX

Various forms of ECM exist in all animal tissues. During growth, development, and throughout the lifespan of an organism, ECM components are secreted, absorbed, and remodeled by resident cells that are spatially associated with the matrix. In most connective tissues, these cells are part of the fibroblast family. The molecular structure of the ECM is highly complex. Completion of the genome sequences for humans and other model organisms has shown that the ECM is formed by approximately 300 proteins [4]. Together, these ECM proteins form the so-called matrisome. Key components of the matrisome can be subclassified as fibrous proteins, proteoglycans, and glycoproteins [5]. The relative composition of these components within an ECM determines its form and function. This results in a wide spectrum of different types of ECM, ranging from the calcified ECM of bone to the elastic ECM of skin and the delicate ECM of renal glomeruli.

FIBROUS PROTEINS

Fibrous proteins are the most abundant proteins in the ECM and include the collagen and elastin families. Collagens form between 25% and 35% of the total mammalian protein content. The mammalian genome contains genes for over 40 different collagen subunits that are located on over a dozen different chromosomes [5]. The defining molecular characteristic of collagen subunits is a Gly-X-Y triplet repeat, where X is frequently proline and Y is frequently 4-hydroxyproline. Collagen subunits are synthesized by fibroblasts. After transcription of collagen mRNA on the ribosomes of the rough endoplasmic reticulum, the precursor polypeptides undergo extensive posttranslational modifications in the lumen of the endoplasmic reticulum. These posttranslational modifications include hydroxylation of proline and lysine residues, which requires vitamin C as cofactor. Three collagen subunits subsequently join to form a triple helix, known as the procollagen molecule. Procollagen is secreted by vesicles of the Golgi apparatus into the ECM. In the extracellular space, the procollagen are cleaved to form tropocollagen. Tropocollagen molecules then spontaneously aggregate to form higher order 3-D collagen structures that can be classified into different categories [6].

Fibrillar collagens include types I, II, III, V, XI, XXIV, and XXVII. These collagens are characterized by long triple-helical segments with continuous Gly-X-Y repeats over their full length. This allows them to assemble into cross-striated fibers.

The network-forming collagens include types IV, VIII, and X. These collagens contain sections of Gly-X-Y repeats that are interrupted by other motifs that allow them to assemble into supercoiled net-like structures [7]. Fibril-associated collagens with interrupted triple helices (FACIT) include types IX, XII, XIV, XVI, XX, and XXI. These collagens have characteristic triple-helical segments that are interspersed with nonhelical domains. These collagens attach to the surface of fibrillar collagens [8]. Collagens with transmembrane domains include types XIII, XVII, XXIII, and XXV. These collagens participate in cellular adhesions and are found in hemidesmosomes of the skin, for example [9]. Multiplexin collagens include types XV and XVIII. These collagens have highly interrupted triple helices and large globular domains at their terminal ends. Finally, filamentous and anchoring fibrillar collagens include Types VI, VII, XXVI, and XXVIII. The functions of these collagens include linking the basement membrane to the underlying ECM. The most abundant types of collagens found in the ECM are types I, II, III, IV, and V [6]. Table 13.1 provides a summary of these collagens.

The function of collagen molecules is to provide structural strength to the ECM. Collagen fibers are organized in different patterns depending on the functional requirements of the tissues. For example, type I collagen fibrils in human tendons are arranged in a linear fashion to maximally resist longitudinal tension. In contrast, type IV collagen in renal glomeruli is arranged as networks to

Table 13.1 List of the Most Abundant Types of Collagens [10]

Collagen Type	Genes	Notes
I	COL1A1 and COL1A2	Fibrillar collagen that forms the main protein component of skin and bone. This is by far the most abundant type of all collagens. Genetic defects cause osteogenesis imperfectal.
II	COL2A1	Fibrillar collagen that forms the main protein component of cartillage.
III	COL3A1	Fibrillar collagen that is found in elastic tissues such as lung and blood vessel walls. Genetic defects cause Ehlers–Danlos syndrome.
IV	COL4A1, COL4A2, COL4A3, COL4A4, COL4A5, and COL4A6	Network-forming collagen that is primarily found in the basement membrane. Genetic defects cause Alport syndrome.
V	COL5A1, COL5A2, and COL5A3	Fibrillar collagen that has a broad tissue distribution. Genetic defects cause Ehlers–Danlos syndrome.

withstand the mechanical force of capillary blood flow and to participate in filtration of urine. These functions are reflected in the diverse disorders caused by genetic defects of collagen genes. These disorders range from brittle bone disease in osteogenesis imperfecta [11] to end-stage renal disease in Alport syndrome [12].

Another type of fibrous protein in the ECM is elastin. In contrast to collagen, elastin is encoded in a single gene localized to chromosome 7. The elastin gene has 36 exons that allow extensive alternative splicing of different isoforms [13]. Elastin mRNA is translated by ribosomes of the rough endoplasmic reticulum into elastin precursor polypeptides called tropoelastin. This molecule undergoes posttranslational modifications including hydroxylation. Tropoelastin is then secreted into the ECM [14]. Similar to collagen, several elastin precursors then aggregate to form a 3-D mature elastin molecule. The elastin precursors are covalently cross-linked to each other. It is thought that elastin molecules adopt a coiled confirmation that allows it to expand and recoil in response to tensile stress [15]. This allows elastin to fulfill its function of endowing the ECM with elastic recoil. The function of elastin is reflected in its abundance in connective tissues that require elastic expansion and contraction, including the conducting arteries. Genetic defects of the elastin gene thus result in defective function of these tissues. For example, supravalvular aortic stenosis causes a significant narrowing of the large conduction arteries [16].

PROTEOGLYCANS

Another major component of the ECM is formed by proteoglycans. These form a hydrated ground substance that embeds associated cells and ECM fibrous proteins. Proteoglycans consist of very diverse ECM core proteins that are associated with glycosaminoglycans (GAGs). This distinguishes them from other glycoproteins. GAGs are unbranched carbohydrate polymers that are formed by repeating disaccharide subunits. One of the two saccharides is always an *N*-acetylglucosamine or *N*-acetylgalactosamine, and frequently this saccharide is sulfated. The other saccharide is usually glucuronic acid or induronic acid. The polysaccharide chain is also modified by epimerization and sulphation. These possible modifications result in a huge diversity of possible GAG chains [17]. The most common types of GAGs include hyaluronan, heparan sulfate, keratan sulfate, dermatan sulfate, and chondroitin sulfate. The size of these GAGs varies between dozens to thousands of saccharide repeats. An important characteristic of GAGs is their high negative charge. The negative charge attracts positively charged electrolytes and water molecules follow via osmosis. As a result, proteoglycans form gels that expand to a very large volume relative to their mass.

The structural functions of proteoglycans include hydration of the ECM, expansion of its volume, and resisting compressive forces [18]. For example, aggrecan, which forms the major constituent of cartilage, associates with hyaluronan to form aggregates at micrometer scale. This allows cartilage in joints to withstand the compressive forces of hundreds of kilograms. The structural function of proteoglycans contrast with the function of collagens, which resist tensile stress. Due to their function in hydrating the ECM, proteoglycans also provide lubrication.

In addition to their structural functions, proteoglycans also actively participate in the regulation of the activity of other extracellular molecules. This can occur by a number of different mechanisms. For example, proteoglycans can bind specific paracrine mediators in order to locally concentrate them in the ground substance. This mechanism is involved in the regulation of chemokines, for example. The chemokines bind to proteoglycans in inflamed tissues, which locally increases their concentration and allows them to attract immune cells. Another mechanism for the regulation of extracellular molecules by proteoglycans is by inhibition. This mechanism is used in the regulation of transforming growth factor, which is inhibited by the proteoglycan decorin.

GLYCOPROTEINS

The third major component of the ECM is formed by the glycoproteins [19]. The glycoproteins are a diverse group of molecules whose functions are legion. Glycoproteins contribute to ECM assembly, cellular adhesion, and signaling.

One example of a well-characterized ECM glycoprotein is fibronectin. This molecule is secreted as a dimer of two similar monomers. The monomers are linked by a pair of disulfide bonds on their C-terminal end. Each monomer has a molecular weight of 220–250 kDa and consists predominantly of three motifs. These motifs repeat and are organized into distinct functional domains. The structure of fibronectin includes binding domains that participate in the interaction of fibronectin with specific receptors such as integrins and collagens [20]. Binding of fibronectin to its target results in conformational changes that subsequently expose cryptic binding sites within fibronectin. These binding functions allow fibronectin to interact with other ECM proteins and participate in cellular adhesion.

Another example of well-characterized ECM glycoproteins is the laminin family. The molecular weight of laminin is approximately 400 kDa. Laminins are heterotrimeric proteins consisting of alpha, beta, and gamma subunits. This results in a variety of over a dozen different laminins. Electron microscopy showed that laminins have a cruciform shape. One arm of the cross is longer than the others and formed by a coil composed of all three laminin subunits. The other three arms of the cross are formed by one subunit each [21]. Laminin is first produced in the eight-cell stage embryo. During later stages of development, laminins are predominantly localized to the basal lamina. Within basal lamina, laminins enable interactions with resident and transient cells and harbor various signaling molecules. Cellular receptors attach to laminin at distinct domains, which have specific functions. For example, receptors with mitogenic function attach to domains in the short arms of the laminin molecule. In contrast, receptors promoting neurite outgrowth attach to the long arm of the laminin molecule.

FUNCTIONS OF NATIVE EXTRACELLULAR MATRIX

STRUCTURAL FUNCTION OF THE EXTRACELLULAR MATRIX

The most obvious function of the native ECM is its role as a structural scaffold. This function of the ECM may have been one of the key innovations that allowed the evolution of multicellular life [22]. The structural functions of the ECM are dependent on its material properties. The material properties of ECM include its physical properties and its chemical properties. Together, these physical properties and the chemical properties of ECM determine its mechanical properties. Typical forces that act on materials include axial forces, transverse forces, and torsional forces. Force acting on materials results in a stress on the material. The SI unit of stress is pascal, which is defined as 1 N per square meter. Compressive stress acts to reduce the volume of the material. Tensile stress acts to increase the volume of the material. Finally, shear stress acts in opposing directions through the cross-section of the material. Stress placed on materials results in strain. Strain is a description of deformation of the material. Strains that reverse after the stress is removed are called elastic strains. If a stress is greater than the elastic limit of a material, irreversible strain results. Such irreversible strains are called plastic strains. Strain eventually results in material failure. In material science, material failure is the loss of the ability of the material to resist strain. The relationship between stress and strain is known as the stress–strain curve. This curve is characteristic for each material. Ductile materials such as cartilage are characterized by progressive strain before the material fails in response to progressive stress. In contrast, brittle materials, such as bones, are characterized by only limited strain before the material fails in response to progressive stress.

The material properties of extracellular matrices are determined by the sum of its different components and their structure, which differ considerably in different tissues. This results in very different material properties in different tissues. For example, the strength of bone depends on the morphology of the bone ultrastructure as well as the molecular composition of the bone ECM, including its collagens and mineralization. Due to these specializations, bones have strengths greater than 160 MPa [23]. Other biomaterials are able to achieve much higher strengths still. Spider silk, for example, can reach almost 2000 MPa, which is greater than steel [24]. Tendons have a high proportion of collagens that are longitudinally arranged that provide tensile strength that is comparable to bone in the longitudinal direction of the tendon. In contrast, collagen in the skin is structured as a network to provide tensile strength in multiple directions. The tensile strength of skin is approximately 20 MPa. Furthermore, the relative proportion of collagens and elastins determines the ECM ductility. Other tissues, such as the lungs and the walls of blood vessels, contain a high proportion of elastins that give them the ability to stretch without material failure.

REGULATION OF THE ACTIVITY OF OTHER EXTRACELLULAR MOLECULES

In addition to their structural functions, the ECM also serves important biological functions. Since the ECM evolved very early in metazoan history as a scaffold that allowed multicellular life, many structural molecules in the matrisome, such as type IV collagen and laminins, are highly conserved among metazoa. However, as described above, the ECM contains not only structural proteins such as the collagens and elastins but also hundreds of other molecules. Many of these other vertebrate ECM proteins have evolved much more recently. In addition, many ECM proteins have complex structures with multiple distinct domains. It is thought that the newly evolved ECM proteins with their complex domain structures have important biological regulatory functions [2].

Regulation of growth factor signaling

Some of these biological regulatory functions relate to the regulation of growth factor signaling. Many growth factors bind to the negatively charged ECM proteoglycans. In particular, binding of growth factors to heparin and heparan sulfate side chains of proteoglycans is well characterized. This allows the ECM to function as a reservoir for growth factors. Subsequent degradation of ECM proteins releases these bound growth factors in a soluble form. This mechanism can establish well-defined concentration gradients. These concentration gradients can be modulated by the affinity of ECM molecules for the respective growth factors. For example, fibroblast growth factor 10 (FGF10) is bound by ECM proteoglycans with high affinity. This high affinity binding results in a highly focused concentration gradient. In contrast, FGF7 is bound by ECM proteoglycans with low affinity. This binding with low affinity results in a broad concentration gradient. One example for the function of such growth factor gradients is the regulation of branching morphogenesis during the development of organs such as lung or mammary tissue. The focused concentration gradient serves to induce growth by branching morphogenesis that is focused toward the ECM. In contrast, the broad concentration gradient may induce growth by branching morphogenesis that is not directed in any one direction but instead occurs in multiple directions [25].

Regulation of proteolytic enzymes

The ECM regulates the activity of several other extracellular molecules. One example of this is the regulation of enzyme activity by the ECM by local activation. Many extracellular proteases exist in an inactive precursor form. This precursor form is activated locally in the desired tissues by other enzymes that are specifically associated with the ECM. This serves to spatially restrict the activation of these proteins to the desired location only. One example of this mechanism is the restriction of plasmin activity to certain areas of the circulation only. Conversely, ECM proteins can also inhibit certain secreted enzymes.

FUNCTIONAL INTERACTIONS OF THE EXTRACELLULAR MATRIX WITH EMBEDDED CELLS

The ECM not only interacts with extracellular molecules but also with the cells that are embedded in it. The interaction between the ECM and its embedded cells is bidirectional. On the one hand, cells maintain and modify the architecture of the ECM. On the other hand, the ECM can influence cellular function by activating cellular signaling pathways. One example of this is regulation of cellular survival and apoptosis. Activation of cellular signaling pathways by the ECM explains the observation that many tissue cells are not viable in suspension. Instead, they depend on anchorage to an extracellular solid to survive [26].

The ECM interacts with cells via specific receptors

Embedded cells interact with the ECM via specific receptors. Among the receptors that allow cells to interact with the ECM are the integrins. Integrins are heterodimeric receptor proteins. There are two different types of subunits that are named alpha and beta subunits. Mammals have 18 alpha and 8 beta subunits. Additional diversity is generated by differential RNA splicing. The integrin subunits are transmembrane proteins with small cytoplasmic domains. The cytoplasmic domains typically consist of 40–70 amino acids. The total weight of the integrin subunits varies between 90 and 160 kDa. Different combinations of the subunits result in the generation of over 20 different integrins [27]. These integrins have specific ligands. Ligands for the integrins include collagens, laminins, fibronectins, growth factors, and other glycoproteins. By interacting with their ligands, integrins can transmit signals from the ECM to the cell. Signaling from the ECM to the cell depends on downstream signaling pathways. For example, integrin binding activates the protein kinase B (AKT) and extracellular signal-regulated kinase (ERK) pathways that allow cells to survive and multiply. In addition, interactions of integrins with their ECM ligands also result in transmission of signals from the cell to the ECM. This depends on linkage of the integrins to the cellular actin cytoskeleton via adhesion complexes. The actin cytoskeleton can thus effect physical changes in the ECM.

ECM physical properties can affect stem cell fate

Through their interaction with the embedded cells, the ECM can also determine stem cell fate. Stem cells are known to circulate and differentiate in situ during development and during tissue regeneration after injuries. It was found that the mechanical properties of the local ECM are involved in determining the lineage of such stem cells. Mesenchymal stem cells were cultured with polyacrylamide gel matrices of different elasticities. The elasticity of these matrices resulted in different lineage phenotypes. Soft matrices that mimicked brain were neurogenic. In contrast, stiffer matrices that mimicked muscle were myogenic. Finally, rigid matrices that mimicked bone were osteogenic. This shows that matrix elasticity can direct stem cell lineage specification [28].

ECM physical properties regulate branching morphogenesis in development

The ECM also plays other important roles during development. One example of this is the role of ECM in branching morphogenesis of the lungs. Branching morphogenesis involves repetitive formation of epithelial branches that grow into the surrounding ECM [29]. The ECM is an active participant in this process by providing a structural scaffold and by serving biological functions that regulate cellular gene expression. One example of the structural role of ECM in branching morphogenesis is provided by the role of elastin and type III collagen in lung development. Elastin and type III collagen are among the most abundant ECM proteins in the lungs. During development, remodeling of these molecules at the leading edge of the growing branches during lung morphogenesis is important in the formation of mature alveoli [30]. This was demonstrated by inhibition of elastin and type III collagen expression, which in turn caused inhibition of alveolar morphogenesis [31].

TISSUE-DERIVED MATRICES FOR TISSUE ENGINEERING

The special properties and complex functions of ECM described earlier make ECM a promising substrate for use in tissue engineering. Tissue engineering involves the manipulation of cells and biomaterials to construct, functionalize, and maintain living tissues [32]. The first step in preparing ECM for applications in tissue engineering is to isolate the ECM. This requires removal of all cells from the donor tissue.

METHODS FOR THE REMOVAL OF CELLS FROM TISSUE-DERIVED MATRICES

A number of different methods have been described to decellularize donor tissue. These methods involve physical protocols, chemical protocols, and biological protocols [33].

Physical protocols to decellularize tissues

One way to decellularize tissues is by physical means. The most commonly used physical protocol to decellularize tissues is freeze–thaw decellularization [34]. Freezing results in the formation of ice crystals, which have a greater volume than the original volume of their constituent liquids and therefore disrupt tissues. Cells are particularly vulnerable to this type of damage because of the small, enclosed cytoplasmic spaces and fragile cell membranes. However, freezing may also damage the ECM. Therefore the freeze–thaw cycles need to be carefully titrated to avoid damage to the ECM. Another physical protocol to decellularize tissues is the application of mechanical force. Such mechanical forces result in pressure on cells that causes rupture of their membranes. However, mechanical pressure also damages the ECM. Therefore this method is poorly suitable for tissues with fragile ECM, such as lung. Yet another physical protocol for decellularizing tissues involves sonication. This results in disruption of cellular membranes but also has the potential to damage the ECM.

Chemical methods to decellularize tissues

Chemical protocols to decellularize tissues include detergent decellularization [35]. Such detergents can be classified as nonionic, ionic, or zwitterionic. Nonionic detergents work by disrupting lipid interactions but do not affect protein–protein interactions. This results in preferential damage to cell membranes. In contrast, the ECM is largely left intact. As a result, nonionic detergents are relatively gentle on the ECM. Therefore nonionic detergents are frequently used to generate tissue-derived matrices. The most widely studied nonionic detergent for decellularization is Triton X-100. The required duration of exposure with Triton X-100 ranges from hours to days, depending on the target tissue. Nonionic detergents are contrasted with ionic detergents. Ionic detergents affect cellular membranes but also have an effect on protein–protein interactions. Among the most commonly used ionic detergents is sodium dodecyl sulfate (SDS). SDS is particularly potent at removing cellular remnants from tissues. However, protocols based on SDS tend to disrupt the ECM with a decrease in GAG concentrations and loss of collagen integrity. Finally, zwitterionic detergents have intermediate properties between nonionic and ionic detergents. A zwitterion is an electrically neutral molecule with both positive and negative electric charges. These detergents have a greater tendency to denature proteins than nonionic detergents but do so to a less extent than ionic detergents. One example for a zwitterionic detergent is 3-[(3-cholamidopropyl) dimethylammonio]-1-propanesulfonate (CHAPS).

Biological methods to decellularize tissues

Biological protocols to decellularize tissues include enzymatic decellularization [36]. The enzymes used in these protocols typically are proteases and nucleases. Trypsin is one of the most commonly used proteases in such protocols. Trypsin is a serine endopeptidase that is produced in the pancreas as an inactive precursor. After activation in the digestive tract, trypsin specifically cleaves peptides at the carboxyl side of lysine or arginine residues, except when either amino acid is followed by a proline residue. The mechanism of trypsin proteolysis involves a catalytic triad consisting of histidine, aspartate, and serine. The aspartate in the catalytic triad specifically attracts the target lysine or arginine amino acids. Furthermore, histidine and aspartate form a charge relay that increases the nucleophilicity of the serine. This allows serine to attack the peptide carbonyl carbon of the target lysine or arginine amino acids and catalyze peptide cleavage at their carboxyl side. The optimal activity of trypsin occurs at 37°C and pH 8. Additionally, nucleases are used to catalyze the degradation of RNA and DNA. Nucleases catalyze the cleavage of phosphodiester bonds of nucleotides. Nucleases are classified as endonucleases and exonucleases. Endonucleases cleave phosphodiester bonds within a nucleic acid chain. In contrast, exonucleases cleave nucleotides from the end of a nucleic acid chain. Enzymatic protocols for decellularization affect both cellular proteins and proteins of the ECM. Therefore the enzyme concentration and duration of enzymatic treatment need to be carefully titrated to optimize the desired effects.

In practice, progressive protocols that involve multiple decellularization protocols in sequential steps are frequently used to achieve optimal results. Furthermore, protease inhibitors are often added to protect the ECM from proteases leaked by the lysed cells. Frequently used protease inhibitors include phenylmethylsulfonylfluoride, aprotinin, and leupeptin. Additionally, buffered solutions can inhibit undesirable proteolysis of the ECM. The ultimate choice of an optimal decellularization protocol also depends on the source tissue and the intended use of the ECM. Therefore different protocols are used for different tissues and different applications.

Delivery of decellularizing solutions

Delivery of the decellularizing solutions should ideally bring each cell into close contact with the decellularizing solution. Depending on the type of tissue, submersion may be sufficient. However, one of the most promising methods for ensuring close contact of each cell with the decellularizing solution is perfusion decellularization. This method makes use of the tissue's endogenous vascular channels. In vivo, the vascular channels ensure the supply of each cell with nutrients and oxygen. Crucially, perfusion decellularization allows the generation of whole organ-derived matrices. A number of different protocols for perfusion decellularization have been described. The protocol used in our laboratory is briefly outlined in the following [37]. The source organ should ideally be freshly collected or preserved on ice for no longer than 24 h. Procurement and subsequent handling of the tissue should involve aseptic techniques to minimize bacterial contamination. Bacterial contamination is known to contribute to the degradation of the ECM by proteinase action. In order to preserve the ability to perfuse the vasculature with the decellularizing solutions, thrombosis and air embolization need to be minimized. To this effect, blood is flushed from the source organ with a suitable isotonic solution. Heparin is also added to minimize thrombosis. The arterial and venous vasculature is then connected to appropriate perfusion lines. Arterial leaks are surgically repaired to ensure adequate perfusion pressure for decellularization. Next, the source organ is mounted into a decellularization chamber (Fig. 13.1).

The decellularization chamber is filled with SDS solution, and the SDS solution is also pumped through the perfusion lines. The pump rate varies depending on the source species and organ [37]. The organs are perfused with SDS between 2 and 12 h, depending on the source organ. Next, the SDS detergent is washed from the organ by perfusion with distilled water. Another step in the protocol involves

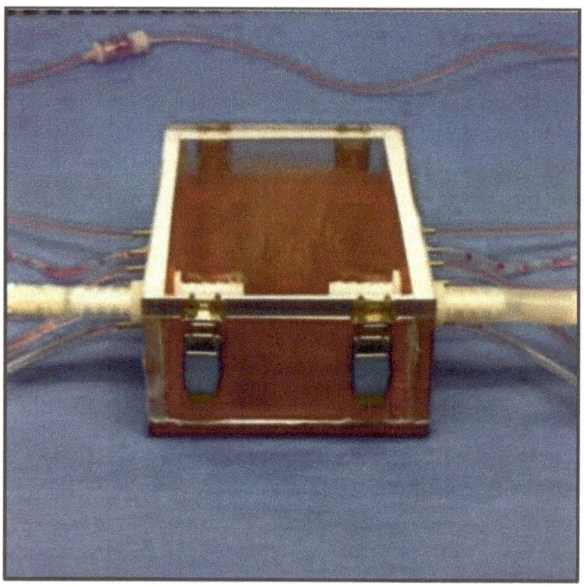

FIGURE 13.1

Photograph of an experimental small animal organ decellularization chamber.

perfusion with Triton X-100 solution. The final wash step consists of perfusion with phosphate buffered saline. This completes decellularization of the organ.

DESIRABLE PROPERTIES OF TISSUE-DERIVED MATRICES

Regardless of the method that is used, the resulting tissue-derived matrices should be nontoxic and biocompatible. Toxicity refers to the degree to which a material damages an organism. The damage can act at the level of the cell, tissue, or entire organism. Biocompatibility refers to the degree to which a material can be implanted into a host organism without causing undesirable local or systemic effects. In addition, the tissue-derived matrices should retain the desirable structural and biological functions of the source tissue ECM. Together, these properties make tissue-derived matrices suitable for applications in tissue engineering.

CURRENT CLINICAL APPLICATIONS FOR TISSUE-DERIVED MATRICES

Tissue-derived matrices have a wide range of clinical applications. The most commonly used tissue-derived matrices in clinical practice include dermal-derived matrices for body wall reconstruction, pericardial-derived matrices for vascular reconstruction, and tissue-derived matrices for heart valve replacement. These applications are briefly outlined in the following section.

DERMAL-DERIVED MATRICES FOR SOFT TISSUE RECONSTRUCTION

More than 10% of patients undergoing abdominal surgical procedures develop incisional hernias [38]. Since there are over 1 million laparotomies performed annually in the United States, at least 100,000 patients develop such hernias every year [39]. Reconstruction of the body wall to treat these hernias using endogenous tissue is frequently not possible. Furthermore, synthetic meshes are contraindicated in infected and contaminated surgical fields. Therefore biologic meshes that are made from dermal-derived matrix grafts are routinely used for body wall reconstructions in contaminated or infected surgical fields. The dermis used to produce these matrices usually originates from human, porcine, or bovine donors. The matrix is derived by decellularizing the dermis as described earlier. These acellular matrices may also be further treated by cross-linking to increase their durability by blocking collagenase binding sites [40].

Human acellular dermal matrix was first introduced for the treatment of full-thickness burn wounds. Subsequently, body wall reconstruction has become a major field for the application of such grafts. The major clinical advantage of dermal-derived matrices over conventional synthetic mesh is the ability to use dermal-derived matrices in a contaminated or infected field [41]. The reason for this is that dermal-derived matrices are revascularized and incorporated into host tissue. Furthermore, decellularization retains the structural strength of the dermal ECM. This prevents failure of the body wall reconstruction and early recurrence of the hernia.

A large number of dermal-derived matrices for abdominal wall reconstruction are clinically available. The most commonly used products include AlloDerm human dermal matrix and XenMatrix porcine dermal matrix (Fig. 13.2).

A number of other clinically available tissue-derived matrices that are used for body wall reconstruction are listed in Table 13.2.

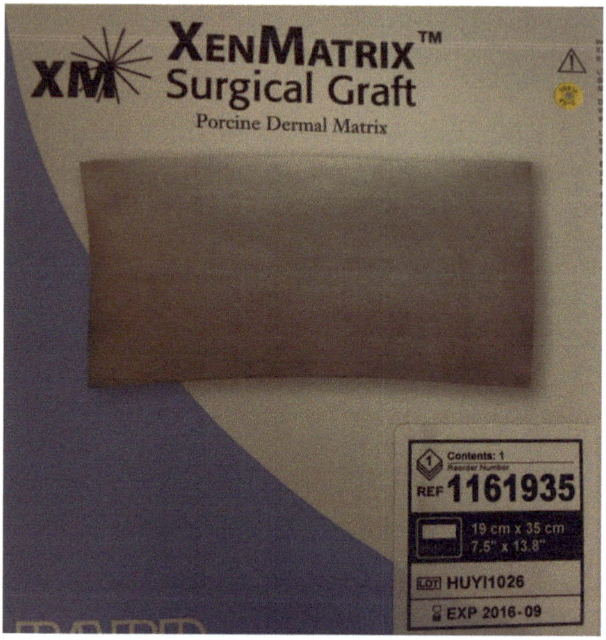

FIGURE 13.2

XenMatrix is a porcine dermal-derived matrix for human clinical application.

Table 13.2 Examples for Clinically Available Tissue-Derived Matrices Products for Body Wall Reconstructions [40]

Name of Product	Manufacturer	Species	Tissue
AlloDerm	LifeCell	Human	Dermis
Strattice	LifeCell	Porcine	Dermis
XenMatrix	Bard	Porcine	Dermis
Surgisis	Cook	Porcine	Small intestine

PERICARDIAL-DERIVED MATRICES FOR VASCULAR RECONSTRUCTIONS

Bovine pericardial-derived matrix is commonly used clinically as a patch in cardiovascular reconstructions.

In order to generate a pericardial-derived matrix, the native bovine pericardium is processed using detergent and enzymatic processes [42]. This results in an acellular pericardium-derived matrix (Fig. 13.3).

Frequently, arterial stenoses are relieved by incorporating a bovine pericardial patch into the vessel wall to increase the vessel diameter. This includes the surgical treatment of carotid stenoses. Bovine pericardial-derived matrix was first described for surgical treatment of carotid stenoses in 1996 [43]. Now, bovine pericardial-derived matrices are used routinely in the surgical treatment of carotid stenoses [44]. Arteriotomies of other vessels are also frequently closed using a bovine patch to avoid stenosis at the arteriotomy site (Fig. 13.4).

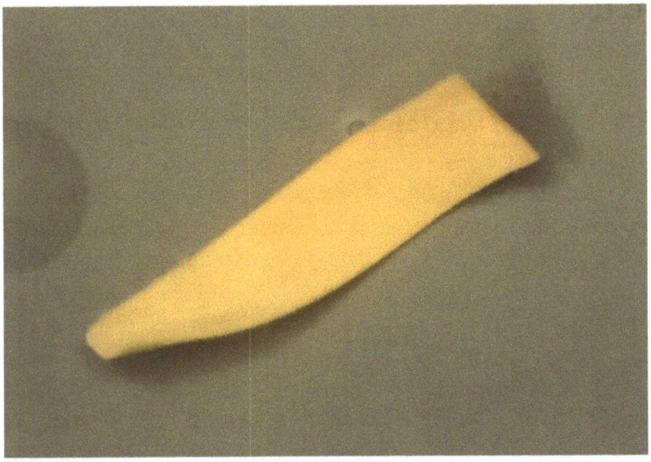

FIGURE 13.3

Photo of bovine pericardial patch being washed in saline prior to use.

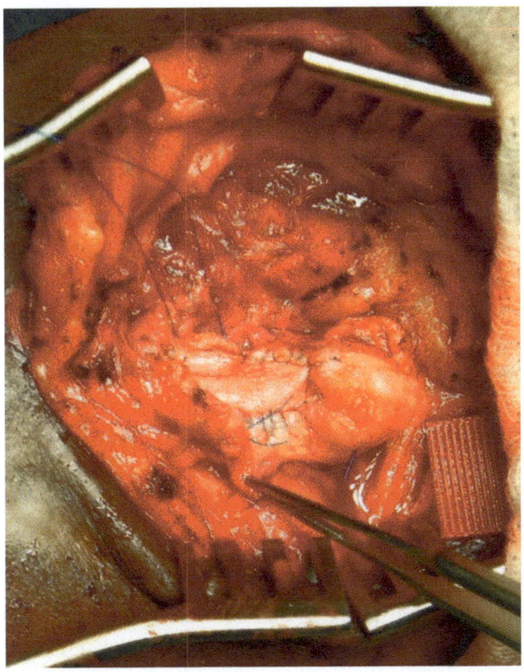

FIGURE 13.4

Intraoperative photograph of bovine pericardial-derived matrix used in a human patient to reconstruct the brachial artery after excision of a pseudoaneurysm.

The advantages of bovine pericardial-derived matrix include easy intraoperative handling, minimal suture line bleeding, low thrombogenicity, and low infection rates.

TISSUE-DERIVED MATRICES FOR HEART VALVE REPLACEMENTS

Heart valves have a hemodynamic function that ensures unidirectional blood flow through the heart. Heart valves also have additional biological functions, including avoiding thrombosis and avoiding infection. The average blood flow across each heart valve is approximately 5 L per minute. During the same time, heart valves open and close over 60 times. Over the course of a human lifetime, this approximates to over 3,000,000,000 cycles. During each of these cycles, the heart valves are subjected to tension from blood pressure and shear stress from blood flow. This can lead to wear and tear of the heart valves over time. Additionally, the heart valves are affected by congenital disorders. Congenital disorders of the heart valves include bicuspid aortic valves or congenital stenoses. Heart valves are also affected by acquired disorders. Acquired disorders of heart valves include rheumatic heart disease and infections leading to endocarditis. Such disorders can seriously affect patients' health. Therefore over 90,000 Americans require replacement of a native heart valve with a prosthetic heart valve every year. Currently available heart valve replacements include mechanical heart valve prostheses, homografts, and biological heart valve prostheses. Mechanical heart valves were historically the first prosthetic valves to be implanted. In 1960, the first successful mitral valve replacement was performed by Starr in Portland [45]. This was followed in the same year by the first successful aortic valve replacement by Harken in Boston [46]. Modern mechanical heart valves have a bileaflet, tilting disk design that provides excellent hemodynamic function and durability. However, despite the application of advanced materials such as alloys and ceramics, mechanical valves remain associated with thromboembolic complications. Therefore patients require lifelong anticoagulation. Another strategy to replace diseased heart valves involves the implantation of homografts. Homografts are effectively allotransplants of cadaveric heart valves. Homograft heart valve replacement using a freeze-dried aortic valve was first carried out in 1962 by Ross in London [47]. However, due to the scarcity of homografts, this is not an option for most patients. Clinically successful biological heart valves were first introduced in the 1960s and 1970s by Carpentier in Paris and Ionescu in Leeds. These valves are made from porcine heart valve-derived matrix or bovine pericardium-derived matrix. The immunogenicity of these xenografts is reduced by treatment with glutaraldehyde. Glutaraldehyde results in cross-linking of collagen in the matrix. The bovine bioprosthetic valve is constructed from bovine pericardial-derived matrix. Sheets of this matrix are arranged such that they form a trileaflet valve. This valve is fixed to a stent that provides a stable scaffold. Additionally, the valves are provided with a sewing ring that allows surgeons to implant the valve. The porcine bioprosthetic valve is created from decellularized porcine aortic matrix. This matrix is also preserved in glutaraldehyde and constructed with a stent and a sewing cuff. Hundreds of thousands of these valves are implanted worldwide every year.

FUTURE DIRECTIONS FOR TISSUE-DERIVED MATRICES

The discussion in the previous section illustrates that tissue-derived matrices currently have widespread applications in clinical medicine. These applications will increase with further progress of the field in the future. This progress will result in quantitative and qualitative advances. Quantitative advances will result in further improvements of currently available clinical products. In contrast, qualitative advances will result in the development of new clinical products.

FUTURE ADVANCES RELATING TO TISSUE-DERIVED MATRICES

One example for future quantitative advances relating to tissue-derived matrices is lower costs. This decrease in costs will be achieved in multiple ways. One way in which the cost of tissue-derived matrices will decrease is refinement of the production processes. Another way is economies of scale that will be realized when more tissue-derived matrices are used clinically. Currently, tissue-derived matrices are very expensive. In a recent study of dermal-derived matrices, the average cost of the biological matrix for abdominal wall reconstruction was $5630 per patient. In contrast, synthetic meshes cost only one-twentieth of the biological matrices [48]. Other examples for quantitative advances relating to tissue-derived matrices will include an increase in the variety of the available products from different companies. This will include a spectrum of tissue-derived matrices with different sizes and material properties.

FUNCTIONALIZATION OF TISSUE-DERIVED MATRICES BY CELLULAR RESEEDING

In the future, tissue-derived matrices will also be further functionalized by reseeding the matrices with cells. This will result in qualitative advances that result in completely new clinical applications for tissue-derived matrices. Tissue-derived matrices that are functionalized with reseeded cells consist of two components. The first component consists of a matrix scaffold. The matrix scaffold is generated by decellularizing donor tissues [37]. The function of the matrix scaffold is to determine the structural properties of the construct, including its size and shape. The second component of such matrices is formed by reseeded cells [49]. The function of the reseeded cells is to endow the construct with additional biological functionality that extends beyond its mere structure. There are two approaches for cellular reseeding of tissue-derived matrix scaffolds. Firstly, the decellularized matrix scaffolds can be reseeded with specific stem cells in vitro before implantation. Secondly, a bare decellularized matrix scaffold without reseeded cells can be implanted into the recipient. Subsequently, this bare matrix scaffold is reseeded in vivo with cells that originate from the recipient bloodstream. These two strategies are described in the following section.

IN VITRO RESEEDING OF TISSUE-DERIVED MATRICES

In vitro reseeding of tissue-derived matrices involves the use of stem cells. Stem cells are characterized by their ability to differentiate into specialized cells and to produce more stem cells by cell division. Based on their ability to differentiate into other cell types, such stem cells can be classified as totipotent, pluripotent, multipotent, or unipotent. Totipotent stem cells are able to produce all differentiated cells in an organism. Pluripotent stem cells are able to produce cells of all three germ layers. Multipotent stem cells are able to produce cells of a limited number of different lineages. Unipotent stem cells are able to differentiate into one type of cell only. Such stem cells for in vitro reseeding tissue-derived matrices could potentially come from a number of different sources. These sources include embryonic stem cells, adult stem cells, and induced stem cells.

Embryonic stem cells

Embryonic stem cells were first derived from mouse embryos in 1981 [50]. Embryonic stem cells are obtained from early embryos at the blastocyst stage. The blastocyst stage of development starts approximately 4 days after fertilization. At this time, the embryo consists of approximately 100 cells. The embryonic stem cells are able to proliferate indefinitely in an undifferentiated state. Moreover, embryonic stem cells are pluripotent and able to differentiate into any of the germ layers involved in embryogenesis. These germ layers ultimately form all organs of the organism. For example, endoderm forms the lungs and gastrointestinal tract, mesoderm forms muscles and blood, and ectoderm forms the dermis and the nervous system. Thus embryonic stem cells are able to differentiate via the formation of precursor cells into virtually any type of cell. This makes them promising candidates for use in tissue engineering. However, harvesting embryonic stem cells destroys the embryo. This has led to major ethical concerns about their use.

Adult stem cells

Adult stem cells can be obtained without major harm to the donor. Therefore there are no ethical concerns about their use. Ideally, the intended recipient patient would donate his own adult stem cells for use in tissue engineering. Adult stem cells are found in small numbers in a wide range of adult tissues. The adult heart contains cardiac stem cells. Evidence for the existence of these stem cells was revealed by a number of important findings. Firstly, myocardial infarction leads to limited myocyte replication and myocardial regeneration [51]. Secondly, female hearts transplanted into male recipients were found to be chimeras that contain engrafted male cells [52]. Finally, measurement of the incorporation of atmospheric carbon-14 generated by nuclear bomb tests during the Cold War provided evidence for continuous renewal of cardiomyocytes with fewer than 50% of cardiomyocytes exchanged during a lifetime [53]. Skeletal muscles contain skeletal myoblasts. These cells were first described in 1961 [54]. Their function is to regenerate skeletal muscle cells after injury. Bone marrow contains three different types of stem cells. The first type is hematopoietic stem cells. These stem cells give rise to blood cells. The second type is mesenchymal stem cells. These stem cells give rise to a number of different cell types, including adipocytes and osteoblasts. The third type is endothelial stem cells. These stem cells participate in the formation of endothelium in new blood vessels. The mammary glands contain mammary stem cells. These cells participate in the growth of the mammary gland during puberty and gestation. However, mammary stem cells are also thought to play a role in the development of breast cancer. The intestine contains intestinal stem cells [55]. These cells are located at the base of the crypts of Lieberkuhn and are responsible for the constant renewal of the intestinal mucosa. However, it is thought that intestinal stem cells also play a role in the development of colon cancer [56]. The neural tissues contain neural stem cells. Such stem cells are found in the brain as well as the peripheral nervous system [57]. In addition to the tissues mentioned previously, adult stem cells can be found in many other tissues. Unlike pluripotent embryonic stem cells, adult stem cells usually are multipotent. This describes their potential to differentiate into multiple different cell types but not all cell types.

Induced pluripotent stem cells

Human somatic cells can also be induced to become stem cells. The induction of pluripotent stem cells was first demonstrated by Shinya Yamanaka in Kyoto in 2006 [58]. Such cells are typically derived by the expression of specific transcription factors such as octamer-binding transcription factor 4 (OCT4), sex determining region Y-box 2 (SOX2), kruppel-like factor 4 (KLF4), avian myelocytomatosis viral oncogene homolog (c-MYC), homebox protein NANOG, and micro-RNA binding protein LIN28 [59,60]. Induced pluripotent stem cells can subsequently differentiate into a number of different cellular lineages. However, some of transcription factors that are used to induce pluripotency can also function as oncogenes. For example the Myc protein plays a role in cell cycle progression, apoptosis, and cellular transformation. Mutation of this gene is responsible for most cases of Burkitt lymphoma in man [61]. Mutations in Myc are also implicated in a number of other cancers, including cervix, colon, breast, and lung. This raises concern for carcinogenesis from implantation of induced pluripotent stem cells.

In vivo reseeding of tissue-derived matrices

Disadvantages of the approach of in vitro reseeding of tissue-derived matrices include the fact that it requires a large number of suitable cells that need to be seeded into the matrix before it can be implanted. Obtaining a large number of such suitable cells has been one of the main challenges of this approach. Another potential strategy to functionalize tissue-derived matrices with cells involves reseeding matrices in vivo by extravasation of host circulating stem cells into the implanted matrix. This approach relies on effective recruitment of appropriate host cells into the implanted matrix. As a result, high requirements are placed on the matrix. Firstly, the matrix needs to incorporate targeting cues that result in the recruitment of appropriate host progenitor cells. Secondly, the matrix needs to provide a microenvironment that allows these progenitor cells to lodge and proliferate. Thirdly, the matrix needs to provide further cues that direct differentiation of the progenitor cells into appropriate tissue types. In order to achieve this, it may be necessary to modify tissue-derived matrices in vitro. Such modifications might include enriching the matrix with specific chemokines and growth factors, for example.

The host cells for in vivo reseeding may come from a number of different sources. It is well established that adult stem cells circulate in the blood. Many of these stem cells remain quiescent until they are activated by specific stimuli. The specific stimuli that activate quiescent stem cells include injury as well as ordinary wear and tear. Once the stem cells become activated, they divide and contribute to repair of the injury. In addition, the bone marrow is known to host multiple populations of stem cells. These populations of stem cells include hematopoietic stem cells, mesenchymal stem cells, and endothelial progenitor cells. Hematopoietic stem cells are derived from mesoderm. These cells give rise to all other blood cells, including the myeloid and lymphoid lineages of cells. Mesenchymal stem cells are stromal cells that can differentiate into a number of different lineages, including myocytes, osteoblasts, and adipocytes. Mesenchymal cells are also found in other tissues, such as adipose tissue and fat. Endothelial progenitor cells participate in the formation of the endothelial lining of blood vessels. Bone marrow-derived endothelial progenitor cells were shown to localize to injured blood vessels and participate in angiogenesis. All of these stem cell populations are potential players in reseeding tissue-derived matrices in vivo. The ability of implanted matrices to be reseeded with cells has been proven experimentally. For example, implantation of bare allogeneic decellularized matrix scaffolds in the orthotopic position in lambs aged 10–12 weeks resulted in recellularization with interstitial cells from the bloodstream after 3 months [62].

APPLICATIONS FOR RESEEDED TISSUE-DERIVED MATRICES

Regardless of the method for reseeding the matrices, such functionalization has a number of potential clinical applications. On the one hand, reseeded tissue-derived matrices will serve generic functions, such as growth in pediatric applications and self-repair. On the other hand, reseeded tissue-derived matrices will serve organ-specific functions, such as gas exchange in bioengineered lungs or generation of pump function in bioengineered hearts.

Adaptive growth of tissue-derived matrices

One of the key functions of reseeded tissue-derived matrices will be adaptive growth in pediatric applications. Approximately 3% of newborn babies have congenital malformations that seriously interfere with their well-being [63]. Surgical treatments that involve prosthetic implants are currently inadequate because commercially available prostheses are unable to grow adaptively with the babies' somatic growth. One clinical area where this problem is particularly acute is the treatment of congenital defects of heart valves. Children with prosthetic heart valves frequently need multiple reoperations to implant successively larger prostheses as they grow [64]. As a result, the affected children suffer from morbidity and mortality [65], the affected families suffer from psychological stress [66], and society suffers from high costs [67]. Therefore there is an urgent need for heart valve prostheses with the ability to grow adaptively with recipient children.

Tissue engineering using generic decellularized matrix scaffolds that are reseeded with appropriate cells is promising to deliver such heart valve prostheses [68]. Each component of these tissue-engineered heart valve constructs has well-defined functions. The function of the matrix scaffold is to determine the structural properties of the construct, including its size and shape. These structural properties of the tissue-engineered construct allow it to serve its hemodynamic function as a valve. The function of the reseeded cells is to endow the construct with active functionality that extends beyond its mere structure. This active functionality includes the ability to grow adaptively with the rest of the heart during ontogenesis. Growth of the tissue-engineered heart valve construct depends critically on changes in the matrix scaffold, since the matrix determines the overall size and shape of the tissue-engineered constructs. Therefore the reseeded cells need to affect this change by remodeling the matrix. Such adaptive growth of decellularized reseeded heart valve constructs has already been demonstrated in a pilot human trial [69].

Organ-derived matrices for organ engineering

Currently, tissue-derived matrices serve to fulfill the function of specific tissues. This includes body wall reconstructions with dermal-derived matrices, vascular reconstructions with bovine pericardium-derived matrices, and heart valve replacements with bioprosthetic heart valves. Tissues are collections of cells that derive from a similar origin that represent an intermediate level of biological organization between cells and complete organs. Organs refer to a collection of tissues that are spatially colocated to serve specific functions. In the future, further progress in tissue engineering will result in the availability of organ-derived matrices for organ engineering. The generation of organ-derived matrices by perfusion decellularization is described previously. These organ-derived matrices will be used to fulfill organ-specific functions. Together with reseeding of these organ-derived matrices with cells, this will lead to major new clinical applications. One of these applications will be in organ transplantation.

Bioartificial organs for transplantation

A particularly important unsolved problem in clinical medicine relates to solid organ transplantation. In most countries, demand for organs far outweighs the available supply. As a result, donor organs need to be rationed. Most countries have formal systems for rationing the allocation of donor organs. In the United States, deceased donor organs are primarily allocated by the United Network for Organ Sharing. The criteria used for allocation include the medical urgency for transplantation, waiting time, compatibility including immunobiology of ABO blood group antigens and organ size, the ability of the recipient to recover from surgery, and physical distance between deceased donor and recipient. Due to this need for rationing, over 100,000 patients are currently awaiting organs for transplantation in the United States alone. This represents a fourfold increase in the past 20 years [70]. Advances in organ engineering are promising a solution to this problem. Currently, many donor organs are discarded because of poor quality. Many of these organs could theoretically be rescued by means of organ engineering. Proteolysis is known to occur within 4–6 h after death [71]. Within this timeframe, there is a window to harvest the organ and generate an organ-derived matrix. Subsequent regeneration of viable organs by organ engineering would yield many additional grafts for transplantation. Additional sources for organ-derived matrices could also come from animals. Decellularization of the animal organs would remove a large proportion of the xenogeneic antigens that mediate rejection. The few xenogeneic antigens that remain could potentially be eliminated by a number of different strategies. One example for an antigen that is known to cause acute rejection of xenografts is galactosyl-alpha(1,3)galactose. This antigen can be eliminated by enzymatic processing [72]. Another strategy to eliminate such antigens in donor animals involves the use of genetic engineering [73].

CONCLUSION

In summary, tissue-derived matrices are biomaterials that are generated from the ECM of specific tissues. The molecular structure of the ECM is very complex and involves approximately 300 proteins. These proteins form a dynamic 3-D structure that exists in all tissues and fulfills important functions. On the one hand, the ECM serves structural functions as a scaffold. On the other hand, the ECM serves additional biological functions that include the regulation of the activity of extracellular molecules and interaction with embedded cells. These ECM properties make tissue-derived matrices promising substrates for use in tissue engineering and biomaterial design. Tissue-derived matrices are generated by decellularizing specific tissues. Whole organ matrices can be isolated by perfusion decellularization. Current clinical applications for tissue-derived matrices include pericardium-derived matrices for cardiovascular reconstructions, dermal-derived matrices for body wall reconstructions, and tissue-derived matrices for heart valve replacements. In the future, tissue-derived matrices will be further functionalized by reseeding with specific cells that can fulfill additional biological functions. These functions may be generic, such as growth and self-repair. Alternatively, these functions may be organ-specific, such as gas exchange for bioengineered lungs or generation of pump function for bioengineered hearts.

GLOSSARY

Matrisome The ensemble of ECM and ECM-associated proteins.

Organ engineering Manipulation of cells, matrix scaffolds, and biomaterials to construct, functionalize, and maintain living organs.

Tissue engineering Manipulation of cells and biomaterials to construct, functionalize, and maintain living tissues.

LIST OF ACRONYMS AND ABBREVIATIONS

CHAPS 3-[(3-cholamidopropyl)dimethylammonio]-1-propanesulfonate
c-MYC Avian myelocytomatosis viral oncogene homolog
ECM Extracellular matrix
FACIT Fibril-associated collagens with interrupted triple helices
GAGs Glycosaminoglycans
KLF4 Kruppel-like factor 4
OCT4 Octamer-binding transcription factor 4
SDS Sodium dodecyl sulfate
SOX2 Sex determining region Y-box 2

REFERENCES

[1] Mecham RP. Overview of extracellular matrix. Current protocols in cell biology. Wiley-Blackwell; 2001.
[2] Hynes RO. The extracellular matrix: not just pretty fibrils. Science 2009;326(5957):1216–9.
[3] Song JJ, Ott HC. Organ engineering based on decellularized matrix scaffolds. Trends Mol Med 2011;17(8):424–32.
[4] Naba A, Clauser KR, Hoersch S, Liu H, Carr SA, Hynes RO. The matrisome: in silico definition and in vivo characterization by proteomics of normal and tumor extracellular matrices. Mol Cell Proteomics 2011;11(4). http://dx.doi.org/10.1074/mcp.M111.014647.
[5] Hynes RO, Naba A. Overview of the matrisome–an inventory of extracellular matrix constituents and functions. Cold Spring Harb Perspect Biol 2011;4(1):a004903.
[6] Ricard-Blum S, Ruggiero F. The collagen superfamily: from the extracellular matrix to the cell membrane. Pathol Biol 2005;53(7):430–42.
[7] Khoshnoodi J, Pedchenko V, Hudson BG. Mammalian collagen IV. Microsc Res Tech 2008;71(5):357–70.
[8] Olsen BR, Winterhalter KH, Gordon MK. FACIT コラーゲンとその生物学的機能. Trends Glycosci Glycotechnol 1995;7(34):115–27.
[9] Franzke C-W, Tasanen K, Schumann H, Bruckner-Tuderman L. Collagenous transmembrane proteins: collagen XVII as a prototype. Matrix Biol 2003;22(4):299–309.
[10] Mouw JK, Ou G, Weaver VM. Extracellular matrix assembly: a multiscale deconstruction. Nat Rev Mol Cell Biol 2014;15(12):771–85.
[11] Rauch F, Glorieux FH. Osteogenesis imperfecta. Lancet 2004;363(9418):1377–85.
[12] Alport AC. Hereditary familial congenital haemorrhagic nephritis. BMJ 1927;1(3454):504–6.
[13] Indik Z, Yeh H, Ornstein-Goldstein N, et al. Alternative splicing of human elastin mRNA indicated by sequence analysis of cloned genomic and complementary DNA. Proc Natl Acad Sci 1987;84(16):5680–4.
[14] Debelle L, Tamburro AM. Elastin: molecular description and function. Int J Biochem Cell Biol 1999;31(2):261–72.
[15] Hoeve CAJ, Flory PJ. The elastic properties of elastin. Biopolymers 1974;13(4):677–86.
[16] Curran M. The elastin gene is disrupted by a translocation associated with supravalvular aortic stenosis. Cell 1993;73(1):159–68.
[17] Esko JD, Selleck SB. Order out of chaos: assembly of ligand binding sites in heparan sulfate. Annu Rev Biochem 2002;71(1):435–71.
[18] Yanagishita M. Function of proteoglycans in the extracellular matrix. Pathol Int 1993;43(6):283–93.
[19] Labat-Robert J, Robert L. Fifty years of structural glycoproteins. Pathol Biol 2012;60(1):66–75.
[20] Singh P, Carraher C, Schwarzbauer JE. Assembly of fibronectin extracellular matrix. Annu Rev Cell Dev Biol 2010;26(1):397–419.
[21] Hunter I, Schulthess T, Bruch M, Beck K, Engel J. Evidence for a specific mechanism of laminin assembly. Eur J Biochem 1990;188(2):205–11.
[22] Whittaker CA, Bergeron K-F, Whittle J, Brandhorst BP, Burke RD, Hynes RO. The echinoderm adhesome. Dev Biol 2006;300(1):252–66.
[23] Gosline J, Guerette P, Ortlepp C, Savage K. Molecular and mechanical design of spider's silks. Comp Biochem Physiol Part A Mol Integr Physiol 1999;124:S34.
[24] Agnarsson I, Kuntner M, Blackledge TA. Bioprospecting finds the toughest biological material: extraordinary silk from a giant riverine orb spider. PLoS One 2010;5(9):e11234.
[25] Makarenkova HP, Hoffman MP, Beenken A, et al. Differential interactions of FGFs with heparan sulfate control gradient formation and branching morphogenesis. Sci Signal 2009;2(88):ra55.
[26] Discher DE. Tissue cells feel and respond to the stiffness of their substrate. Science 2005;310(5751):1139–43.
[27] Hynes RO. Integrins. Cell 2002;110(6):673–87.
[28] Engler AJ, Sen S, Sweeney HL, Discher DE. Matrix elasticity directs stem cell lineage specification. Cell 2006;126(4):677–89.

[29] Kim HY, Nelson CM. Extracellular matrix and cytoskeletal dynamics during branching morphogenesis. Organogenesis 2012;8(2):56–64.
[30] Bonnans C, Chou J, Werb Z. Remodelling the extracellular matrix in development and disease. Nat Rev Mol Cell Biol 2014;15(12):786–801.
[31] Mammoto T, Jiang E, Jiang A, Mammoto A. Extracellular matrix structure and tissue stiffness control postnatal lung development through the lipoprotein receptor–related protein 5/Tie2 signaling system. Am J Respir Cell Mol Biol 2013;49(6):1009–18.
[32] Langer R, Vacanti JP. Tissue engineering. Science 1993;260(5110):920–6.
[33] Gilbert T, Sellaro T, Badylak S. Decellularization of tissues and organs. Biomaterials 2006;27.
[34] Burk J, Erbe I, Berner D, et al. Freeze-thaw cycles enhance decellularization of large tendons. Tissue Eng Part C Methods 2014;20(4):276–84.
[35] Cebotari S, Tudorache I, Jaekel T, et al. Detergent decellularization of heart valves for tissue engineering: toxicological effects of residual detergents on human endothelial cells. Artif Organs 2010;34(3):206–10.
[36] Yang M, Chen C-Z, Wang X-N, Zhu Y-B, Gu YJ. Favorable effects of the detergent and enzyme extraction method for preparing decellularized bovine pericardium scaffold for tissue engineered heart valves. J Biomed Mater Res 2009;91B(1):354–61.
[37] Guyette JP, Gilpin SE, Charest JM, Tapias LF, Ren X, Ott HC. Perfusion decellularization of whole organs. Nat Protoc 2014;9(6):1451–68.
[38] Mudge M, Hughes LE. Incisional hernia: a 10 year prospective study of incidence and attitudes. Br J Surg 1985;72(1):70–1.
[39] Flum DR, Horvath K, Koepsell T. Have outcomes of incisional hernia repair improved with time? Ann Surg 2003;237(1):129–35.
[40] Shankaran V, Weber DJ, Reed RL, Luchette FA. A review of available prosthetics for ventral hernia repair. Ann Surg 2011;253(1):16–26.
[41] Diaz JJ. Human acellular dermal matrix for ventral hernia repair in the compromised surgical field. Hernia repair sequelae. Springer Science + Business Media; 2010. p. 103–11.
[42] Courtman DW, Pereira CA, Kashef V, McComb D, Lee JM, Wilson GJ. Development of a pericardial acellular matrix biomaterial: biochemical and mechanical effects of cell extraction. J Biomed Mater Res 1994;28(6):655–66.
[43] Biasi G, Sampaolo A, Ferrari S, Baronio L, Mingazzini P. Bovine pericardium patch angioplasty in carotid surgery. Cardiovasc Surg 1995;3:90.
[44] Ho KJ, Nguyen LL, Menard MT. Intermediate-term outcome of carotid endarterectomy with bovine pericardial patch closure compared with Dacron patch and primary closure. J Vasc Surg 2012;55(3):708–14.
[45] Starr A, Edwards ML. Mitral replacement. Ann Surg 1961;154(4):726.
[46] Harken DE, Taylor WJ, Lefemine AA, et al. Aortic valve replacement with a gaged ball valve. Am J Cardiol 1962;9(2):292–9.
[47] Ross DN. Homograft replacement of the aortic valve. Lancet 1962;280(7254):487.
[48] Blatnik J, Jin J, Rosen M. Abdominal hernia repair with bridging acellular dermal matrix—an expensive hernia sac. Am J Surg 2008;196(1):47–50.
[49] Robertson MJ, Dries-Devlin JL, Kren SM, Burchfield JS, Taylor DA. Optimizing recellularization of whole decellularized heart extracellular matrix. PLoS One 2014;9(2):e90406.
[50] Evans MJ, Kaufman MH. Establishment in culture of pluripotential cells from mouse embryos. Nature 1981;292(5819):154–6.
[51] Beltrami AP, Urbanek K, Kajstura J, et al. Evidence that human cardiac myocytes divide after myocardial infarction. N Engl J Med 2001;344(23):1750–7.
[52] Quaini F, Urbanek K, Beltrami AP, et al. Chimerism of the transplanted heart. N Engl J Med 2002;346(1):5–15.
[53] Bergmann O, Bhardwaj RD, Bernard S, et al. Evidence for cardiomyocyte renewal in humans. Science 2009;324(5923):98–102.
[54] Mauro A. Satellite cell of skeletal muscle fibers. J Cell Biol 1961;9(2):493–5.

[55] van der Flier LG, Clevers H. Stem cells, self-renewal, and differentiation in the intestinal epithelium. Annu Rev Physiol 2009;71(1):241–60.
[56] Barker N, Ridgway RA, van Es JH, et al. Crypt stem cells as the cells-of-origin of intestinal cancer. Nature 2008;457(7229):608–11.
[57] Lewis PD. Mitotic activity in the primate subependymal layer and the genesis of gliomas. Nature 1968;217(5132):974–5.
[58] Takahashi K, Yamanaka S. Induction of pluripotent stem cells from mouse embryonic and adult fibroblast cultures by defined factors. Cell 2006;126(4):663–76.
[59] Takahashi K, Tanabe K, Ohnuki M, et al. Induction of pluripotent stem cells from adult human fibroblasts by defined factors. Cell 2007;131(5):861–72.
[60] Yu J, Vodyanik MA, Smuga-Otto K, et al. Induced pluripotent stem cell lines derived from human somatic cells. Science 2007;318(5858):1917–20.
[61] Finver SN, Nishikura K, Finger LR, et al. Sequence analysis of the MYC oncogene involved in the t(8;14)(q24;q11) chromosome translocation in a human leukemia T-cell line indicates that putative regulatory regions are not altered. Proc Natl Acad Sci 1988;85(9):3052–6.
[62] Lichtenberg A. Preclinical testing of tissue-engineered heart valves re-endothelialized under simulated physiological conditions. Circulation 2006;114(Suppl. 1):I-559–65.
[63] Kalter H, Warkany J. Congenital malformations. N Engl J Med 1983;308(8):424–31.
[64] Ackermann K, Balling G, Eicken A, Günther T, Schreiber C, Hess J. Replacement of the systemic atrioventricular valve with a mechanical prosthesis in children aged less than 6 years: late clinical results of survival and subsequent replacement. J Thorac Cardiovasc Surg 2007;134(3):750–6.
[65] Jacobs ML, O'Brien SM, Jacobs JP, et al. An empirically based tool for analyzing morbidity associated with operations for congenital heart disease. J Thorac Cardiovasc Surg 2013;145(4):1046–57e1.
[66] Lawoko S, Soares JJF. Psychosocial morbidity among parents of children with congenital heart disease: a prospective longitudinal study. Heart Lung J Acute Crit Care 2006;35(5):301–14.
[67] Pasquali SK, Jacobs ML, He X, et al. Variation in congenital heart surgery costs across hospitals. Pediatrics 2014;133(3):e553–60.
[68] Ott HC. Engineering tissues for children: building grafts that grow. Lancet 2012;380(9846):957–8.
[69] Cebotari S. Clinical application of tissue engineered human heart valves using autologous progenitor cells. Circulation 2006;114(Suppl. 1):I-132–7.
[70] Soto-Gutierrez A, Wertheim JA, Ott HC, Gilbert TW. Perspectives on whole-organ assembly: moving toward transplantation on demand. J Clin Invest 2012;122(11):3817–23.
[71] Tomita Y, Nihira M, Ohno Y, Sato S. Ultrastructural changes during in situ early postmortem autolysis in kidney, pancreas, liver, heart and skeletal muscle of rats. Leg Med 2004;6(1):25–31.
[72] Stone KR, Ayala G, Goldstein J, Hurst R, Walgenbach A, Galili U. Porcine cartilage transplants in the cynomolgus monkey. Transplantation 1998;65(12):1577–83.
[73] Lila N, McGregor CGA, Carpentier S, Rancic J, Byrne GW, Carpentier A. Gal knockout pig pericardium: new source of material for heart valve bioprostheses. J Heart Lung Transplant 2010;29(5):538–43.

PART

5

TISSUE-SPECIFIC APPLICATIONS

CHAPTER

SYNOVIAL JOINT: IN SITU REGENERATION OF OSTEOCHONDRAL AND FIBROCARTILAGINOUS TISSUES BY HOMING OF ENDOGENOUS CELLS

14

S. Tarafder, C.H. Lee

Columbia University Medical Center, New York, NY, United States

CHAPTER OUTLINE

INTRODUCTION

A synovial joint is the most common joint in mammals, and it allows for more movement of articulating bones than other joints such as synarthroses, sutures, syndesmoses, or gomphoses. Anatomically, a *synovial joint* is a solid organ consisting of articular cartilage, synovium, perichondrium,

In Situ Tissue Regeneration. http://dx.doi.org/10.1016/B978-0-12-802225-2.00014-3

and subchondral bone, including all cell types in bone marrow. The smooth and slippery lubricated surface of the articular cartilage covers the ends of bones, allowing the sliding of bones at the joint without rubbing each other. Load transfer with a minimum frictional coefficient and shock absorption is the principal function of the articular cartilage during movement [1]. Articular cartilage is hyaline cartilage, which is avascular, aneural, and alymphatic. The dense extracellular matrix (ECM) is sparsely populated by highly specialized cells known as chondrocytes. ECM is largely composed of water (up to 80% of the wet weight) and collagen (up to 60% of the dry weight, of which 90% is type II collagen) with other noncollagenous proteins and glycoproteins (10–15% of the wet weight) [1]. The fibrils and fibers formed by type II collagen are intertwined with proteoglycan aggregates.

Osteoarthritis (OA) is one of the most common forms of arthritis and represents chronic degeneration of the synovial joints, which is the leading cause of chronic disabilities worldwide [2–4]. OA is also known as degenerative joint disease or degenerative arthritis [5,6]. It is a chronic condition that breaks down cartilage, the material that cushions the joints. Cartilage breakdown causes bones to rub against each other, causing joint stiffness, pain, swelling, and reduced movement [5,7]. Multiple tissues including articular cartilage, subchondral bone, synovium, meniscus, and joint capsule can be involved in OA, although articular cartilage is frequently the focus of attention due to its breakdown and loss of function [8]. It is estimated that about 27 million people in the United States have OA afflicting about 14% of the US adult population aged 25 years and older, and about 34% of those adults are aged over 65 years [6]. Common symptoms of OA include pain, swelling, sore or stiff joints, and decreased mobility.

A healthy articular cartilage tolerates intensive and repetitive physical stress, but surprisingly it cannot self-heal or repair, even with the most minor injury. When damaged, the articular cartilage does not spontaneously repair due to a paucity of progenitor cells [9], a lack of blood vessels [9], a low cell-to-matrix ratio (~5%) [10,11], and low metabolic activity of mature chondrocytes [10,11]. The limited spontaneous repair of cartilage lesions leads to a progressive loss in joint function, together with the continuing destabilization of tissue matrix [8,12].

Total joint arthroplasty (TJA) is the predominant therapy for late stage OA using synthetic prosthesis of metal, plastic, and ceramics. Despite its reported clinical success, TJA has significant limitations, including wear debris, aseptic loosening, metal allergy, and infections. With an average service life of 10–15 years, TJA necessitates an inevitable revision in many patients; revision surgeries are technically challenging and costly [13–16]. Since current synthetic prosthesis cannot remodel with native bone that undergoes physiologically necessary remodeling, there has been a great deal of effort to develop biological therapies for cartilage and synovial joint regeneration, including abrasion arthroplasty, autologous chondrocyte implantation (ACI), and mosaicplasty [17]. However, few therapies are effective or commercially viable; they have drawbacks such as limited integration, suboptimal conformity of cartilage surface, altered cartilage phenotype, and donor site morbidity [13–16]. Additionally, the existing biological therapies are only applicable to focal cartilage lesions but not the entire articular surface of the synovial joint. To date, no biological therapies exist for resurfacing of the entire articular cartilage of the synovial joint.

Articular cartilage consists of chondrocytes and ECM that is rich in type II collagen fibrils and proteoglycans. Chondrocytes, despite their indispensible role in cartilage morphogenesis and maintenance, only account for 5% of the total cartilage volume in the adult [10,18]. Chondrocytes receive nutrients by diffusion exchange with perichondrium, synovial fluid, and subchondral bone, since articular cartilage is devoid of vascular supply [10]. The hydrated ECM, which accounts for the bulk of cartilage volume, provides structural stability under mechanical stress exerted by load bearing and locomotion. Since articular cartilage is a structural material, scaffolds have been designed and fabricated to incorporate chondrocytes or progenitor cells within a 3-D structure.

In addition to articular cartilage, knee meniscus plays essential roles in joint function and stability. Knee meniscus is C-shaped fibrocartilaginous tissue in the knee that sits on the top surface of the tibia. The menisci allow smooth load transfer from femur to tibia. Bone-to-bone friction would otherwise cause inflammation or arthritis without these wedge-shaped shock-absorbing cartilage pads. The lateral meniscus is generally wider than the medial meniscus. The peripheral borders of the fibrocartilaginous menisci are thick, convex, and well vascularized from capillaries branching off the fibrous capsule and synovial membrane [19], whereas the inner borders are thin, concave, and avascular.

Highly hydrated meniscus is composed of almost 72% water, and the remaining 28% is ECM and cells [20,21]. Meniscus ECM contains about 75% collagens, 17% glycosaminoglycans, <1% adhesion glycoproteins, and <1% elastin [21,22]. Collagen type II (about 80% of the dry weight) is predominantly present at the thick outer side of the meniscus with the presence of other collagen variants (<1% of the dry weight) [21]. Both type I (60%) and type II (40%) collagen make up the 70% collagen of the dry weight of the thin inner part of the meniscus. The cells in the outer thick region exhibit the characteristics of fibroblast and can be described as fibrochondrocytes, whereas cells in the inner region are characteristically more like both fibrocytes and chondrocytes and can be described as fibrochondrocytes or chondrocyte-like cells [19].

CURRENT TREATMENTS AND BIOLOGICALLY BASED APPROACHES

ARTICULAR CARTILAGE LESIONS

When articular cartilage defects are diagnosed to require intervention, microabrasion or microfracture is frequently considered as a first-line treatment for focal cartilage defects [23]. The surgeon abrades the damaged cartilage surface down to bleeding bone marrow and removes any softened or loose bits and osteophytes in arthroscopy. The underlying idea is to induce cells from the bleeding bone marrow to populate articular cartilage defects. Whereas cells from bone marrow do populate articular cartilage defects following microabrasion, the regenerating tissue is frequently fibrous tissue or fibrocartilage instead of hyaline cartilage [23]. Fibrocartilage has mechanical properties that are a fraction of hyaline cartilage in several aspects, and therefore it does not function nearly as well [24,25]. Therefore it is not a surprise that progressive matrix degeneration is associated with microabrasion, and focal defects frequently deteriorate to end-stage OA [23].

Mosaicplasty or autologous osteochondral grafting is performed to treat focal defects in articular cartilage. Cartilage or osteochondral cylinders are removed from nonloading areas of synovial joint and transplanted into the load-bearing defect site. Mosaicplasty is designed to fill the defects with mature, hyaline articular cartilage. Previous reports show the survival of the transplanted hyaline cartilages with good repair tissue filling [8,26,27]. However, transplantation of multiple cylindrical grafts in a focal defect inevitably leaves voids between the grafts, which may lead to tissue inhomogeneity and fibrocartilage formation [24]. Donor site morbidity and its failure to regenerate normal hyaline cartilage are other shortcomings of mosaicplasty [8,26,27].

Instead of cartilage grafts, chondrocytes are isolated from harvested tissues of the nonloading area of articular cartilage and processed for cell-based therapy for focal defects. This method, known as autologous chondrocyte implantation (ACI), has been applied in focal cartilage defects [28,29]. The isolated chondrocytes are culture-expanded in vitro and in a commercial entity and shipped to surgeons for delivery in focal articular cartilage defects with a periosteal flap sutured to surrounding articular cartilage. In a second surgical procedure, the surgeon fills the defect by injecting the expanded chondrocytes into the defect. A periosteal flap is sewed over the defect to secure the chondrocytes at the implanted site [30]. Despite encouraging short- or middle-term clinical outcomes, ACI has several intrinsic drawbacks including two-stage procedures, donor site trauma, the leakage of transplanted chondrocytes, uneven distribution of injected chondrocytes, periosteal hypertrophy, unavoidable suturing on the healthy surrounding cartilage, and loss of chondrogenic phenotype during in vitro cell manipulation [29,31].

To date, existing biologically based therapies including microabrasion, mosaicplasty, and ACI are applicable to focal cartilage defects and have an unpredictable clinical outcome. Given that focal defects have a tendency to deteriorate to end-stage OA, there is a clinical need for regeneration or resurfacing of the entire articular surface of the synovial joint.

Cell delivery matrices and scaffolds

The delivery of cell suspension into articular cartilage defects covered by a periosteum or a synthetic membrane is limited by an uneven cell distribution, leakage of the transplanted cells, and loss of chondrogenic phenotype. To overcome these deficiencies, various biomaterials have been studied as carrier vehicles to improve the maintenance of cells and chondrocyte phenotypes. Biomaterials can also be used to construct scaffolds for cartilage tissue engineering that enable 3-D culture of chondrogenic cells and support the structural integrity of the engineered tissues [32].

Matrix-induced autologous chondrocytes implantation

Matrix-induced ACI (MACI) (Genzyme Biosurgery, MA) is a clinically available approach to deliver autologous chondrocytes in a biopolymer membrane [31]. Chondrocytes are isolated from a nonloading area of articular cartilage, culture-expanded in vitro, and seeded within a bilayered membrane of collagen types I and III. The cell-seeded membrane is then transplanted to the cartilage defect and fixed using fibrin glue without a need of cover or sewing. Primary benefits of MACI include the even distribution of chondrocytes in the transplanted site and removal of suturing into healthy cartilage [28,31,33]. However, MACI failed to prevent fibrocartilaginous healing (the *goal* is *hyaline cartilage*), one of the critical shortcomings of current biological treatments [28,29,31,33]. Other MACI membranes include Maix (Matricel, Germany) and Chondro-Gide (Geistlich Biomaterials, Switzerland), consisting of porcine collagen types I–III with a mechanically stable outer layer and porous inner layer [29]. The multilayered membranes showed appropriate cell attachment, homogenous cell distribution, maintenance of chondrocytes phenotype over time, and security of the implanted cells in the defect site [29]. Nonetheless, the integration of de novo tissue into host hyaline cartilage is still unsatisfactory due to the intrinsic features of fully differentiated chondrocytes with their poor capability of tissue remodeling [8,29].

Hydrogels

3-D matrices in the form of hydrogels have been frequently used as cell delivery vehicles or scaffolds for cartilage tissue engineering, combined with autologous chondrocytes or bone marrow-derived mesenchymal stem cells (MSCs) or their derivatives [34–41]. Hydrogels are a class of biomaterials capable of absorbing biological fluids while maintaining a 3-D structure [38]. Hydrogels provide chondrocytes or chondrocyte precursor cells with a scaffold that simulates the formation of cartilaginous ECM comprised of type II collagen fibers residing within hydrated proteoglycan macromolecules [42,43]. Biomaterials constructing the hydrogels include, but are not limited to, collagen, hyaluronic acid (HA), fibrin, and polyethylene glycol (PEG) [9,29,32,37]. Although some of the biomaterials can be prepared in the form of both sponge and gel as scaffolds for cartilage tissue engineering, 3-D gels are considered to provide a more propitious structural environment for cartilage regeneration, also enabling a high cell density that is a critical factor for chondrogenic differentiation in an engineered cartilage tissue [44,45].

Collagen is the most abundant biopolymer in the body that can be processed to form a macroporous sponge or a microporous gel [46,47]. Clinically available collagen-based treatments include Atelocollagen (Koken Co. Ltd, Japan) that is a type I collagen gel modified to suppress immunorejection from the host [47]. Chondrocytes transplanted within the atelocollagen gel successfully maintained their phenotype and an even distribution without a leakage [31,46,47]. However, the attachment of the implanted cell–gel construct by a periosteal cover is still an issue [8,48,49]. Although type II collagen is a major component of native hyaline cartilage [11,18,32], both type I and type II collagen gels have been investigated as cultivate systems of chondrocytes or their progenitors [50–54]. Traditionally, several studies directly compared type I and type II collagen gels and revealed the superiority of type II collagen in maintaining chondrocyte phenotype and cartilage matrix formation as compared to type I collagen [53,54]. Nonetheless, it is still controversial whether the type of collagen is a critical factor to determine the fate of chondrocytes in a 3-D collagen construct [51]. Multiple previous works have reported that chondrogenic cells cultivated in type I collagen gel maintained their phenotype and expressed cartilage-related genes [41,46,55,56]. These findings, together with the fast remodeling rate of collagen in vivo, may suggest that a collagen gel primarily serves as a temporary matrix supporting chondrogenic cells, rather than as a sustained structural matrix.

Hyaluronan, commonly known as hyaluronic acid (HA), a polysaccharide-based biological polymer found in cartilage tissue, plays a pivotal role in cartilage homeostasis and is involved in cellular processes such as proliferation, migration, morphogenesis, and differentiation [57–60]. HA-based scaffolds can be prepared in the form of hydrogels, sponges, and meshes [29,46]. MSC-laden HA hydrogels appeared to be promising for regenerating hyaline-like cartilage with zonal architecture in rabbit osteochondral defects [61]. Hyalograft-C (Fidia Advanced Biopolymers Laboratories, Abano Terme, Italy), a chondrocyte-seeded nonwoven HA-based mesh (Hyaff-11), has been transplanted in patients [60]. Midterm clinical follow-ups revealed an improved repair of cartilage lesions in comparison with preoperative evaluations [60]. Recently reported photo-crosslinked HA hydrogels that are seeded with MSCs may serve as a minimally invasive approach to treat cartilage lesions [62].

Fibrin, a naturally occurring protein involved in the clotting of blood, has been widely used as tissue glue in surgeries. Given the rapid polymerization process of fibrinogen by the reaction with thrombin, fibrin received attention in cartilage repair as a minimally invasive cell delivery vehicle [34]. Chondrocytes or MSCs can be arthroscopically transplanted into the cartilage defect with injectable fibrin-based gels or glues. In addition, fibrin glue may be a suitable material to achieve an initial adhesion with host tissue. Indeed, recently reported 1-year clinical results showed that fibrin glue improved the integration of tissue-engineered cartilage constructs with surrounding tissues [63]. However, previous in vivo studies demonstrated that fibrin may not be an appropriate scaffold for cartilage tissue engineering due to the poor cell migration and tissue genesis into the matrix, in addition to the possible immune response [29,64,65].

PEG is a notable example of hydrogel, which is highly hydrophilic, biocompatible, and intrinsically resistant to protein adsorption and cell adhesion [36]. PEG hydrogel is frequently photo-crosslinked by UV light for several minutes, enabling a minimally invasive injection of cell–gel solution followed by polymerization in vivo [66,67] or a straightforward procedure to fabricate anatomically shaped tissue-engineered constructs using a mold [4,35,68]. The light-initiated polymerization of PEG can be utilized for engineering a multilayered construct [35,68], as further described in the following. PEG hydrogels encapsulated with chondrocytes or MSC-derived chondrogenic cells were able to maintain the original shape as generating cartilage-like matrix in vitro and in vivo [4,35,68]. Despite the advantages, clinical use of PEG hydrogels may be limited by the slow biodegradation rate, poor tissue ingrowth, and lack of interaction with host cells and tissues. Efforts have been made to improve the fixation of PEG hydrogel in vivo, and a chondroitin sulfate-based glue [69] was recently tested in a clinical setting to secure the PEG-cartilage bonding (Cartilix, Inc., Foster City, CA).

Major shortcomings of hydrogels as a scaffold for cartilage tissue engineering include poor mechanical strength, significant shrinkage of cell-laden hydrogel, and limited integration with host cartilage tissue. A recent study on hydrogels reported the compressive strength of a hydrogel, which can meet or exceed native cartilage [62,70,71]. A tissue-engineered construct needs to be remodeled in vivo to a mature tissue. In that point of view, the suboptimal mechanical strength, likely due to a more penetrable structure, may be more desirable than a dense tissue construct. Nevertheless, an engineered tissue graft should obtain the initial structural stability corresponding to that of native tissue, especially for the articular cartilage that is subjected to a substantial magnitude of loadings [72,73].

Cell-laden hydrogels also suffer from volumetric shrinkage in response to biochemical environments [74]. Given that most of the hydrogels are biodegradable, cell-mediated matrix degradation and remodeling may be one of the causes of the shrinkage. One must control the shrinkage to engineer tissue grafts to fit in the implantation sites. Additionally, the biological fixation of cell–hydrogel constructs in the implanted sites has been unsatisfactory [15,25,63,69]. Fibrin glue or a molecular adhesive have been investigated to improve the initial bonding between the engineered construct and host tissues [63,69]. However, it is still questionable whether a long-lasting biological integration can be followed by the interim biochemical bonds [63,69].

Hybrid scaffolds: a combination of hydrogels and solid polymers

Use of hydrogel alone, despite the 3-D hydrated structure promising for chondrogenesis, may be insufficient to engineer a cartilage construct of clinical relevance, primarily due to its poor mechanical strength. Accordingly, efforts have been made to improve the mechanical properties of cell–hydrogel constructs with use of physical stimulations or biochemical modifications [70,71,73]. More recently, hybrid scaffolds, a composite of hydrogels and porous polymeric scaffolds, started to draw attention. Synthetic copolymers, including poly(lactic acid) (PLA), poly(glycolic acid) (PGA), poly(lactic-co-glycolic acid) (PLGA), and poly(caprolactone) (PCL), have been widely used to fabricate porous scaffolds for tissue engineering applications. Such synthetic polymers are adequate to manufacture scaffolds with precisely controlled porosity, elasticity, and custom designed external shape [4,75,76]. They can also be efficiently modified for a specific hydrophilicity or biodegradation rate, depending on the application [77,78]. However, the polymeric porous scaffolds are often associated with low cell-seeding density and loss of chondrogenic phenotype over time [77]. Taken together, a combination of hydrogels and synthetic polymers was proposed to obtain both the chondrogenesis-favorable 3-D cultivation and the mechanical integrity in a scaffold system [44,77]. Collagen, fibrin, HA, alginate, and chitosan gels, loaded with chondrocytes or MSCs, have been infused into the pores of PGA-, PLA-, or PCL-based scaffolds to engineer cartilage constructs in vitro and in vivo [44,55,77]. A comparative study demonstrated that PCL/HA and PCL/chitosan hybrids were superior in promoting neocartilage formation and initial cell retention in vitro, as compared to other hybrids, including PCL/collagen and PCL/fibrin [55].

Bilayered scaffold for osteochondral tissue engineering

Chondral constructs for a treatment of partial- or full-thickness cartilage defects, despite the modest success in neocartilage formation, are challenged by the unsatisfactory integration of de novo cartilage in vivo [79]. As a relevant strategy to improve the cartilage integration, bilayered scaffolds comprised of cartilage and bone phases have been devised for osteochondral tissue engineering [49,79]. Subchondral bone is a highly vascularized tissue allowing recruitment of progenitor cells and therefore is more likely regenerative than avascular cartilage [17,49,79]. Thus osteochondral grafts may yield improved host-to-engineered cartilage integration, supported by bony integration in the subchondral construct [17,49,79]. In addition, creation of an osteochondral defect leads to formation of a fibrin clot that may assist to establish initial fixation of cartilage grafts, and the recruited chondrocytes progenitor cells (eg, MSC) from local bone marrow have potentials to facilitate cartilage regeneration [17,49].

Bilayered osteochondral grafts have been constructed by (1) layering chondrocytes or engineered cartilage tissue on a bone scaffold; (2) assembling two distinct cartilage and bone scaffolds; or (3) bioengineering cartilage and bone tissue layers in an integrated biphasic scaffold [49,79]. Bioceramics, hydrogel–ceramic composites, or decellularized bones have been used to build bone scaffolds, and cartilage scaffolds have been manufactured with polymeric sponges, meshes, or hydrogels [25,49,79,80]. Porous polymeric scaffolds, with varying internal microarchitectures, have been adopted both for bone and cartilage regions [81–83]. Bonding between the cartilage and bone layers was established by fibrin glue, suturing, press fitting, or in situ polymerization of hydrogels [49], but the mechanical integrity of layered or assembled cartilage is still questionable [25,69]. Accordingly, biphasic osteochondral tissues were engineered in an integrated scaffold system. For this, two distinct types of cells, MSC-derived or isolated chondrocytes and osteoblasts, were seeded in different layers of an integrated scaffold [35,48,68,84]. Previously, bone and cartilage layers were fabricated with two different compositions of materials using novel technologies, including 3-D printing, 3-D fibers deposition, and fused deposition modeling [81,85]. In other studies, two different compositions of hydrogels or a single hydrogel loaded with two different cells were cross-linked layer-by-layer to create an integrated osteochondral construct [35,68]. Recently, a concentration gradient (CG) of microencapsulated growth factors, including bone morphogenetic protein 2 (BMP2) and insulin-like growth factor 1 (IGF1), was incorporated in an MSC-loaded alginate gel [86]. MSCs exhibited osteogenic and chondrogenic differentiation along the CG of BMP2 and IGF1 [86], suggesting a new method to create an osteochondral construct. However, the coexistence of chondrogenic and osteogenic cues in the osteochondral interface may weaken the maturity of regenerating tissues [86,87].

Tissue-engineered osteochondral grafts have been examined in vivo, mainly for localized osteochondral defects in dimensions of 5–11 mm in diameter and 3–7 mm in height [35,48,49,68,84]. When implanted in osteochondral defects in animal models, new bone ingrowth and integration were observed in subchondral regions, and articular cartilage was adequately resurfaced [81,83,88]. However, no previous work appeared to avoid the formation of a fibrous interface between the implanted cartilage and adjacent host cartilage [81,83,88,89]. The incongruity at the graft interface can generate stress concentrations on the articular surface that may lead to graft loosening or progressive cartilage degeneration [24,25]. Therefore the incomplete integration of cartilage still remains as a critical issue, despite the promising concept of bilayered osteochondral construct.

Anatomically shaped 3-D scaffolds for the regeneration of the entirearticular surface of synovial joint

Current biological treatments, including the majority of previous tissue-engineered grafts, are designed for localized cartilage or osteochondral lesions, not for the entire synovial joints condyles. Unfortunately, the localized cartilage lesions frequently deteriorate into more severe OA that warrants TJA [13]. Accordingly, biologically based cartilage resurfacing or replacement of the entire synovial joint condyle has been proposed [15,17,49,90]. Tissue-engineered grafts for entire synovial joint condyles need only integration with the subchondral bone, therefore overcoming the limited integration of cartilage grafts. Previously, stratified layers of cartilage and bone were regenerated in dimensions of an entire human synovial joint in vitro and in vivo [35,45,68,48,84]. For example, our group has regenerated human-shaped temporomandibular joint (TMJ) condyles ectopically in vivo using a two-step photo-crosslinking of polyethylene glycol diacrylate (PEGDA) hydrogels, loaded with MSC-derived chondrocytes and osteoblasts in different layers [35,68]. Others have engineered anatomically shaped patellar condylar constructs by layering chondrocytes-laden agarose gel on a bony scaffold machined from devitalized native trabecular bone [25,80].

A key challenge in regenerating the entire synovial joint condyle is scaling-up the engineered grafts [4]. Regenerating tissue over 100–200 μm requires vascularization for nutrient diffusion and waste removal [91], which is essential for subchondral bone rather than avascular cartilage [17,49]. Recently, human- shaped TMJ condylar bone graft was engineered in vitro in dimensions of $15 \times 15 \times 5\,mm^3$ [80]. Decellularized bovine trabecular bone was machined to create an anatomically correct bony scaffold, and human bone marrow-derived MSCs (hMSCs) were culture-differentiated in the scaffold using a perfusion bioreactor [80]. It appeared that use of a bioreactor is unavoidable to provide efficient exchange of nutrients and metabolites for new tissue formation in the large engineered tissue [80]. Interestingly, our recent work demonstrated that tissue formation and vascularization in a large construct can be enabled only by precisely controlled internal microarchitecture of scaffolds [4]. An anatomically-shaped human tibial condyle with stratified layers of bone and cartilage was regenerated in vivo in dimensions of $20 \times 15 \times 15\,mm^3$, representing 25% of the original size [4]. Layer-by-layer fabricated poly(caprolactone)–hydroxyapatite (PCL-HA) scaffolds with repeating units of 400-μm interlaid strands and microchannels were used to engineer subchondral bone using osteogenic progenies of hMSCs. PEGDA hydrogel encapsulating hMSC-derived chondrogenic cells was molded as articular cartilage layer and infused into microchannels of the PCL-HA scaffold. Upon 6 weeks subcutaneous implantation, de novo tissue formation and angiogenesis were discovered in the large condylar constructs even without cell transplantation, suggesting the potentials of refined internal microstructure in regenerating large complex tissues [75,92–94]. Similarly to our approach, a recent work engineered rabbit-shaped knee joint condyles using layer-deposited poly(ethylene glycol)–terephthalate/poly(butylene terephthalate) scaffolds [95]. Chondrocyte-seeded scaffolds surgically replaced entire tibial and femoral condyles of rabbits for 6 weeks, and bony ingrowth and integration were superior in the 3-D-fiber deposited scaffolds in comparison with the porous scaffolds prepared by particle precipitating [95]. However, the regenerating cartilage failed to achieve a satisfactory tissue maturity and a full coverage of articular surface [95]. Table 14.1 presents a summary of cartilage regeneration modalities.

MENISCUS INJURY

Meniscus lesions are one of the most frequent intraarticular knee injuries that eventually lead to degeneration of the knee articular cartilage. The complex inflammatory responses caused by a partial or total injured meniscus might cause progressive chronic joint degeneration and OA [96,97]. Tears in the thick peripheral vascularized outer zone have greater healing capacity than the thin inner avascular regions [19].

Meniscectomy

Although a subtotal or total meniscectomy was the gold standard in the old days, nowadays this procedure is only rarely performed because this eventually leads to OA through chronic degeneration of the joint [19,96]. It was then advised that only the unrepairable portion of the meniscus tissue should be excised, preserving as much meniscus tissue as possible [98]. Torn part removal of the meniscus through partial meniscectomy has gained popularity due to the increase in popularity of arthroscopic surgery. This is only a short-term remedy because the load bearing and load distribution capacity is greatly compromised with the presence of decreased amount of meniscus. Therefore the patient will suffer from severe pain caused by cartilage degradation in the longer run [97]. Autrografts such as fat pad, tendon, cartilage, periosteum, synovial flap, and perichondrium have been tested for improved meniscus healing and functionality with no satisfactory outcome. Some of the major disadvantages are that these tissues have low mechanical properties and are not suitable for varying structure geometry [19].

Table 14.1 Comparison Cartilage Regeneration Modalities

	Cartilage Alone	Osteochondral Plugs	Entire Synovial Joint Condyle
Clinical relevance	Focal cartilage defects	Focal cartilage/osteochondral defects	End-stage OA
No. of tissue types	1 (cartilage alone)	2 (cartilage and subchondral bone)	2 (cartilage and subchondral bone)
Graft-to-host integration	By cartilage	By cartilage and subchondral bone	By subchondral bone
Vascularization	Not required	Required (potential bone marrow contribution to regeneration)	Important (potential bone marrow contribution to regeneration)
Anatomic shape	Cartilage surface conformity not specified	Cartilage surface conformity not specified	Important
Type of scaffolds	Not required (microabrasion), hydrogels, sponges, meshes, hybrids	Cylindrical bilayered scaffolds	Anatomical dimensioned scaffolds

Meniscus allograft transplantation (MAT)

Meniscus allograft transplantation (MAT) is generally performed on patients with pain following total or subtotal meniscectomy. Cryopreserved meniscus allografts (CryoLife Orthopedics, Marietta, GA) are the most widely used for MAT [99,100]. Young and active patients with minimal degenerative changes are suitable candidates for MAT [99]. Relief from the preoperative pain is the most common benefit reported in patients from clinical trials. Although decellularized meniscus allografts transplantation can lead to short-term clinical success in terms of functionality and retention of biomechanical properties, these allografts come with high processing cost, potential for infectious disease transmission, immunogenic reactions, difficult sizing, shrinkage, and potential incongruence [96]. There is also lack of standardized graft processing, surgical techniques, and long-term follow-up data for MAT procedure. It is also not substantiated by evidence that meniscus allograft can prevent progressive degenerative arthritis at the knee joint.

Biomaterials-assisted meniscal regeneration

A collagen scaffold was the first tissue-engineered construct used for meniscal tissue in clinical practice [19,101]. This is now commercially available as collagen meniscus implant (CMI) (Ivy Sports Medicine, Gräfelfing, Germany) in Europe [22]. A second meniscus implant that is commercially available also in Europe is a polyurethane polymeric implant (Actifit) (Orteq Sports Medicine, London, UK) [102]. None of these implants have been granted the US Food and Drug Administration approval. Highly porous CMI scaffold is made of type I collagen fibers. Although satisfactory clinical results are reported on CMI scaffolds, there are some concerns raised over their use. Both short and long follow-up extending up to 10 years showed a significant shrinkage of CMI scaffolds, and it forms a scar tissue instead of native tissue-like fibrocartilage [19,103,104]. Highly interconnected porous synthetic polyurethane polymeric implant (Actifit) can be a suitable alternative biomaterial for partial meniscectomy. There are no mid- and long-term clinical data available for Actifit. Short-term follow-up clinical results showed significant pain reduction, better tissue in growth, and improved functionality for Actifit. A 19-month follow-up indicated a nonfibrocartilage tissue regeneration [104]. However, long-term randomized clinical results are necessary on safety and effectiveness to claim Actifit a valid alternative to be used in partial meniscectomy.

Polyvinyl alcohol hydrogel (PVA-H) implant was tested in a rabbit model [105, 106]. A 2-year follow-up showed compressive strength and viscoelastic behavior similar to that of the native tissue with successful chondroprotection but failed to show meniscal tissue regeneration [106]. HA and PCL matrix augmented with circumferential PLA acid fibers showed good tissue ingrowth and chondroprotection after 4 months when tested in sheep model [107–109]. Hyaluronan–gelatin [110,111], PGA–PLGA [112], and Silk [113] also have been tested for meniscal tissue regeneration. No short- and long-term clinical data are still available for these materials to compare with the existing ones. Other techniques such as needling, gluing, synovial flaps, meniscal wrapping, and fibrin glue techniques also provide only short-term results for repairing of the meniscal tear.

REGENERATION OF SYNOVIAL JOINTS BY ENDOGENOUS STEM/PROGENITOR CELL HOMING

As described above, transplantation of cells with a regenerative capacity, such as mesenchymal stem/progenitor cells (MSCs) either from bone marrow, synovium, or adipose tissue, has been extensively investigated for regeneration of articular cartilage and knee meniscus. Despite being a meritorious approach, cell transplantation has encountered several critical barriers within the realm of current medicine. Technological and economic viability of cell transplantation, especially if it requires substantial ex vivo cell manipulation, has been questioned [114–116]. In some cases, transplanted stem/progenitor cells from an exogenous source fail to incorporate into host tissues in spite of their beneficial effects [117,118]. As summarized in Table 14.2, immune rejection, pathogen transmission, potential tumorigenesis, packaging/storage/shipping, and anticipated difficulties in clinical adoption and regulatory approval are among some of the roadblocks for cell delivery therapy.

Given the shortcomings related to cell delivery, there is a growing interest to regenerate tissues by homing endogenous cells, including stem/progenitor cells, rather than transplanting cells [119,120]. The recruited host cells may be then guided to release signaling cues and/or to participate in tissue healing. In the stem cell biology field, the term "homing" has been used to describe stem cells' ability to find their way to an anatomic destination or a niche via the bloodstream that has been extensively studied in the hematopoietic society. Recently, the concept of cell homing has been extended to recruitment of local stem/progenitor cells into implanted scaffolds or defect sites by chemotactic signals [117,121–123]. The new therapeutic option by harnessing the host's innate capacity for regeneration will likely cost less than the cell delivery-based therapy and potentially overcome the issues related to clinical safety and technical shortcomings. In addition, since this technology catalyzes the endogenous regenerative capacity without a need of ex vivo-cultured stem cells, the regulatory approval for clinical application and the commercialization of cell homing-based therapy may be facilitated in comparison with cell delivery approaches [121–123].

In earlier works, cell-free biomaterial scaffolds with growth factors have been implanted in vivo in the hope to regenerate cartilage or osteochondral defects from endogenous cells despite the lack of understanding of cell sources and homing mechanism [81,121,124]. For example, a layer-deposited cylindrical osteochondral scaffold ($6 \times 6 \times 3\,mm^3$), consisting of an ultra-high molecular weight polyethylene fiber and a hydroxyapatite coating, was impregnated with a type I collagen gel with or without basic fibroblast growth factor (bFGF) [81]. Upon 48 weeks in vivo implantation, bFGF delivery promoted neocartilage formation and subchondral bone regeneration. Although the incongruence still remained at the graft boundary, scaffold with growth factor delivery without any

Table 14.2 Comparison of Cell Delivery and Homing Approaches for Synovial Joint Regeneration

	Cell Transplantation		
	Autologous Cells	**Allogeneic Cells**	**Cell Homing**
No. of surgeries including both cell isolation and therapy	2	1	1
Ex vivo cell manipulation	Yes	Yes	No
Cell shipping and storage	Yes	Yes	No
Off-the-shelf product	Difficult	Difficult	Possible
Potential immunorejection	No	Possible	No
Pathogen contamination	Possible	Possible	No
Costs of development and therapy	High	High	Not as high

cell transplantation showed potentials in osteochondral regeneration [49,81]. CG collagen gels, designed for promoting cell recruitment via haptotaxis, were implanted in a full-thickness cartilage defect (5 mm × 5 mm) in rabbit model [124]. Up to 12 weeks in vivo, the CG collagen gels recruited significantly more MSC-like bromodeoxyuridine (BrdU) positive cells and promoted neocartilage formation as compared to homogenous collagen gels [124]. In another study, PEG hydrogel was tested in a clinical setting (ChonDux) (Cartilix, Inc., Foster City, CA) to secure blood clot derived from an abrasion arthroplasty. Upon creating a microfracture in the articular cartilage defect, PEG solution was applied in the defect site and then polymerized by UV light. The PEG hydrogels were consequently mixed with the blood derived from bone marrow, which contains chondrocyte precursor cells [17,125,126]. Fixation of the PEG hydrogel to the surrounding tissues was promptly achieved by a chondroitin sulfate-based adhesive [69].

The previously mentioned works, despite the enhanced healing, lacked identification of the cell sources responsible for endogenous cartilage regeneration and the mechanism of homing and regeneration. Thus far, MSCs from synovium and bone marrow and chondrogenic progenitor cells (CPCs) have been suggested as potential candidates to guide endogenous cartilage/osteochondral regeneration [17,121]. Accordingly, more sophisticated strategies are being developed to target specific populations of endogenous stem/progenitor cells. For example, fibrin/hyaluronic acids (HA) gel loaded with stromal derived factor-1 (SDF-1) was applied in cartilage defect in an explant model to improve healing by recruiting migratory CPCs [127]. Similarly, a combination of mechano growth factor and transforming growth factor beta 3 (TGFβ3) loaded in silk fibroin scaffolds successfully promoted healing of a focal cartilage defect in rabbit by recruiting and differentiating endogenous cells [128]. Radially oriented collagen scaffolds loaded with SDF-1 also showed improved healing of osteochondral defects in rabbit model [129]. However, these studies were limited in regeneration of focal cartilage or osteochondral defects.

REGENERATION OF ENTIRE ARTICULAR SURFACE BY ENDOGENOUS CELL HOMING

Besides the aforementioned focal defect regenerations, cell homing-based approaches have been applied for a regeneration of entire synovial joint condyle. We have recently demonstrated that functional entire articular surface of a synovial joint can be regenerated without cell transplantation using a layer-deposited PCL-HA scaffold with two distinct inner microstructures: 400 and 200 μm repeats of interlaid strands and microchannels for cartilage and bone regions, respectively [121]. TGFβ3-loaded collagen gel was infused into the microchannels of the cartilage layer. The bioengineered grafts surgically replaced the entire rabbit humeral condyles and induced promising regeneration of hyaline cartilage and vascularized subchondral bone, fully integrated with host tissues [121]. Analysis of recruited cells in scaffolds revealed that regenerated cartilage and subchondral bone were from synovial cells and bone marrow MSCs, respectively. Fully layered articular surface and functional restoration of the operated joints were obtained in TGFβ3-infused grafts, lending support to the idea that precisely controlled scaffold design combined with biological cues can lead to the functional regeneration of large complex tissues in vivo [121,123]. Nonetheless, long-term functionality and homeostasis of the regenerating cartilage, especially in larger animal models or patients, may warrant a prolonged release of the biological cues to maintain the tissue maturity and perhaps cell transplantation. Delivery vehicles made of biodegradable synthetic or biological polymers are incorporable in cell-free scaffold systems [87,130,131]. Whether this approach will be realized in preclinical animal models and in OA patients warrants separate investigations.

KNEE MENISCUS REGENERATION BY ENDOGENOUS CELL HOMING

More recently, we have applied spatiotemporal delivery system incorporated in the state-of-art 3-D printed scaffolds for knee meniscus regeneration [122]. Anatomically correct sheep meniscus scaffolds were fabricated by layers deposition of PCL using a 3-D printer (Fig. 14.1). Then connective tissue growth factor (CTGF) and TGFβ3 were spatially delivered in the scaffold to recapitulate the zone-specific matrix phenotypes: primarily type I collagen in the outer zone, and type II collagen in the inner zone, reminiscent of the native meniscus (Fig. 14.1).

When released from microchannels of 3-D printed, human meniscus scaffolds, CTGF and TGFβ3 induced endogenous stem/progenitor cells to differentiate and synthesize zone-specific type I and II collagens. We then replaced sheep meniscus with anatomically correct, 3-D printed scaffolds that incorporated spatially delivered CTGF and TGFβ3. At 12 days postop, the majority of the recruited cells into the scaffolds were positive for synovium MSC markers, including CD44 and CD90, indicating the cell source for meniscus regeneration (Fig. 14.2).

After 3 months, endogenous cells successfully regenerated the meniscus with zone-specific matrix distribution and cell phenotypes. Spatiotemporally delivered CTGF and TGFb3 also restored inhomogeneous mechanical properties in the regenerated sheep meniscus without any noticeable defects in femoral condyle and tibia plateau (Fig. 14.3).

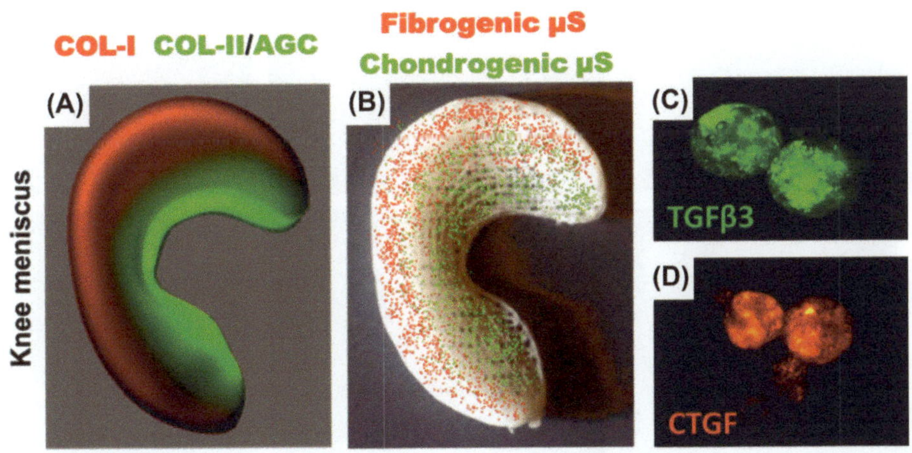

FIGURE 14.1

3-D printed anatomically correct knee meniscus scaffolds with spatiotemporal delivery of growth factors. Native knee meniscus exhibits multiphase fibrocartilaginous matrix distribution with more collagen I toward outer region and dominant collagen II in inner region and mixed fibrocartilaginous in middle region (A). To recapitulate the native multiphase matrix distribution, CTGF- and TGFβ3-encapsulated microspheres were spatially incorporated in the scaffold (B). Distribution of the two different growth factors was visualized by encapsulating dextran conjugated with fluorescein isothiocyanate (FITC) and Rhodamine (C, D).

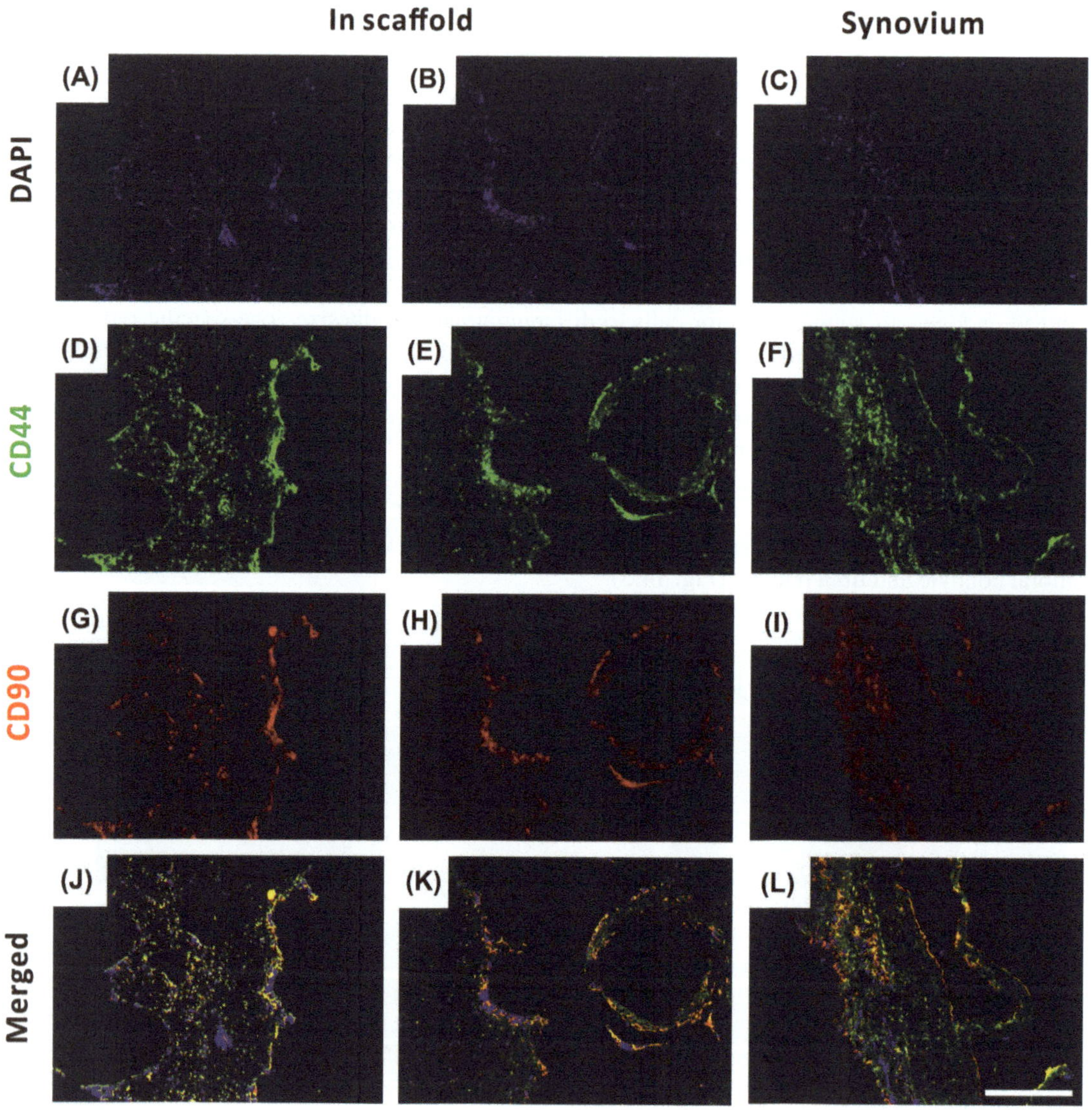

FIGURE 14.2

Identification of the recruited cells into the implanted meniscus scaffolds in vivo at day 12. The majority of cells recruited into the scaffolds expressed CD44 and CD90 (A, B, D, E, G, H, J, K) that is consistent with synovium MSCs (C, F, I, L). Scale = 200 μm.

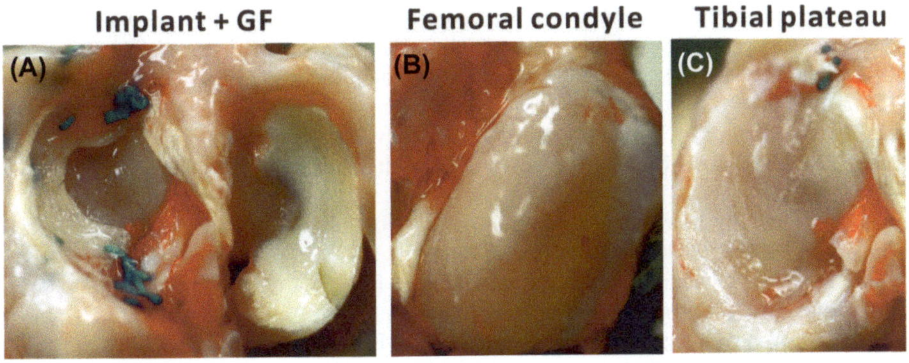

FIGURE 14.3

Functional regeneration of sheep meniscus. After 3 months implantation, the implanted scaffolds were fully integrated with host tissues (A) with no sign of cartilage breakdown on femoral condyle and tibia plateau (B, C).

SUMMARY AND PERSPECTIVES

Regeneration of articular cartilage and knee meniscus will benefit millions of patients who suffer from problems in synovial joints, and therefore is one of the key challenges for regenerative medicine. The recent scientific advances in cell homing-based approaches made a significant step toward development of therapeutics to regenerate articular cartilage and knee meniscus. We expect that our journey to regenerate a functional and sustainable articular cartilage and knee meniscus in patients with OA or sports injuries will be feasible by incorporating novel concepts and existing approaches that are consistent with regulatory and commercialization realities.

REFERENCES

[1] Sophia Fox AJ, Bedi A, Rodeo SA. The basic science of articular cartilage: structure, composition, and function. Sports Health 2009;1:461–8.

[2] Kraus VB. Pathogenesis and treatment of osteoarthritis. Med Clin North Am 1997;81:85–112.

[3] Lawrence RC, Helmick CG, Arnett FC, Deyo RA, Felson DT, Giannini EH, et al. Estimates of the prevalence of arthritis and selected musculoskeletal disorders in the United States. Arthritis Rheum 1998;41:778–99.

[4] Lee CH, Marion NW, Scott HJ, Mao J. Tissue formation and vascularization of anatomically shaped human tibial condyle in vivo. Tissue Eng Part A 2009;15.

[5] http://www.arthritis.org/; A.F. 2015.

[6] http://www.cdc.gov/; C.f.D.C.a.P. 2015.

[7] http://www.nlm.nih.gov/; N.L.o.M. 2015.

[8] Mano JF, Reis RL. Osteochondral defects: present situation and tissue engineering approaches. J Tissue Eng Regen Med 2007;1:261–73.

[9] Temenoff JS, Mikos AG. Review: tissue engineering for regeneration of articular cartilage. Biomaterials 2000;21:431–40.

[10] Hunziker EB. Growth-factor-induced healing of partial-thickness defects in adult articular cartilage. Osteoarthritis Cartilage 2001;9:22–32.

[11] Pacifici M, Koyama E, Iwamoto M, Gentili C. Development of articular cartilage: what do we know about it and how may it occur? Connect Tissue Res 2000;41:175–84.
[12] Aigner T, McKenna L. Molecular pathology and pathobiology of osteoarthritic cartilage. Cell Mol Life Sci 2002;59:5–18.
[13] Buckwalter JA, Martin JA. Osteoarthritis. Adv Drug Deliv Rev 2006;58:150–67.
[14] Goldberg VM, Caplan AI. Biological resurfacing: an alternative to total joint arthroplasty. Orthopedics 1994;17:819–21.
[15] Grayson WL, Chao PH, Marolt D, Kaplan DL, Vunjak-Novakovic G. Engineering custom-designed osteochondral tissue grafts. Trends Biotechnol 2008;26:181–9.
[16] Tuan RS. A second-generation autologous chondrocyte implantation approach to the treatment of focal articular cartilage defects. Arthritis Res Ther 2007;9:109.
[17] Mao JJ. Stem-cell-driven regeneration of synovial joints. Biol Cell 2005;97:289–301.
[18] Archer CW, Francis-West P. The chondrocyte. Int J Biochem Cell Biol 2003;35:401–4.
[19] Scotti C, Hirschmann MT, Antinolfi P, Martin I, Peretti GM. Meniscus repair and regeneration: review on current methods and research potential. Eur Cell Mater 2013;26:150–70.
[20] Herwig J, Egner E, Buddecke E. Chemical changes of human knee joint menisci in various stages of degeneration. Ann Rheum Dis 1984;43:635–40.
[21] Makris EA, Hadidi P, Athanasiou KA. The knee meniscus: structure-function, pathophysiology, current repair techniques, and prospects for regeneration. Biomaterials 2011;32:7411–31.
[22] Rongen JJ, van Tienen TG, van Bochove B, Grijpma DW, Buma P. Biomaterials in search of a meniscus substitute. Biomaterials 2014;35:3527–40.
[23] Mithoefer K, Williams 3rd RJ, Warren RF, Potter HG, Spock CR, Jones EC, et al. Chondral resurfacing of articular cartilage defects in the knee with the microfracture technique. Surgical technique. J Bone Joint Surg Am 2006;88(Suppl. 1 Pt. 2):294–304.
[24] Ahmad CS, Cohen ZA, Levine WN, Ateshian GA, Mow VC. Biomechanical and topographic considerations for autologous osteochondral grafting in the knee. Am J Sports Med 2001;29:201–6.
[25] Hung CT, Lima EG, Mauck RL, Takai E, LeRoux MA, Lu HH, et al. Anatomically shaped osteochondral constructs for articular cartilage repair. J Biomech 2003;36:1853–64.
[26] Kish G, Hangody L. A prospective, randomised comparison of autologous chondrocyte implantation versus mosaicplasty for osteochondral defects in the knee. J Bone Joint Surg Br 2004;86:619. author reply 619–20.
[27] Kish G, Modis L, Hangody L. Osteochondral mosaicplasty for the treatment of focal chondral and osteochondral lesions of the knee and talus in the athlete. Rationale, indications, techniques, and results. Clin Sports Med 1999;18:45–66. vi.
[28] Gooding CR, Bartlett W, Bentley G, Skinner JA, Carrington R, Flanagan A. A prospective, randomised study comparing two techniques of autologous chondrocyte implantation for osteochondral defects in the knee: Periosteum covered versus type I/III collagen covered. Knee 2006;13:203–10.
[29] Iwasa J, Engebretsen L, Shima Y, Ochi M. Clinical application of scaffolds for cartilage tissue engineering. Knee Surg Sports Traumatol Arthrosc 2009;17:561–77.
[30] Mobasheri A, Kalamegam G, Musumeci G, Batt ME. Chondrocyte and mesenchymal stem cell-based therapies for cartilage repair in osteoarthritis and related orthopaedic conditions. Maturitas 2014;78:188–98.
[31] Zheng MH, Willers C, Kirilak L, Yates P, Xu J, Wood D, et al. Matrix-induced autologous chondrocyte implantation (MACI): biological and histological assessment. Tissue Eng 2007;13:737–46.
[32] Vinatier C, Mrugala D, Jorgensen C, Guicheux J, Noel D. Cartilage engineering: a crucial combination of cells, biomaterials and biofactors. Trends Biotechnol 2009;27:307–14.
[33] Krishnan SP, Skinner JA, Carrington RW, Flanagan AM, Briggs TW, Bentley G. Collagen-covered autologous chondrocyte implantation for osteochondritis dissecans of the knee: two- to seven-year results. J Bone Joint Surg Br 2006;88:203–5.

[34] Ahmed TA, Dare EV, Hincke M. Fibrin: a versatile scaffold for tissue engineering applications. Tissue Eng Part B Rev 2008;14(2):199–215.
[35] Alhadlaq A, Elisseeff JH, Hong L, Williams CG, Caplan AI, Sharma B, et al. Adult stem cell driven genesis of human-shaped articular condyle. Ann Biomed Eng 2004;32:911–23.
[36] Buxton AN, Zhu J, Marchant R, West JL, Yoo JU, Johnstone B. Design and characterization of poly(ethylene glycol) photopolymerizable semi-interpenetrating networks for chondrogenesis of human mesenchymal stem cells. Tissue Eng 2007;13:2549–60.
[37] Drury JL, Mooney DJ. Hydrogels for tissue engineering: scaffold design variables and applications. Biomaterials 2003;24:4337–51.
[38] Lee KY, Mooney DJ. Hydrogels for tissue engineering. Chem Rev 2001;101:1869–79.
[39] Ng KW, Mauck RL, Statman LY, Lin EY, Ateshian GA, Hung CT. Dynamic deformational loading results in selective application of mechanical stimulation in a layered, tissue-engineered cartilage construct. Biorheology 2006;43:497–507.
[40] Park JS, Yang HN, Woo DG, Chung HM, Park KH. In vitro and in vivo chondrogenesis of rabbit bone marrow-derived stromal cells in fibrin matrix mixed with growth factor loaded in nanoparticles. Tissue Eng Part A 2009;15:2163–75.
[41] Schagemann JC, Erggelet C, Chung HW, Lahm A, Kurz H, Mrosek EH. Cell-laden and cell-free biopolymer hydrogel for the treatment of osteochondral defects in a sheep model. Tissue Eng Part A 2009;15:75–82.
[42] Oxley HR, Corkhill PH, Fitton JH, Tighe BJ. Macroporous hydrogels for biomedical applications: methodology and morphology. Biomaterials 1993;14:1064–72.
[43] Peppas NA, Huang Y, Torres-Lugo M, Ward JH, Zhang J. Physicochemical foundations and structural design of hydrogels in medicine and biology. Annu Rev Biomed Eng 2000;2:9–29.
[44] Hannouche D, Terai H, Fuchs JR, Terada S, Zand S, Nasseri BA, et al. Engineering of implantable cartilaginous structures from bone marrow-derived mesenchymal stem cells. Tissue Eng 2007;13:87–99.
[45] Troken A, Marion N, Hollister S, Mao J. Tissue engineering of the synovial joint: the role of cell density. Proc Inst Mech Eng H 2007;221:429–40.
[46] Kerker JT, Leo AJ, Sgaglione NA. Cartilage repair: synthetics and scaffolds: basic science, surgical techniques, and clinical outcomes. Sports Med Arthrosc 2008;16:208–16.
[47] Ochi M, Uchio Y, Kawasaki K, Wakitani S, Iwasa J. Transplantation of cartilage-like tissue made by tissue engineering in the treatment of cartilage defects of the knee. J Bone Joint Surg Br 2002;84:571–8.
[48] Isogai N, Landis W, Kim TH, Gerstenfeld LC, Upton J, Vacanti JP. Formation of phalanges and small joints by tissue-engineering. J Bone Joint Surg Am 1999;81:306–16.
[49] Martin I, Miot S, Barbero A, Jakob M, Wendt D. Osteochondral tissue engineering. J Biomech 2007;40:750–65.
[50] Breinan HA, Minas T, Hsu HP, Nehrer S, Shortkroff S, Spector M. Autologous chondrocyte implantation in a canine model: change in composition of reparative tissue with time. J Orthop Res 2001;19:482–92.
[51] Freyria AM, Ronziere MC, Cortial D, Galois L, Hartmann D, Herbage D, et al. Comparative phenotypic analysis of articular chondrocytes cultured within type I or type II collagen scaffolds. Tissue Eng Part A 2009;15:1233–45.
[52] Lee CR, Breinan HA, Nehrer S, Spector M. Articular cartilage chondrocytes in type I and type II collagen-GAG matrices exhibit contractile behavior in vitro. Tissue Eng 2000;6:555–65.
[53] Nehrer S, Breinan HA, Ramappa A, Shortkroff S, Young G, Minas T, et al. Canine chondrocytes seeded in type I and type II collagen implants investigated in vitro. J Biomed Mater Res 1997;38:95–104.
[54] Nehrer S, Breinan HA, Ramappa A, Young G, Shortkroff S, Louie LK, et al. Matrix collagen type and pore size influence behaviour of seeded canine chondrocytes. Biomaterials 1997;18:769–76.
[55] Schagemann JC, Chung HW, Mrosek EH, Stone JJ, Fitzsimmons JS, O'Driscoll SW, et al. Poly-epsilon-caprolactone/gel hybrid scaffolds for cartilage tissue engineering. J Biomed Mater Res A 2010;93(2):454–63.

[56] Yamaoka H, Tanaka Y, Nishizawa S, Asawa Y, Takato T, Hoshi K. The application of atelocollagen gel in combination with porous scaffolds for cartilage tissue engineering and its suitable conditions. J Biomed Mater Res A 2010;93(1):123–32.
[57] Chen WY, Abatangelo G. Functions of hyaluronan in wound repair. Wound Repair Regen 1999;7:79–89.
[58] Gobbi A, Kon E, Berruto M, Filardo G, Delcogliano M, Boldrini L, et al. Patellofemoral full-thickness chondral defects treated with second-generation autologous chondrocyte implantation: results at 5 years' follow-up. Am J Sports Med 2009;37:1083–92.
[59] Gobbi A, Kon E, Berruto M, Francisco R, Filardo G, Marcacci M. Patellofemoral full-thickness chondral defects treated with Hyalograft-C: a clinical, arthroscopic, and histologic review. Am J Sports Med 2006;34:1763–73.
[60] Marcacci M, Berruto M, Brocchetta D, Delcogliano A, Ghinelli D, Gobbi A, et al. Articular cartilage engineering with Hyalograft C: 3-year clinical results. Clin Orthop Relat Res 2005:96–105.
[61] Liu Y, Shu XZ, Prestwich GD. Osteochondral defect repair with autologous bone marrow-derived mesenchymal stem cells in an injectable, in situ, cross-linked synthetic extracellular matrix. Tissue Eng 2006;12:3405–16.
[62] Erickson IE, Huang AH, Sengupta S, Kestle S, Burdick JA, Mauck RL. Macromer density influences mesenchymal stem cell chondrogenesis and maturation in photocrosslinked hyaluronic acid hydrogels. Osteoarthritis Cartilage 2009;17(12):1639–48.
[63] Visna P, Pasa L, Cizmar I, Hart R, Hoch J. Treatment of deep cartilage defects of the knee using autologous chondrograft transplantation and by abrasive techniques – a randomized controlled study. Acta Chir Belg 2004;104:709–14.
[64] Brittberg M, Sjogren-Jansson E, Lindahl A, Peterson L. Influence of fibrin sealant (Tisseel) on osteochondral defect repair in the rabbit knee. Biomaterials 1997;18:235–42.
[65] van Susante JL, Buma P, Schuman L, Homminga GN, van den Berg WB, Veth RP. Resurfacing potential of heterologous chondrocytes suspended in fibrin glue in large full-thickness defects of femoral articular cartilage: an experimental study in the goat. Biomaterials 1999;20:1167–75.
[66] Bryant SJ, Anseth KS. The effects of scaffold thickness on tissue engineered cartilage in photocrosslinked poly(ethylene oxide) hydrogels. Biomaterials 2001;22:619–26.
[67] Kretlow JD, Young S, Klouda L, Wong M, Mikos AG. Injectable biomaterials for regenerating complex craniofacial tissues. Adv Mater 2009;21:3368–93.
[68] Alhadlaq A, Mao JJ. Tissue-engineered osteochondral constructs in the shape of an articular condyle. J Bone Joint Surg Am 2005;87:936–44.
[69] Wang DA, Varghese S, Sharma B, Strehin I, Fermanian S, Gorham J, et al. Multifunctional chondroitin sulphate for cartilage tissue-biomaterial integration. Nat Mater 2007;6:385–92.
[70] Byers BA, Mauck RL, Chiang IE, Tuan RS. Transient exposure to transforming growth factor beta 3 under serum-free conditions enhances the biomechanical and biochemical maturation of tissue-engineered cartilage. Tissue Eng Part A 2008;14:1821–34.
[71] Lima EG, Bian L, Ng KW, Mauck RL, Byers BA, Tuan RS, et al. The beneficial effect of delayed compressive loading on tissue-engineered cartilage constructs cultured with TGF-beta3. Osteoarthritis Cartilage 2007;15:1025–33.
[72] Butler DL, Goldstein SA, Guilak F. Functional tissue engineering: the role of biomechanics. J Biomech Eng 2000;122:570–5.
[73] Hung CT, Mauck RL, Wang CC, Lima EG, Ateshian GA. A paradigm for functional tissue engineering of articular cartilage via applied physiologic deformational loading. Ann Biomed Eng 2004;32:35–49.
[74] Kim SJ, Spinks GM, Prosser S, Whitten PG, Wallace GG, Kim SI. Surprising shrinkage of expanding gels under an external load. Nat Mater 2006;5:48–51.
[75] Hollister SJ. Porous scaffold design for tissue engineering. Nat Mater 2005;4:518–24.
[76] Williams JM, Adewunmi A, Schek RM, Flanagan CL, Krebsbach PH, Feinberg SE, et al. Bone tissue engineering using polycaprolactone scaffolds fabricated via selective laser sintering. Biomaterials 2005;26:4817–27.

[77] Eyrich D, Wiese H, Maier G, Skodacek D, Appel B, Sarhan H, et al. In vitro and in vivo cartilage engineering using a combination of chondrocyte-seeded long-term stable fibrin gels and polycaprolactone-based polyurethane scaffolds. Tissue Eng 2007;13:2207–18.
[78] Hutmacher DW. Scaffold design and fabrication technologies for engineering tissues – state of the art and future perspectives. J Biomater Sci Polym Ed 2001;12:107–24.
[79] O'Shea TM, Miao X. Bilayered scaffolds for osteochondral tissue engineering. Tissue Eng Part B Rev 2008;14:447–64.
[80] Grayson WL, Frohlich M, Yeager K, Bhumiratana S, Chan ME, Cannizzaro C, et al. Engineering anatomically shaped human bone grafts. Proc Natl Acad Sci USA 2010;107(8):3299–304.
[81] Fukuda A, Kato K, Hasegawa M, Hirata H, Sudo A, Okazaki K, et al. Enhanced repair of large osteochondral defects using a combination of artificial cartilage and basic fibroblast growth factor. Biomaterials 2005;26:4301–8.
[82] Shao X, Goh JC, Hutmacher DW, Lee EH, Zigang G. Repair of large articular osteochondral defects using hybrid scaffolds and bone marrow-derived mesenchymal stem cells in a rabbit model. Tissue Eng 2006;12:1539–51.
[83] Shao XX, Hutmacher DW, Ho ST, Goh JC, Lee EH. Evaluation of a hybrid scaffold/cell construct in repair of high-load-bearing osteochondral defects in rabbits. Biomaterials 2006;27:1071–80.
[84] Weng Y, Cao Y, Silva CA, Vacanti MP, Vacanti CA. Tissue-engineered composites of bone and cartilage for mandible condylar reconstruction. J Oral Maxillofac Surg 2001;59:185–90.
[85] Cao T, Ho KH, Teoh SH. Scaffold design and in vitro study of osteochondral coculture in a three-dimensional porous polycaprolactone scaffold fabricated by fused deposition modeling. Tissue Eng 2003;9(Suppl. 1):S103–12.
[86] Wang X, Wenk E, Zhang X, Meinel L, Vunjak-Novakovic G, Kaplan DL. Growth factor gradients via microsphere delivery in biopolymer scaffolds for osteochondral tissue engineering. J Control Release 2009;134:81–90.
[87] Moioli EK, Hong L, Guardado J, Clark PA, Mao JJ. Sustained release of TGFbeta3 from PLGA microspheres and its effect on early osteogenic differentiation of human mesenchymal stem cells. Tissue Eng 2006;12:537–46.
[88] Swieszkowski W, Tuan BH, Kurzydlowski KJ, Hutmacher DW. Repair and regeneration of osteochondral defects in the articular joints. Biomol Eng 2007;24:489–95.
[89] Yoshioka T, Mishima H, Ohyabu Y, Sakai S, Akaogi H, Ishii T, et al. Repair of large osteochondral defects with allogeneic cartilaginous aggregates formed from bone marrow-derived cells using RWV bioreactor. J Orthop Res 2007;25:1291–8.
[90] Moutos FT, Freed LE, Guilak F. A biomimetic three-dimensional woven composite scaffold for functional tissue engineering of cartilage. Nat Mater 2007;6:162–7.
[91] Jain RK, Au P, Tam J, Duda DG, Fukumura D. Engineering vascularized tissue. Nat Biotechnol 2005;23:821–3.
[92] Hutmacher DW, Cool S. Concepts of scaffold-based tissue engineering – the rationale to use solid free-form fabrication techniques. J Cell Mol Med 2007;11:654–69.
[93] Langer R, Tirrell DA. Designing materials for biology and medicine. Nature 2004;428:487–92.
[94] Lutolf MP, Hubbell JA. Synthetic biomaterials as instructive extracellular microenvironments for morphogenesis in tissue engineering. Nat Biotechnol 2005;23:47–55.
[95] Woodfield TB, Guggenheim M, von Rechenberg B, Riesle J, van Blitterswijk CA, Wedler V. Rapid prototyping of anatomically shaped, tissue-engineered implants for restoring congruent articulating surfaces in small joints. Cell Prolif 2009;42:485–97.
[96] Liu C, Toma IC, Mastrogiacomo M, Krettek C, von Lewinski G, Jagodzinski M. Meniscus reconstruction: today's achievements and premises for the future. Arch Orthop Trauma Surg 2013;133:95–109.
[97] Buma P, Ramrattan NN, van Tienen TG, Veth RP. Tissue engineering of the meniscus. Biomaterials 2004;25:1523–32.

[98] McGinity JB, Geuss LF, Marvin RA. Partial or total meniscectomy: a comparative analysis. J Bone Joint Surg Am 1977;59:763–6.
[99] Stollsteimer GT, Shelton WR, Dukes A, Bomboy AL. Meniscal allograft transplantation: a 1- to 5-year follow-up of 22 patients. Arthroscopy 2000;16:343–7.
[100] Hommen JP, Applegate GR, Del Pizzo W. Meniscus allograft transplantation: ten-year results of cryopreserved allografts. Arthroscopy 2007;23:388–93.
[101] Stone KR, Steadman JR, Rodkey WG, Li ST. Regeneration of meniscal cartilage with use of a collagen scaffold. Analysis of preliminary data. J Bone Joint Surg Am 1997;79:1770–7.
[102] Vrancken AC, Buma P, van Tienen TG. Synthetic meniscus replacement: a review. Int Orthop 2013;37:291–9.
[103] Martinek V, Ueblacker P, Braun K, Nitschke S, Mannhardt R, Specht K, et al. Second generation of meniscus transplantation: in-vivo study with tissue engineered meniscus replacement. Arch Orthop Trauma Surg 2006;126:228–34.
[104] Spencer SJ, Saithna A, Carmont MR, Dhillon MS, Thompson P, Spalding T. Meniscal scaffolds: early experience and review of the literature. Knee 2012;19:760–5.
[105] Kobayashi M, Toguchida J, Oka M. Preliminary study of polyvinyl alcohol-hydrogel (PVA-H) artificial meniscus. Biomaterials 2003;24:639–47.
[106] Kobayashi M, Chang YS, Oka M. A two year in vivo study of polyvinyl alcohol-hydrogel (PVA-H) artificial meniscus. Biomaterials 2005;26:3243–8.
[107] Chiari C, Koller U, Dorotka R, Eder C, Plasenzotti R, Lang S, et al. A tissue engineering approach to meniscus regeneration in a sheep model. Osteoarthritis Cartilage 2006;14:1056–65.
[108] Kon E, Chiari C, Marcacci M, Delcogliano M, Salter DM, Martin I, et al. Tissue engineering for total meniscal substitution: animal study in sheep model. Tissue Eng Part A 2008;14:1067–80.
[109] Kon E, Filardo G, Tschon M, Fini M, Giavaresi G, Marchesini Reggiani L, et al. Tissue engineering for total meniscal substitution: animal study in sheep model – results at 12 months. Tissue Eng Part A 2012;18:1573–82.
[110] Angele P, Johnstone B, Kujat R, Zellner J, Nerlich M, Goldberg V, et al. Stem cell based tissue engineering for meniscus repair. J Biomed Mater Res A 2008;85:445–55.
[111] Zellner J, Mueller M, Berner A, Dienstknecht T, Kujat R, Nerlich M, et al. Role of mesenchymal stem cells in tissue engineering of meniscus. J Biomed Mater Res A 2010;94:1150–61.
[112] Kang SW, Son SM, Lee JS, Lee ES, Lee KY, Park SG, et al. Regeneration of whole meniscus using meniscal cells and polymer scaffolds in a rabbit total meniscectomy model. J Biomed Mater Res A 2006;78:659–71.
[113] Mandal BB, Park SH, Gil ES, Kaplan DL. Multilayered silk scaffolds for meniscus tissue engineering. Biomaterials 2011;32:639–51.
[114] Ahsan T, Nerem RM. Bioengineered tissues: the science, the technology, and the industry. Orthod Craniofac Res 2005;8:134–40.
[115] Fodor WL. Tissue engineering and cell based therapies, from the bench to the clinic: the potential to replace, repair and regenerate. Reprod Biol Endocrinol 2003;1:102.
[116] Muschler GF, Nakamoto C, Griffith LG. Engineering principles of clinical cell-based tissue engineering. J Bone Joint Surg Am 2004;86-A:1541–58.
[117] Chen FM, Wu LA, Zhang M, Zhang R, Sun HH. Homing of endogenous stem/progenitor cells for in situ tissue regeneration: promises, strategies, and translational perspectives. Biomaterials 2011;32:3189–209.
[118] Yoshikawa T, Mitsuno H, Nonaka I, Sen Y, Kawanishi K, Inada Y, et al. Wound therapy by marrow mesenchymal cell transplantation. Plast Reconstr Surg 2008;121:860–77.
[119] Chamberlain G, Fox J, Ashton B, Middleton J. Concise review: mesenchymal stem cells: their phenotype, differentiation capacity, immunological features, and potential for homing. Stem Cells 2007;25:2739–49.
[120] Laird DJ, von Andrian UH, Wagers AJ. Stem cell trafficking in tissue development, growth, and disease. Cell 2008;132:612–30.

[121] Lee CH, Cook JL, Koch PD, Moioli EK, Xin X, Mao JJ. Functional regeneration of total synovial joint condyle without cell transplantation. In: 55th Annual Meeting of the Orthopaedic Research Society, Las Vegas, NV. 2009.
[122] Lee CH, Rodeo SA, Fortier LA, Lu C, Erisken C, Mao JJ. Protein-releasing polymeric scaffolds induce fibrochondrocytic differentiation of endogenous cells for knee meniscus regeneration in sheep. Sci Transl Med 2014;6:266ra171.
[123] Mao JJ, Stosich MS, Moioli EK, Lee CH, Fu SY, Bastian B, et al. Facial reconstruction by biosurgery: cell transplantation vs. cell homing. Tissue Eng Part B Rev 2010;16(2):257–62.
[124] Mimura T, Imai S, Kubo M, Isoya E, Ando K, Okumura N, et al. A novel exogenous concentration-gradient collagen scaffold augments full-thickness articular cartilage repair. Osteoarthritis Cartilage 2008;16:1083–91.
[125] Caplan AI. Mesenchymal stem cells. J Orthop Res 1991;9:641–50.
[126] Prockop DJ. Marrow stromal cells as stem cells for nonhematopoietic tissues. Science 1997;276:71–4.
[127] Yu Y, Brouillette MJ, Seol D, Zheng H, Buckwalter JA, Martin JA. Use of recombinant human stromal cell-derived factor 1α-loaded fibrin/hyaluronic acid hydrogel networks to achieve functional repair of full-thickness bovine articular cartilage via homing of chondrogenic progenitor cells. Arthritis Rheumatol 2015;67(5):1274–85.
[128] Luo Z, Jiang L, Xu Y, Li H, Xu W, Wu S, et al. Mechano growth factor (MGF) and transforming growth factor (TGF)-beta3 functionalized silk scaffolds enhance articular hyaline cartilage regeneration in rabbit model. Biomaterials 2015;52:463–75.
[129] Chen P, Tao J, Zhu S, Cai Y, Mao Q, Yu D, et al. Radially oriented collagen scaffold with SDF-1 promotes osteochondral repair by facilitating cell homing. Biomaterials 2015;39:114–23.
[130] Lu L, Stamatas GN, Mikos AG. Controlled release of transforming growth factor beta1 from biodegradable polymer microparticles. J Biomed Mater Res 2000;50:440–51.
[131] Lu L, Yaszemski MJ, Mikos AG. TGF-beta1 release from biodegradable polymer microparticles: its effects on marrow stromal osteoblast function. J Bone Joint Surg Am 2001;83-A(Suppl. 1):S82–91.

CHAPTER

BIOENGINEERED STRATEGIES FOR TENDON REGENERATION

15

A.I. Gonçalves, M.T. Rodrigues, R.L. Reis, M.E. Gomes
University of Minho, Guimarães, Portugal

CHAPTER OUTLINE

INTRODUCTION

Their important mechanical function predisposes tendons to injury and rupture, becoming a worldwide clinical problem. Commonly injured tendons include the rotator cuff, finger flexors, patellar, and Achilles tendon [1]. As poor cellular and vascular tissues [2], tendons present some healing constraints, typically requiring surgical intervention. Available reparative surgeries rely on tissue replacement with auto- or allografts [3], which are often accompanied with donor site morbidity, pain, inferior functionalities, and eventually graft failure.

Due to the market demand, commercial substitutes for tendon repair have been developed as biological and synthetic scaffolds. Despite being Food and Drug Administration approved, both positive

In Situ Tissue Regeneration. http://dx.doi.org/10.1016/B978-0-12-802225-2.00015-5

and negative results have been reported in clinical applications. Among biological devices, *Restore*, *TissueMend*, *OrthoMend*, and *GraftJacket* are some of the most used products for tendon repair. *Restore* implant is composed of porcine small intestine submucosa, predominantly collagen types I and III and has controversial outcomes in rotator cuff tendon repair [4,5]. The devices *TissueMend* and *OrthoMend Soft Tissue Repair Matrix*, both made of collagen matrix derived from bovine skin, are thin sheets used to wrap around and reinforce the repaired area during healing of Achilles tendon [6]. GraftJacket is another commercial scaffold obtained from cadaver human skin that has been recently used in rotator cuff [7,8] and Achilles tendon rupture [6,9].

Alternatively to biological scaffolds, synthetic ones are also available in the surgical market. *Surgi-Wrap MAST Tendon Sheet* is a polymeric surgical mesh for tendon augmentation that functions as a resorbable implant in a sheet form manufactured from poly (L-lactide-co-D,L-lactide) 70:30. Although less reported in clinical trials, *Sportmesh Artelon fibers* (polycaprolactone-based poly(urethane urea) material) are also used in tendon reparative surgeries [10,11]. Independently of the origin, biological and synthetic scaffolds can cause adverse events, such as noninfectious effusion and synovitis, that ultimately may result in the failure of surgery [12].

These surgical approaches are not successful to consistently restore the original properties of a functional tissue. Tendon tissue engineering (TTE) strategies might overcome these limitations, providing the ultimate solution to restore the damaged tendon to its preinjured state, improving the functionality outcomes while reducing healing time and medical complications due to surgery and follow-up care. TTE approaches have sought to augment the injured tissue with cells, scaffolds, bioactive agents, and mechanical stimulation to stimulate an efficient natural healing response. Furthermore, due to the particular nature of tendon as mechanoresponsive tissues and the limited cell and vascular density in these tissues to promote healing, the key tools for restoring full tendon functions following injury will likely include an optimal combination of these agents.

One of the major difficulties of recreating tendon functional substitutes is to mimic the highly organized matrix of this tissue, which is mainly responsible for tendon biomechanical functions. Thus the biomaterial fabrication technology should envision the development of biomimetic scaffolds for supporting and directing cell behavior, as well as for accommodating other predefined and reproducible features enabling multiple functionalities to synergistically enhance tissue regeneration capacity. Hence, the scaffold should guide cell proliferation and differentiation toward a specialized type of cells, the tenocyte, via physical and biochemical cues similar to the ones available in the native cellular environment. The differentiation into tendon cells will allow the cells to respond to the surrounding milieu similarly to tenocytes in native tendons. To achieve this, TTE constructs should be able to simultaneously induce cellular alignment and orientation and respond accordingly toward stimulated environments. Because tendons are mechanoresponsive tissues dynamic loading modulates the synthesis and remodeling of the extracellular matrix (ECM) through mechanotransduction signaling, promoting biochemical signals responsible for cell proliferation, differentiation, and ECM synthesis [13].

It is widely accepted that environmental biochemical factors such as growth factors (GFs) are potential agents to target specific tissue responses because of their regulatory roles in cellular functions, including adhesion, proliferation, migration, matrix synthesis, and cell differentiation [14,15]. Due to GFs' role in cellular behavior, they have been attracting attention in tendon studies as a mean to promote tenogenic differentiation and ultimately guide injured tissue regeneration.

Nanotechnology has also arisen instrumental as a tool for future developments in tissue engineering (TE) and TE regenerative medicine (TERM) approaches. In particular, there is an increasing interest regarding the use of magnetic nanoparticles (MNPs) in TERM applications, which will be further debated in this chapter. MNPs may enable multifunctionality of TE strategies, as they can be used in the tagging, tracking, and activation of stem cells, both in vitro and in vivo [16].

In this chapter, we discuss efforts and achievements to identify topographical, mechanical, and chemical factors in guiding stem cells to recapitulate critical aspects of tenogenesis and discuss the role these works may have in the future of TTE.

BIOLOGICAL STRUCTURE AND EXTRACELLULAR MATRIX ROLE, MECHANICAL DEMANDS, AND BIOACTIVE MOLECULES IN TENDON TISSUE

TENDON DEVELOPMENT AND PHYSIOLOGY

Healthy tendons are strong bands of brilliant white and fibroelastic tissue, connecting muscles to bones, allowing the anatomic alignment of the skeleton and transmission of tensile forces with great resistance to applied mechanical loads [17], while providing connective flexibility, which permits body locomotion and joint stability/movement [2,18].

Distinctly to other skeletal tissues as bone, muscle, or cartilage, tendon morphogenesis is less known and understood. Human tendons appear in the mesenchyme of the limb bud at 6–8 weeks of fetal life and join with the muscles originated from the somites. Embryonic tendons are highly cellular and begin with a sparse, disorganized collagen fiber matrix. Throughout growth to adulthood, as matrix elements are synthesized [19], mature functional tendons become highly aligned, structurally closely packed, and composed of collagen fibers that are integral to their uniquely high tensile strength and function [20]. Collagen fibers are arranged in bundles and primarily aligned in the direction of the long axis of the tendon. Bundles of fibers form tendon fascicles, which, in turn, bind together by a thin layer of connective tissue named endotenon. Several fiber bundles and endotenon are encompassed by the epitenon, which is covered by another layer of connective tissue named paratenon. Together, the paratenon and the epitenon are called peritenon [2]. Besides the dense network of collagen type I fibers, the tendons are comprised of few blood vessels, a limited number of spindle-shaped cells (tenoblasts/tenocytes) found in rows between the collagen bundles, and water. Of the tendon dry weight, 60–85% is collagen, predominantly collagen type I (~60%) arranged in tensile-resistant fibers [21]. Collagen type III copolymerizes with collagen I, and despite its low amount in the ECM, it provides tissue elasticity and is essential for normal fibrillogenesis. Besides collagen, tendons also contain proteoglycans, among them aggrecan and decorin (DCN), and other glycoproteins, such as collagen oligomeric matrix protein (COMP), lubricin, and tenascin-C. The primary role of proteoglycans and glycoproteins is to guide and maintain the organization of fibrous connective tissue. Aggrecan holds water and resists compression, while DCN, the most abundant tendon proteoglycan, facilitates fibrillar slippage and regulates tendon structure by stabilizing and aligning collagen fibrils [22,23], having a mediator role in the process of collagen fibrillogenesis, and is involved in the development of a tendon-like fibril profile. COMP is involved in the repair and remodeling processes of the tendon [24,25] as collagen III and is particularly synthesized in response to, and to resist, loading [26]. Lubricin, another glycoprotein found in the tendon matrix, enables sliding and recoil between adjacent fascicles playing an important role in interfascicular lubrication [27] and tendon gliding function [28]. Tenascin-C is an ECM protein present in developing and mature tendons [29], and the transcription of its gene is directly associated with mechanical loading

[30–32]. The relaxation of the cytoskeleton was found to suppress the induction of the tenascin-C gene by cyclic stretch [30]. Also, scleraxis (Scx) has been described as a specific molecular marker of tendon and ligaments [33], a basic helix–loop–helix transcription factor, which regulates tendon formation and collagen type I, DCN, fibromodulin (Fmod), and tenomodulin in tendon ECM.

TENDON EXTRACELLULAR MATRIX: A CRITICAL PARTICIPANT IN TENDON FUNCTIONALITY

Tendons' functional capacity is directly related to the composition of this unique ECM arranged in a highly organized hierarchy of parallel, cross-linked collagen fibrils assembled from nano- to macro-structures. This organization allows tendons to handle high unidirectional tensile loads and regulates cell behavior [34] (Fig. 15.1).

Tenocytes are responsible to maintain tendon homeostasis [35] and, in response to mechanical loads, initiate controlled responses that particularly result in the production of biomolecules, mainly glycosaminoglycans and glycoproteins that play specific yet interactive roles in tendon adaptation to the tensile forces applied.

Tenascin-C, fibronectin, and elastin enhance mechanical stability, allowing tendons to return to their prestretched lengths after physiological loading [35]. Additionally, elastin (2% of the dry weight) within the matrix forms cross-linked sheets allowing the tissue to stretch and coil, thus recovering after stimulus. ECM reorganization generates functional tissue with enhanced mechanical properties to withstand loading [13]. The direction of loading, intensity, frequency, and type of stimuli also influences the synthesis and organization of the ECM niche.

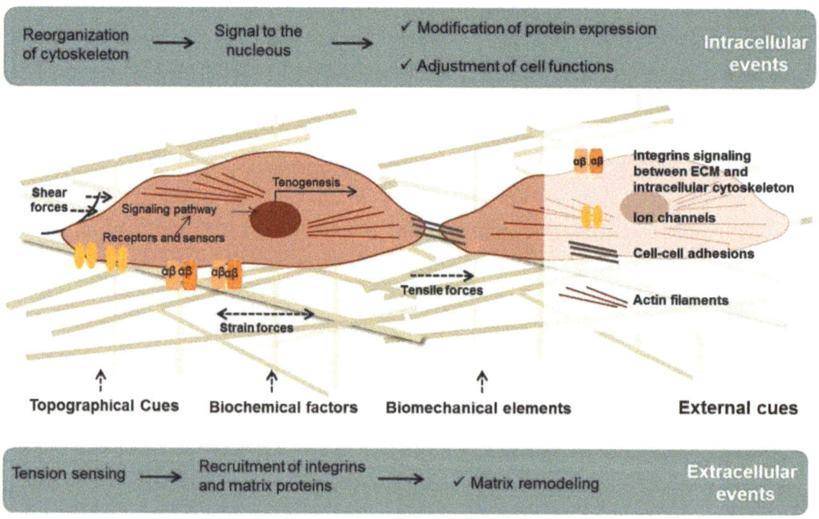

FIGURE 15.1 Schematic representation of cell–ECM interactions.

Cell responses via the application of external cues from the extracellular environment regulate a series of intracellular signalings achieving tenogenic differentiation.

MECHANICAL BEHAVIOR OF TENDONS

Tendon fiber patterns and viscoelastic characteristics contribute to their unique mechanical behavior [35] when subjected to dynamic mechanical forces, making tendon tissues highly efficient in response to constant loadings of variable transmittal forces in daily routine activities. Collagens and proteoglycans are primarily responsible for the viscoelasticity, while the collagen fibers resist tension forces to the tissue. Structural integrity and normal mechanical function of the tendon depends on precise alignment of collagen type I fibrils to confer longitudinal deformation and a high tensile strength to tendons and also on proteoglycans that regulate collagen fibrillogenesis and thus, indirectly, tendon function [23]. Proteoglycans, such as aggrecan and versican, members of large modular proteoglycans or lecticans, provide tendon tissues with a high capacity to resist high compressive and tensile forces associated with loading and mobilization [23]. As distinct tendons have different functions by responding to different loading stresses, they differ in matrix composition and mechanical properties related to their location in the body. So, it is not surprising that tendons exhibit strain rate values according to the anatomical distribution.

The Achilles tendon is the thickest and the strongest tendon in the human body, as it sustains the body weight and has a major impact on postural orientation. Being approximately 15 cm long, human Achilles experiences higher in vivo stresses than any other tendons, with a failure load of 5098 ± 1199 N and a modulus value of 819–870 MPa [36,37]. In contrast, the dynamic modulus of the supraspinatus was found to be the stiffest (17.3 ± 8.9 MPa) of the rotator cuff tendons followed by the subscapularis (15.2 ± 6.9 MPa) and infraspinatus (12.4 ± 8.2 MPa) [38,39]. These tendons are active participants in shoulder movement and in maintaining the shoulder joint (glenohumeral) stability. Load-bearing tendons, such as the patellar tendon (PT) that connects the patella to the tibia and is involved in the ability of the knee to flex and extend, showed values of 3855 ± 550 N (max. stress 40.6 MPa) [40], and modulus values were found between 300 and 660 MPa [41,42].

Despite the similar location of flexor and extensor tendons of the hand, their specific function influences the pressure that these tendons withstand. Human flexor digitorum profundus presents elastic modulus values of 1000 MPa, while human extensor digitorum longus exhibits 1600 MPa values [42].

Independently of the anatomical location, tendons are mechanoresponsive tissues that require specific stimulation to be healthy and thus maintain their intricate functionality. Among the various types of mechanical stimulation, tensile loading seems to be the most appropriate for subjecting constructs aimed at tendon approaches, as native tendon's primary function is to resist and transmit tension forces caused by muscle contractions.

BIOACTIVE MOLECULES

Unraveling the regulation mechanisms of tendon tissue differentiation remains a critical question required to develop efficient therapies [43]. Some studies propose the use of embryonic signaling factors as cues to promote tendon regeneration [20,44,45]. These environmental biomolecules that are present during embryonic tendon formation will induce a developmental response from progenitor cells, guiding them to regenerate new functional tissue [46].

Although there is limited knowledge on the precise mechanisms of action of signaling molecules, numerous GFs are described to participate in both tendon development and healing. These biomolecules powerfully regulate the cell response; their exogenous addition can further stimulate stem cells into the tenogenic lineage. Among GFs studied, fibroblastic growth factor 4 and TGF-β2 (transforming growth factor beta 2) appear to be important tenogenic factors [44] upregulating tendon progenitor marker Scx expression in tendon mesenchymal progenitor cells. Moreover, TGF-β signaling was reported to be a potent inducer of Scx [33,47,48], and its disruption or receptor inactivation resulted in the loss of most tendons and ligaments in the limbs, trunk, tail, and head [48] of mouse embryos. Interestingly, after short-term exposure to bone morphogenetic proteins (BMP), such as BMP4, BMP2, or BMP7, Scx expression was shown to be downregulated in manipulated limbs [33]. Although TGF-β1 was not detected in tendon on days 13–16, TGF-β2 and -β3 were present in patterns that were dynamic with time and distinct from one another, suggesting independent roles of TGF-β isoforms in tendon development [45]. Not only are the TGF-β isoforms involved in the process of tenogenesis but growth and differentiation factors −5, −6, and −7, were described to induce neotendon/ligament formation when implanted at ectopic sites in a rat model [49], highlighting the critical role of TGF-β superfamily in tendon strategies. Despite the knowledge gathered in the last few years, the use of GFs in clinical tendon repair remains challenging. Little is known about the synergistic and antagonist interactions or the optimal spatial and temporal distribution of GFs that could produce optimal results [50]. Nevertheless, a few clinical studies report the application of cocktails of GFs, mainly in the form of platelet-rich plasma or platelet lysates to stimulate tendon regeneration [51–55].

INTEGRATED APPROACHES TOWARD TENDON REPAIR

TTE strategies often address the challenge to explore stem cell commitment toward the tenogenic lineage, which can be induced through the provision of cellular cues and stimulation. Therefore biological [56–58] and mechanical stimuli [59–61] have been employed for the differentiation of stem cells toward tendon cells. TE protocols are well defined and established for investigating skeletal tissues as bone or cartilage. A very good example is the standardization of differentiation culture media for bone and cartilage, supplemented with regulatory factors that became part of the routine in worldwide cell culture labs. These include TGF-β for chondrogenic differentiation, dexamethasone, ascorbic acid, and B-glycerophosphate for inducing the osteogenic phenotype. However, concerning tendon approaches, this basic information remains elusive. Studies on differentiation cocktails are dispersed, and the outcomes are not requiring additional validation before obtaining the consensus of the scientific community. Moreover, the fact that tendon-specific markers are also not fully established is another critical factor resulting in debatable and apprehensible outcomes. A more detailed description on potential tenogenic differentiation culture media will be discussed in section "Stem Cells and Their Role in Tendon Tissue Engineering". Thus considerable challenges remain to be addressed regarding the innate complexity of natural tendon tissue and the limited research in this area.

The necessary steps in developing functional TE substitutes include cells, which can maintain good proliferation and differentiation toward tenogenic lineage; a scaffold, which can provide a 3-D environment for cell growth; and appropriate mechanical and/or chemical stimulation providing appropriate behavioral instructions for stimulating the new tissue formation. Since the 1990s, a significant expansion and maturation of the TERM field has occurred, translated into promising tissue-engineered and cell-based products. Nevertheless, TERM continues to grow and design innovative multifunctional biomaterials with complex features and controlled biological activity that more closely recapitulate tendon morphogenesis towards functional tendon substitutes. Some strategies focus on developing biomimetic materials to recreate the delicate microenvironment of tendons, in which mechanical properties and efficient gliding are pivotal elements to completely restore the damaged tissue. Other approaches target on engineering smart surfaces to which cells interact to being stimuli-responsive structures with key functionalities to evoke oriented biological responses, enhancing the tissue regeneration capacity. Based on their biomechanical demands, native geometry, and anatomical properties, tendon regenerative investigation may enable the orchestration of coordinated strategies that would nourish tenogenic achievement.

STEM CELLS AND THEIR ROLE IN TENDON TISSUE ENGINEERING

The human body presents a number of endogenous mechanisms for the repair and regeneration of damaged tissues in which stem cells play a major role.

The discovery of tendon stem cells with regenerative capabilities [62] opened new possibilities to treat injured tendon tissues. In an attempt to answer if tendon-derived cells possess multiple differentiation capacities, Yanming Bi and coworkers [62] investigated the commonly used criteria that define stem cells (clonogenicity, multipotency, and self-renewal) in adult tendon cells and pursued to identify critical components of the tendon stem cell niche. Outcomes revealed that the isolated cell populations from both human and mouse tendons possess clonogenicity, self-renewal, and multidifferentiation potentials. Also, tendon stem/progenitor cells (TSPCs) could regenerate tendon-like tissues after extended expansion in vitro and transplantation in vivo, residing in a unique niche predominantly comprised of an ECM being mainly organized by two proteoglycans, biglycan and Fmod. The depletion of these molecules affected the differentiation of TSPCs by modulating BMP signaling and impaired tendon formation in vivo. On completion, an ECM-rich niche may control the self-renewal and differentiation of TSPCs, and its alteration in terms of composition leads to tendon malformation and pathologic ossification [62]. This is in agreement that ECM directly influences the proliferation and differentiation of stem cells, playing an important role in stem cell niche [34].

Although stem/progenitor tendon cells have not been fully explored for TTE applications, their application in regenerative approaches is limited by the associated morbidity of healthy tendon tissue, from where these cells are harvested. Therefore finding the optimal conditions that will induce other sources of stem cells with less detrimental effects in healthy tissues, such as the adipose tissue, into tendon-forming cells is crucial for the development of stem cell-based tendon regeneration. To date, these conditions have not been established, but several studies suggest [63,64] that it may require (1) biochemical signals; (2) mechanical signals; or (3) an adequate combination of both, provided by either the culturing environment and/or scaffold material. Moreover, tendon-associated markers are barely explored and difficult to establish beyond developmental biology. Nevertheless, Scx [33,65,66], tenascin-C [31,66], DCN [31,67], and tenomodulin [66,68–70] are regarded as generally accepted tendon-specific markers.

Moreover, and despite the effort, no differentiation media with specific supplementation toward the tenogenic lineage has been standardized or established, but some attempts are being carried out [56,63]. Combining the exogenous addition of GFs to the cellular microenvironment could provide a trigger to assist the differentiation of multipotent cells into a tenogenic lineage, enhancing the expression of tendon-related markers and the synthesis of tendon-like ECM [63]. Recent advances in basic biology have shown the enormous potential of stem cell technologies for therapeutic approaches in the clinics [71]. The application of stem cells in tendon regenerative strategies is of key importance to restore tissue functionality, as these cells stimulate the repair, maintain homeostasis, and in some cases, reduce the inflammation process. Cell-based therapies have been employed in veterinary medicine specifically by direct cell applications for the treatment of equine tendon injuries [72–74].

TENDON TISSUE ENGINEERING STRATEGIES WITH AND WITHOUT EXOGENOUS SCAFFOLDS

In order to meet the tendon requirements from a cellular, physical, and biomechanical point of view, strategies are being developed where biomimetic concepts are being investigated, as well as the cellular response to environmental cues (Table 15.1).

Being highly organized and mechanically responsive tissues, the envisioned biomimetic systems must induce cellular alignment and orientation and simultaneously respond in a precise manner to defined environment stimuli, considering the anatomical region and type of tendon to regenerate. Hypothesizing that tensile stimulation in combination with a biomimetic alignment would direct human mesenchymal stem cells (hMSCs) differentiation toward a ligament fibroblast-like phenotype, Subramony and coworkers [59] developed an aligned nanofiber matrix seeded with hMSCs and cultured into a custom high-throughput bioreactor, which applied uniaxial tensile strain. The importance of coupled effects was verified, as unaligned constructs cultured with mechanical loading only modulate cell attachment morphology without subsequent induction of cell differentiation.

Also, the structural characteristics of the connective tissue, such as collagen fibril diameter and organization, are crucial design parameters for biomimetic scaffolds intended for tendon or ligament regeneration [75]. A study on cell–material interactions was carried out by Erisken et al. [75], which focused on scaffold fiber diameter effect on the response of human tendon cells. PLGA [poly(lactic-co-glycolic acid)] scaffolds with different fiber diameters were produced by electrospinning and used to test the response of human rotator cuff tendon fibroblasts. Cells were significantly more aligned on scaffolds with larger fibers (1.80 μm) and could more readily spread on nanofiber scaffolds as compared to microfiber ones due to smaller depth of grooves with a higher fiber density. Also, fibroblasts synthesized more collagen and proteoglycans on scaffolds with a smaller fiber diameter (320 nm). They hypothesized that the scaffolds with a smaller fiber diameter resemble a matrix in the state of injury, and the cells, therefore, initiated a healing response by producing more matrix components. While scaffolds with larger fibers likely approximate the fiber diameter of a healthy tendon matrix, the cells would, therefore, minimize excess matrix deposition [75]. Moreover, the largest fiber diameter scaffolds favored the formation of a more tendon-like matrix. Therefore it is probable that the interaction between microfiber scaffolds and fibroblasts more closely resembles native environment, better mimicking the collagen fibers of the native tendon.

In order to achieve a multiscale architecture evolving to meet the biomechanical, biochemical, and topographical requirements, favorable topographical cues with either biochemical cues (eg, GFs) or mechanical forces would reinforce the performance of constructs in successful TTE strategies. The importance of topographical control and incorporation of GFs in biomaterials for stem cell proliferation and differentiation was demonstrated in the work of Cheng and colleagues [76], which focused on the development of poly(lactic-co-glycolic acid)-monomethoxy-poly(ethylene glycol) nanoparticles inserted into aligned collagen fiber scaffolds. This combination promoted the tenogenic differentiation of ADSCs from two different cues, topographical and chemical [76]. Likewise, the development of a mechanovariant platform, which created localized regions of tenogenic cell differentiation mediated through the combination of substrate mechanics and ligand gradients (fibronectin and collagen type I, as ECM representatives), was reported by Sharma et al. [77].

Table 15.1 Summary of In Vitro and In Vivo Studies on TTE Approaches, From 2010

Material / Approach	Cells / Culture Method	Main Outcomes	References
• PLGA-m-PEG NPs • Collagen-NPs composite fibers loaded with PDGF Topographical (aligned collagen fiber) and chemical (PDGF release) cues investigation on tenogenic differentiation of ADSCs.	ADSCs Static In vitro	Controlled and sustained release of PDGF from biocompatible PDGF-containing collagen–NP fibers that enhanced the proliferation and promoted the tenogenic differentiation of ADSCs from two different cues.	[76]
• PHBHHx tubes • PHBHHx fibers • PHBHHx/collagen gel hybrids Collagen gels reinforced by polymer fibers inserted into the lumen of scaffold tubes for implantation to repair an induced Achilles tendon defect.	Rat tenocytes In vivo rat Achilles tendon repair model	PHBHHx in conjunction with collagen and tenocytes showed an accelerated return of function when compared to control, with no prolonged immunological or inflammatory response in the rat model, over 40 days. Cells migrate into the PHBHHx–collagen core and become organized along the fiber surface within the PHBHHx fiber–collagen core in vivo.	[96]
• Collagen ELAC threads, mimicking native tendon, used to study the effect of collagen orientation on cell morphology, proliferation, and tenogenic differentiation.	hMSCs Static culture	The anisotropically oriented dense collagen matrix (substrate densely packed and uniformly aligned) promoted tenogenic differentiation of hMSCs, even in the absence of bioinductive cues.	[66]
• Silk fibroin (SF) Investigation of a synergistic effect of 3-D mechanical conditioning and aligned contact guidance.	MSCs Static and dynamic culture	Hybrid SF scaffold showed favorable topographical and surface chemistry for cellular alignment. High amounts of ligament-related proteins indicated ligament fibroblast differentiation.	[97]
• RGD-coupled alginate Codelivery system based on TGF-β3-loaded RGD-coupled alginate microspheres encapsulating periodontal ligament and gingival stem cells.	Human PDLSCs, GMSCs, and hBMMSCs In vitro and in vivo (subcutaneous transplant into immunocompromised mice)	The MSC and alginate constructs were shown to effectively differentiate and organize their ECM into tendon tissue. Important role of the microenvironment as well as of inductive signals (TGF-β3) for the viability and differentiation of dental MSCs into tendon-like tissue.	[98]
• Poly(L-lactic acid) Aligned braided bundles of electrospun PLLA nanofibers capable of supporting both stem cell expansion and tenogenic differentiation.	hMSCs Cyclic tensile strain	The mechanical properties of braided nanofibrous scaffolds mimicked the triphasic mechanical behavior of native T/L when loaded. Seeded with hMSCs, the scaffolds were able to support cell attachment, proliferation, and tenogenic differentiation when mechanically stimulated in a bioreactor.	[99]

Continued

Table 15.1 Summary of In Vitro and In Vivo Studies on TTE Approaches, From 2010—cont'd

Material / Approach	Cells / Culture Method	Main Outcomes	References
• Poly(lactide-co-glycolide) Investigation on the role of nanofiber matrix alignment and mechanical stimulation on MSC differentiation.	hMSCs Bioreactor (uniaxial tensile strain)	MSCs differentiate into ligament fibroblast-like cells when cultured on aligned nanofibers and subjected to tensile loading. On unaligned nanofibers, mechanical loading only modulates cell attachment morphology without subsequent induction of fibroblastic differentiation.	[59]
• Poly(e-caprolactone) Multilayered electrospun scaffolds coated with tendon-derived ECM, potential for rotator cuff TE.	hASCs Static culture	TDM-coated scaffolds showed increased levels of collagen accumulation by hASCs as compared to FN- or PBS-coated scaffolds. Gene expression of type I collagen, decorin, and tenascin-C increased over time, with no effect of scaffold coating, as well as sulfated glycosaminoglycan and dsDNA.	[100]
• Silk fibers and type I collagen Knitted silk–collagen sponge scaffold–hESC-derived mesenchymal stem cells construct in promoting tendon regeneration.	hESCs-MSCs In vitro dynamic mechanical stress and in vivo mechanical loading	hESCs-MSCs differentiated into the tenogenic lineage, evaluated both in vitro and in a rat Achilles tendon injury model. In ectopic transplantation, the TE tendon under mechanical stimulus displayed more regularly aligned cells and larger collagen fibers. Dynamic mechanical stimulation is beneficial to TE tendons.	[101]
• Poly(ethylene glycol)-based hydrogel material oligo(poly(ethylene glycol) fumarate) OPF hydrogels as hMSC carriers under cyclic tensile strain bioreactor in promoting tendon/ligament fibroblast phenotype.	hMSCs Custom tensile culture bioreactor	Cyclic strain significantly upregulated all tendon/ligament fibroblastic genes examined by day 21, whereas genes for other pathways (osteogenic, chondrogenic, and adipogenic) did not increase. Novel system in examining cellular differentiation under tensile loading in response to controlled physicochemical changes in the extracellular environment.	[102]
• Acrylamide (4–12%) and bisacrylamide (3.8–5%) gels Substrate system with a gradient of stiffness, mechanical compliances, and ligand chemistry, creating local regions of tenogenic differentiation on a single substrate.	hBMSCs Static culture	Increased osteogenic fate was observed on FN substrates and tenogenic differentiation observed on collagen substrates, and these responses further depended on the stiffness of the substrate. Mechanovariant substrates offer a platform to engineer cell differentiation into targeted lineages without the necessary use of exogenous biochemical stimulation apart from cell culture growth medium.	[77]

PLGA-m-PEG, *Poly(lactic-co-glycolic acid)-monomethoxy-poly(ethylene glycol);* NPs, *nanoparticles;* PDGF, *platelet-derived growth factor;* ADSCs, *adipose-derived stem cells;* PHBHHx, *poly(3-hydroxybutyrate-co-3-hydroxyhexanoate);* hMSCs, *human mesenchymal stem cells;* ELAC, *electrochemically aligned collagen;* RGD, *arginine–glycine–aspartic acid tripeptide;* PDLSCs, *periodontal ligament stem cells;* GMSCs, *gingival mesenchymal stem cells;* hBMMSCs, *human bone marrow mesenchymal stem cells;* ECM, *extracellular matrix;* TGF-*β*, *transforming growth factor-beta;* hMSCs, *human mesenchymal stem cells;* PLLA, *poly(L-lactic acid);* T/L, *tendon and ligament;* hASCs, *human adipose stem cells;* TDM, *tendon-derived matrix;* FN, *fibronectin;* PBS, *phosphate-buffered saline;* dsDNA, *double-stranded DNA;* TE, *tissue-engineered;* hESCs, *human embryonic stem cells;* OPF, *oligo(poly(ethylene glycol) fumarate);* hBMSCs, *human bone marrow stromal cells.*

Although scaffold mechanics and ECM cues are important factors to be considered when designing a biomimetic system, alternative scaffold-free approaches have been also investigated. A bioengineered strategy using sheets of hMSCs to revitalize cryopreserved tendon grafts was studied by Ouyang and colleagues [78]. The hMSC sheets were well incorporated within the peritenon, around the tendon, and adopted the characteristic spindle-shaped morphology of tenocyte-like cells. Another study reported neotendon formation in a nude mouse model using an engineered tendon composed of tendon-derived stem cells and connective tissue growth factor without exogenous scaffolds [79]. Cell sheet approaches also resulted in the development of functional periosteal progenitor cell (PPC) sheets using polymerized fibrin-coated dishes for osteo–tendon interface [80]. The bioengineered PPC sheets were evaluated in an extra-articular bone tunnel model in rabbit, aiming at enhancing tendon–bone healing. The results demonstrated improvement of healing by applying the PPC sheet at the tendon–bone interface. An increased amount of glycosaminoglycans and perpendicular collagen fibers at the insertion was also observed, as well as fibrocartilage tissue that was formed by PPC sheets between the tendon and bone 4 weeks postimplantation. After 8 weeks, the PPC sheet treatment revealed fibrocartilage and new bone regeneration. The PPC sheet showed to possess a powerful inductive ability between tendon and bone to incorporate healing, as the PPC monolayer maintains the differentiated capacity and the osteochondral potential in order to promote fibrocartilage formation [80]. Also, these studies evidenced that cell sheets may be an interesting alternative approach for engineering tendon and tendon interfaces.

MECHANOTRANSDUCTION AND MECHANICAL STIMULI IN TENDON TISSUE ENGINEERING

It is known that loading modulates ECM synthesis and tissue remodeling through mechanotransduction mechanisms, promoting biochemical signals responsible for cell proliferation, differentiation, and ECM synthesis [13]. In recent years, mechanical cues are being successfully employed to promote stem cell differentiation and functional tissue formation in musculoskeletal-engineered strategies. The ability of cells to sense and respond to their mechanical environment is critical for cell and tissue rearrangement. As neotissue forms in TE constructs, mechanical loading modulates ECM synthesis and remodeling through mechanotransduction. Mechanotransduction defines cellular mechanisms that convert mechanical stimuli into biochemical signals responsible for cell proliferation, differentiation, and ECM synthesis [13]. Mechanical stimuli in the extracellular environment activate mechanosensitive receptors and sensors at the surface of the cells, namely ion channels, caveolae, integrins, cadherins, growth factor receptors, and others that have a contribution in the mechanotransduction response by triggering intracellular signaling mechanisms (Fig. 15.1). The major cell–cell and cell–ECM sites of mechanotransduction may be integrin-dependent. Integrins are adhesion receptor proteins and transmembrane components involved in cell sensing and response to external forces of their surroundings, therefore establishing the connection and communication between the extracellular environment to the intracellular cytoskeleton (Fig. 15.1). The activation of signaling events results in cytoskeletal reorganization, cell shape, mechanotransduction, and ultimately tenogenic differentiation. In this sense, tenogenic differentiation might be achieved by activating the mitogen-activated protein kinase (MAPK) signaling pathway [81]. Moreover, a recent study by Havis and coworkers demonstrated that TGF-β and MAPK are two important signaling pathways involved in tendon gene expression in late limb explants during tendon differentiation [82]. Also, RhoA/ROCK (small G-protein) and focal adhesion kinase are signaling events that sense mechanical stretching and drive tenogenic differentiation [61].

Since tendon cells use force as a mechanical signal to sense and respond to the surrounding microenvironment, the application of mechanical stimuli becomes imperative in TTE approaches. In a recent study, Yuan Xu and coworkers [31] assessed the efficacy of tendon-derived stem cells (TDSCs) in a poly(L-lactide-co-ε-caprolactone)/collagen scaffold under mechanical stimulation both in vitro and in vivo and evaluated the efficacy of the transplanted construct to promote rabbit PT defect regeneration. TDSCs upregulated the expression of tenogenic differentiation-related mRNA while downregulating the expression of osteogenic and chondrogenic differentiation-related mRNA under a mechanical traction stimulation system.

As tensile strain is one of the major mechanical stimulus that tendons are subjected to, an investigation performed by Bayer and colleagues [83] proposed to observe the response of human tendon cells to release of tension. The loss of tension leads to a decrease in phenotypical markers for tendon; normal tendon architecture was disturbed, and expression of proinflammatory mediators was induced.

In addition, the mechanical parameters must also be considered when designing a material support for cells. An in situ cell–matrix strains study was carried out by Duncan and colleagues [84] in which they applied tension in tendon fascicles and contrasted with cell–collagen gel constructs. This work suggests that the collagen type I gel strings did not replicate the nonuniform strain pattern of native tendon fascicles. Houssen et al. [85] continuously monitor tendon microstructure during multiple loading cycles, stating that mechanical preconditioning mostly arises from sliding and is reversible on long timescales, thus supporting the notion that the mechanical behavior of a tendon fascicle relies on its microstructure remodeling. Loading was also verified to act on tendon gene expression. Legerlotz et al. [86] showed significantly higher expression of collagen, type I, alpha 1, and interleukin 6 in fatigue-loaded specimens of isolated tendon fascicles compared with controls.

In summary, all studies using stimulation highlight the requirement for mechanical loading of tendon substitutes in order to maintain normal tendon structure and biochemical phenotype.

MECHANICAL STIMULATION USING MAGNETIC FORCE FIELDS

Recently, a growing interest in another distinct field is emerging, resulting from the combination of nanotechnology and MNPs in TE strategies.

MNPs biomedical applications include (1) imaging contrast agents for MRI; (2) localization of therapy/targeted drug release; and more recently, (3) utilization of nanoparticles for cell labeling/internalization and the development of micro–nano engineered scaffolds.

Furthermore, the idea of using magnetic fields to remotely control magnetic responsive systems has recently been examined in the general TE field with likewise high potential for tendon approaches, including (1) 3-D magnetic scaffolds, which can provide unique capabilities not available with other methods and materials [87]; (2) magnetic hydrogels with a magnetic component embedded in the matrix [88]; and (3) assembling of magnetically labeled cells into larger tissue prototypes through magnetic force appliance.

An example of an in vitro loading system using an applied magnetic field to produce time-varying loading in rat-tail tendon fascicles was investigated by Adekanmbi et al. [89]. The effect of high frequency low magnitude (HFLM) loads on tendon mechanobiology was studied [89]. HFLM in vitro loading was found to maintain the elastic moduli of cultured tendon fascicles after 7 days, while the moduli of unloaded tendons decreased twofold. HFLM-loaded tendon fascicles showed higher tensile strength than unloaded and fresh fascicles, and differences between groups were not statistically significant. Further, although HFLM-loaded tendons displayed higher modulus and tensile strength than fresh controls, static loaded tendons did not, suggesting that HFLM loading provides greater stimulation.

Furthermore, the incorporation of MNPs within 3-D scaffolds or hydrogels may constitute an attractive approach to achieve magnetically responsive systems, enabling remote control over TE constructs in vitro and in vivo [90]. The functionalization of inert scaffolds with MNPs influences the creation of magnetic forces capable of attracting and retaining cells within the material through a rather simplistic, fast, and cost-effective approach [90].

In a previous work, we developed magnetic polymer scaffolds with aligned architecture aimed at applications in TTE (Fig. 15.2). Aligned fibrous scaffolds were obtained from a biodegradable blend of 30% starch and 70% polycaprolactone (starch and polycaprolactone, SPCL) by rapid prototyping through the incorporation of iron oxide particles in SPCL matrix in a 0.018:1 weight ratio. Tenascin-C protein was detected by immunolocation assays in scaffolds seeded with human adipose stem cells (hASCs) for 7 days and exposed to a magnetic field, as shown in Fig. 15.2. Main results suggest that the effect of the magnetic-aligned scaffolds structure combined with magnetic stimulation influences stem cell behavior toward the tenogenic phenotype and consequently with potential to impact the field of TTE.

The magnetic force can also contribute for a uniform distribution of the cells within the 3-D template [90]. Various methods have been developed to fabricate magnetic hydrogels, including a blending method, an in situ precipitation method, and the grafting-onto method [88]. Also, MNPs can be associated with stem cells, presenting an advantage as cells naturally respond to magnetic forces, and consequently, the application of a magnetic field may enhance cell biological performance and ultimately stimulate cell proliferation, migration, and differentiation. Moreover, MNPs have been used for controlled cell assembly through magnetic force appliance in order to achieve 3-D multilayer constructs [91].

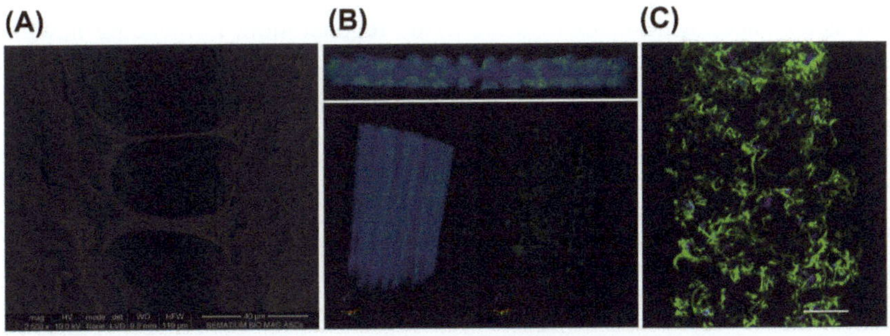

FIGURE 15.2 Magnetic polymer scaffolds developed by rapid prototyping technology.

(A) Scanning electron microscope micrograph of an aligned magnetic scaffold cultured with hASCs in basal medium for 7 days under magnetic stimulation. (B) 3-D representation of the developed magnetic scaffolds by micro-CT analysis. The polymeric matrix is represented in *blue* (SPCL), and MNPs are observed in gray. (C) Tenascin-C immunolocation in hASCs: mag-SPCL constructs after 1 week under magnetic stimulation. DAPI (4,6-Diamidino-2-phenylindole, dilactate; *blue*) stains cell nuclei and tenascin-C (*green*) is a typical protein present in tendon ECM. Scale bar represents 100 μm.

In fact, magnetic responsive materials have already been investigated for in vitro and in vivo bone TE applications [92–94]. Another novel technique that makes use of magnetic force and functionalized MNPs is the magnetic forced-based TE methodology proposed by Ito et al. [95] for production of magnetic cell sheets. Herein, cells are labeled with ferrous-based nanoparticles being then manipulated using magnets. Up to date, no adequate system proposed to study the application of simultaneous topographical and magnetic stimuli on stem cells' behavior toward the tenogenic phenotype, but all these magnetically based approaches can also be envisioned to engineer tendon substitutes.

CONCLUSIONS AND FUTURE PERSPECTIVES

Efforts to differentiate stem cells toward the highly specialized tendon cells have been challenged by paucity of tenogenic cues as well as a lack of benchmarks to assess tenogenic lineage commitment. Future directions on TTE should conceive highly efficient and multifunctional tendon constructs fulfilling the currently unmet requirements for tendon regeneration.

An envisioned functionalized cell scaffold construct would be stimuli-responsive where incorporated cells could be governed by their ability to respond to scaffold surface, sensing and responding to their surroundings, and guided into the tenogenic phenotype. Also, not less important is the function and characteristics of the ECM in cueing stem cell behavior. Beyond that, as load-bearing tissues, mechanosignaling is a critical component in new tissue formation and ECM organization of engineered tissue substitutes, underlying the importance of bioreactors in TTE strategies. Despite the many described methodologies to fabricate tendon-oriented scaffolds, a functional and translational TE construct is not available yet. Thus novel approaches are required to fill the gap in tendon tissue replacement.

The ability to tailor the microenvironment at a nano- and microscale, thus spatially controlling the localization of cells and other biological factors, would assist the development of tailored structures with precise architectures. The utilization of MNPs and application of magnetic stimulation are currently regarded as advanced techniques to drive tissue regeneration, influencing new biological and engineering solutions. Thus these magnetic strategies envision greater mechanical stimulation of the seeded cells, improved cell seeding, and the means of assembling a scaffold in the desired configuration.

LIST OF ACRONYMS AND ABBREVIATIONS

ADSCs Adipose-derived stem cells
Bgn Biglycan
bHLH Basic helix–loop–helix
BMP Bone morphogenetic protein
COL1A1 Collagen, type I, alpha 1
COMP Collagen oligomeric matrix protein
DCN Decorin
ECM Extracellular matrix
FAK Focal adhesion kinase

FDA Food and Drug Administration
FGF Fibroblastic growth factor
Fmod Fibromodulin
GDFs Growth and differentiation factors
GFs Growth factors
HFLM High frequency low magnitude
IL6 Interleukin 6
MAPK Mitogen-activated protein kinase
MNPs Magnetic nanoparticles
MPa Megapascal
MRI Magnetic resonance imaging
mRNA Messenger RNA
MSCs Mesenchymal stem cells
N Newton
P(LLA-CL)/Col Poly(L-lactide-co-ε-caprolactone)/collagen
PDGF Platelet-derived growth factor
PLA Poly(L-lactide-co-D,L-lactide)
PLGA Poly(lactic-co-glycolic acid)
PLGA-m-PEG Poly(lactic-co-glycolic acid)-monomethoxy-poly(ethylene glycol)
PPC Periosteal progenitor cell
PT Patellar tendon
RhoA/ROCK Ras homolog family member A/Rho kinase
Scx Scleraxis
SIS Small intestine submucosa
SPCL Starch and polycaprolactone
TDCs Tendon-derived cells
TDSCs Tendon-derived stem cells
TE Tissue engineering
TERM Tissue engineering and regenerative medicine
TGFβ Transforming growth factor beta
TSPCs Tendon stem/progenitor cells
TTE Tendon tissue engineering

REFERENCES

[1] Shearn JT, et al. Tendon tissue engineering: progress, challenges, and translation to the clinic. J Musculoskelet Neuronal Interact 2011;11(2):163–73.
[2] Liu CF, et al. What we should know before using tissue engineering techniques to repair injured tendons: a developmental biology perspective. Tissue Eng Part B Rev 2011;17(3):165–76.
[3] Rodrigues MT, et al. Engineering tendon and ligament tissues: present developments towards successful clinical products. J Tissue Eng Regen Med 2013;7(9):673–86.
[4] Walton JR, et al. Restore orthobiologic implant: not recommended for augmentation of rotator cuff repairs. J Bone Jt Surg 2007;89(4):786–91.
[5] Metcalf MH, et al. Surgical technique for xenograft (SIS) augmentation of rotator-cuff repairs. Op Tech Orthop 2002;12(3):204–8.
[6] Song L, et al. Biomechanical evaluation of a cellular collagen matrix augmented Achilles tendon repair in sheep. J Foot Ankle Surg 2010;49(5):438–41.

[7] Johnson S, et al. Twenty-four month ultrasonographic and clinical follow-up of graft Jacket augmented rotator cuff repair: is it effective? Bone Jt J Orthop Proc Suppl 2014;96(Suppl. 14):2.
[8] Smith R, et al. 95 An in vitro comparative analysis of scaffolds for the augmentation of rotator cuff repair. Br J Sports Med 2014;48(Suppl. 2):A62-A.
[9] Barber FA, et al. A biomechanical study of Achilles tendon repair augmentation using GraftJacket matrix. Foot Ankle Int 2008;29(3):329–33.
[10] Barber FA, et al. Biomechanical testing of commercially available soft-tissue augmentation materials. Arthrosc J Arthrosc Relat Surg 2009;25(11):1233–9.
[11] Shea KP, et al. Human tendon cell response to 7 commercially available extracellular matrix materials: an in vitro study. Arthrosc J Arthrosc Relat Surg 2010;26(9):1181–8.
[12] Chen J, et al. Scaffolds for tendon and ligament repair: review of the efficacy of commercial products. Expert Rev Med Devices 2009;6(1):61–73.
[13] Benhardt HA, et al. The role of mechanical loading in ligament tissue engineering. Tissue Eng Part B Rev 2009;15(4):467–75.
[14] Yun YR, et al. Fibroblast growth factors: biology, function, and application for tissue regeneration. J Tissue Eng 2010;2010:218142.
[15] Guilak F, et al. Control of stem cell fate by physical interactions with the extracellular matrix. Cell Stem Cell 2009;5(1):17–26.
[16] Wimpenny I, et al. Orthopaedic applications of nanoparticle-based stem cell therapies. Stem Cell Res Ther 2012;3.
[17] Zeugolis DI, et al. Tendons: engineering of functional tissues. In: Pallua N, Suscheck CV, editors. Tissue engineering. Berlin Heidelberg: Springer; 2011. p. 537–72.
[18] Sharma P, et al. Basic biology of tendon injury and healing. The Surgeon J R Coll Surg Edinb Irel 2005;3(5):309–16.
[19] Maffulli N. Tendon injuries. Springer; 2005.
[20] Marturano JE, et al. Characterization of mechanical and biochemical properties of developing embryonic tendon. Proc Natl Acad Sci USA 2013;110(16):6370–5.
[21] Kjaer M. Role of extracellular matrix in adaptation of tendon and skeletal muscle to mechanical loading. Physiol Rev 2004;84(2):649–98.
[22] Zhang G, et al. Decorin regulates assembly of collagen fibrils and acquisition of biomechanical properties during tendon development. J Cell Biochem 2006;98(6):1436–49.
[23] Yoon JH, et al. Tendon proteoglycans: biochemistry and function. J Musculoskelet Neuronal Interact 2005;5(1):22–34.
[24] Sodersten F, et al. Immunolocalization of collagens (I and III) and cartilage oligomeric matrix protein in the normal and injured equine superficial digital flexor tendon. Connect Tissue Res 2013;54(1):62–9.
[25] DiCesare P, et al. Cartilage oligomeric matrix protein (COMP) is an abundant component of tendon. FEBS Lett 1994;354(2):237–40.
[26] Smith R, et al. The distribution of cartilage oligomeric matrix protein (COMP) in tendon and its variation with tendon site, age and load. Matrix Biol 1997;16(5):255–71.
[27] Kohrs RT, et al. Tendon fascicle gliding in wild type, heterozygous, and lubricin knockout mice. J Orthop Res 2011;29(3):384–9.
[28] Hayashi M, et al. The effect of lubricin on the gliding resistance of mouse intrasynovial tendon. PLoS One 2013;8(12):e83836.
[29] Tucker RP, et al. The regulation of tenascin expression by tissue microenvironments. Biochim Biophys Acta 2009;1793(5):888–92.
[30] Chiquet M, et al. How do fibroblasts translate mechanical signals into changes in extracellular matrix production? Matrix Biol 2003;22(1):73–80.
[31] Xu Y, et al. The effect of mechanical stimulation on the maturation of TDSCs-poly(L-lactide-co-e-caprolactone)/collagen scaffold constructs for tendon tissue engineering. Biomaterials 2014;35(9):2760–72.

[32] Subramony SD, et al. Combined effects of chemical priming and mechanical stimulation on mesenchymal stem cell differentiation on nanofiber scaffolds. J Biomech 2014;47(9):2189–96.
[33] Schweitzer R, et al. Analysis of the tendon cell fate using Scleraxis, a specific marker for tendons and ligaments. Development 2001;128(19):3855–66.
[34] Gattazzo F, et al. Extracellular matrix: a dynamic microenvironment for stem cell niche. Biochim Biophys Acta 2014;1840(8):2506–19.
[35] Wang JH, et al. Tendon biomechanics and mechanobiology–a minireview of basic concepts and recent advancements. J Hand Ther 2012;25(2):133–40. quiz 141.
[36] Wren TA, et al. Mechanical properties of the human achilles tendon. Clin Biomech 2001;16(3):245–51.
[37] Lichtwark GA, et al. In vivo mechanical properties of the human Achilles tendon during one-legged hopping. J Exp Biol 2005;208(Pt 24):4715–25.
[38] Nightingale EJ, et al. Mechanical properties of the rotator cuff: response to cyclic loading at varying abduction angles. Knee Surg Sports Traumatol Arthrosc 2003;11(6):389–92.
[39] Silldorff MD, et al. Effect of supraspinatus tendon injury on supraspinatus and infraspinatus muscle passive tension and associated biochemistry. J Bone Jt Surg 2014;96(20):e175.
[40] Handl M, et al. Reconstruction of the anterior cruciate ligament: dynamic strain evaluation of the graft. Knee Surg Sports Traumatol Arthrosc 2007;15(3):233–41.
[41] Johnson GA, et al. Tensile and viscoelastic properties of human patellar tendon. J Orthop Res 1994;12(6):796–803.
[42] Wong JY, et al. Balance of chemistry, topography, and mechanics at the cell–biomaterial interface: issues and challenges for assessing the role of substrate mechanics on cell response. Surf Sci 2004;570(1):119–33.
[43] Lorda-Diez CI, et al. Divergent differentiation of skeletal progenitors into cartilage and tendon: lessons from the embryonic limb. ACS Chem Biol 2014;9(1):72–9.
[44] Brown JP, et al. Embryonic mechanical and soluble cues regulate tendon progenitor cell gene expression as a function of developmental stage and anatomical origin. J Biomech 2014;47(1):214–22.
[45] Kuo CK, et al. Spatiotemporal protein distribution of TGF-betas, their receptors, and extracellular matrix molecules during embryonic tendon development. Dev Dyn 2008;237(5):1477–89.
[46] Glass ZA, et al. Informing tendon tissue engineering with embryonic development. J Biomech 2014;47(9):1964–8.
[47] Lorda-Diez CI, et al. Transforming growth factors beta coordinate cartilage and tendon differentiation in the developing limb mesenchyme. J Biol Chem 2009;284(43):29988–96.
[48] Pryce BA, et al. Recruitment and maintenance of tendon progenitors by TGFbeta signaling are essential for tendon formation. Development 2009;136(8):1351–61.
[49] Wolfman NM, et al. Ectopic induction of tendon and ligament in rats by growth and differentiation factors 5, 6, and 7, members of the TGF-beta gene family. J Clin Invest 1997;100(2):321–30.
[50] Yang G, et al. Tendon and ligament regeneration and repair: clinical relevance and developmental paradigm. Birth Defects Res Part C Embryo Today Rev 2013;99(3):203–22.
[51] Creaney L, et al. Growth factor-based therapies provide additional benefit beyond physical therapy in resistant elbow tendinopathy: a prospective, single-blind, randomised trial of autologous blood injections versus platelet-rich plasma injections. Br J Sports Med 2011;45(12):966–71. p. bjsports82503.
[52] de Jonge S, et al. One-year follow-up of platelet-rich plasma treatment in chronic achilles tendinopathy a double-blind randomized Placebo-controlled trial. Am J Sports Med 2011;39(8):1623–9.
[53] De Vos R, et al. Autologous growth factor injections in chronic tendinopathy: a systematic review. Br Med Bull 2010;95:63–77. p. ldq006.
[54] Kon E, et al. Platelet-rich plasma (PRP) to treat sports injuries: evidence to support its use. Knee Surg Sports Traumatol Arthrosc 2011;19(4):516–27.
[55] Ruiz-Moneo P, et al. Plasma rich in growth factors in arthroscopic rotator cuff repair: a randomized, double-blind, controlled clinical trial. Arthrosc J Arthrosc Relat Surg 2013;29(1):2–9.

[56] Tan S, et al. The effect of growth differentiation Factor-5 (GDF-5) on the proliferation and tenogenic differentiation potential of human mesenchymal stem cells in vitro. J Health Transl Med 2013:45.
[57] Manning CN, et al. Controlled delivery of mesenchymal stem cells and growth factors using nanofiber scaffold for tendon repair. Acta Biomater 2013;9:6905–14.
[58] Lee JY, et al. BMP-12 treatment of adult mesenchymal stem cells in vitro augments tendon-like tissue formation and defect repair in vivo. PLoS One 2011;6(3):e17531.
[59] Subramony SD, et al. The guidance of stem cell differentiation by substrate alignment and mechanical stimulation. Biomaterials 2013;34(8):1942–53.
[60] Yang G, et al. Enhancement of tenogenic differentiation of human adipose stem cells by tendon-derived extracellular matrix. Biomaterials 2013;34:9295–306.
[61] Xu B, et al. RhoA/ROCK, cytoskeletal dynamics, and focal adhesion kinase are required for mechanical stretch-induced tenogenic differentiation of human mesenchymal stem cells. J Cell Physiol 2012;227(6):2722–9.
[62] Bi Y, et al. Identification of tendon stem/progenitor cells and the role of the extracellular matrix in their niche. Nat Med 2007;13(10):1219–27.
[63] Goncalves AI, et al. Understanding the role of growth factors in modulating stem cell tenogenesis. PLoS One 2013;8(12):e83734.
[64] Qiu Y, et al. Development of a refined tenocyte differentiation culture technique for tendon tissue engineering. Cells Tissues Organs 2013;197(1):27–36.
[65] Dyment NA, et al. The paratenon contributes to scleraxis-expressing cells during patellar tendon healing. PLoS One 2013;8(3):e59944.
[66] Kishore V, et al. Tenogenic differentiation of human MSCs induced by the topography of electrochemically aligned collagen threads. Biomaterials 2012;33(7):2137–44.
[67] Lorda-Diez CI, et al. *Decorin* gene expression in the differentiation of the skeletal connective tissues of the developing limb. Gene Expr Patterns 2014;15(1):52–60.
[68] Shukunami C, et al. Scleraxis positively regulates the expression of tenomodulin, a differentiation marker of tenocytes. Dev Biol 2006;298(1):234–47.
[69] Jelinsky SA, et al. Tendon-selective genes identified from rat and human musculoskeletal tissues. J Orthop Res 2010;28(3):289–97.
[70] Docheva D, et al. Tenomodulin is necessary for tenocyte proliferation and tendon maturation. Mol Cell Biol 2005;25(2):699–705.
[71] Centeno CJ. Clinical challenges and opportunities of mesenchymal stem cells in musculoskeletal medicine. PM R 2014;6(1):70–7.
[72] Godwin EE, et al. Implantation of bone marrow-derived mesenchymal stem cells demonstrates improved outcome in horses with overstrain injury of the superficial digital flexor tendon. Equine Veterinary J 2012;44(1):25–32.
[73] Renzi S, et al. Autologous bone marrow mesenchymal stromal cells for regeneration of injured equine ligaments and tendons: a clinical report. Res Veterinary Sci 2013;95:272–7.
[74] de Mattos Carvalho A, et al. Use of adipose tissue-derived mesenchymal stem cells for experimental tendinitis therapy in equines. J Equine Veterinary Sci 2011;31(1):26–34.
[75] Erisken C, et al. Scaffold fiber diameter regulates human tendon fibroblast growth and differentiation. Tissue Eng Part A 2013;19(3–4):519–28.
[76] Cheng X, et al. Platelet-derived growth-factor-releasing aligned collagen-nanoparticle fibers promote the proliferation and tenogenic differentiation of adipose-derived stem cells. Acta Biomater 2014;10(3):1360–9.
[77] Sharma RI, et al. Biochemical and biomechanical gradients for directed bone marrow stromal cell differentiation toward tendon and bone. Biomaterials 2010;31(30):7695–704.
[78] Ouyang HW, et al. Mesenchymal stem cell sheets revitalize nonviable dense grafts: implications for repair of large-bone and tendon defects. Transplantation 2006;82(2):170–4.

[79] Ni M, et al. Engineered scaffold-free tendon tissue produced by tendon-derived stem cells. Biomaterials 2013;34(8):2024–37.
[80] Chang CH, et al. Bioengineered periosteal progenitor cell sheets to enhance tendon-bone healing in a bone tunnel. Biomed J 2012;35(6):473–80.
[81] Cai T-Y, et al. Fibroblast growth factor 2 induces mesenchymal stem cells to differentiate into tenocytes through the MAPK pathway. Mol Med Rep 2013;8(5):1323–8.
[82] Havis E, et al. Transcriptomic analysis of mouse limb tendon cells during development. Development 2014;141(19):3683–96.
[83] Bayer ML, et al. Release of tensile strain on engineered human tendon tissue disturbs cell adhesions, changes matrix architecture, and induces an inflammatory phenotype. PLoS One 2014;9(1):e86078.
[84] Duncan NA, et al. In situ cell-matrix mechanics in tendon fascicles and seeded collagen gels: implications for the multiscale design of biomaterials. Comput Methods Biomech Biomed Eng 2014;17(1):39–47.
[85] Houssen YG, et al. Monitoring micrometer-scale collagen organization in rat-tail tendon upon mechanical strain using second harmonic microscopy. J Biomech 2011;44(11):2047–52.
[86] Legerlotz K, et al. Cyclic loading of tendon fascicles using a novel fatigue loading system increases interleukin-6 expression by tenocytes. Scand J Med Sci Sports 2013;23(1):31–7.
[87] Sensenig R, et al. Magnetic nanoparticle-based approaches to locally target therapy and enhance tissue regeneration in vivo. Nanomedicine 2012;7(9):1425–42.
[88] Li Y, et al. Magnetic hydrogels and their potential biomedical applications. Adv Funct Mater 2013;23(6):660–72.
[89] Adekanmbi I, et al. A novel in vitro loading system for high frequency loading of cultured tendon fascicles. Med Eng Phys 2013;35(2):205–10.
[90] Santo VE, et al. Contributions and future perspectives on the use of magnetic nanoparticles as diagnostic and therapeutic tools in the field of regenerative medicine. Expert Rev Mol Diagn 2013;13(6):553–66.
[91] Lee EA, et al. Application of magnetic nanoparticle for controlled tissue assembly and tissue engineering. Archiv Pharmacal Res 2014;37(1):120–8.
[92] Meng J, et al. Super-paramagnetic responsive nanofibrous scaffolds under static magnetic field enhance osteogenesis for bone repair in vivo. Sci Rep 2013;3.
[93] Zeng XB, et al. Magnetic responsive hydroxyapatite composite scaffolds construction for bone defect reparation. Int J Nanomed 2012;7:3365–78.
[94] Panseri S, et al. Magnetic hydroxyapatite bone substitutes to enhance tissue regeneration: evaluation in vitro using osteoblast-like cells and in vivo in a bone defect. PLoS One 2012;7(6).
[95] Ito A, et al. Construction and harvest of multilayered keratinocyte sheets using magnetite nanoparticles and magnetic force. Tissue Eng 2004;10(5–6):873–80.
[96] Webb WR, et al. The application of poly(3-hydroxybutyrate-co-3-hydroxyhexanoate) scaffolds for tendon repair in the rat model. Biomaterials 2013;34(28):6683–94.
[97] Teh TKH, et al. Aligned hybrid silk scaffold for enhanced differentiation of mesenchymal stem cells into ligament fibroblasts. Tissue Eng – Part C Methods 2011;17(6):687–703.
[98] Moshaverinia A, et al. Application of stem cells derived from the periodontal ligament or gingival tissue sources for tendon tissue regeneration. Biomaterials 2014;35(9):2642–50.
[99] Barber JG, et al. Braided nanofibrous scaffold for tendon and ligament tissue engineering. Tissue Eng Part A 2013;19(11–12):1265–74.
[100] Chainani A, et al. Multilayered electrospun scaffolds for tendon tissue engineering. Tissue Eng Part A 2013;19(23–24):2594–604.
[101] Chen JL, et al. Efficacy of hESC-MSCs in knitted silk-collagen scaffold for tendon tissue engineering and their roles. Biomaterials 2010;31(36):9438–51.
[102] Doroski DM, et al. Cyclic tensile culture promotes fibroblastic differentiation of marrow stromal cells encapsulated in poly(ethylene glycol)-based hydrogels. Tissue Eng Part A 2010;16(11):3457–66.

CHAPTER

IN SITU VOLUMETRIC MUSCLE REPAIR

16

L.E. Shapiro, J.H. Kim, S.J. Lee, J.J. Yoo, A. Atala, I.K. Ko
Wake Forest School of Medicine, Winston-Salem, NC, United States

CHAPTER OUTLINE

INTRODUCTION

Skeletal muscle tissue constitutes 45% of the total body weight and functions in the body to provide movement, stability, heat production, glycemic control, as well as expansion and contraction of orifices [1]. It is a metabolically active tissue that requires an abundance of nutrients and metabolites, which are provided by an extensive capillary network forming an organized branching pattern throughout the fibers [2]. Groups of functionally related muscles or muscle compartments are located in the pelvic floor, abdominal wall, thoracic wall, and limbs. Whereas mild injury and stress on the skeletal muscle can be healed by a robust and natural regeneration process, extensive muscle damage due to trauma or tumor ablation requires reconstructive procedures to restore normal muscle function [3]. Severe muscle injury that is associated with irrecoverable loss of muscle function is referred to as volumetric muscle loss (VML) [4].

In Situ Tissue Regeneration. http://dx.doi.org/10.1016/B978-0-12-802225-2.00016-7

VML can be defined as loss of muscle functionality due to external trauma or surgical insult as a result of treatment [5]. VML is clinically challenging, not only for military medicine, but also for civilian medicine. It is often seen with penetrating trauma (ie, bullets, explosions) and high-energy motor vehicle accidents; furthermore, it is commonly a result of surgical treatment for extremity compartment syndrome, where debridement and excision of dead tissue may be necessary [6]. In many cases, more than 20% of muscle loss is critically challenging [3] for functional muscle restoration since the damaged muscle tissue is incapable of being regenerated by natural healing capacity and fails to repair the defect. The outcome is muscle atrophy, scar formation, and denervation of the entire muscle tissue. While the current standard of care for such severe muscle defects involves autologous muscle flaps and physical therapy, there remains significant donor site morbidity associated with this surgical procedure due to the limited tissue available for large muscle defects [7]. Recent advances in skeletal muscle tissue engineering present promising new approaches to address the current limitations involved with structural and functional recovery of volumetric muscle injury. Engineering of functional muscle tissue constructs in vitro with cultured muscle cells seeded on scaffolds followed by implantation in vivo may provide a solution to this unmet medical need. Rapid progress has been made in the development of engineered skeletal muscle using biodegradable synthetic polymers and gel-based matrices; however, donor tissue biopsy and ex vivo cell manipulation are required prior to implantation for this therapy to be successful. In addition, a reduction in cell viability within the scaffolding system after implantation is a critical limiting factor for cell-based tissue constructs [8]; thus the development of new strategies will be necessary to eliminate cell manipulation prior to implantation.

In situ tissue regeneration has risen to the forefront of tissue engineering to address the limitation of cell-based strategies [9–12]. Since in situ regeneration often relies on the body's ability to repair itself, efficient infiltration of host cells into the muscle-specific scaffolding system is a critical factor for functional muscle restoration. Therefore an ideal strategy is to enrich the infiltrates with host stem/progenitor cells. Furthermore, providing a microenvironment for in situ functional muscle regeneration would allow for the ability to control the fate of the host cell populations. Such an approach includes development of a muscle target-specific scaffolding system and identification of biochemical cues for accelerating regeneration. This chapter describes basic components of in situ muscle regeneration such as endogenous cells, scaffolding systems, and bioactive factors as well as a summary of current preclinical and clinical approaches and therapies for treatment of VML of various types of muscle tissues.

BASIC COMPONENTS FOR IN SITU MUSCLE REGENERATION

The basic concept of muscle regeneration in situ involves harnessing the native regenerative capacity of the host by recruiting stem or progenitor cells to the injury site. Unlike minimal muscle injury, the muscle regeneration from VML requires a template that occupies the defected void and provides an appropriate microenvironment for the recruited cells to facilitate such cellular behaviors as growth and differentiation. In addition, acceleration of muscle regeneration, which requires activating infiltration and growth of endogenous cells, will prevent further complications (Fig. 16.1A). Exogenously administered bioactive cues may be used to achieve implementation of muscle regeneration.

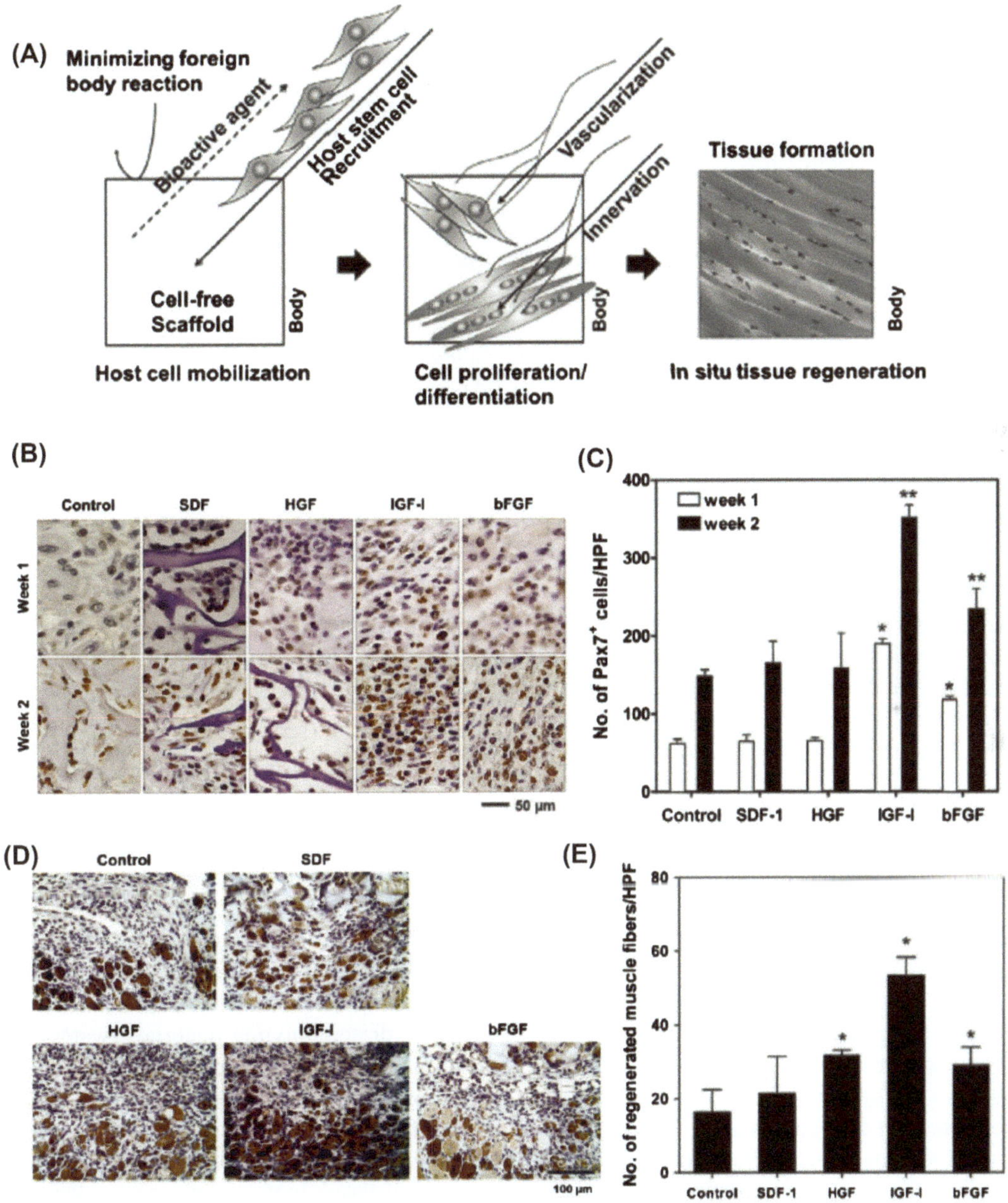

FIGURE 16.1

In situ regeneration of skeletal muscle tissue through host cell recruitment. (A) Schematic representation of the strategy of in situ muscle tissue regeneration using a target-specific scaffolding system. (B–E) Immunohistological analysis demonstrates that recruitment of Pax7 positive satellite cells and formation of MHC positive muscle fibers into the implanted scaffold at 1 and 2weeks after implantation are most prominent in the IGF-1-loaded scaffold among other growth factors.

Data from Ju YM, Atala A, Yoo JJ, Lee SJ. In situ regeneration of skeletal muscle tissue through host cell recruitment. Acta Biomater 2014;10(10):4332–9 were used with permission.

ENDOGENOUS CELLS

Primary cell components that comprise normal muscle structures include skeletal muscle cells, stromal cells, endothelial cells, and neural cells, and the roles of those cell types are myogenesis, angiogenesis, and innervation, respectively [13,14]. Satellite cells, which are skeletal muscle cellular components, play a significant role in muscle regeneration. Satellite cells are located on the surface of muscle fibers and remain in a quiescent state. Once the muscle tissue is injured, regeneration signaling will activate satellite cells to proliferate and differentiate to form new muscle fibers. In addition, other cell types adjacent to the basal lamina are involved in muscle regeneration. Pericytes, or mesenchymal stem cells (MSCs), are an important cell population that possesses myogenic potency and nonmyogenic function. Pericytes or MSCs have a broad range of roles to maintain myogenesis [15], angiogenesis [16], and secretion of trophic factors [15,17]. Nonmyogenic regeneration includes vascularization and innervation and is critical to supporting functional muscle regeneration. During the regenerating process, hematopoietic stem cells (HSCs), endothelial progenitor cells (EPCs), and neural progenitor cells initiate angiogenesis and innervation [13]. Thus the functional muscle regeneration from VML relies on an efficiently coordinated recruitment of various cell types in a timely and spatial manner.

SCAFFOLDING SYSTEM

For a successful outcome of this approach, development of an appropriate muscle-specific scaffolding system is vital to achieve functional muscle regeneration. Such scaffolding systems should provide appropriate environments for host cell infiltration to promote growth and further functional muscle tissue formation within the implanted scaffolds. Therefore it is desirable that the scaffolds have the following features: 3-D porous structures to provide ample space with efficient nutrients and oxygen supply for the seeded cells to reside, biodegradability to allow for tissue growth within the scaffold, appropriate biological properties to stimulate and direct tissue growth and formation of functional tissues and/or organs, and mechanical properties to maintain the engineered tissue formation during in vitro culture and in vivo implantation.

To date, numerous biomaterials created with various fabrication methods have been used for muscle regeneration. Both natural and synthetic biomaterials are used for tissue engineering purposes. Naturally derived polymers, including collagen, hyaluronic acid, alginate, agarose, chitosan, fibrin, and gelatin, facilitate the ability to support cell adhesion, proliferation, and differentiation within the materials. Most natural biomaterials belong to a class of highly hydrated polymer materials (water content ≥30% by weight) and are compatible with native tissue. Synthetic polymers, particularly biodegradable materials such as poly(glycolic acid), poly(lactic acid), and poly(lactic-*co*-glycolic acid), have been widely used in tissue engineering. Unlike nondegradable synthetic polymers that are not physiological and show less favorable interactions with the body, these degradable materials have several advantages: they yield nontoxic degradation products, they promote good tissue ingrowth during biodegradation in vivo, and they relate to natural metabolites. Moreover, the degradation rate of the biodegradable materials can be controlled from several weeks to several years for specific purposes.

Naturally derived biologic materials are considered promising scaffolding materials in tissue engineering [18]. In most cases, the biologic materials are derived from decellularization of native tissue or organs, and the acellular collagen-rich matrices maintain their structural and mechanical similarity to native tissues. Of note, these tissue matrices have been used for a number of tissue engineering applications as tissue-specific scaffolding and have provided a greater understanding of the physicochemical properties of ECM. For example, by harnessing the cell matrix interactions that are crucial for cell adhesion, proliferation, and differentiation, several studies have promoted tissue formation by combining cells with tissue-specific ECM from decellularized heart, urinary bladder, liver, lung, and small intestinal submucosa (SIS). In addition, these ECM proteins play an important role in tissue maintenance and regeneration of skeletal muscle, and they can modulate cell adhesion and migration, growth factor storage and release, and satellite cell activation and differentiation.

An essential step in engineering functional skeletal muscle tissue involves the ability to mimic the structure of native muscle tissue, which is comprised of highly oriented myotubes formed from numerous fused mononucleated muscle cells. It is well known that the structure and organization of muscle fibers dictate tissue function. Thus muscle cell alignment that permits organized myotube formation is a crucial step in musculoskeletal myogenesis. Recently, several reports demonstrated fabrication of an acellular muscle scaffold by decellularization of native muscle tissue [7,19]. The decellularized skeletal muscle matrices maintained the mechanical and structural integrity of the original tissue with minimal disruption to the ECM. Upon implantation, the muscle scaffold allowed for the infiltration of host cells and tissue formation with the implant. A possible challenge, however, is inefficient cell infiltration on the inner side of the scaffold that may delay the muscle tissue formation and limit further functional muscle regeneration [7,19].

BIOACTIVE FACTORS

A key to in situ tissue regeneration in the initial stage is proficient recruitment of host stem or progenitor cells into an implanted scaffold. Adult stem cell populations in the body are generally too low in number to have a significant impact on accelerated tissue regeneration. Depending on the cell population targeted to recruit, the choice of bioactive cues varies. Several growth factors and cytokines have been identified and characterized in terms of myogenic cell population. Insulin-like growth factor-1 (IGF-1) is a mitogenic growth factor for myoblasts [20–22] as well as for muscle progenitor cells [23,24]. Also, IGF-1 was reported to improve contractility in vivo [25]. In addition, several growth fac tors are related to muscle regeneration through satellite cell migration and proliferation by hepatocyte growth factor (HGF) [26] and stromal cell-derived factor 1α (SDF-1α) [27,28]. Fibroblast growth factor-2 (FGF-2) [29] and vascular endothelial growth factor (VEGF) [30] are pleiotropic factors that modulate muscle cell growth and apoptosis.

Various bioactive factors have been reported to facilitate recruitment and migration of stem or progenitor cells during injury. In most cases, bone marrow-derived cells, which include MSCs, HSCs, and EPCs, have been shown to contribute to muscle regeneration events. Substance P (SP), a neurotransmitter and neuromodulator, plays a significant role in inducing stem or progenitor cells during injury. A recent report showed strong evidence that injury-derived and exogenously administered SP increased the $CD29^+$ MSC-like cell population in the bloodstream and mobilized those cells to the injury site [31]. Another report showed the positive contribution of SP to vascularization. In this study, the patients with myocardial infarction maintained a high level of SP in the blood and resulted in improved recruitment of host cells into the damaged site [32]. A recent study also described the therapeutic effects of SP on skeletal muscle regeneration that most likely occurred through the recruitment of host therapeutic cells and stimulating nervous system [33]. Granulocyte-colony stimulating factor (G-CSF), another stem or progenitor cell-inducing factor, has been widely used in clinical trials [34]. The function of G-CSF was reported to be the mobilization of $CD34^+$, $CD133^+$ EPCs that contributed to vascularization at the injury site [35]. When G-CSF is combined with AMD3100 which is an antagonist of C-X-C chemokine receptor 4, the recruitment of HSCs and progenitor cells was improved compared with the use of a single agent [36]. Recently, G-CSF has shown effects on muscle regeneration through multiple stages of regenerated myocytes in a genetic muscle disease (Duchenne muscular dystrophy) [37]. Other factors that are involved in stem cell recruitment include stem cell factor [38] and monocyte chemotactic proteins (MCPs) [39] and are known to enhance migration and recruitment of HSCs and MSCs to injury sites. A recent report also showed the contribution of a member of the MCP family, chemokine ligand 2, to muscle regeneration through the activation of intramuscular macrophages in an acute muscle injury model [40]. A key factor that is closely related to efficient muscle regeneration is the acceleration of angiogenesis and innervation. Such factors that promote angiogenesis and innervation have been identified and include VEGF [41], FGF-2 [42], platelet-derived growth factor composed of two B chains (PDGF-BB) [14,43], angiopoietins [44], brain-derived neurotropic factor [45], glial cell line-derived neurotropic factor [46], and agrin [47]. These factors are closely related to muscle regeneration through direct or indirect activation of myogenesis.

BIOACTIVE FACTORS DELIVERY SYSTEM

One significant criterion for developing a biomaterial scaffold, especially for in situ muscle regeneration, is delivery of bioactive factors and regulatory signals in a precise temporal and spatial manner for effective tissue regeneration. When bioactive factors are exogenously administered to the injury site, they tend to lose their activity before they can act on the targeting cell population. To overcome this issue, a controlled and sustained delivery system of the bioactive factors has been developed to facilitate efficient muscle tissue regeneration [48]. The idea behind this technique requires encapsulating the factors within the scaffolding system through physical and chemical binding and allowing the encapsulated factors to be released in a temporal and spatial manner. The release patterns will be influenced by scaffold fabrication through changes of physical properties, pH, and scaffold degradability as well as the microenvironment of the implant site. Since skeletal muscle regeneration is a highly orchestrated event, various factors contribute to the regeneration process in response to the injury. For instance, a recent study reported various delivery methods of bioactive cues for controlled release over time [48]. Sustained release of multiple factors mimics tissue regeneration profiles in vivo that contribute to efficient and functional tissue regeneration. In one study, researchers developed a multiple protein delivery system for accelerating muscle regeneration through efficient vascularization [49]. They developed an injectable scaffolding system using alginate gel to deliver VGEF and IGF-1 for treatment of ischemic leg muscle tissue in mice. The controlled release of IGF-1 and VEGF significantly improved muscle regeneration through enhanced muscle fiber formation and vascularization, respectively. This study suggests that delivery of multiple factors in a simultaneous manner was effective to target distinct aspects of the muscle regenerative process. Similarly, another study developed a sustained delivery system of four growth factors, VEGF, angiopoietin 1, keratinocyte growth factor, and PDGF, which, when released, promoted angiogenesis with a potential for efficient tissue regeneration [50]. While this approach resulted in successful outcomes in terms of the efficacy of a multiple molecule delivery system, such systems are limited to local delivery at the implantation site and cause accumulation of the recruited cells at the periphery site of the scaffold that would delay cell infiltration to the inner site. Consequently, this unbalanced cell localization may prevent efficient tissue regeneration.

To address this issue, our group developed a novel delivery method that incorporated a combined approach of systemic with local delivery of multiple factors (SP and SDF-1a, respectively) to enhance infiltration of host stem cells (MSCs and HSCs) into the implant [10]. The strategy is composed of a two-step delivery: (1) increase of mobilization of bone marrow-derived MSCs and HSCs by systemic administration of SP intravenously; and (2) enhance recruitment of the mobilized MSCs and HSCs population from the circulating blood to the implant via localized release of SDF-1 from the scaffold. The results demonstrated that the combination delivery significantly promoted recruitment of the $CD29^+CD45^-$ MSC-like cell population, $CD146^+\alpha$-SMA^+ pericyte population, and c-kit^+-included HSC population into the implanted scaffold and suggested the effectiveness of the delivery system for in situ tissue regeneration. In a parallel study by our group, a myogenic factor deliver system was developed that allowed examination of the level of host cell recruitment by various myogenic factors such as SDF-1α, HGF, IGF-1, and FGF-2 [12]. The bioactive molecules were incorporated into the gelatin-based scaffold, and the single factor-contained scaffold was implanted into the VML rat model for 2 weeks. The histological analysis of the retrieved implant demonstrated that local release of IGF-1 significantly enhanced $Pax7^+$ muscle satellite cells recruitment (Fig. 16.1B and C) and myosin heavy chain $(MHC)^+$ muscle fibers into the scaffold implant (Fig. 16.1D and E) that led to accelerated efficient muscle regeneration in situ when compared to other factors. This study suggested that implantable scaffolds could be incorporated with myogenic accelerating factors for efficient recruitment of muscle host cells, and the recruited cells underwent growth and differentiation events within the scaffold for muscle regeneration in situ. Further studies are expected to incorporate the myogenic factor into the combination delivery system for acceleration of muscle regeneration in situ.

VARIOUS APPLICATIONS OF VOLUMETRIC MUSCLE REGENERATION IN SITU

The concept of tissue regeneration in situ has been applied to various applications for treatment of volumetric muscle regeneration in situ. Depending on the skeletal muscle and injury type, various types of scaffolding systems and combinations with bioactive cues have been developed for functional muscle regeneration (see Table 16.1). While many technologies are still in the early investigative stages, several techniques have been applied to preclinical animal models and clinical trials with satisfactory results. Although a number of engineered muscle constructs composed of scaffolds seeded with cultured cells have been extensively developed and applied to treat the VML, those studies will not be described in this chapter.

LEG MUSCLE REGENERATION

ANTERIOR MUSCLE

The muscles of the anterior leg are the tibialis anterior (TA), extensor digitorum longus (EDL), fibularis tertius, and extensor hallucis longus. These muscles are innervated by the common or deep nerves or by both, and they dorsiflex the foot. Impairment of skeletal muscle tissue function in the leg could cause instability of the entire body posture and difficulty moving and standing, which affects activities of daily life and independence [51]. Common injuries of skeletal muscle in the leg include strains, tears,

Table 16.1 Various Approaches to VML Repair Using In Situ Muscle Regeneration

Muscle Type	Animal Model	Defect Model	Biomaterials	Bioactive Factors	References
Tibialis anterior (TA)	Rat	VML (20% laceration)	RAMM (rat acellular muscle matrix)	–	Wu et al. [7]
	Rat	VML	Atelocollagen gel	Double-stranded miR-1, miR-133, miR-206	Nakasa et al. [52]
	Rat	VML (30% laceration)	PLLA	HGF, SDF-1α, IGF-1, bFGF	Ju et al. [12]
	Mouse	Ischemia	Alginate gel	VEGF, IGF-1	Borselli et al. [49]
Extensor digitorum longus (EDL)	Rabbit	VML	SIS	–	Crow et al. [54]
Thigh	Human	VML (trauma by explosion)	SIS–ECM	–	Mase et al. [56]
Quadriceps	Mouse	VML	SIS	–	Sicari et al. [4] Sicari et al. [55]
	Human	Skiing accident; exercise-induced	Urinary bladder ECM scaffold	–	Sicari et al. [55]
Vastus lateralis	Rabbit	VML (1 cm × 1 cm × 0.5 cm)	Cross-linked atelocollagen	–	Kin et al. [57]
Gastrocnemius (GA)					Ma et al. [78]
	Mouse	VML	–	bFGF, IGF-1, NGF	Menetrey et al. [25]
	Rat	Laceration; small and large defect	Homologous decellularized muscle ECM	–	Merritt et al. [19]
Diaphragm	Pig	VML (left hemidiaphragm defect)	ePTFE, SIS–ECM	–	Gonzalez et al. [68]
	Rat	VML (70% of left diaphragm defect)	Electrospun fiber with PCL and collagen	–	Zhao et al. [70]
	Rat	VML	Porous collagen sponge with heparin	VEGF, HGF	Brouwer et al. [73]
Abdominal wall defect	Rat	VML (full-thickness)	SIS-ECM	–	Ma et al. [78]
	Human	VML	Surgisis, Permacol, Allo-derm	–	Beale et al. [77]
	Rat	VML (partial-thickness defect)	SIS-ECM	NELL1 (cell signaling protein for growth and differentiation)	Turner et al. [81]

bFGF, *Basic fibroblast growth factor;* ePTFE, *expanded polytetrafluoroethylene;* HGF, *hepatocyte growth factor;* IGF-1, *insulin-like growth factor-1;* NGF, *nerve growth factor;* PLLA, *Poly(L-lactic acid);* SDF-1α, *stromal cell-derived factor 1;* SIS-ECM, *small intestine submucosa extracellular matrix;* VEGF, *vascular endothelial growth factor;* VML, *Volumetric muscle loss. AlloDerm—human acellular dermal matrix; Permacol—cross-linked porcine acellular dermal matrix; Surgisis—porcine SIS.*

and lacerations due to sports; however, severe traumatic injury to the anterior lower leg muscles is uncommon in either the sporting or nonsporting populations [51]. In particular, there have been very few reports of traumatic injury leading to rupture of the TA muscle [51]. Due to limitations such as the low level of clinical relevance, technical complexity, and nonreproducibility, most studies have focused on developing animal models for treatment of VML in the leg muscle injury [7].

In attempts to develop accurate VML animal models, TA muscle tissue has been considered a desirable type of skeletal muscle tissue due to the ease of accessibility to isolate from adjacent muscle tissues. Initially, the VML model was created by simple excision (~20% of total TA weight) of large volume of TA [7]. Wu et al. attempted to develop VML models that are technically simple, reliable, and clinically relevant (Fig. 16.2A). Muscle function analysis demonstrated that the volumetric excision led to an incomplete recovery of muscle weight and peak isometric tetanic force up to 4 months. The length of muscle recovery time from this model is adequate to evaluate the effects of therapeutic treatment on functional muscle regeneration. In addition, the regeneration ability was demonstrated by the implantation of a muscle-derived rat extracellular matrix scaffold (Fig. 16.2A), which suggested the possible application of this VML model to develop an in situ muscle tissue regeneration model to treat VML in the TA muscle tissue.

Using the similar excision model, Nakasa et al. tested the effects of microRNA (miRNA) on muscle regeneration [52]. The defect was wedge-shaped and was approximately 6 mm length by 4 mm wide by 5 mm depth. To treat the skeletal muscle injury, local injection of muscle-specific miRNA was applied. A mixture of double-stranded miRNAs, miR-1, miR-133, and miR-206 in a collagen gel was injected into the lacerated rat TA muscles. At 1 week after injection, the histological analysis confirmed enhanced muscle regeneration as evidenced by the expression of myogenic markers, MyoD1, myogenin, and Pax7 in the muscle tissue. Also, reduced fibrosis was observed compared to the control and the single injection groups. Similar experimental outcomes for miRNA on the muscle regeneration in vivo were observed when using the muscle cell line (C2C12). The results suggest that local administration of miRNA molecules, which retain therapeutic effects on the muscle regeneration, could be a novel strategy in the treatment of skeletal muscle injury in situ.

Another muscle tissue in the anterior part of the leg with large muscle volume, EDL muscle, has been used for VML model creation on animal [53]. A study by Garrett et al. compared the effect of the degree of laceration to EDL muscle in a rabbit model on the functional muscle recovery. Partially or completely lacerated muscle belly recovered to between 50% and 60% of normal function at 12 weeks after the injury. Histological analysis revealed that the laceration resulted in anatomic changes of muscle fiber atrophy and formation of new muscle fiber based on nuclear centralization and dense scar due to increased fibrosis. The results demonstrated that EDL muscle could recover following laceration, and normal functional outcome was obtained, which suggested that appropriate interventions are necessary for the treatment of VML of EDL muscle tissue.

Using the same VML model, Crow et al. examined a biomaterial-based intervention for the treatment of complete EDL laceration in a rabbit model [54]. They utilized SIS, which is a naturally derived biomaterial that has been extensively used in a wide application [18]. SIS graft was implanted into the completely lacerated EDL muscle, and then they compared the structural and functional recovery with controls such as unrepaired and suture-only groups (current standard treatment). SIS implantation of complete muscle lacerations resulted in recovery of normal muscle in terms of morphology and function (79% recovery of normal function) when compared to controls. This would suggest that SIS augmentation might have important clinical advantages over current standards of treatment and warrants further clinical study.

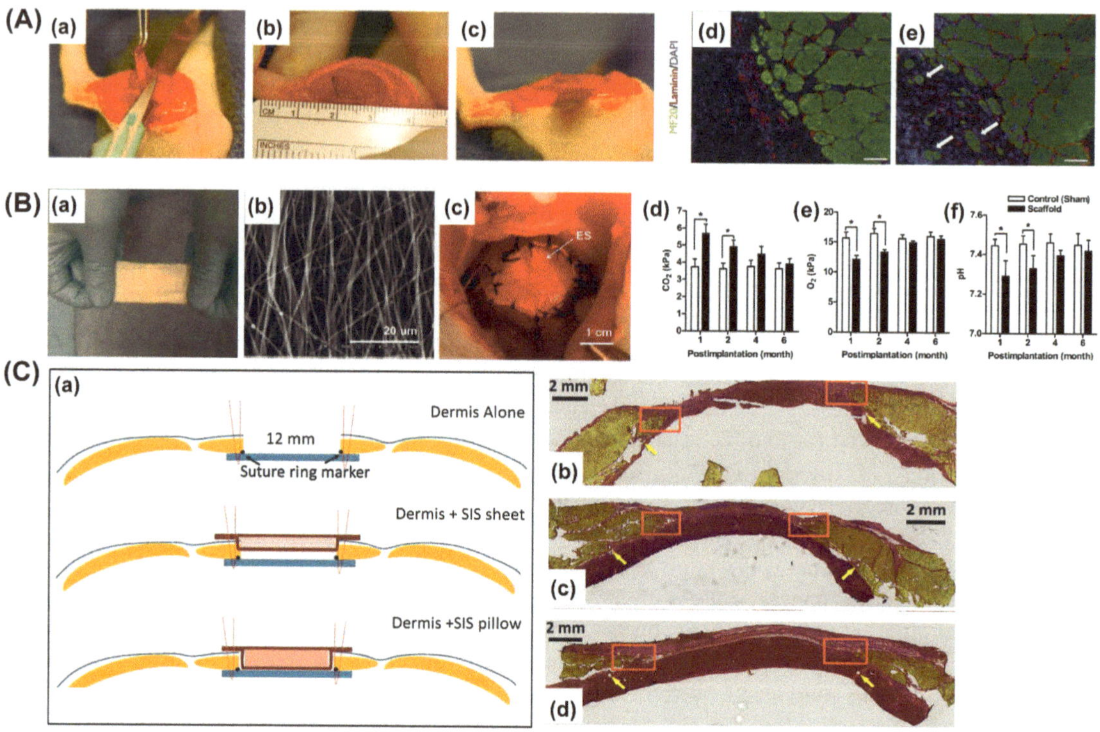

FIGURE 16.2

Several approaches to VML repair using in situ muscle regeneration. (A) Leg muscle regeneration. Illustration of rat TA muscle surgical procedure (a–c) and formation of higher number of MHC positive at the site of implantation with scaffold (e) compared with no implantation (d) *(Data were used from Wu X, Corona BT, Chen X, Walters TJ. A standardized rat model of volumetric muscle loss injury for the development of tissue engineering therapies. Biores Open Access 2012;1(6):280–90 with permission.)* (B) Diaphragm muscle regeneration. Gross appearance (a) and SEM image (b) of the electrospun aligned PCL/collagen scaffolds. (c) The scaffold was implanted in the left side of the diaphragm in the rats. ES indicates the electrospun scaffold. Blood gas analyses of control (sham operation) and scaffold implanted groups: (d) CO_2, (e) O_2, and (f) pH (*$p<.05$). *(Data from Zhao W, Ju YM, Christ G, Atala A, Yoo JJ, Lee SJ. Diaphragmatic muscle reconstruction with an aligned electrospun poly(epsilon-caprolactone)/collagen hybrid scaffold. Biomaterials 2013;34(33):8235–40 were used with permission.)* (C) Abdominal wall muscle regeneration with a full-thickness defect. (a) A 12 mm × 12 mm full-thickness, midline, abdominal wall defect was created in the rectus muscles of the rat, centered on the linea alba. In all groups, a 20 mm × 20 mm dermis graft was implanted in an underlay fashion with epidermal side toward the viscera. Representative sections of 16-week explanted repair constructs from the Dermis group (b), Sheet group (c), and Pillow group (d) (Herovici staining; yellow: muscle fibers; red/purple: collagen). In all groups, muscle fibers appeared to be distributed near the defect edge but not in the center of the defect (b). *(Data from Ma J, Sahoo S, Baker AR, Derwin KA. Investigating muscle regeneration with a dermis/small intestinal submucosa scaffold in a rat full-thickness abdominal wall defect model. J Biomed Mater Res B Appl Biomater 2015;103(2):355–64 were used with permission.)*

The quadriceps muscle is a large muscle belly that can easily be accessed in the anterior part of the leg. Sicari et al. developed a murine model of VML using the mouse quadriceps muscle by making a full-thickness unilateral excision of a 4 mm × 3 mm in the muscle. Histological examination demonstrated that the lateral laceration resulted in an appropriate VML model having irrecoverable muscle recovery up to 56 days. As an appropriate treatment, SIS–ECM augmentation was evaluated, and the histological and functional results showed that the implantation of SIS–ECM at the site of the defect prevented scar tissue formation and facilitated innervation and vascularization on the regenerated skeletal muscle.

Biologic ECM matrix has been used to treat VML in patients. Before a clinical trial, the therapeutic effect of urinary bladder ECM scaffold was confirmed in a rodent model [55]. Subsequently, porcine urinary bladder ECM scaffolds were used as a surgical treatment for VML in five male patients (anterior tibial compartment injury in two patients, quadriceps in two patients, and anterior/lateral tibial compartment in one patient) [55]. The clinical translation showed that ECM scaffolds promoted remodeling of muscle with de novo formation of skeletal muscle cells and vascularization at the site of injury. Interestingly, muscle function was improved in three patients. The outcomes of this translational clinical trial showed that biological ECM scaffolds might serve as inductive templates that promote recovery of muscle tissue in VML. Thus the concept of in situ tissue regeneration using acellular scaffold to treat VML in patients is worthy of further study.

In a similar way, SIS–ECM was applied to a young marine who presented with a large VML of the right thigh due to an explosion [56]. A multilayered SIS–ECM was surgically implanted and resulted in restoration of a portion of the lost vastus medialis muscle, which resulted in a gain in isokinetic performance at 4 months after surgery and new tissues at the implant site. Data from this clinical trial suggest a promising indicator of the use of biologic ECM for the treatment of VML in leg muscles.

Another type of biomaterial has been used to treat VML of thigh muscles using a cross-linked atelocollagen sponge as a scaffold to regenerate skeletal muscle by in situ tissue engineering in a rabbit model [57]. Vastus lateralis muscle (the largest part of the quadriceps muscle) defects (1.0 cm × ~1.0 cm × ~0.5 cm) were created, and an acellular collagen sponge was implanted into the injured site. Regenerating myofibers with mild concavity were observed at 24 weeks after surgery in the implanted group only.

POSTERIOR LEG MUSCLE

A leg muscle tissue that has also been used for VML preclinical models is the gastrocnemius (GA) muscle. GA muscle is located in the posterior part of the lower leg and functions in the fast movements of the leg for running and jumping through planar flexing of the foot. This fast movement is supported by white muscle fibers that are characterized by type II fast twitch. As a large muscle belly in the posterior part of the lower leg, laceration of the GA resulted in sustained severe function loss when left unrepaired [58]; therefore, this VML model has been considered as appropriate muscle type for preclinical studies. Recently, Merritt et al. developed a lateral GA-damage model in Sprague–Dawley rats [19]. A small defect (0.5 cm × 1.0 cm) and a large defect (1.0 cm × 1.0 cm) were created, and the function was not recovered until 28 days after the defect was made. A homologous, decellularized muscle ECM was implanted into the lateral GA defect sites (1.0 cm × 1.0 cm) of Lewis rats, and vessel ingrowth and myofiber formation into the ECM were observed after 42 days, although muscle function was not recovered. Thus it was demonstrated that acellular ECM scaffolds from skeletal muscle tissue could be used to support muscle and blood vessel regeneration.

DIAPHRAGM REGENERATION

The diaphragm is a dome-shaped tissue composed of skeletal muscle cells and fibrous cells. It functions as the primary muscle tissue of respiration and provides a physical barrier between the thoracic and abdominal cavities. A congenital abnormality called diaphragmatic hernia (CDH) is characterized by perforations in the corner of the diaphragm and is a life-threatening pathology in newborns and infants. The incidence of CDH is as high as 1 in 2500 births [59,60], and immediate surgical treatment for severe CDH pathology is needed. Current treatments include the use of prosthetic materials and autologous muscle grafts. Prosthetic patch repairs have been developed as a relatively simple method for primary closure of diaphragmatic defects. Expanded polytetrafluoroethylene (ePTFE) patches, reinforced silastic sheets, and polypropylene (PP) meshes are the most popular biomaterials chosen for this procedure [61–65]. Disadvantages of these synthetic nonabsorbable biomaterial patches include a failure to degrade in the body, which may lead to granulation without host tissue formation within the implant, immune reaction, infection, restricted chest wall development, mechanical mismatch with native tissue, and recurrent herniation. Consequently, autologous muscle flaps have been developed to repair large diaphragmatic defects and minimize the possibility of complications associated with synthetic nondegradable materials [65,66]. The surgical approach used to obtain and implant autologous muscle flap, however, is rather complex and invasive and requires prolonged operating times that may lead to bleeding, infection, necrosis, and other complications with higher morbidity and mortality. Therefore a degradable material-based patch that allows host cell infiltration, tissue ingrowth, and functional tissue formation has become a promising scaffold to repair CDH defects [67].

Gonzalez et al. compared the level of diaphragmatic tissue repair between a nonabsorbable mesh (ePTFE) and an absorbable biologic scaffold (SIS) over a 6-month period using a left hemidiaphragm model in a developing porcine model [68]. Histological analysis revealed that the SIS mesh provided better integration to the chest wall tissue with an increase in new formation of muscle growth within the diaphragmatic tissue and less fibrotic tissue formation than ePTFE. These results suggest that biodegradable SIS matrix is a more appropriate prosthetic material than a nondegradable material in the treatment of diaphragmatic defects in a growing animal. In another study, SIS matrix was tested in a diaphragmatic defect in a young cat model [69]. CT imaging demonstrated that the SIS graft facilitated restoration of normal function without restriction of chest wall development during growth of young cats, which suggested that biodegradable materials could be used for the treatment of diaphragmatic defects.

Using different biodegradable materials and fabrication techniques, our group developed a biodegradable sheet-shaped scaffold for a diaphragmatic muscle reconstruction [70] (Fig. 16.2B). The fabrication of a hybrid scaffold is based on an electrospinning technique composed of a combination of poly(ε-caprolactone) (PCL) and collagen protein [71] that provides a unidirectional orientation to guide host cell alignment and enhances myotube formation in vitro [72]. To develop a diaphragmatic model, 70% of the diaphragmatic tissue on the left side in rats was excised, and the hybrid scaffolds were implanted into a central left hemidiaphragmatic defect. Radiographic and MRI analysis demonstrated no evidence of herniation or retraction up to 6 months after implantation. Histological and immunohistochemical analysis revealed host cell infiltration and ingrowth of muscle tissue into the implanted scaffolds. The mechanical properties of the retrieved scaffolds were similar to those of normal diaphragm tissue at the designated time periods. The results show that the biodegradable hybrid scaffolds allowed muscle cell migration and tissue formation and may provide implantable functional muscle tissues for patients with diaphragmatic muscle defects [70].

In a recent report, Brouwer et al. [73] developed a porous collagen scaffold to improve cellular infiltration for diaphragmatic reconstruct. For this purpose, several growth factors, such as VEGF and HGF, were incorporated through immobilized heparin on the collagen scaffold and tested in a diaphragmatic model of rats. At 2 weeks after implantation, gross and histological analysis demonstrated that the incorporated growth factors enhanced vascularization at the lung site and did not show any difference in terms of immune cell infiltration. These cell types were, however, decreased in number at 12 weeks. Based on these results, the incorporation of growth factors into the scaffold did not influence cellular response to the implant; therefore, further optimization of the dosage used and release profile criteria are required.

ABDOMINAL MUSCLE REGENERATION

The abdominal wall consists of several types of tissues such as skin, superficial fascia, fat, skeletal muscle, and connective tissue [74]. Particularly, the abdominal muscle is composed of four paired muscle tissues that include rectus abdominis, internal and external oblique, transversus abdominis, and pyramidalis muscle. The abdominal muscle aids the breathing process; movements including flexion, extension, and rotation of the trunk; protection of inner organs; postural support; defecation; urination; and prevention of hyperextension. Defects in the abdominal wall often cause ventral hernias due to volumetric defects such as severe tissue loss by trauma, edema, or tumor resection, as well as massive infection or radiation necrosis [75]. Current treatment includes open primary tissue closure, bioprosthetic mesh placement, and autologous flap grafting. Particularly, the mesh placement is the standard treatment for patients with a defect greater than 2 cm [75]. Two common mesh materials include PP and ePTFE, which have been clinically used for a long time. Synthetic nondegradable materials, however, often result in complications such as scar formation and chronic immune response that can lead to bowel obstruction and enterocutaneous fistula [76,77]. To address this issue, biodegradable mesh materials have been considered as an alternative and reliable option to treat abdominal defects. The degradable mesh can reduce adhesion and scar formation while mechanical stability is maintained. Particularly, acellular collagen matrix has been shown to promote host cell infiltration and tissue ingrowth within the implant and is superior to nondegradable materials. The disadvantages of using degradable mesh include cost-ineffectiveness and the lack of long-term follow-up studies [75,77].

Among such degradable meshes, SIS matrix has been widely used as an appropriate option for the treatment of abdominal defects. Ma et al. investigated whether SIS grafts can be applied to repair a full-thickness abdominal wall defect in a rat model [78] (Fig. 16.2C). Interestingly, this study utilized the dermis layer as a supporting material to mechanically bridge the defect, as SIS graft is easily degraded in the short term. After 16 weeks of implantation, histological analysis demonstrated that the combined prosthetic approach of the SIS and dermis graft could not promote muscle regeneration in the severe VML model and led to incomplete abdominal closure. Thus further investigations using a combination of cellular components and bioactive factors are needed to improve functional muscle regeneration.

A comparative study conducted by Beale et al. examined the impact of the type of biologic matrix, allograft, or xenograft on hernia recurrence and surgical site complications [79]. Allografts or xenograft materials used included Permacol (cross-linked porcine acellular dermal matrix), Surgisis (porcine SIS), or AlloDerm (human acellular dermal matrix). The results showed that allograft acellular dermal matrix had a higher recurrence rate when compared to xenograft materials; moreover, this would support the current trend of using xenografts as prosthetic meshes in hernia repair [79]. In a similar study, the effect of cross-linking of the biologic acellular matrix was examined by histological methods and biomechanical properties [80]. Histological analysis revealed that the noncross-linked matrix showed faster degradation, cell infiltration, and vascularization than the cross-linked product.

As mentioned earlier, the ability to control remodeling of biological tissue is necessary to improve repairs to tissue function following a defect. Turner et al. hypothesized that the addition of NELL1, a cell signaling protein that controls cell growth and differentiation, would enhance the tissue remodeling of two collagen-based scaffolds (pure or SIS–ECM) [81]. To test the hypothesis, a partial-thickness abdominal wall defect rodent model was used to compare the effect of NELL1 on constructive remodeling. Histological analysis demonstrated that incorporation of NELL1 protein improved the constructive remodeling of pure collagen scaffolds but not SIS–ECM scaffolds. Muscle functional analysis showed that addition of NELL1 into the collagen-treated group increased the contractile force of the remodeled skeletal muscle and yielded a fast-to-slow muscle composition similar to native muscle tissue, while NELL1 did not influence the effect by SIS–ECM. This group suggested that NELL1 protein does contribute to the enhanced constructive remodeling of skeletal muscle.

CONCLUSION AND FUTURE PERSPECTIVES

Recent advances in the fabrication of functional biomaterials-based scaffolding systems, an understanding of biological, molecular, and physiological aspects of skeletal muscle regeneration, and identification of novel bioactive cues for acceleration of muscle regeneration have allowed the field of in situ muscle regeneration to make promising advances toward repairing and restoring muscle functions following muscle injury. Particularly, VML from leg muscle, diaphragm, and abdominal wall tissue has been considered to be among the most critical challenges due to the development of serious complications from entire loss of muscle function, dysfunction of other tissue and organs, and life-threatening symptoms. Many experimental approaches utilizing functional scaffolding systems and incorporation of bioactive cues have been performed to test new strategies for the repair of VML, and several have become clinically applicable.

While previous treatments have resulted in successful outcomes in the improvement of muscle function from VML, several obstacles delay the acceleration of functional muscle regeneration. Indeed, the recapitulation of the normal skeletal muscle function in terms of its structural and functional complexity will ultimately require a master system capable of successfully mimicking all key aspects of muscle physiology. To achieve this goal, multidisciplinary research in this field should be conducted in a well-balanced manner. Such studies should include more sophisticated fabrication of a scaffolding system, application of appropriate mechanical stimuli [2], prevention of severe scar formation from VML [82,83], identification of stem cell inducing and proliferation factors in vivo [31], and the development of an accelerated approach to vascularization and innervation of the implanted scaffolding system with the host environments.

ACKNOWLEDGMENT

We wish to thank Dr. Heather Hatcher for editorial assistance with this manuscript.

REFERENCES

[1] Huard J, Li Y, Fu FH. Muscle injuries and repair: current trends in research. J Bone Joint Surg 2002;84-A(5).
[2] Cittadella Vigodarzere G, Mantero S. Skeletal muscle tissue engineering: strategies for volumetric constructs. Front Physiol 2014;5:362.
[3] Turner NJ, Badylak SF. Regeneration of skeletal muscle. Cell Tissue Res 2012;347(3):759–74.
[4] Sicari BM, Agrawal V, Siu BF, Medberry CJ, Dearth CL, Turner NJ, et al. A murine model of volumetric muscle loss and a regenerative medicine approach for tissue replacement. Tissue Eng Part A 2012;18(19–20):1941–8.
[5] Grogan BF, Hsu JR. Volumetric muscle loss. J Am Acad Orthop Surg 2011;19(Suppl. 1):S35–7.
[6] MacKenzie EJ, Bosse MJ, Kellam JF, Burgess AR, Webb LX, Swiontkowski MF, et al. Characterization of patients with high-energy lower extremity trauma. J Orthop Trauma 2000;14(7):455–66.
[7] Wu X, Corona BT, Chen X, Walters TJ. A standardized rat model of volumetric muscle loss injury for the development of tissue engineering therapies. Biores Open Access 2012;1(6):280–90.
[8] Beauchamp JR, Morgan JE, Pagel CN, Partridge TA. Dynamics of myoblast transplantation reveal a discrete minority of precursors with stem cell-like properties as the myogenic source. J Cell Biol 1999;144(6):1113–22.
[9] Lee SJ, Van Dyke M, Atala A, Yoo JJ. Host cell mobilization for in situ tissue regeneration. Rejuvenation Res 2008;11(4):747–56.
[10] Ko IK, Ju YM, Chen T, Atala A, Yoo JJ, Lee SJ. Combined systemic and local delivery of stem cell inducing/recruiting factors for in situ tissue regeneration. FASEB J 2012;26(1):158–68.
[11] Ko IK, Lee SJ, Atala A, Yoo JJ. In situ tissue regeneration through host stem cell recruitment. Exp Mol Med 2013;45:e57.
[12] Ju YM, Atala A, Yoo JJ, Lee SJ. In situ regeneration of skeletal muscle tissue through host cell recruitment. Acta Biomater 2014;10(10):4332–9.
[13] Tedesco FS, Dellavalle A, Diaz-Manera J, Messina G, Cossu G. Repairing skeletal muscle: regenerative potential of skeletal muscle stem cells. J Clin Invest 2010;120(1):11–9.
[14] Karalaki M, Fili S, Philippou A, Koutsilieris M. Muscle regeneration: cellular and molecular events. In Vivo 2009;23(5):779–96.
[15] Crisan M, Yap S, Casteilla L, Chen CW, Corselli M, Park TS, et al. A perivascular origin for mesenchymal stem cells in multiple human organs. Cell Stem Cell 2008;3(3):301–13.
[16] Crisan M, Deasy B, Gavina M, Zheng B, Huard J, Lazzari L, et al. Purification and long-term culture of multipotent progenitor cells affiliated with the walls of human blood vessels: myoendothelial cells and pericytes. Methods Cell Biol 2008;86:295–309.
[17] Caplan AI, Dennis JE. Mesenchymal stem cells as trophic mediators. J Cell Biochem 2006;98(5):1076–84.
[18] Badylak SF, Freytes DO, Gilbert TW. Extracellular matrix as a biological scaffold material: structure and function. Acta Biomater 2009;5(1):1–13.
[19] Merritt EK, Hammers DW, Tierney M, Suggs LJ, Walters TJ, Farrar RP. Functional assessment of skeletal muscle regeneration utilizing homologous extracellular matrix as scaffolding. Tissue Eng Part A 2010;16(4).
[20] Damon SE, Haugk KL, Birnbaum RS, Quinn LS. Retrovirally mediated overexpression of insulin-like growth factor binding protein 4: evidence that insulin-like growth factor is required for skeletal muscle differentiation. J Cell Physiol 1998;175(1):109–20.
[21] Engert JC, Berglund EB, Rosenthal N. Proliferation precedes differentiation in IGF-I-stimulated myogenesis. J Cell Biol 1996;135(2):431–40.
[22] Florini JR, Ewton DZ, Coolican SA. Growth hormone and the insulin-like growth factor system in myogenesis. Endocr Rev 1996;17(5):481–517.
[23] Allen RE, Boxhorn LK. Regulation of skeletal muscle satellite cell proliferation and differentiation by transforming growth factor-beta, insulin-like growth factor I, and fibroblast growth factor. J Cell Physiol 1989;138(2):311–5.

[24] Florini JR, Magri KA. Effects of growth factors on myogenic differentiation. Am J Physiol 1989;256 (4 Pt 1):C701–11.
[25] Menetrey J, Kasemkijwattana C, Day CS, Bosch P, Vogt M, Fu FH, et al. Growth factors improve muscle healing in vivo. J Bone Joint Surg Br 2000;82(1):131–7.
[26] Gal-Levi R, Leshem Y, Aoki S, Nakamura T, Halevy O. Hepatocyte growth factor plays a dual role in regulating skeletal muscle satellite cell proliferation and differentiation. Biochim Biophys Acta 1998;1402(1):39–51.
[27] Odemis V, Boosmann K, Dieterlen MT, Engele J. The chemokine SDF1 controls multiple steps of myogenesis through atypical PKCzeta. J Cell Sci 2007;120(Pt 22):4050–9.
[28] Fibbi G, D'Alessio S, Pucci M, Cerletti M, Del Rosso M. Growth factor-dependent proliferation and invasion of muscle satellite cells require the cell-associated fibrinolytic system. Biol Chem 2002;383(1):127–36.
[29] Stratos I, Madry H, Rotter R, Weimer A, Graff J, Cucchiarini M, et al. Fibroblast growth factor-2-overexpressing myoblasts encapsulated in alginate spheres increase proliferation, reduce apoptosis, induce adipogenesis, and enhance regeneration following skeletal muscle injury in rats. Tissue Eng Part A 2011;17(21–22):2867–77.
[30] Arsic N, Zacchigna S, Zentilin L, Ramirez-Correa G, Pattarini L, Salvi A, et al. Vascular endothelial growth factor stimulates skeletal muscle regeneration in vivo. Mol Ther 2004;10(5):844–54.
[31] Hong HS, Lee J, Lee E, Kwon YS, Lee E, Ahn W, et al. A new role of substance P as an injury-inducible messenger for mobilization of CD29(+) stromal-like cells. Nat Med 2009;15(4):425–35.
[32] Amadesi S, Reni C, Katare R, Meloni M, Oikawa A, Beltrami AP, et al. Role for substance p-based nociceptive signaling in progenitor cell activation and angiogenesis during ischemia in mice and in human subjects. Circulation 2012;125(14):1774–86. S1-19.
[33] Khattak MJ, Ahmad T, Rehman R, Umer M, Hasan SH, Ahmed M. Muscle healing and nerve regeneration in a muscle contusion model in the rat. J Bone Joint Surg Br 2010;92(6):894–9.
[34] Petit I, Szyper-Kravitz M, Nagler A, Lahav M, Peled A, Habler L, et al. G-CSF induces stem cell mobilization by decreasing bone marrow SDF-1 and up-regulating CXCR4. Nat Immunol 2002;3(7):687–94.
[35] Zhou M, Liu Z, Li K, Qiao W, Jiang X, Ran F, et al. Beneficial effects of granulocyte-colony stimulating factor on small-diameter heparin immobilized decellularized vascular graft. J Biomed Mater Res A 2010;95(2):600–10.
[36] Capoccia BJ, Shepherd RM, Link DC. G-CSF and AMD3100 mobilize monocytes into the blood that stimulate angiogenesis in vivo through a paracrine mechanism. Blood 2006;108(7):2438–45.
[37] Hayashiji N, Yuasa S, Miyagoe-Suzuki Y, Hara M, Ito N, Hashimoto H, et al. G-CSF supports long-term muscle regeneration in mouse models of muscular dystrophy. Nat Commun 2015;6:6745.
[38] McNiece IK, Briddell RA. Stem cell factor. J Leukoc Biol 1995;58(1):14–22.
[39] Schenk S, Mal N, Finan A, Zhang M, Kiedrowski M, Popovic Z, et al. Monocyte chemotactic protein-3 is a myocardial mesenchymal stem cell homing factor. Stem Cells 2007;25(1):245–51.
[40] Lu H, Huang D, Ransohoff RM, Zhou L. Acute skeletal muscle injury: CCL2 expression by both monocytes and injured muscle is required for repair. FASEB J 2011;25(10):3344–55.
[41] Cao Y, Langer R. A review of Judah Folkman's remarkable achievements in biomedicine. Proc Natl Acad Sci USA 2008;105(36):13203–5.
[42] Cross MJ, Claesson-Welsh L. FGF and VEGF function in angiogenesis: signalling pathways, biological responses and therapeutic inhibition. Trends Pharmacol Sci 2001;22(4):201–7.
[43] Xue Y, Lim S, Yang Y, Wang Z, Jensen LD, Hedlund EM, et al. PDGF-BB modulates hematopoiesis and tumor angiogenesis by inducing erythropoietin production in stromal cells. Nat Med 2012;18(1):100–10.
[44] Mofarrahi M, McClung JM, Kontos CD, Davis EC, Tappuni B, Moroz N, et al. Angiopoietin-1 enhances skeletal muscle regeneration in mice. Am J Physiol Regul Integr Comp Physiol 2015;308(7):R576–89.
[45] Clow C, Jasmin BJ. Brain-derived neurotrophic factor regulates satellite cell differentiation and skeletal muscle regeneration. Mol Biol Cell 2010;21(13):2182–90.

[46] Suzuki H, Hase A, Kim BY, Miyata Y, Nonaka I, Arahata K, et al. Up-regulation of glial cell line-derived neurotrophic factor (GDNF) expression in regenerating muscle fibers in neuromuscular diseases. Neurosci Lett 1998;257(3):165–7.

[47] Bentzinger CF, Barzaghi P, Lin S, Ruegg MA. Overexpression of mini-agrin in skeletal muscle increases muscle integrity and regenerative capacity in laminin-alpha2-deficient mice. FASEB J 2005;19(8):934–42.

[48] Chen FM, Zhang M, Wu ZF. Toward delivery of multiple growth factors in tissue engineering. Biomaterials 2010;31(24):6279–308.

[49] Borselli C, Storrie H, Benesch-Lee F, Shvartsman D, Cezar C, Lichtman JW, et al. Functional muscle regeneration with combined delivery of angiogenesis and myogenesis factors. Proc Natl Acad Sci USA 2010;107(8):3287–92.

[50] Elia R, Fuegy PW, VanDelden A, Firpo MA, Prestwich GD, Peattie RA. Stimulation of in vivo angiogenesis by in situ crosslinked, dual growth factor-loaded, glycosaminoglycan hydrogels. Biomaterials 2010;31(17):4630–8.

[51] Constantinou M, Wilson A. Traumatic tear of tibialis anterior during a Gaelic football game: a case report. Br J Sports Med 2004;38(6):e30.

[52] Nakasa T, Ishikawa M, Shi M, Shibuya H, Adachi N, Ochi M. Acceleration of muscle regeneration by local injection of muscle-specific microRNAs in rat skeletal muscle injury model. J Cell Mol Med 2010;14(10):2495–505.

[53] Garrett Jr WE, Seaber AV, Boswick J, Urbaniak JR, Goldner JL. Recovery of skeletal muscle after laceration and repair. J Hand Surg 1984;9(5):683–92.

[54] Crow BD, Haltom JD, Carson WL, Greene WB, Cook JL. Evaluation of a novel biomaterial for intrasubstance muscle laceration repair. J Orthop Res 2007;25(3):396–403.

[55] Sicari BM, Rubin JP, Dearth CL, Wolf MT, Ambrosio F, Boninger M, et al. An acellular biologic scaffold promotes skeletal muscle formation in mice and humans with volumetric muscle loss. Sci Transl Med 2014;6(234).

[56] Mase Jr VJ, Wolf SE, Wenke J, Baer DG, Owens J, Badylak SF, et al. Clinical application of an acellular biologic scaffold for surgical repair of a large, traumatic quadriceps femoris muscle defect. Orthopedics 2010;33(7):511.

[57] Kin S, Hagiwara A, Nakase Y, Kuriu Y, Nakashima S, Yoshikawa T, et al. Regeneration of skeletal muscle using in situ tissue engineering on an acellular collagen sponge scaffold in a rabbit model. ASAIO J 2007;53(4):506–13.

[58] Menetrey J, Kasemkijwattana C, Fu FH, Moreland MS, Huard J. Suturing versus immobilization of a muscle laceration. A morphological and functional study in a mouse model. Am J Sports Med 1999;27(2):222–9.

[59] Irish MS, Holm BA, Glick PL. Congenital diaphragmatic hernia. A historical review. Clin Perinatol 1996;23(4):625–53.

[60] Logan JW, Rice HE, Goldberg RN, Cotten CM. Congenital diaphragmatic hernia: a systematic review and summary of best-evidence practice strategies. J Perinatol 2007;27(9):535–49.

[61] Newman BM, Jewett TC, Lewis A, Cerny F, Khan A, Karp M, et al. Prosthetic materials and muscle flaps in the repair of extensive diaphragmatic defects: an experimental study. J Pediatr Surg 1985;20(4):362–7.

[62] Lally KP, Cheu HW, Vazquez WD. Prosthetic diaphragm reconstruction in the growing animal. J Pediatr Surg 1993;28(1):45–7.

[63] Kimber CP, Dunkley MP, Haddock G, Robertson L, Carey FA, Cuschieri A. Patch incorporation in diaphragmatic hernia. J Pediatr Surg 2000;35(1):120–3.

[64] Saltzman DA, Ennis JS, Mehall JR, Jackson RJ, Smith SD, Wagner CW. Recurrent congenital diaphragmatic hernia: a novel repair. J Pediatr Surg 2001;36(12):1768–9.

[65] Koot VC, Bergmeijer JH, Molenaar JC. Lyophylized dura patch repair of congenital diaphragmatic hernia: occurrence of relapses. J Pediatr Surg 1993;28(5):667–8.

[66] Masumoto K, Nagata K, Souzaki R, Uesugi T, Takahashi Y, Taguchi T. Effectiveness of diaphragmatic repair using an abdominal muscle flap in patients with recurrent congenital diaphragmatic hernia. J Pediatr Surg 2007;42(12):2007–11.
[67] Gasior AC, St Peter SD. A review of patch options in the repair of congenital diaphragm defects. Pediatr Surg Int 2012;28(4):327–33.
[68] Gonzalez R, Hill SJ, Mattar SG, Lin E, Ramshaw BJ, Smith CD, et al. Absorbable versus nonabsorbable mesh repair of congenital diaphragmatic hernias in a growing animal model. J Laparoendosc Adv Surg Tech Part A 2011;21(5):449–54.
[69] Andreoni AA, Voss K. Reconstruction of a large diaphragmatic defect in a kitten using small intestinal submucosa (SIS). J Feline Med Surg 2009;11(12):1019–22.
[70] Zhao W, Ju YM, Christ G, Atala A, Yoo JJ, Lee SJ. Diaphragmatic muscle reconstruction with an aligned electrospun poly(epsilon-caprolactone)/collagen hybrid scaffold. Biomaterials 2013;34(33):8235–40.
[71] Ju YM, Choi JS, Atala A, Yoo JJ, Lee SJ. Bilayered scaffold for engineering cellularized blood vessels. Biomaterials 2010;31(15):4313–21.
[72] Choi JS, Lee SJ, Christ GJ, Atala A, Yoo JJ. The influence of electrospun aligned poly(epsilon-caprolactone)/collagen nanofiber meshes on the formation of self-aligned skeletal muscle myotubes. Biomaterials 2008;29(19):2899–906.
[73] Brouwer KM, Wijnen RM, Reijnen D, Hafmans TG, Daamen WF, van Kuppevelt TH. Heparinized collagen scaffolds with and without growth factors for the repair of diaphragmatic hernia: construction and in vivo evaluation. Organogenesis 2013;9(3):161–7.
[74] Ahluwalia SH, Burger JP, Quinn TH. Anatomy of the anterior abdominal wall. Oper Tech Gen Surg 2004;6(3):147–55.
[75] Garrido-Delgado R, Aponte YM, Behnam AB, Keeshin T, Sinha V, Evans KK, et al. Updates in abdominal wall reconstruction. Anal Bioanal Chem 2013;2(1):10000104.
[76] Butler CE, Campbell KT. Minimally invasive component separation with inlay bioprosthetic mesh (MICSIB) for complex abdominal wall reconstruction. Plast Reconstr Surg 2011;128(3):698–709.
[77] Beale EW, Hoxworth RE, Livingston EH, Trussler AP. The role of biologic mesh in abdominal wall reconstruction: a systematic review of the current literature. Am J Surg 2012;204(4):510–7.
[78] Ma J, Sahoo S, Baker AR, Derwin KA. Investigating muscle regeneration with a dermis/small intestinal submucosa scaffold in a rat full-thickness abdominal wall defect model. J Biomed Mater Res B Appl Biomater 2015;103(2):355–64.
[79] Gucciardo L, Ozog Y, Rusconi S, Lories R, Damink LO, Deprest J. Full thickness abdominal wall defect in growing rats as a model for congenital diaphragmatic hernia prosthetic repair. J Pediatr Surg 2014;49(10):1458–65.
[80] Deeken CR, Melman L, Jenkins ED, Greco SC, Frisella MM, Matthews BD. Histologic and biomechanical evaluation of crosslinked and non-crosslinked biologic meshes in a porcine model of ventral incisional hernia repair. J Am Coll Surg 2011;212(5):880–8.
[81] Turner NJ, Londono R, Dearth CL, Culiat CT, Badylak SF. Human NELL1 protein augments constructive tissue remodeling with biologic scaffolds. Cells Tissues Organs 2013;198(4):249–65.
[82] Mietz H, Chevez-Barrios P, Lieberman MW, Wendt M, Gross R, Basinger SF. Decorin and suramin inhibit ocular fibroblast collagen production. Graefes Arch Clin Exp Ophthalmol 1997;235(6):399–403.
[83] Chan YS, Li Y, Foster W, Horaguchi T, Somogyi G, Fu FH, et al. Antifibrotic effects of suramin in injured skeletal muscle after laceration. J Appl Physiol 2003;95(2):771–80.

CHAPTER

MENDING THE HEART THROUGH IN SITU CARDIAC REGENERATION

17

J.C.M. Teo[1], S.M. Boularaoui[1], N.S.A. AlWahab[1], N. Christoforou[1,2]
[1]*Khalifa University, Abu Dhabi, United Arab Emirates;* [2]*Duke University, Durham, NC, United States*

CHAPTER OUTLINE

INTRODUCTION

The heart's capacity to continually function uninterrupted and efficiently defines an individual's quality of life. Congenital and acquired cardiac diseases can have deleterious effects on the life of the individual, ultimately leading to their death [1,2]. Diminished functional cardiac output can occur as a result of multiple factors, including ischemic heart disease, diabetes, hypertension, viral infections, and chemotherapy. Myocardial infarction in particular occurs when the blood supply to the heart muscle is reduced or entirely blocked due to effects of cardiovascular disease (CVD) and clot formation. The subsequent transient loss of oxygen supply causes ischemia/reperfusion injury, which in turn leads to a large-scale loss of myocardial tissue followed by fibrosis and scarring. The normal healing response (6–8 weeks) involves an inflammation phase, followed by the formation of granulation tissue, and concludes with scar tissue formation [3,4]. This is partly due to ventricular remodeling caused by the replacement of the healthy myocardium with scar tissue, which is unable to withstand the pressure–volume load on the heart muscle. Heart muscle necrosis and scar formation may also lead to cardiac arrhythmias and sudden death [5]. Ultimately, the injury leads to heart failure, as characterized by the ineffectiveness of the heart to pump blood to the body.

Traditionally, it was understood that the adult mammalian heart lacks the intrinsic potential to regenerate, and adult mammalian cardiomyocytes that exit from the cell cycle cannot undergo

In Situ Tissue Regeneration. http://dx.doi.org/10.1016/B978-0-12-802225-2.00017-9

proliferation in the mature heart. However, recent multiple independent lines of evidence have demonstrated that nascent cardiomyogenesis is still possible in the postnatal and adult heart [6]. This, in turn, has ignited an intense interest by multiple research groups worldwide that are trying to understand the intrinsic regenerative capacity of the heart with the ultimate goal of manipulating it for the purpose of returning sufficient cardiac functional output and significantly improving the life quality and expectancy of the patient. Current strategies being undertaken for this purpose include: (1) inducing cardiomyocytes to proliferate and generate nascent functional contractile cells; (2) delivering stem cells or progenitor cells with the capacity to differentiate into either cardiomyocytes or vasculature; (3) activating the intrinsic population of cardiac progenitor cells or recruiting system stem cells to the myocardium; (4) transdifferentiating cardiac nonmyocytes into cardiomyocytes; and (5) using biomaterials to mechanically support the ailing myocardium [6].

In this chapter, we aim to describe specific state-of-the-art tools that are currently being developed for the purpose of inducing a robust cardiac regenerative response. We start by analyzing the current understanding concerning the intrinsic regenerative capacity of the mammalian heart, both under physiological and pathophysiological conditions and in the absence of any therapeutic interventions. We continue by describing various populations of both resident and remote progenitor cells that have been shown to have a therapeutic regenerative potential in the myocardium. We then describe protein therapeutics that have been used to achieve various proregenerative effects including vascularization, increased recruitment of cell progenitors to the myocardium, induction of proliferation in existing cardiomyocytes, and increased differentiation of progenitor cells. We also briefly discuss methods that focus on the delivery of such protein therapeutics to the in vivo environment. Additionally, we describe molecular pathways that, once manipulated through the use of gene overexpression, gene knockdown, microRNAs, or novel genetic engineering tools, can have a significant proregenerative effect on the myocardium. Finally, we discuss the induction of in situ cardiac regeneration via the epigenetic reprogramming of nonmyocytes into cardiomyocytes.

INTRINSIC REGENERATIVE CAPACITY OF THE MAMMALIAN HEART

The intrinsic regenerative capacity of the mammalian heart is small when compared to other organs, suggesting that injury to the myocardium can have long-term deleterious effects [7]. A single major myocardial infarction incident can quickly lead to the elimination of up to 25% of the 2–4 billion cardiomyocytes that comprise the contractile machinery of the left ventricle [8]. Additionally, aging or long-term cardiac overburden as a result of chronic disease, such as hypertension, can also induce a significant loss of cardiomyocytes [9,10]. Thus in the absence of a significant induction of regeneration in the injured, ailing, or aging myocardium, the end result is heart failure and eventual death. Importantly, though, by understanding the small but definitive innate capacity of the heart to regenerate as well as the mechanisms that prevent it from doing so robustly, we can engineer tools that would ultimately allow us to otherwise induce a strong in situ cardiac regeneration, potentially allowing the complete functional recovery of the organ.

During development, both the human and rodent fetal hearts grow through proliferation of diploid mononucleated cardiomyocytes. Cardiomyocytes in human hearts continue to proliferate for the first months following birth, while in rodents, cardiomyocytes withdraw from the cell cycle within the first few days. In both species, this is followed by a significant increase in size of the cell cycle-withdrawn cardiomyocytes. The majority of rodent cardiomyocytes are binucleated with diploid nuclei as a result of a final nuclear division without undergoing cytokinesis [11]. Human cardiomyocytes, however, remain mononucleated and tetraploid, as the final nuclear division is not followed by cytokinesis [12]. This usually changes upon exposure to a pathophysiology, such as hypertension or cardiac overload due to myocardial infarction. Although the human cardiomyocytes remain mononucleated, they initiate DNA synthesis without undergoing division or proliferation leading to polyploid cells [12].

Unlike the mammalian heart, the zebrafish heart is capable of complete regeneration following surgical amputation. Cardiac regeneration in the zebrafish is due to the induction of proliferation of preexisting cardiomyocytes and not due to the generation of new cells from a population of progenitor cells [13]. The capacity of preexisting cardiomyocytes to proliferate following injury is almost completely absent in the mammalian rodent heart, and a recent study has revealed that only ~0.008% of cardiomyocytes undergo division in the boundary region of the injured myocardium [14]. However, another possibility is that the rodent myocardium could regenerate due to the presence of a stem cell or progenitor cell population capable of differentiating into nascent cardiomyocytes. Studies have demonstrated that although such an effect does not take place during normal aging, following myocardial injury, a limited endogenous regenerative mechanism is indeed activated and is dependent on the presence of a progenitor cell population, rather than the induction of proliferation of preexisting cardiomyocytes [15]. Interestingly, a recent study has shown that the rodent heart can indeed completely regenerate following induction of injury similar to that performed in zebrafish, but this capacity is lost within the first 7 days following birth, suggesting that molecular events activated early in the mammalian life prevent future innate cardiac regeneration [16].

Human cardiac regeneration has been difficult to be confirmed definitively, due to the fact that macroscopically regeneration has not been observed, and at the cellular level, cardiomyocytes reinitiate DNA synthesis without undergoing cytokinesis following injury or overload. This translates into more or less the same number of cardiomyocytes but with increasing nuclear ploidy levels. When attempting to meticulously quantify the cardiomyocyte content in the human myocardium, it becomes apparent that the number of cardiomyocyte nuclei in the healthy heart is constant, and it only increases linearly following induction of hypertrophy, thus suggesting that human cardiac regeneration does occur at low levels due to pathological events [7,17,18]. A recent study elegantly attempted to accurately measure the amount of cardiomyocyte nuclei by taking advantage of the transient spike of atmospheric C^{14} concentrations, which occurred during the Cold War [19]. They determined that approximately 55% of human cardiomyocytes persist throughout the life of an individual, whereas 45% gets renewed.

Taken together, this evidence suggests that a baseline level of regeneration in the human heart does occur, although clearly this is insufficient to achieve full functional recovery to the organ due to the effects of aging, chronic disease, or injury. Moreover, it is not clear whether this is a result of proliferation of an existing population of cardiomyocytes or through the differentiation of a particular intrinsic stem cell or progenitor cell population. This, however, suggests that it is possible to engineer specific therapeutic tools that could either significantly enhance the existing baseline levels of human cardiac regeneration or inhibit the molecular mechanisms that prevent it from occurring more robustly with the ultimate goal of achieving complete organ regeneration and full functional recovery.

SYSTEMIC AND RESIDENT CARDIAC STEM OR PROGENITOR CELLS

Since the focus of this chapter is on in situ cardiac regeneration, we covered adult stem or progenitor cell populations that either reside within the heart itself or are found systemically and have been shown to have a cardiac proregenerative therapeutic potential. It is important, however, to mention that embryonic stem cells (ESCs) and induced pluripotent stem (iPS) cells also have a significant cardiomyogenic differentiation capacity, in addition to the fact that efficient protocols have been developed, allowing their differentiation into the various cardiac cell lineages efficiently [20]. This makes them an ideal cell source for the derivation of cell lineages necessary for cardiac tissue engineering applications and the development of robust models of human cardiac physiology and pathophysiology [21,22].

One of the earliest reports focusing on the utilization of adult stem cells for the treatment of myocardial infarction injury described the use of bone marrow-derived Lin^{-}/c-Kit^{+} cells [23]. Remarkably, within 9days following injection in the mouse infarcted myocardium, the authors reported ~70% regeneration. CD117, or c-Kit, is a receptor tyrosine kinase expressed on a variety of adult cells, including hematopoietic stem cells, endothelial cells, and immature cardiomyocytes [24]. Interestingly, subsequently other groups reported that they were unable to replicate these results, even though they tried to accurately emulate all aspects of the original study [25,26]. The same group also reported the derivation and characterization of a resident cardiac progenitor cell, which was also Lin^{-}/c-Kit^{+}. The cells were reported to be capable of self-renewal, clonogenic, multipotent, and capable of differentiating in vitro into cardiomyocytes, smooth muscle cells, and endothelial cells [27]. When injected in the infarcted mouse heart, c-Kit^{+} cardiac progenitor cells formed functional vasculature and differentiated into cardiomyocytes [27–29]. Once again, however, subsequent studies have questioned the original findings focusing on the in vitro capacity of the cardiac resident c-Kit^{+} cells to differentiate into cardiomyocytes and their potential to regenerate the adult infarcted myocardium [30,31]. What seems to be clear is that c-Kit^{+} cardiac progenitors are having a small but significant positive effect on the functional output of treated patients [Stem Cell Infusion in Patients with Ischemic Cardiomyopathy (SCIPIO) clinical trial] [32,33]; however, the mode of action is still unclear, especially since their capacity to form cardiomyocytes at the scale needed to regenerate the myocardium is contentious.

A second resident cardiac progenitor cell population was reported based on the expression of the mouse cell surface stem cell antigen 1 (Sca-1). Sca-1 encodes for an 18-kDa glycosyl phosphatidylinositol-anchored cell surface protein and is a common marker used to enrich for a population of adult mouse hematopoietic stem cells [34]. The authors demonstrate that Sca-1^{+} cardiac progenitors were able to differentiate into cardiomyocytes following exposure to 5-azacytidine in vitro. Moreover, following intravenous cell delivery postinduction of myocardial infarction in the murine heart, the authors determined that the cells migrated to the injured myocardium and differentiated into cardiomyocytes [35,36]. Importantly, there is no human homologue for the mouse Sca-1 cell surface marker, making it unlikely that this technique can be emulated for isolation of human cardiac progenitor cells.

The Abc transporter protein (Abcg2) allows cells to quickly export the DNA dye Hoechst, thus making them identifiable via flow cytometry. Its expression is a characteristic of a third resident cardiac progenitor cell population [37]. Further analysis has shown that a particular subgroup of the cardiac side population ($CD31^{-}$/Sca-1^{+}) is capable of differentiating into functional cardiomyocytes, and this process was dependent on their coupling to preexisting mature cardiomyocytes [38]. Finally, following intravenous injection in adult rats with induced myocardial infarcts, the cells migrated to the injured region and differentiated into cardiomyocytes, endothelial cells, and smooth muscle, thus demonstrating their in vivo cardiac regenerative potential [39].

The capacity of a subpopulation of cardiac cells to grow as self-adherent clusters following in vitro culture of human or mouse cardiac biopsies has also been used to derive the now called cardiosphere-derived cells. These cells were determined to be clonogenic, capable of self-renewal, and were shown to differentiate both in vitro and in vivo into cardiomyocytes and vascular cells [40,41]. Based on preclinical evidence demonstrating that cardiosphere-derived cells were capable of inducing scar reduction, increase in the amount of viable myocardium, and functional recovery boost, this work was translated into a clinical trial [CArdiosphere-Derived aUtologous StemCElls to reverse ventricUlar dySfunction (CADUCEUS)] demonstrating that intracoronary administration of these cells did not induce any significant safety issues. Moreover, the group reported a decrease in scar size, an increase in the amount of viable myocardium, and an improvement in cardiac function as far as 1 year post cell administration [42,43]. Interestingly though, a recent study has demonstrated that mouse cardiosphere-derived cells primarily resembled cardiac fibroblasts and lacked both cardiomyogenic and endothelial differentiation potential, a finding that contradicts previous reports [44].

During development, the epicardium migrates to the surface of the developing myocardium and ultimately covers the entire heart. It forms a uniform epithelial layer, and some of its cells undergo an epithelial-to-mesenchymal transition, becoming a population of epicardium-derived cells (EPDCs), which, in turn, contribute to the vascular smooth muscle and fibroblastic component of the myocardium [45]. It is believed that EPDCs also contribute to the endothelial and cardiomyocyte cell lineages, although this hypothesis is still contested. EPDCs can be tracked via the expression of proteins Wt1, Tbx18, Tcf21, and Raldh2. In the adult organism, the epicardium becomes dormant and does not seem to have an active role in the physiology of the heart. Interestingly, following myocardial infarction injury, the epicardium is quickly reactivated in a manner that resembles its embryonic origins, and it proceeds to expand and cover the exposed injured myocardium [46]. $Wt1^+$ EPDCs emerge from the reactivated epicardium and are primarily responsible for providing fibroblasts to the injured myocardium, although it has been shown that these cells are capable of also differentiating into vasculature and de novo cardiomyocytes [47,48]. This finding, however, has been questioned by another study, which has reported that although the epicardium does not contribute to cardiomyocytes or endothelial cells following myocardial infarction injury, it does secrete proangiogenic paracrine signals [49]. It is thus hypothesized that the regenerative induction capacity of the reactivated epicardium depends on the epicardial synthesis of retinoic acid, which, in turn, has a robust proregenerative effect in the neonatal mouse myocardium and the adult zebrafish myocardium, an effect lost in the adult mammalian heart [45].

Endothelial progenitor cells (EPCs) are characterized based on the expression of the cell surface markers CD34, CD133, and KDR, and their main role in the adult is reendothelialization and neovascularization [50]. In one of the first reports describing the utilization of EPCs for the treatment of myocardial infarction injury ex vivo, expanded EPCs accumulated in the injured region of the rat myocardium and participated in the process of neovascularization that ultimately induced a significant functional recovery of the injured myocardium [51]. Similar results were also reported when human EPCs were utilized in a porcine model of myocardial infarction injury. The authors reported significant functional improvement, which they attributed to an increase in regional blood flow and a higher capillary density at the site of injury [52]. Based on this preliminary information, a clinical study was established to examine the potential therapeutic effect of human EPCs [Transplantation of progenitor cells and regeneration enhancement in acute myocardial infarction (TOPCARE-AMI)]. The authors reported that within 4 months, EPC transplantation resulted in a significant increase in cardiac functional output as well as an increase in cardiomyocyte cell viability when compared to the control group [53].

Mesenchymal stem cells (MSCs) are another adult stem cell population, which has been widely investigated for its ability to induce regeneration in the myocardium. The International Society of

Stem Cell Research defines MSCs as cells that (1) adhere to plastic in standard culture conditions; (2) express the cell surface markers CD73, CD90, and CD105 and do not express CD34, CD45, HLA-DR, CD14 or CD11b, CD79a, or CD19; and (3) are able to differentiate into osteocytes, adipocytes, and chondrocytes [54]. The cells reside in a variety of adult tissues; however, their primary source of isolation for the purpose of regenerative applications has been bone marrow, adipose tissue, and umbilical cord [55]. There has been a significant amount of literature reports describing the pro-regenerative inductive effect MSCs have on the injured myocardium, and this effect can be attributed to a variety of factors, including the reduction of fibrotic tissue formation, the stimulation of angiogenesis, and through the activation of endogenous cardiac stem cells, ultimately leading to a restoration of cardiac functional output [55]. Preliminary data focusing on MSC utilization for regenerative therapy applications has been extremely promising, and the cells have been tested in different clinical trials: PROMETHEUS [56], AC-HFT [57], and POSEIDON [58]. In general, it has been determined that MSCs are safe to use in therapeutic applications and induced a small but significant functional recovery of the ailing heart.

Heart failure due to myocardial infarction injury is caused due to the loss of roughly 25% of ventricular cardiomyocytes (~10^9 cells) [59]. Complete regeneration and functional recovery would then mean the complete replacement and adequate distribution of these cells within the existing myocardium [8,59]. It is also important to consider that (1) the efficiency of the aforementioned populations of stem cells or progenitor cells to differentiate into functional cardiomyocytes is very small; and (2) their survival/engraftment in the myocardium following intracoronary or intramuscular injection is also very low (2–3% at 1 month postinjection [60]). How is it possible to reconcile the low cardiomyocyte differentiation potential and long-term engraftment capacity with the significant functional improvement observed following delivery of these cells in the ailing heart?

It has been hypothesized that the proregenerative therapeutic effect and functional output recovery observed following delivery of some of the stem or progenitor cells described above is due to the "paracrine effect": spatiotemporal secretion of protein ligands that, in turn, promote cardiac repair and regeneration. This may act in a variety of ways, including the enhancement of cardiomyocyte survival, induction of existing cardiomyocyte proliferation, promotion of vascularization, activation of the resident progenitor cell populations, and rearrangement of the extracellular matrix component [61]. Thus it is conceivable that by understanding the exact nature of the molecular signals secreted by the cells and which are inducing myocardial regeneration and functional recovery, we will be able to emulate and even significantly enhance their proregenerative effect by engineering their controlled spatiotemporal delivery in the ailing myocardium. In the next section, we focus on particular protein ligands and their capacity to induce significant regeneration in the myocardium.

PROTEIN LIGANDS FOR INDUCING CARDIAC REGENERATION

The in vivo delivery of protein ligands as therapeutic tools can directly activate particular signaling pathways, which, in turn, may induce a significant regenerative effect. Ultimately, protein ligand-induced organ regeneration may improve clinical function to a sufficient degree that would significantly improve the life quality of the patient. In regard to the ailing myocardium, protein ligands can induce a significant amount of functional recovery through four main mechanisms: (1) induction of in situ angiogenesis and revascularization of the organ; (2) increased recruitment of stem cells or progenitor cells to the myocardium; (3) prevention of cell death or induction of proliferation in existing populations of cardiomyocytes; and (4) increased growth and induction of differentiation of resident stem cell or progenitor cells. In this section, we aim to describe protein ligands that have been demonstrated to have such therapeutic effects when delivered to the myocardium (see Fig. 17.1 and Table 17.1).

Vascular endothelial growth factor (**VEGF**) is a survival factor for endothelial cells; it activates growth in endothelial cells in vitro and induces a potent angiogenic response in vivo. Atherosclerosis leads to coronary vessel occlusion and damage of the myocardial microvasculature [68]. It is thus conceivable that neovascularization in the myocardium significantly increases the cardiac perfusion volume, which, in turn, preserves functional output [69]. VEGF was utilized to treat the ischemic myocardium of either dogs or pigs, and the degree of collateral blood supply was measured. It was determined that VEGF administration significantly improved the level of collateral blood supply, which, in turn, improved cardiac function [70,71].

Interestingly, when delivered in vivo, VEGF is associated with the induction of nitric oxide-mediated hypotension, which, in turn, limits the amount that can be safely used for therapeutic purposes. When used at the maximum allowed dose, VEGF did not induce a sufficient level of cardiac output due to an increase of collateral blood supply [72–74]. Additionally, uncontrolled VEGF delivery produces unstable and leaky blood vessels due to the fact that VEGF is only one of the components active during the process of neovascularization, and its activity must usually be eventually countered by antiangiogenic signals that help induce neo-vessel maturation [74].

The **stromal cell-derived factor 1 alpha** (**SDF-1α** or **CXCL12**) is a secreted small protein ligand and chemoattractant for hematopoietic stem cells ($CD34^+$) and EPCs [75,76]. SDF1α expression levels are upregulated in the myocardium following myocardial infarction injury; however, the durations of temporal upregulation and ligand concentration are not sufficient to induce the level of neovascularization needed to produce a significant improvement in functional cardiac output [77]. Forced overexpression of SDF1α via transplantation of genetically engineered fibroblasts in the infarcted myocardium induced a significant increase in vasculature density and cardiac function [78]. To ensure long-term delivery of an active protease-resistant variant of SDF1α, Segers et al. genetically engineered the protein ligand and delivered it in the ischemic myocardium with self-assembling peptide nanofibers, ultimately demonstrating increased recruitment of $CXCR4^+$/c-Kit^+ stem cells, higher coronary vessel density, and improvement of cardiac function [79].

The **granulocyte-colony stimulating factor** (**G-CSF**) is also a small protein ligand, which stimulates progenitor cells residing in the bone marrow to differentiate into granulocytes and activates mobilization of hematopoietic stem cells in the bloodstream [80,81]. Previously, the same protein ligand had been approved by the US Food and Drug Administration for clinical trial application in other disease phenotypes. As it was previously demonstrated that bone marrow c-Kit^+ progenitor cells are capable of significant heart regeneration following myocardial infarction injury, G-CSF was tested for its capacity to regenerate the human infarcted heart in clinical trials [82,83]. Although no significant functional improvement was measured at the completion of these studies, additional meta-analysis of the acquired data suggested that G-CSF was indeed capable of inducing a significant functional improvement in the cohort of patients where it was administered early following the infarction injury [84]. It is hypothesized that since the cardiomyocyte differentiation potential of c-Kit^+ hematopoietic progenitor cells is debatable, the activity of G-CSF could be attributed to its capacity to protect cardiomyocytes from apoptosis due to ischemia/reperfusion injury [85].

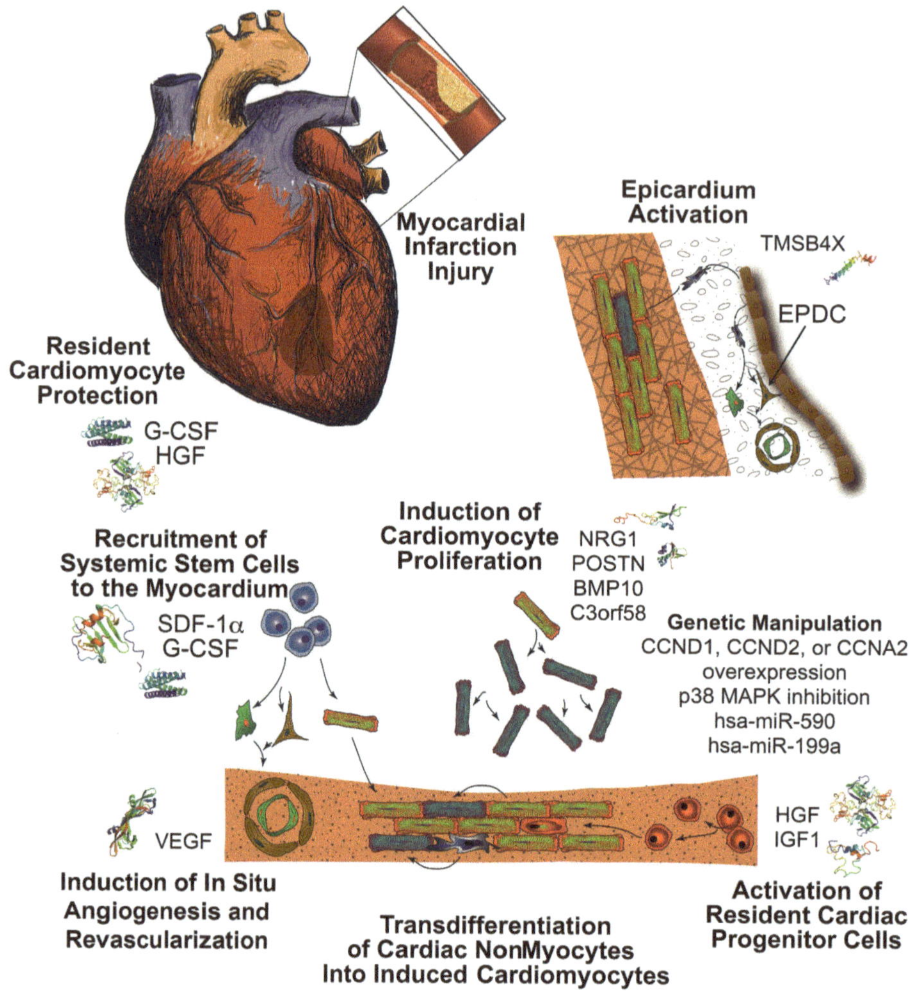

FIGURE 17.1 Induction of in situ cardiac regeneration via protein ligand delivery or genetic manipulation of signaling pathways.

Myocardial infarction injury occurs when the blood supply to the heart muscle is reduced or entirely blocked due to effects of cardiovascular disease and clot formation. The subsequent transient loss of oxygen supply causes ischemia/reperfusion injury, which leads to a large-scale loss of myocardial tissue followed by fibrosis and scarring. Traditionally, it was understood that the adult mammalian heart lacks the intrinsic potential to regenerate; however, recent reports have demonstrated that cardiac regeneration is still possible in the postnatal and adult heart. Current strategies undertaken focus on the controlled delivery of protein ligands or the genetic manipulation of intrinsic cardiac cells in order to induce a robust regenerative response, which would ultimately significantly improve the functional output of the heart. Cardiac regeneration can be achieved via multiple mechanisms of action, including: (1) protection of existing cardiomyocytes from undergoing apoptosis or necrosis; (2) protein ligand-based recruitment of systemic stem cells to the injured myocardium, where they can differentiate into cardiomyocytes or vascular cells; (3) induction of in situ angiogenesis and

The **hepatocyte growth factor** (**HGF**) is a protein ligand that regulates cell growth and proliferation through receptor kinase activating signaling (c-Met receptor). HGF is capable of inducing proliferation in hepatocytes, and it also protects cells from undergoing apoptosis [69,86,87]. Following delivery of recombinant HGF in the infarcted rat myocardium, it was determined that the size of the infarct area was reduced, and cardiomyocyte apoptosis was suppressed, possibly through an induced increase in the expression of Bcl-xL by the affected cardiomyocytes [88]. An alternative mechanism of action for HGF was also proposed following observations that it may also act by activating mobilization of resident cardiac stem cells. In particular, it was hypothesized that resident progenitor cells express on their surface the c-Met receptor and that HGF itself may act by mobilizing them to the site of injury [89]. In that study, HGF was delivered in conjunction with IGF1, whose role was to induce survival and proliferation in the mobilized progenitor cells. The authors of the particular study reported that following the delivery of the two growth factors, they observed nascent myocardium formation, which was vascularized and matured over time, ultimately increasing the survival of the animals [89]. Clearly though, this dual growth factor combination therapy did not delineate the exact mechanism of action of each of the two delivered growth factors.

Neuregulin 1 (**NRG1**) is a member of the epidermal growth factor family of receptor tyrosine kinase protein ligands (ERBB2, ERBB3, ERBB4), and its activity includes the activation of proliferation, survival, and differentiation of cells in many tissue types, including epithelium, neurons, and myocytes [90]. NRG1 is expressed by endothelial cells in the adult heart, and its receptors (ERBB2, ERBB4) are expressed on cardiomyocytes. In vitro NRG-1 has been shown to induce induction of cardiomyocyte survival and hypertrophy. It also modulates the level of cardiomyocyte contractility and electromechanical coupling [90]. In vivo NRG1 signaling improves cardiac function in various models of cardiomyopathies including ischemic, toxic, and dilated [90]. In 2009, Bersell et al. clearly demonstrated that NRG1 signaling can induce myocardial regeneration and improve functional cardiac output by specifically inducing cardiomyocyte division through the ERBB4 receptor [91]. Two more recent reports suggested that NRG1 administration in the mouse neonatal heart is very effective in inducing cardiomyocyte proliferation and protection against apoptosis via the ERBB2 receptor only if given immediately following cryoinjury induction [92,93]. Moreover, ERBB2 cardiomyocyte expression gradually decreases, correlating with the diminished response of cardiomyocytes to NRG1 signaling. Interestingly, overexpression of the ERBB2 receptor in adult cardiomyocytes was sufficient in inducing proliferation and reactivating the regenerative potential only previously observed in the neonatal heart [92].

◀ revascularization; (4) activation of resident cardiac stem cells followed by a transient proliferation and differentiation into cardiomyocytes or vascular cells; (5) induction of proliferation of preexisting cardiomyocytes; (6) activation of the epicardium, derivation of epicardium-derived progenitor cells (EPDCs) and their subsequent differentiation into fibroblasts, vascular cells, and cardiomyocytes; and (7) transdifferentiation of resident non-myocytes into cardiomyocytes. Protein ligands that have been shown to have a proregenerative cardiac effect include: granulocyte colony stimulating factor (G-CSF), stromal cell-derived factor 1 alpha (SDF1α), vascular endothelial growth factor (VEGF), hepatocyte growth factor (HGF), neuregulin 1 (NRG1), Periostin (POSTN), bone morphogenic protein 10 (BMP10), C3orf58, thymosin β4 (TMSB4X), and insulin-like growth factor 1 (IGF1). Genes that, when overexpressed, have been shown to induce cardiomyocyte proliferation include: cyclin D1 (CCND1), cyclin D2 (CCND2), and cyclin A2 (CCNA2). Delivery of microRNA mimics hsa-miR-590, and hsa-miR-199a and inhibition of p38 MAPK has also been shown to induce cardiomyocyte proliferation.

Table 17.1 Protein Ligands for Cardiac Regeneration

Therapeutic Protein Ligand	Delivery Method	Animal Model Used	Comments and Observations	References
Neuregulin 1 (NRG1)	Protein ligand encapsulation in a hyaluronic acid (HA) hydrogel. Peri-infarct intramyocardial injections.	Mouse (2-month-old): left anterior descending coronary artery ligation. Four experimental groups: Saline only, NRG1 only, HA only, NRG1+HA.	• Detection of cardiomyocyte proliferation in the NRG1 + HA treated group: $H3P^+$ and $Ki67^+$ cells in histological heart sections • Cardioprotection: activated caspase-3 is significantly lower in the NRG1 + HA group (NRG1 + HA: 1.5±0.29 cells, NRG1: 3.5±0.29 cells, HA: 6.2±0.97 cells, Saline: 5.6±0.8 cells), number of positive cells per 10×high-powered field • LVEF: significantly greater in the NRG1 + HA treated animals (NRG1 + HA: 37.5±3.6%, NRG1: 20.1±4.7%, HA: 17.2±3.7%, Saline: 20.2±3.2%) • Left ventricular chamber area: significantly lower in the NRG1 + HA group (NRG1 + HA: 0.18±0.02 cm^2, NRG1: 0.33±0.04 cm^2, HA: 0.26±0.05 cm^2, Saline: 0.29±0.02 cm^2) • Myocardium border zone thickness is significantly higher in the NRG1 + HA group (NRG1 + HA: 0.65±0.07 mm, NRG1: 0.30±0.05 mm, HA: 0.26±0.05 mm, Saline: 0.27±0.04 mm)	A bioengineered hydrogel system enables targeted and sustained intra-myocardial delivery of neuregulin, activating the cardiomyocyte cell cycle, and enhancing ventricular function in a murine model of ischemic cardiomyopathy [62]
Neuregulin 1 (NRG1) and fibroblast growth factor 1 (FGF1)	Intramyocardial injection of microparticles (MP) loaded with FGF1 and NRG1.	Rat (female Sprague–Dawley): permanent left anterior descending coronary artery occlusion. 4 experimental groups: control (MP only), NGR1–MP, FGF1–MP, and NGR1/FGF1–MP.	• LVEF: Significantly greater in the FGF1/NRG1 treated group (FGF1/NRG1: 13.0±1.9%, control: 1.1±3.6%) • Significant improvement in LVED volume and LVES volume, as well as LV mass in FGF1/NRG1 group • Significant reduction in infarct size in FGF1/NRG1 treated group as compared to control (FGF1/NRG1: 11.7±3.8%, control: 16.8±2.8%) • Significant increased LV thickness in FGF1/NRG1 treated group (FGF1/NRG1: 1.93±0.14 mm, control: 1.55±0.14 mm) • Significant increase: SMA^+ vessel density in FGF1/NRG1 treated group • Significant increase in capillaries found in the infarct and peri-infarct zone in FGF1/NRG1 treated group	Controlled delivery of FGF-1 and NRG1 from biodegradable microparticles promotes cardiac repair in a rat myocardial infarction model through activation of endogenous regeneration [63]

Periostin (POSTN)	Intrapericardial injection of drug-eluting hydrogel (recombinant POSTN delivered within gelfoam hydrogel).	Pig (female Yorkshire pig): left anterior descending coronary artery occlusion. Two experimental groups: Gelfoam loaded with and without POSTN.	• Cardiomyocyte proliferation in the POSTN group: fivefold PCNA$^+$ cardiomyocyte increase over control and 6.5-fold H3P$^+$ cardiomyocyte increase • Higher number of CD31$^+$ vessels within the border zone in POSTN-treated animals over control • No significant difference in the mitotic activity of nonmyocytes • No difference in the degree of inflammation	Intrapericardial delivery of gel foam enables the targeted delivery of POSTN peptide after myocardial infarction by inducing fibrin clot formation [64]
Insulin-like growth factor (IGF1) and hepatocyte growth factor (HGF)	NOGA catheter-guided intramyocardial injection of IGF-1/HGF incorporated in UPy hydrogel.	Pig (female Dalland Landrace pigs): Intracoronary occlusion of the left circumflex followed by reperfusion. Experimental groups: IGF-1/HGF in 0.9% saline, IGF-1/HGF in UPy hydrogel, and UPy hydrogel (control).	• Significant increase in c-kit$^+$ epCSC (endogenous porcine cardiac stem cells) number in UPy + IGF1 + HGF (0.24 ± 0.06%) compared to IGF1 + HGF (0.14 ± 0.06) and control (0.12 ± 0.01%) • Increase in the number of capillaries in the infarct border zone in UPy + IGF1 + HGF (8.6 ± 0.9 per 0.2 mm^2) versus IGF1 + HGF (7.8 ± 0.9 per 0.2 mm^2) versus control (6.3 ± 0.8 per 0.2 mm^2) • Significant improvement of the LVED volumes relative to baseline in UPy + IGF1 + HGF (−1.1 ± 2.3) compared to IGF1 + HGF (−10.3 ± 9.9) and control (−9.5 ± 4.6 mL) • Reduction is fibrosis in UPy + IGF1 + HGF and IGF1 + HGF compared to control • Attenuated cardiomyocyte hypertrophy in UPy + IGF1 + HGF and IGF1 + HGF compared to control	Sustained delivery of IGF1/HGF stimulates endogenous cardiac repair in the chronic infarcted pig heart [65]

Continued

Table 17.1 Protein Ligands for Cardiac Regeneration—cont'd

Therapeutic Protein Ligand	Delivery Method	Animal Model Used	Comments and Observations	References
Vascular endothelium growth factor (VEGF)	Epicardial delivery system of VEGF and cardiac stem cells using a poly(L-lactic acid) (PLLA) mat.	Rat (10-week-old male Sprague–Dawley rats): Acute myocardium infarction. Ligation of the proximal left anterior descending coronary artery. Four experimental groups: control (no implantation), mat (PLLA mat only), mat+VEGF (VEGF-loaded PLLA mat), and mat+VEGF+CSC (implanted VEGF-loaded PLLA mat populated with c-Kit$^+$ cardiac stem cells).	• LV wall thickness preserved in treated hearts (Mat+VEGF+CSC: 0.6±0.1 mm, Mat+PLLA: 0.3±0.1 mm, control: 0.3±0.1 mm) • Reduced scar in treated hearts (Mat+VEGF+CSC: 18.3±3.8%, Mat+PLLA: 26±2.2%, control: 24.3±3.7%) • EF and FS significantly higher in treated hearts (Mat+VEGF+CSC: 47.4±2.5% and 21.9±1.4%, Mat+PLLA: 38.0±3.7% and 16.0±1.7%) • Significant increase in the density of SMA$^+$ blood vessels in treated group (Mat+VEGF+CSC: 38.6±3.8/mm^2, Mat+PLLA: 26.0±2.8/mm^2) • PCNA$^+$ proliferating cardiomyocytes (Mat+VEGF+CSC: 18.6±2.1/mm^2, Mat+PLLA: 6.7±1.8/mm^2, control: 7.2±1.8/mm^2)	Epicardial delivery of VEGF and cardiac stem cells guided by 3-D PLLA mat enhancing cardiac regeneration and angiogenesis in acute myocardial infarction [66]
VEGF and HGF	Bioactive hydrogels with a protease-degradable cross-linker loaded with HGF and VEGF.	Rat (adult Sprague–Dawley rats): Either subjected to sham surgery or induction of myocardial infarction via ischemia/reperfusion (IR) surgery. Experimental groups: untreated animals, VEGF, HGF, VEGF+HGF, PEG, PEG+VEGF, PEG+HGF, and PEG+VEGF+HGF.	• Significant increase in the level of vascularization in treated animals (PEG+VEGF+HGF: 16.3±0.6 vessels/mm^2, control: 8.3±0.5 vessels/mm^2) • Significant decrease in the size of the fibrotic area (PEG+VEGF+HGF: 13.9±3.5%, control: 41.5±3.3%) • Significant increase in c-Kit$^+$ cells in treated animals (PEG+VEGF+HGF: 10.6 c-Kit$^+$/1000 nuclei, control: 3.1 c-Kit$^+$/1000 nuclei) • Significant improvement in LVED in PEG+VEGF+HGF treated animals • Significant improvement in LVED pressure, LVES volume, and LVED volume in PEG+VEGF+HGF	Dual delivery of hepatocyte and vascular endothelial growth factors via a protease-degradable hydrogel improves cardiac function in rats [67]

LVEF, *left ventricular ejection fraction;* LVED, *left ventricular end diastolic;* LVES, *left ventricular end systolic;* LV, *left ventricular;* PLLA, *poly-L-lactic acid;* EF, *ejection fraction;* FS, *functional shortening;* Ki67, *nuclear protein associated with cellular proliferation;* PCNA, *proliferating cell nuclear antigen. Marks proliferating cells, H3P—phospho-histone H3, marks cells undergoing the G2/M transition.*

Periostin (POSTN) is a small extracellular matrix protein expressed by cardiac fibroblasts, and it is active both during cardiac development and during the epithelial-to-mesenchymal transition process [69,94]. Although POSTN expression levels are low in the adult heart, its expression is quickly upregulated following myocardial infarction injury. Its main function is the induction of remodeling of extracellular matrix [94]. When used in a model of myocardial infarction injury, POSTN induced cardiomyocyte cell cycle reentry and mitosis, which ultimately improved the degree of ventricular remodeling, improved myocardial function, reduced fibrosis and infarct size, and increased angiogenesis [95]. This finding, however, has come into question by a subsequent study where it was reported that POSTN does not stimulate DNA synthesis, mitosis, or cytokinesis of cardiomyocytes in vitro or in vivo and ultimately had no obvious effect on myocardial regeneration [96].

Bone morphogenetic proteins belong to the transforming growth factor beta (TGF-β) superfamily of protein ligands and play important roles during development by regulating morphogenesis of a variety of organs, including the eye, the heart, and skin. **Bone morphogenic protein 10** (BMP10) is a 48-KDa protein ligand with a diverse range of functions during development [97]. BMP10 is essential in regulating cardiac growth, embryonic survival, and chamber maturation, and once silenced in mice, it reduces embryonic cardiomyocyte proliferative activity [98]. Sun et al. investigated the cardiac regenerative capacity of BMP10. Following exposure to BMP10, both neonatal and adult rat cardiomyocytes activated DNA synthesis and decreased the cell cycle inhibitor p57. This ultimately translated into cardiomyocyte mitosis and cytokinesis [97]. Importantly, the therapeutic capacity of BMP10 to treat the in vivo infarcted myocardium still needs to be determined.

C3orf58 is a 49.5-kDa protein ligand that was recently identified as a novel paracrine factor secreted by MSCs [99]. When cardiomyocytes are exposed to C3orf58 both in vitro and in vivo, they are protected from apoptosis via activation of protein kinase C epsilon [100]. Moreover, C3orf58 treated neonatal cardiomyocytes exhibit a 60% increase in DNA synthesis, which translates to a 50–100% increase in the number of cardiomyocytes in the mitotic and cytokinesis phases [99]. Interestingly, when overexpressed in vivo, C3orf58 results in an increased amount of DNA synthesis and cytokinesis in cardiomyocytes via modulation of the phosphoinositide 3-kinase–protein kinase B–cycle-dependent kinase 7 pathway [99].

Growth differentiation factor 11 (GDF11) or BMP11 is another member of the TGF-β superfamily of protein ligands that was recently identified as being responsible for the reversal of age-related cardiac hypertrophy using a model of heterochronic parabiosis [101]. The authors determined that blood circulation parabiosis led to a reversal of cardiac myocyte hypertrophy and that this reduced cardiomyocyte size and translated into a reduction in global cardiac mass. Via proteomic analysis, the authors identified the GDF11 protein ligand as the main mediator of systemic antihypertrophic activity [101]. No reports have yet been made concerning the capacity of GDF11 to induce regeneration of the injured myocardium.

Thymosin β4 (TMSB4X) is a 43-amino acid (5-kDa) G-actin-sequestering polypeptide expressed in the embryonic heart, able to stimulate in vitro cardiomyocyte migration and increase cardiac function while promoting the survival of adult cardiomyocytes in vivo [102]. It was demonstrated that TMSB4X was capable of stimulating outgrowth in quiescent adult epicardial explants and triggering proliferation and differentiation of cardiac fibroblasts, smooth muscle, and endothelial cells, concluding that it is a potent signal for the induction of neovascularization in the injured myocardium [47]. It was then demonstrated that systemic administration of TMSB4X in addition to stimulating myocardial neovascularization was also capable of inhibiting cardiomyocyte cell death and activating a resident stem cell population, which ultimately led to both myocardial and vascular regeneration [103]. A subsequent study suggested that priming the myocardium with TMSB4X activates a population of $Wt1^+$ epicardium-derived progenitor cells, which differentiate into nascent cardiomyocytes without fusing with existing cells [48]. The most recent finding, however, has been brought into question by another study, which demonstrated that although TMSB4X treatment induces an increase in the epicardial thickness and coronary capillary density of the infarcted mouse myocardium, it does not induce differentiation of the epicardium-derived progenitor cells into cardiomyocytes [49]. It is thus important to consider that for successful translation to clinical application of a protein ligand such as TMSB4X, a clearly defined primary mechanism of action and exact definition of its pharmacokinetic properties is necessary for the development of the protein as a therapeutic tool.

Insulin-like growth factor 1 (IGF1) is a secreted protein ligand that functions through a receptor tyrosine kinase signaling mechanism. In particular, IGF1 activates the AKT signaling pathway, which induces cellular growth and proliferation while inhibiting cellular apoptosis. It was previously demonstrated that IGF1 induced cardiac progenitor cell division ($c\text{-}Kit^+$), upregulation of telomerase activity, and inhibition of progenitor cell aging [104]. Delivery in the infarcted rat myocardium of IGF1 in conjunction with $c\text{-}Kit^+$ cardiac progenitor cells significantly increased the level of myocardial regeneration as related to progenitors or IGF1 alone, demonstrating its capacity to further activate and mobilize the cell progenitors [105].

PROTEIN DELIVERY SYSTEMS FOR IN SITU CARDIAC REGENERATION

Peptide-based stimulation of in vivo cardiac regeneration requires accurate spatiotemporal release kinetics of the protein ligand in order to minimize the required therapeutic dose and potential off-target undesirable effects. In general, proteins are considered as poor therapeutic candidates due to their decreased oral bioavailability and lack of long-term stability [106]. Drug delivery systems are designed after taking into consideration the characteristics of the drug being delivered, the organ system in which it is administered, and the disease being treated. Proteins are labile molecules with primary, secondary, tertiary, and sometimes quaternary structures. Peptide bioactivity depends on the macromolecule being properly folded; however, proper protein folding can be easily destabilized, leading to protein denaturation due to external physical factors, including temperature changes, pH changes, pressure changes, the presence of metal ions and denaturing molecules, and the presence of proteases that can readily degrade the therapeutic peptides. Thus the ideal protein delivery system for in situ cardiac regeneration would warrant the delivery of a properly folded peptide (1) for the appropriate amount of time; (2) at the right concentration; and (3) at the appropriate location in order to induce maximal organ regeneration and sufficient cardiac functional output recovery. In this section, we will discuss particular state-of-the-art methods used to deliver therapeutic peptides in vivo.

A novel and elegant protein delivery system used is based on the principle of protease-demanded liberation whose premise is the tethering of the growth factors to be delivered on the hydrogel backbone via a protease cleavable tether. Salimath et al. used a polyethylene glycol hydrogel (PEG) on which they tethered VEGF, HGF, and RGD (arginylglycylaspartic acid) via a protease-degradable peptide sequence. Hydrogel injections were performed into the perimeter of the ischemic zone immediately after ischemia/reperfusion injury in rat hearts [67]. The authors reported a significant increase in angiogenesis and stem cell recruitment while not detecting any acute effects as a result of the biomaterial injection itself.

Moreover, they reported a decrease in the level of fibrosis, and this effect was significantly higher when dual growth factor delivery was performed, ultimately translating to improved functional cardiac output.

In a similar approach, Zhang et al. engineered a PEGylated fibrin hydrogel on which they attached, through covalent bonding, mouse recombinant SDF-1α, which is a systemic c-Kit$^+$ stem cell-mobilizing peptide. Following induction of hydrogel polymerization, they placed the fibrin patch containing the growth factor on the surface of the infarcted mouse myocardium. They detected a significant increase in the cardiac recruitment of c-Kit$^+$ cells within 2 weeks post myocardial infarction injury as compared to untreated animals. SDF-1α release was sustained for up to 28 days postdelivery, correlating to increased levels of stem cell homing and significant left ventricular functional recovery [107].

Cohen et al. attempted to circumvent issues associated with daily NRG1β systemic infusions and off-target exposure by encapsulating the growth factor in a hydrogel system delivered directly into the infarcted myocardium [62]. The NRG1β-containing hydrogel was delivered via intramyocardial injections in the infarcted mouse myocardium. NRG1β was detected in myocardium within 6 days following delivery injection without evidence of off-target exposure. Within 2 weeks, the treated animal group exhibited significant functional improvement, as determined by left ventricular ejection fraction and increased border zone thickness [62].

Rubinov et al. attempted to sequentially deliver in the infarcted rat myocardium IGF1 followed by HGF using an injectable affinity-binding alginate biomaterial. First, they determined that the hydrogel protected the delivered growth factors from proteolysis. Intramyocardial injection of the growth factor-loaded alginate hydrogel preserved scar thickness, reduced infarct enlargement, and reduced fibrosis. This was concurrent with increased neovascularization. Finally, they reported detection of cardiomyocyte cell cycle reentry and increased incidence of GATA4 positive cell clusters, indicative of neomuscularization [108].

TMSB4X was another therapeutic protein ligand that was delivered via a controlled release system. Chiu et al. used a collagen–chitosan controlled release hydrogel system to deliver TMSB4X either subcutaneously or within the infarcted myocardium. When delivered subcutaneously, they detected significant vascularization when compared to protein peptide delivered alone. Importantly, when delivered in the infarcted rat myocardium, the authors reported improved angiogenesis, reduced tissue loss, and retained left ventricular wall thickness [109].

In order to ensure a minimally invasive delivery mechanism, Bastings et al. used a catheter to deliver a pH responsive liquid, which within the physiological pH range, forms a hydrogel as it comes into contact with tissue. The hydrogel was loaded with HGF and IGF1 and injected in the infarcted porcine myocardium, ultimately demonstrating hydrogel biocompatibility and a reduction of scar formation [110].

The studies described previously primarily focused on the delivery of particular growth factors to the infarcted myocardium within a hydrogel matrix and via either intramyocardial or intracoronary injections. Alternatively, protein ligands could be delivered systemically via a delivery vehicle, which would target, carry, and unload them within the injured, where they could activate their respective regenerative pathways. Formiga et al. prepared microparticles using a multiple emulsion solvent evaporation technique and loaded them with NRG1 and fibroblast growth factor 1 (FGF1). The growth factor-loaded microparticles were subsequently injected in the peri-infarct zone of infarcted rat hearts. The microparticles released the two growth factors in a temporally sustained manner, and 3 months postdelivery, the authors detected a significant improvement in cardiac function, smaller infarct size, and induction of revascularization [63].

Scott et al. took advantage of the fact that following myocardial infarction injury, the local vascular endothelium upregulates expression of the cell surface marker P-Selectin. The authors conjugated anti-P-Selectin antibodies on liposomes loaded with the provascularization growth factor VEGF. They demonstrated that their targeting system induced a significant increase in cardiac function and vasculature content in a rat model of myocardial infarction injury, which led to a significant functional improvement of cardiac output. Interestingly, no significant improvement was detected in animals treated with systemically delivered VEGF or nontargeted VEGF-loaded liposomes, suggesting that the targeting device itself is essential for the successful delivery of VEGF [111].

In a more recent elegant study, Nguyen et al. took advantage of the fact that following myocardial infarction injury, the inflammatory response that ensues induces the expression of matrix metalloproteinase proteases for extracellular matrix reorganization. The authors designed a micellar vehicle containing a matrix metalloproteinase-targeting peptide. They first demonstrated using an in vitro assay of matrix metalloproteinase overexpression that the targeting peptide showed 10-fold higher binding efficiency to the cells overexpressing the enzyme. When delivered systemically in a mouse model of myocardial infarction injury, the micelles were detected with macrophages infiltrating the injury site. Although no protein peptide was loaded in the micelles, this is a proof-of-principle study demonstrating a robust delivery system able to target the injury site during the inflammation period [112].

VEGF-A had previously been identified as being sufficient to drive vascular specification of Isl1$^+$ cardiac progenitor cells away from the cardiomyocyte or smooth muscle cell lineages [113]. However, when used therapeutically, VEGF-A failed to achieve consistent results, and this was attributed to a variety of possible factors, including the very short half-life of VEGF-A in plasma, the lack of a controlled release vehicle, and possible off-target effects as a result of the systemic delivery methods used. Thus Zangi et al. examined the capacity of messenger RNA (mRNA) encoding for VEGF-A to induce a proregenerative effect while avoiding the issues, which aroused as a result of systemic growth factor delivery [114]. Since mRNA can induce activation of the innate immunity through recognition of toll-like receptors, they generated a modified RNA molecule, which has been shown to both reduce activation of the innate immunity and increase efficiency of mRNA translation [115,116]. Following intramyocardial injection of the modified mRNA in the infarcted myocardium, they detected a significant improvement in formation of functional vasculature in the peri-infarct region associated specifically with altered activity of epicardial-derived progenitor cells. Importantly, the authors stated that (1) the unique kinetics of modified mRNA delivery were required to obtain the particular therapeutic benefit, permitting pulse-like VEGF-A delivery at precisely the time that myocardial infarction injury activated the Wt1$^+$ epicardial-derived progenitor cells; and (2) the transient nature of the delivery was crucial, as sustained VEGF-A delivery by naked plasmid DNA led to adverse effects on vascular function [114,115].

GENETICALLY ALTERING THE IN SITU REGENERATION CAPACITY OF THE HEART

Traditionally, the functional role of a specific gene was determined using genetic model organisms where the gene of interest is either overexpressed or deleted. Modern genetic manipulation techniques have allowed fine spatiotemporal control of the desired genetic effect, permitting the overexpression or knockdown of the particular gene product specifically in cardiomyocytes at particular time points (ie, post myocardial infarction injury induction). Through this work, gene products have been identified that when overexpressed or deleted have a profound effect on the cell cycle status of cardiomyocytes: DNA synthesis initiation, cytokinesis, cytoskeletal rearrangement, and differentiation. Ultimately, this provides information on particular pathways that play a fundamental role in preventing cardiomyocytes from reentering the cell cycle under physiological conditions and an opportunity to engineer tools that can genetically alter cardiomyocytes in order to induce them to proliferate and ultimately regenerate the injured heart. In this section, we will be discussing studies that have focused on the induction of cardiac regeneration via the genetic manipulation of cardiomyocytes (see Fig. 17.2).

One of the pioneer scientists whose group has focused on the potential induction of adult mammalian cardiomyocyte proliferation via the generic manipulation of the cell cycle genetic network is Dr. Loren Field, and in one of his initial studies, he examined the effect that an overexpressed viral SV40 large T antigen has on cardiomyocytes. Large T antigen overexpression induced hyperplasia in both atrial and ventricular mouse cardiomyocytes, which continued to express sarcomeric myosin, and retained ultrastructural characteristics typically observed in mitotic myocytes in vivo, demonstrating the capacity of this viral oncogene to bypass the molecular hurdles that block cardiomyocyte proliferation under physiological conditions [127]. Subsequently, the same group demonstrated that when overexpressed, the SV40 large T antigen seems to bind and inactivate cell cycle regulators, including the tumor suppressor protein p53, whose function is required for the large T antigen induction of proliferation within cardiomyocytes [128,129]. Although the SV40 large T antigen is a well-known oncogene, which would not be therapeutically translatable, these studies helped demonstrate that it is possible to bypass the physiological cell cycle controls that are otherwise preventing cardiomyocytes from proliferating and ultimately regenerating the heart.

Transition from G1 to the S state of the cell cycle is a highly controlled process, and it signals the initiation of DNA synthesis. Soonpaa et al. attempted to induce DNA synthesis and proliferation of cardiomyocytes by overexpressing cyclin D1 (CCND1), which, in conjunction with cyclin-dependent kinase 4 (CDK4), controls the G1→S transition. Using a transgenic mouse in which CCND1 was being overexpressed in the heart, the authors detected abnormal patterns of cardiomyocyte multinucleation and an increase in the number of cardiomyocyte nuclei in histological sections, demonstrating at least they could bypass the G1→S control point [117]. In a subsequent study, the same group compared the capacity of all three D-type cyclins (CCND1, CCND2, CCND3) to drive cardiomyocyte cell cycle activity. The authors determined that although under physiological conditions, all three cyclins had the same effect at the level of induction of DNA synthesis in the targeted cardiomyocytes, only CCND2 remained active, due to its subcellular organization following myocardial infarction injury induction. Importantly, CCND2 activity in the injured myocardium correlated with a marked regression of the infarct size, suggesting that the cyclin control system may be engineered to promote cardiomyocyte proliferation and sufficient cardiac regeneration [118].

Cyclin A2 (CCNA2) is another gene targeted for its potential in inducing cell cycle reentry and proliferation in adult cardiomyocytes. CCNA2 regulates both the G1→S and G2→M transition and is usually silenced in the postnatal mammalian heart. Constitutive overexpression of CCNA2 in the postnatal mouse heart induced cardiomyocyte hyperplasia associated with nuclear localization of the protein. When examined in a mouse model of myocardial infarction injury, CCNA2 induced cardiomyocyte mitosis in the peri-infarct zone, ultimately translated into a significant improvement in the cardiac ejection fraction as compared to control animals [119]. In a subsequent study, the same group examined the capacity of CCNA2 to induce significant cardiac regeneration in a large animal model of myocardial infarction injury. Occlusion of the left anterior descending artery was induced in pigs, resulting in myocardial infarction

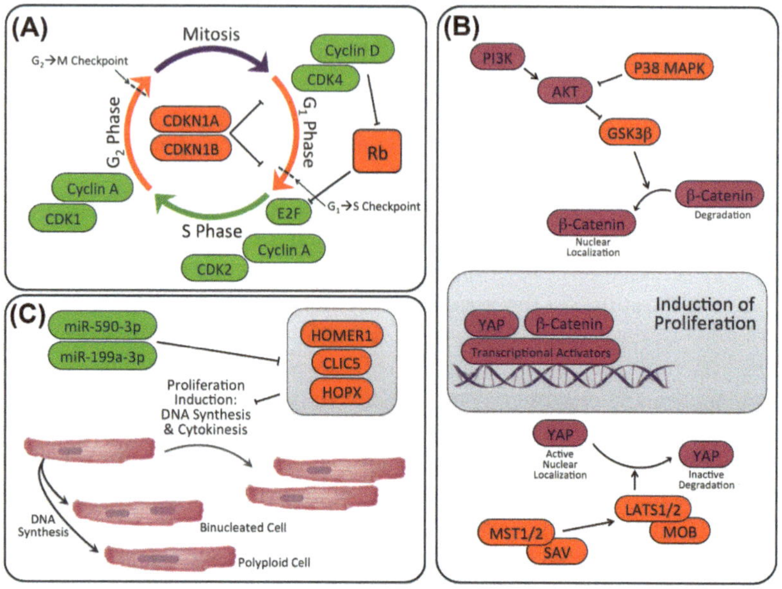

FIGURE 17.2 Genetically altering the in situ regeneration capacity of the heart.

(A) Induced expression of CCND1 in cardiomyocytes is associated with upregulation of cyclin-dependent kinase 4 (CDK4) expression, detection of cardiomyocyte multinucleation, and an increase in the number of cardiomyocyte nuclei, demonstrating passage through the G1→S checkpoint [117]. Following induction of myocardial infarction in the mouse heart, overexpressed CCND2 remains localized in the nucleus, whereas CCND1 and CCND3 relocate in the cytoplasm. CCND2 activity in the injured myocardium correlated with a marked regression of infarct size, suggesting that the cyclin control system may be engineered to promote cardiomyocyte proliferation and sufficient cardiac regeneration [118]. Cyclin D is a retinoblastoma inhibitor, which, in turn, is an inhibitor of the E2F transcription factor. Active E2F is necessary for the induction of cardiomyocyte proliferation. Cyclin A2 (CCNA2) regulates both the G1→S and G2→M transition and is silenced in the postnatal mammalian heart. Constitutive overexpression of CCNA2 in the postnatal mouse heart induced cardiomyocyte hyperplasia associated with nuclear localization of the protein. When examined in a mouse model of myocardial infarction injury, CCNA2 induced cardiomyocyte mitosis in the peri-infarct zone, ultimately translating into a significant improvement in the cardiac ejection fraction as compared to control animals [119]. A subsequent study examined the capacity of CCNA2 to induce cardiac regeneration in a large animal model. One week following induction of myocardial infarction injury, pigs were injected intramyocardially around the circumference of the peri-infarct zone with replication-deficient adenoviral vectors, allowing the constitutive expression of CCNA2. CCNA2 overexpression induced cardiomyocyte cell cycle activation and a significant improvement of cardiac function as determined by left ventricular angiography, 2-D and 3-D echocardiography, and MRI. Expression of CCNA2 was also associated with decreased fibrosis, lack of a hypertrophic response, and significantly increased numbers of cardiomyocytes per unit area [120]. The CDK inhibitors CDKN1A and CDKN1B impede cell proliferation and cell cycle advancement by inhibiting the CDK/cyclin protein complex activity. (B) The enzyme p38 MAPK is capable of inducing cardiomyocyte differentiation and withdrawal from the cell cycle. Its overexpression is associated with inhibition of cardiomyocyte proliferation, whereas its inhibition induces cardiomyocyte apoptosis. It is hypothesized that p38 MAPK inhibition is required for growth factor-mediated induction of cell cycle activation through the phosphatidylinositol-3-kinase injury. One week later, the pigs were injected intramyocardially around the circumference of the peri-infarct zone with replication-deficient adenoviral vectors, allowing the constitutive expression of CCNA2. The authors reported that CCNA2 overexpression induced cardiomyocyte cell cycle activation and a significant improvement of cardiac function as determined by left ventricular angiography, 2-D and 3-D echocardiography, and MRI, in addition to seeing decreased fibrosis, lack of a hypertrophic response, and significantly increased numbers of cardiomyocytes per unit area [120].

The signaling protein p38 mitogen-activated protein kinase (p38 MAPK) has been previously shown to induce cell cycle exit and induction of differentiation in a variety of cell models [121]. Activation of p38 MAPK is also responsible for the induction of cardiomyocyte differentiation and hypertrophy [130]. Engel et al. examined whether manipulation of the p38α MAPK signaling cascade could induce cardiomyocyte cell cycle reentry and proliferation. When using a mouse knockout model of p38α MAPK, the authors demonstrated a 92.3% increase in neonatal cardiomyocyte mitosis and promotion of adult cardiomyocyte cytokinesis [121]. However, when translated in a mouse model of myocardial infarction injury, p38α MAPK inhibitor therapy alone failed to rescue cardiac function, despite increased induction of cardiomyocyte mitosis, whereas when delivered in conjunction with the pro-angiogenic growth factor FGF1, the therapy resulted in reduced scarring and cardiac wall thinning with a significant improvement in cardiac functional output [131].

Genetic screens performed in *Drosophila* for the characterization of abnormal growth regulation phenotypes identified a novel signaling pathway named Hippo/Yap. This pathway is central to in vitro cell–cell contact inhibition and a limitation of cell proliferation. Yap overexpression can overcome contact inhibition, and it stimulates cell proliferation via the activation of cyclins and CDKs [122]. During heart development, the Hippo/Yap signaling pathway participates in limiting trabecular cardiomyocyte proliferation, whereas Yap activation is sufficient to sustain cardiomyocyte cell cycle activity and a delay in cardiomyocyte cell cycle withdrawal [122,123]. Interestingly, when overexpressed in vivo in a neonatal mouse model of myocardial infarction injury, activated Yap was capable of extending the neonatal therapeutic window as determined by the regeneration of the infarcted myocardium and the minimal amount of scar tissue formation [124]. When, however, activated Yap was overexpressed in the infarcted mouse heart at a later stage, it induced a significantly lower level or cardiac regeneration, suggesting that Yap activation alone is insufficient to overcome the barriers to postnatal cardiomyocyte cell cycle activity or that unknown factors may block Yap activity in the adult heart [122,125].

(PI3K)/AKT signaling pathway, which otherwise acts to inhibit glycogen synthase kinase 3 (GSK3β) and allow nuclear localization of β-catenin [2,121]. Activation of the Hippo pathway involves the formation of two enzymatic complexes (SAV/MST1/MST2 and MOB/LATS1/LATS2), which, in turn, phosphorylate the transcriptional coactivator Yes-associated protein (YAP). This causes YAP to remain in the cytoplasm and ultimately be degraded. Inhibition of the Hippo pathway allows the nuclear localization of YAP, which, in conjunction with β-catenin and other transcriptional activators, induces cardiomyocyte proliferation [122–125]. (C) Hsa-miR-590 and hsa-miR-199a are two microRNA mimic molecules identified based on their capacity to induce proliferation in cultures of neonatal rat ventricular myocytes. When delivered in vivo via adeno-associated virus systemically and at 12 days after injection, the hearts of these animals were morphologically normal but significantly enlarged without showing any signs of cardiomyocyte hypertrophy. Importantly, when delivered following myocardial infarction injury, the two microRNAs significantly reduced infarct size and improved cardiac functional output. Their mode of action seems to be through the downregulation of a calcium signaling modulator (HOMER1), a homeodomain protein (HOPX), and a chloride intracellular channel 5 (CLIC5) [2,126].

The techniques described in this section require the genetic manipulation of cells, ultimately translating to the specific overexpression or knockdown of particular gene products in cardiomyocytes. A critical issue pertaining to this approach involves the development of methods that would allow the transduction of a sufficient portion of cardiomyocytes in order to establish functional efficacy within safety limits [132]. This usually involves the use of nonintegrating viral gene delivery systems, including adeno-associated virus or adenovirus. When designing such a delivery system, certain factors should be taken under consideration, including (1) prevention of systemic exposure and restriction of the gene delivery vector to the heart; (2) the potential risk of an immunological response due to the vector capsid itself and its delivery method; (3) delivery of an appropriate transgene for the intended therapeutic aim; (4) sufficient transduction of targeted cardiomyocytes; (5) using a clinically appropriate delivery route; and (6) delivering the minimally effective dose for the induction of functional recovery [132,133].

ROLE OF MICRORNAS IN CARDIAC REGENERATION

MicroRNAs are single-stranded RNA molecules that bind to complementary sequences on mRNA molecules and downregulate their translation into their respective protein products. MicroRNAs are capable of targeting multiple mRNA targets, suggesting that their manipulation can induce significant effects on cellular physiology. Interestingly, microRNAs have significant functions under pathophysiological conditions [134]. There have been numerous studies demonstrating a strong correlation between particular microRNAs and specific cardiovascular disorders, including cardiac hypertrophy, myocardial infarction injury, fibrosis, and vascularization [2,134]. Thus microRNA expression manipulation through its overexpression or inhibition can induce significant phenotypic outcomes, including the induction of cardiac regeneration. In this section, we will be discussing specific microRNAs and how their potential manipulation could induce cardiac regeneration.

Particular components of the miR-15 microRNA family (miR-15a, miR-15b, miR-16-1, miR-16-2, miR-195, miR-497) have been shown to be upregulated in the heart following myocardial infarction injury. MiR-195 overexpression during development induces cardiomyocyte cell cycle arrest, hypoplasia, and congenital heart abnormalities. It also prevents cardiac regeneration following induction of myocardial induction injury [2,135]. Interestingly, inhibition of the miR-15 microRNA family induces a significant improvement in cardiac functional output following myocardial infarction injury and significant enhancement of contractile output following ischemia/reperfusion injury, suggesting that it is an important therapeutic target for cardiac regeneration applications [136,137].

Using high throughput screening, Eulalio et al. screened a library of 875 microRNA mimic molecules for their capacity to induce proliferation in cultures of neonatal rat ventricular cardiomyocytes [126]. The screen identified two microRNA molecules (hsa-miR-590 and hsa-miR-199a), which, once exogenously administered, stimulated postnatal cardiomyocyte proliferation in vitro. MicroRNA mimics were subsequently delivered via adeno-associated virus systemically, and at 12 days after injection, the hearts of these animals were morphologically normal but significantly enlarged without showing any signs of cardiomyocyte hypertrophy. Importantly, when delivered following myocardial infarction injury induction, the two microRNAs significantly reduced infarct size and improved cardiac functional output. This study further demonstrated that exogenously administered microRNAs have the potential to restore cardiac function to almost normal levels following myocardial infarction injury and with a significant therapeutic potential [2,126].

DIRECT IN SITU EPIGENETIC REPROGRAMMING OF NONMYOCYTES INTO CARDIOMYOCYTES

The advent of direct epigenetic reprogramming or transdifferentiation approaches to induce the conversion of one terminally differentiated cell type into another without first generating a pluripotent intermediate is a new approach for potentially producing nascent cardiomyocytes. Although transdifferentiation paradigms were previously evident in the scientific literature, the recent discovery that the transient overexpression of four transcription factors (POU5F1, SOX2, KLF4, MYC) is sufficient to epigenetically reprogram terminally differentiated somatic cells into iPS cells [138,139], which closely resemble embryonic stem cells and hold a significant potential to differentiate into functional cardiomyocytes [140,141], attracting the attention of the scientific community with scientists looking for other potential applications of epigenetic reprogramming. The creation of induced cardiomyocytes through the process of direct reprogramming initiates a new direction toward achieving a robust induction of cardiac regeneration while avoiding the involvement of cell transplantation and through the direct conversion of cardiac fibroblasts into functional integrated cardiomyocytes [142]. In this section, we will first be discussing recent reports describing the in vitro transdifferentiation of nonmyocytes into induced cardiomyocytes, and second, the translation of these technologies in vivo for the in situ induction of transdifferentiation and cardiac regeneration in the ailing myocardium.

Development of the technique for the derivation of induced cardiomyocytes via direct epigenetic reprogramming was pioneered by the group of Dr. Deepak Srivastava, demonstrating that overexpression of three transcription factors (Gata4, Tbx5, Mef2c) rapidly and efficiently reprogrammed postnatal cardiac or dermal mouse fibroblasts into differentiated cardiomyocyte-like cells [143]. Reprogramming efficiency was initially reported as a percentage of GFP^+ cells (20%, αMHC-GFP). Approximately one-third of the GFP^+ cells also expressed cardiac troponin T, with this percentage increasing over time. The authors also reported some degree of spontaneous Ca^{2+} oscillations, characteristic of functional cardiomyocytes and a low frequency of spontaneously contracting induced cardiomyocytes [143]. It is important to note that the effectiveness of the three transcription factors to generate induced cardiomyocytes was questioned in a report by Chen et al., who argued that overexpression of the three genes was not sufficient to induce activation of cardiomyocyte-specific promoters, and although they detected significant upregulation of cardiac troponin, they could not detect functional cardiomyocytes. Certain important differences exist between the two studies, including the developmental stage of the cell source to be reprogrammed, the gene delivery vehicle, and potentially the environment within which the experiment was performed (media, substrate), indicating that the reprogramming process itself may require significant improvement and fine tuning [142,144].

Since the initial report [143] describing the derivation of induced cardiomyocytes, a series of subsequent reports focused on further enhancing the transdifferentiation efficiency of nonmyocytes into induced cardiomyocytes. Song et al. reported that the transcription factor Hand2, when added to the existing three growth factors, led to a significant enhancement in generating induced cardiomyocytes from adult tail-tip fibroblasts and cardiac fibroblasts [145]. Protze et al. reported that the Myocd, Mef2c, and Tbx5 led to greater expression of cardiomyocyte genes than as compared to Gata4, Tbx5, and Mef2c [146]. Jayawardena et al. approached the problem from a different angle, reporting the utilization of a combination of microRNAs (miR-1, miR-133, miR-208, miR-499) and a chemical Janus Kinase (JAK) inhibitor to induce transdifferentiation of neonatal and adult cardiac fibroblasts to induced cardiomyocytes [147]. Additional reports focused on the identification of induced cardiomyocytes based on their functional characteristics (ie, Ca^{2+} oscillations) rather than activation of a transgenic marker in order to identify more accurately real transdifferentiation events [148,149]. Although cardiomyocyte generation via in vitro reprogramming is inefficient as compared to the generation of cardiomyocytes via the differentiation of stem cells when it comes down to in situ cardiac regeneration, transdifferentiation offers a striking advantage over stem cell therapies: the potential to replace lost cardiomyocytes without cell transplantation [142].

The transcription factor combination identified through multiple screenings based on its capacity to induce transdifferentiation of nonmyocytes into induced cardiomyocytes was defined using mouse cells, and in order for this technology to be translated into a human system, it was important to determine whether it could also be effective when overexpressed in human primary cells. Fu et al. quickly determined that overexpression of GATA4, TBX5, and MEF2C in human cardiac fibroblasts was insufficient to induce transdifferentiation. When including the transcription factors ESRRG, MESP1, MYOCD, and ZFPM2, they reported transdifferentiation into human-induced cardiomyocytes based on the detection of sarcomere formation, calcium transients, and action potentials, although their transdifferentiation efficiency remained low [150]. Nam et al. decided to utilize a combination of both transcription factors and microRNAs to induce transdifferentiation of human cardiac fibroblasts into induced cardiomyocytes. Overexpression of GATA4, HAND2, TBX5, MYOCD, MiR-1, and Mir-133 induced formation of reprogrammed cardiomyocytes with sarcomere-like structures and calcium transients. Additionally, a small subset of the derived cells exhibited spontaneous contractions [151].

Importantly, successful generation of in situ cardiac regeneration would depend on whether the transdifferentiation process could be translated to the in vivo environment. Qian et al. designed an elegant study using transgenic mice to demonstrate that in vivo cardiac fibroblasts could be reprogrammed into induced cardiomyocytes. Transcription factors were delivered in the mouse infarcted myocardium using intramyocardial injection of retroviruses. The authors detected binucleated induced cardiomyocytes with assembled sarcomeres and a gene expression pattern resembling bona fide cardiomyocytes. Importantly, the reprogramming process achieved a decrease in infarct size and attenuated cardiac dysfunction [152]. Similarly, Song et al. demonstrated that overexpression of GATA4, HAND2, MEF2C, and TBX5 induced epigenetic reprogramming of dividing nonmyocytes in the mouse infarcted myocardium, improved cardiac functional output, and reduced ventricular remodeling [145]. These reports strongly suggest that the process of direct reprogramming and formation of nascent functional cardiomyocytes in vivo and following myocardial injury is a pragmatic approach with a significant therapeutic potential.

CONCLUSIONS

Worldwide CVD is the main cause of morbidity and mortality, and despite current state-of-the-art therapeutic treatment options, including statins, angiotensin-converting enzyme inhibitors, beta blockers, and other drugs, its prevalence continues to increase, underscoring the need for new therapeutic strategies [134]. Most of the current therapeutic approaches focus on supporting the remaining healthy myocardium rather than attempting to induce its regeneration to a degree that would return a healthy physiological cardiac functional output. This approach was followed partly due to the belief that the myocardium is unable of regenerating itself. Recently, however, multiple independent lines of evidence have demonstrated that neo-cardiomyogenesis is still possible in the postnatal and adult heart [6]. This has ignited an intense interest by multiple research groups attempting to understand the intrinsic regenerative capacity of the heart with the intention of manipulating it for the purpose of returning sufficient cardiac functional output and significantly improving the life quality and expectancy of the patient. Current strategies include (1) inducing cardiomyocytes to proliferate and generate nascent functional contractile cells; (2) delivering in the myocardium stem cells or progenitor cells with the capacity to differentiate into either cardiomyocytes or vasculature; (3) activating the intrinsic population of cardiac progenitor cells or recruiting systemic stem cells to the myocardium; (4) epigenetically reprogramming resident nonmyocytes into cardiomyocytes; and (5) using biomaterials to mechanically support the ailing myocardium [6]. Preliminary in vitro and in vivo data has demonstrated the immense therapeutic potential of these strategies, and some of these approaches are now being translated into clinical trials with promising preliminary results. This has suggested that regeneration-inducing approaches like the ones mentioned in this chapter hold a huge potential for significantly changing the landscape of CVD treatment.

The capacity of preexisting cardiomyocytes to proliferate following injury is almost completely absent in the mammalian rodent heart, as it was reported that only ~0.008% of cardiomyocytes undergo division in the boundary region of the injured myocardium [14]. Moreover, human cardiac regeneration has been difficult to confirm due to the fact that macroscopical regeneration has not been observed, and at the cellular level, cardiomyocytes reinitiate DNA synthesis without undergoing cytokinesis following injury or overload. By taking advantage of the transient spike of atmospheric C^{14} concentrations, which occurred during the Cold War, it was determined that approximately 55% of human cardiomyocytes persist throughout the life of an individual, whereas 45% gets renewed [19]. Additionally, the number of cardiomyocyte nuclei in the healthy heart is more or less constant, and it only increases linearly following induction of hypertrophy, thus suggesting that human cardiac regeneration does occur at low levels due to pathological events [7,17,18]. Interestingly, the rodent heart is capable of complete regeneration, but this capacity is lost within the first 7 days following birth, suggesting that molecular events activated early in the mammalian life prevent future innate cardiac regeneration [16]. Altogether, this suggests that (1) mammalian cardiac regeneration takes place at a very low level, and inherent molecular barriers prevent it from becoming sufficient to achieve full functional recovery to the organ due to the effects of aging, chronic disease, or injury; and (2) it is possible to engineer specific therapeutic tools that could significantly enhance the existing baseline levels of cardiac regeneration or reduce the molecular barriers that inhibit it from ultimately achieving complete organ regeneration and full functional recovery.

A main strategy in attempting to induce in situ cardiac regeneration focuses on either activating the intrinsic population of cardiac progenitor cells, recruiting systemic stem cells to the injured myocardium, or expanding ex vivo these cell populations and then delivering them in the heart. Success of such a strategy depends on a thorough understanding of the target stem cell or progenitor cell population and understanding their therapeutic potential. Based on the work of multiple groups focusing on identifying intrinsic cardiac stem cells or progenitor cells, the mammalian heart seems to be containing more than one type of resident cells: Lin^{-}/c-Kit^{+} cell progenitors [27], Sca-1^{+} cell progenitors [34], side population cell progenitors [37], and cardiosphere-derived cell progenitors [40]. Arguably, it is noteworthy that an organ, which is unable to regenerate itself, may have so many different and unique intrinsic progenitor cell populations. It is important to state, though, that individual unique progenitor cell populations may also express on their cell surface markers used to identify alternative cell progenitors, which may suggest that these markers may be identifying a single resident cell progenitor population at different phenotypic stages. Importantly, although the capacity of these cells to differentiate into nascent cardiomyocytes has been partly demonstrated, it is debatable whether these cells are actively forming nascent cardiac muscle in the heart. What is indeed very significant is the fact that once delivered in the injured myocardium, these cells do exert an effect, which induces a real and significant functional cardiac improvement. It has been hypothesized that this proregenerative therapeutic effect is due to the "paracrine effect": spatiotemporal secretion of protein ligands that, in turn, promote cardiac repair and regeneration. It is thus conceivable that by understanding the exact nature of the molecular signals secreted by the cell progenitors and which are inducing myocardial regeneration, we can emulate and enhance their proregenerative effect.

Emulating the paracrine effect through the engineered delivery of protein ligands can significantly enhance the innate regenerative capacity of the injured myocardium. In situ delivery of protein ligands can induce cardiac regeneration through the following mechanisms of action: (1) induction of in situ angiogenesis and revascularization of the organ; (2) increased recruitment of stem cells or progenitor cells to the myocardium; (3) prevention of cell death or induction of proliferation in existing populations of cardiomyocytes; and (4) increased growth and induction of differentiation of resident stem cell or progenitor cells. Although the protein ligands described in this chapter have exhibited a significant preclinical capacity for inducing myocardial regeneration, the precise understanding of their mechanistic action and knowledge of their exact pharmacokinetic profile, both locally as well as systemically, are too limited for their immediate translation as drug candidates [69].

Peptide-based stimulation of in vivo cardiac regeneration would require accurate spatiotemporal release kinetics of the protein ligand to minimize the required therapeutic dose and potential off-target undesirable effects. Thus the ideal protein delivery system for in situ cardiac regeneration would warrant the delivery of a properly folded peptide (1) for the appropriate amount of time; (2) at the right concentration; and (3) at the appropriate location in order to induce maximal organ regeneration and sufficient cardiac functional output recovery. Current state-of-the-art delivery vehicles include hydrogels, within which protein ligands are either passively suspended or actively conjugated on the polymer backbone through a bioactive linker, which can be degraded due to enzymatic activity. Systemic delivery methods involve the introduction of the protein ligands within particles, which are also tagged with targeting signals, allowing them to accumulate and release their contents at the site of injury.

In addition to the release of protein ligands, genetic manipulation of the heart and its cellular components may be another realistic strategy to induce a sufficient regeneration of the infarcted myocardium. Induction of proliferation of existing cardiomyocytes via a genetic manipulation approach seems to be a likely therapeutic strategy only if the following goals are met: (1) identification of the molecular barriers that prevent cardiomyocytes from initiating DNA synthesis, undergoing cytokinesis, rearrange their cytoskeleton during cell division, differentiate into cardiomyocytes postdivision; (2) identification of molecular tools that would allow the inhibition of the appropriate molecular barriers for the induction of cardiomyocyte proliferation; the role of these tools would include the induction of overexpression of a gene product, the emulation microRNA activity, the silencing of a particular gene from being transcribed or translated, the inhibition of specific microRNA activity; (3) identification of the exact spatiotemporal kinetics that must be emulated in order to achieve maximum proliferation of existing cardiomyocytes while minimizing potential side effects; and (4) development of efficient gene delivery vehicles that would specifically target only the desired cell subpopulations, ensuring accurate spatiotemporal expression of their delivery product while avoiding nonspecific targets.

An alternative novel approach for the induction of cardiac regeneration is the epigenetic reprogramming of nonmuscle cells in the injured heart into induced cardiomyocytes by exploiting developmental gene regulatory networks that have been deciphered over the past two decades [2]. Numerous issues remain to be resolved before this strategy can be therapeutically translated in a human system. The current reprogramming efficiency is extremely low, primarily due to the epigenetic status of the targeted nonmyocyte cells. The derived induced cardiomyocytes are nonproliferative, which would generally translate into a 1:1 ratio in formation of nascent cardiomyocytes, making this approach inadequate in inducing a robust regeneration. Finally, it is necessary that the nascent induced cardiomyocytes must seamlessly integrate within the existing myocardium, the cardiac conduction system, and the vasculature to reestablish a functional tissue and avoid the induction of lethal cardiac arrhythmias [2].

In summary, the regeneration of the mammalian heart represents a major challenge of fundamental significance, given the scale of heart disease and the absence of effective long-term therapies for heart failure. It is highly possible that a future successful cardiac regeneration inducing strategy will be based on one or a combination of the approaches described here.

REFERENCES

[1] Lopez AD, Mathers CD, Ezzati M, Jamison DT, Murray CJ. Global and regional burden of disease and risk factors, 2001: systematic analysis of population health data. Lancet 2006;367(9524):1747–57.

[2] Xin M, Olson EN, Bassel-Duby R. Mending broken hearts: cardiac development as a basis for adult heart regeneration and repair. Nat Rev Mol Cell Biol 2013;14(8):529–41.

[3] Hodgson DM, Behfar A, Zingman LV, Kane GC, Perez-Terzic C, Alekseev AE, et al. Stable benefit of embryonic stem cell therapy in myocardial infarction. Am J Physiol Heart Circ Physiol 2004;287(2):H471–9.

[4] Sun Y, Weber KT. Infarct scar: a dynamic tissue. Cardiovasc Res 2000;46(2):250–6.

[5] Roell W, Lewalter T, Sasse P, Tallini YN, Choi BR, Breitbach M, et al. Engraftment of connexin 43-expressing cells prevents post-infarct arrhythmia. Nature 2007;450(7171):819–24.

[6] Lin Z, Pu WT. Strategies for cardiac regeneration and repair. Sci Transl Med 2014;6(239):239rv1.

[7] Laflamme MA, Murry CE. Heart regeneration. Nature 2011;473(7347):326–35.

[8] Murry CE, Reinecke H, Pabon LM. Regeneration gaps: observations on stem cells and cardiac repair. J Am Coll Cardiol 2006;47(9):1777–85.

[9] Olivetti G, Melissari M, Capasso JM, Anversa P. Cardiomyopathy of the aging human heart. Myocyte loss and reactive cellular hypertrophy. Circ Res 1991;68(6):1560–8.

[10] Whelan RS, Kaplinskiy V, Kitsis RN. Cell death in the pathogenesis of heart disease: mechanisms and significance. Annu Rev Physiol 2010;72:19–44.

[11] Li F, Wang X, Capasso JM, Gerdes AM. Rapid transition of cardiac myocytes from hyperplasia to hypertrophy during postnatal development. J Mol Cell Cardiol 1996;28(8):1737–46.

[12] Olivetti G, Cigola E, Maestri R, Corradi D, Lagrasta C, Gambert SR, et al. Aging, cardiac hypertrophy and ischemic cardiomyopathy do not affect the proportion of mononucleated and multinucleated myocytes in the human heart. J Mol Cell Cardiol 1996;28(7):1463–77.

[13] Poss KD, Wilson LG, Keating MT. Heart regeneration in zebrafish. Science 2002;298(5601):2188–90.

[14] Soonpaa MH, Field LJ. Assessment of cardiomyocyte DNA synthesis in normal and injured adult mouse hearts. Am J Physiol 1997;272(1 Pt 2):H220–6.

[15] Hsieh PC, Segers VF, Davis ME, MacGillivray C, Gannon J, Molkentin JD, et al. Evidence from a genetic fate-mapping study that stem cells refresh adult mammalian cardiomyocytes after injury. Nat Med 2007;13(8):970–4.

[16] Porrello ER, Mahmoud AI, Simpson E, Hill JA, Richardson JA, Olson EN, et al. Transient regenerative potential of the neonatal mouse heart. Science 2011;331(6020):1078–80.

[17] Adler CP, Costabel U. Cell number in human heart in atrophy, hypertrophy, and under the influence of cytostatics. Recent Adv Stud Cardiac Struct Metab 1975;6:343–55.

[18] Herget GW, Neuburger M, Plagwitz R, Adler CP. DNA content, ploidy level and number of nuclei in the human heart after myocardial infarction. Cardiovasc Res 1997;36(1):45–51.

[19] Bergmann O, Bhardwaj RD, Bernard S, Zdunek S, Barnabe-Heider F, Walsh S, et al. Evidence for cardiomyocyte renewal in humans. Science 2009;324(5923):98–102.

[20] Lian X, Hsiao C, Wilson G, Zhu K, Hazeltine LB, Azarin SM, et al. Robust cardiomyocyte differentiation from human pluripotent stem cells via temporal modulation of canonical Wnt signaling. Proc Natl Acad Sci USA 2012;109(27):E1848–57.

[21] Sharma A, Wu JC, Wu SM. Induced pluripotent stem cell-derived cardiomyocytes for cardiovascular disease modeling and drug screening. Stem Cell Res Ther 2013;4(6):150.

[22] Burridge PW, Keller G, Gold JD, Wu JC. Production of de novo cardiomyocytes: human pluripotent stem cell differentiation and direct reprogramming. Cell Stem Cell 2012;10(1):16–28.

[23] Orlic D, Kajstura J, Chimenti S, Jakoniuk I, Anderson SM, Li B, et al. Bone marrow cells regenerate infarcted myocardium. Nature 2001;410(6829):701–5.

[24] Tallini YN, Greene KS, Craven M, Spealman A, Breitbach M, Smith J, et al. c-Kit expression identifies cardiovascular precursors in the neonatal heart. Proc Natl Acad Sci USA 2009;106(6):1808–13.

[25] Balsam LB, Wagers AJ, Christensen JL, Kofidis T, Weissman IL, Robbins RC. Haematopoietic stem cells adopt mature haematopoietic fates in ischaemic myocardium. Nature 2004;428(6983):668–73.

[26] Murry CE, Soonpaa MH, Reinecke H, Nakajima H, Nakajima HO, Rubart M, et al. Haematopoietic stem cells do not transdifferentiate into cardiac myocytes in myocardial infarcts. Nature 2004;428(6983):664–8.

[27] Beltrami AP, Barlucchi L, Torella D, Baker M, Limana F, Chimenti S, et al. Adult cardiac stem cells are multipotent and support myocardial regeneration. Cell 2003;114(6):763–76.

[28] Bearzi C, Rota M, Hosoda T, Tillmanns J, Nascimbene A, De Angelis A, et al. Human cardiac stem cells. Proc Natl Acad Sci USA 2007;104(35):14068–73.

[29] Ellison GM, Vicinanza C, Smith AJ, Aquila I, Leone A, Waring CD, et al. Adult c-kit(pos) cardiac stem cells are necessary and sufficient for functional cardiac regeneration and repair. Cell 2013;154(4):827–42.

[30] Zaruba MM, Soonpaa M, Reuter S, Field LJ. Cardiomyogenic potential of c-Kit(+)-expressing cells derived from neonatal and adult mouse hearts. Circulation 2010;121(18):1992–2000.

[31] Jesty SA, Steffey MA, Lee FK, Breitbach M, Hesse M, Reining S, et al. c-Kit$^+$ precursors support postinfarction myogenesis in the neonatal, but not adult, heart. Proc Natl Acad Sci USA 2012;109(33):13380–5.

[32] Bolli R, Chugh AR, D'Amario D, Loughran JH, Stoddard MF, Ikram S, et al. Cardiac stem cells in patients with ischaemic cardiomyopathy (SCIPIO): initial results of a randomised phase 1 trial. Lancet 2011;378(9806):1847–57.

[33] Chugh AR, Beache GM, Loughran JH, Mewton N, Elmore JB, Kajstura J, et al. Administration of cardiac stem cells in patients with ischemic cardiomyopathy: the SCIPIO trial: surgical aspects and interim analysis of myocardial function and viability by magnetic resonance. Circulation 2012;126(11 Suppl. 1):S54–64.

[34] Holmes C, Stanford WL. Concise review: stem cell antigen-1: expression, function, and enigma. Stem Cells 2007;25(6):1339–47.

[35] Oh H, Bradfute SB, Gallardo TD, Nakamura T, Gaussin V, Mishina Y, et al. Cardiac progenitor cells from adult myocardium: homing, differentiation, and fusion after infarction. Proc Natl Acad Sci USA 2003;100(21):12313–8.

[36] Uchida S, De Gaspari P, Kostin S, Jenniches K, Kilic A, Izumiya Y, et al. Sca1-derived cells are a source of myocardial renewal in the murine adult heart. Stem Cell Rep 2013;1(5):397–410.

[37] Martin CM, Meeson AP, Robertson SM, Hawke TJ, Richardson JA, Bates S, et al. Persistent expression of the ATP-binding cassette transporter, Abcg2, identifies cardiac SP cells in the developing and adult heart. Dev Biol 2004;265(1):262–75.

[38] Pfister O, Mouquet F, Jain M, Summer R, Helmes M, Fine A, et al. CD31− but Not CD31+ cardiac side population cells exhibit functional cardiomyogenic differentiation. Circ Res 2005;97(1):52–61.

[39] Oyama T, Nagai T, Wada H, Naito AT, Matsuura K, Iwanaga K, et al. Cardiac side population cells have a potential to migrate and differentiate into cardiomyocytes in vitro and in vivo. J Cell Biol 2007;176(3):329–41.

[40] Messina E, De Angelis L, Frati G, Morrone S, Chimenti S, Fiordaliso F, et al. Isolation and expansion of adult cardiac stem cells from human and murine heart. Circ Res 2004;95(9):911–21.

[41] Smith RR, Barile L, Cho HC, Leppo MK, Hare JM, Messina E, et al. Regenerative potential of cardiosphere-derived cells expanded from percutaneous endomyocardial biopsy specimens. Circulation 2007;115(7):896–908.

[42] Malliaras K, Makkar RR, Smith RR, Cheng K, Wu E, Bonow RO, et al. Intracoronary cardiosphere-derived cells after myocardial infarction: evidence of therapeutic regeneration in the final 1-year results of the CADUCEUS trial (CArdiosphere-Derived aUtologous stem CElls to reverse ventricUlar dySfunction). J Am Coll Cardiol 2014;63(2):110–22.

[43] Makkar RR, Smith RR, Cheng K, Malliaras K, Thomson LE, Berman D, et al. Intracoronary cardiosphere-derived cells for heart regeneration after myocardial infarction (CADUCEUS): a prospective, randomised phase 1 trial. Lancet 2012;379(9819):895–904.

[44] Andersen DC, Andersen P, Schneider M, Jensen HB, Sheikh SP. Murine "cardiospheres" are not a source of stem cells with cardiomyogenic potential. Stem Cells 2009;27(7):1571–81.

[45] Masters M, Riley PR. The epicardium signals the way towards heart regeneration. Stem Cell Res 2014;13(3 Pt B):683–92.

[46] Huang GN, Thatcher JE, McAnally J, Kong Y, Qi X, Tan W, et al. C/EBP transcription factors mediate epicardial activation during heart development and injury. Science 2012;338(6114):1599–603.

[47] Smart N, Risebro CA, Melville AA, Moses K, Schwartz RJ, Chien KR, et al. Thymosin beta4 induces adult epicardial progenitor mobilization and neovascularization. Nature 2007;445(7124):177–82.

[48] Smart N, Bollini S, Dube KN, Vieira JM, Zhou B, Davidson S, et al. De novo cardiomyocytes from within the activated adult heart after injury. Nature 2011;474(7353):640–4.

[49] Zhou B, Honor LB, Ma Q, Oh JH, Lin RZ, Melero-Martin JM, et al. Thymosin beta 4 treatment after myocardial infarction does not reprogram epicardial cells into cardiomyocytes. J Mol Cell Cardiol 2012;52(1):43–7.

[50] Szmitko PE, Fedak PW, Weisel RD, Stewart DJ, Kutryk MJ, Verma S. Endothelial progenitor cells: new hope for a broken heart. Circulation 2003;107(24):3093–100.

[51] Kawamoto A, Gwon HC, Iwaguro H, Yamaguchi JI, Uchida S, Masuda H, et al. Therapeutic potential of ex vivo expanded endothelial progenitor cells for myocardial ischemia. Circulation 2001;103(5):634–7.

[52] Kamihata H, Matsubara H, Nishiue T, Fujiyama S, Tsutsumi Y, Ozono R, et al. Implantation of bone marrow mononuclear cells into ischemic myocardium enhances collateral perfusion and regional function via side supply of angioblasts, angiogenic ligands, and cytokines. Circulation 2001;104(9):1046–52.

[53] Assmus B, Schachinger V, Teupe C, Britten M, Lehmann R, Dobert N, et al. Transplantation of progenitor cells and regeneration enhancement in acute myocardial infarction (TOPCARE-AMI). Circulation 2002;106(24):3009–17.

[54] Dominici M, Le Blanc K, Mueller I, Slaper-Cortenbach I, Marini F, Krause D, et al. Minimal criteria for defining multipotent mesenchymal stromal cells. The International Society for Cellular Therapy position statement. Cytotherapy 2006;8(4):315–7.

[55] Karantalis V, Hare JM. Use of mesenchymal stem cells for therapy of cardiac disease. Circ Res 2015;116(8):1413–30.

[56] Karantalis V, DiFede DL, Gerstenblith G, Pham S, Symes J, Zambrano JP, et al. Autologous mesenchymal stem cells produce concordant improvements in regional function, tissue perfusion, and fibrotic burden when administered to patients undergoing coronary artery bypass grafting: the Prospective Randomized Study of Mesenchymal Stem Cell Therapy in Patients Undergoing Cardiac Surgery (PROMETHEUS) trial. Circ Res 2014;114(8):1302–10.

[57] Heldman AW, DiFede DL, Fishman JE, Zambrano JP, Trachtenberg BH, Karantalis V, et al. Transendocardial mesenchymal stem cells and mononuclear bone marrow cells for ischemic cardiomyopathy: the TAC-HFT randomized trial. JAMA 2014;311(1):62–73.

[58] Hare JM, Fishman JE, Gerstenblith G, DiFede Velazquez DL, Zambrano JP, Suncion VY, et al. Comparison of allogeneic vs autologous bone marrow-derived mesenchymal stem cells delivered by transendocardial injection in patients with ischemic cardiomyopathy: the POSEIDON randomized trial. JAMA 2012;308(22):2369–79.

[59] Caulfield JB, Leinbach R, Gold H. The relationship of myocardial infarct size and prognosis. Circulation 1976;53(3 Suppl.):I141–4.

[60] Hong KU, Li QH, Guo Y, Patton NS, Moktar A, Bhatnagar A, et al. A highly sensitive and accurate method to quantify absolute numbers of c-kit+ cardiac stem cells following transplantation in mice. Basic Res Cardiol 2013;108(3):346.

[61] Gnecchi M, Zhang Z, Ni A, Dzau VJ. Paracrine mechanisms in adult stem cell signaling and therapy. Circ Res 2008;103(11):1204–19.

[62] Cohen JE, Purcell BP, MacArthur Jr JW, Mu A, Shudo Y, Patel JB, et al. A bioengineered hydrogel system enables targeted and sustained intramyocardial delivery of neuregulin, activating the cardiomyocyte cell cycle and enhancing ventricular function in a murine model of ischemic cardiomyopathy. Circ Heart Fail 2014;7(4):619–26.

[63] Formiga FR, Pelacho B, Garbayo E, Imbuluzqueta I, Diaz-Herraez P, Abizanda G, et al. Controlled delivery of fibroblast growth factor-1 and neuregulin-1 from biodegradable microparticles promotes cardiac repair in a rat myocardial infarction model through activation of endogenous regeneration. J Control Release 2014;173:132–9.

[64] Polizzotti BD, Arab S, Kuhn B. Intrapericardial delivery of gelfoam enables the targeted delivery of Periostin peptide after myocardial infarction by inducing fibrin clot formation. PLoS One 2012;7(5):e36788.

[65] Koudstaal S, Bastings MM, Feyen DA, Waring CD, van Slochteren FJ, Dankers PY, et al. Sustained delivery of insulin-like growth factor-1/hepatocyte growth factor stimulates endogenous cardiac repair in the chronic infarcted pig heart. J Cardiovasc Transl Res 2014;7(2):232–41.

[66] Chung HJ, Kim JT, Kim HJ, Kyung HW, Katila P, Lee JH, et al. Epicardial delivery of VEGF and cardiac stem cells guided by 3-dimensional PLLA mat enhancing cardiac regeneration and angiogenesis in acute myocardial infarction. J Control Release 2015;205:218–30.

[67] Salimath AS, Phelps EA, Boopathy AV, Che PL, Brown M, Garcia AJ, et al. Dual delivery of hepatocyte and vascular endothelial growth factors via a protease-degradable hydrogel improves cardiac function in rats. PLoS One 2012;7(11):e50980.

[68] van der Laan AM, Piek JJ, van Royen N. Targeting angiogenesis to restore the microcirculation after reperfused MI. Nat Rev Cardiol 2009;6(8):515–23.

[69] Segers VF, Lee RT. Protein therapeutics for cardiac regeneration after myocardial infarction. J Cardiovasc Transl Res 2010;3(5):469–77.

[70] Pearlman JD, Hibberd MG, Chuang ML, Harada K, Lopez JJ, Gladstone SR, et al. Magnetic resonance mapping demonstrates benefits of VEGF-induced myocardial angiogenesis. Nat Med 1995;1(10):1085–9.

[71] Banai S, Jaklitsch MT, Shou M, Lazarous DF, Scheinowitz M, Biro S, et al. Angiogenic-induced enhancement of collateral blood flow to ischemic myocardium by vascular endothelial growth factor in dogs. Circulation 1994;89(5):2183–9.

[72] Henry TD, Rocha-Singh K, Isner JM, Kereiakes DJ, Giordano FJ, Simons M, et al. Intracoronary administration of recombinant human vascular endothelial growth factor to patients with coronary artery disease. Am Heart J 2001;142(5):872–80.

[73] Henry TD, Annex BH, McKendall GR, Azrin MA, Lopez JJ, Giordano FJ, et al. The VIVA trial: vascular endothelial growth factor in Ischemia for Vascular Angiogenesis. Circulation 2003;107(10):1359–65.

[74] Epstein SE, Kornowski R, Fuchs S, Dvorak HF. Angiogenesis therapy: amidst the hype, the neglected potential for serious side effects. Circulation 2001;104(1):115–9.

[75] Zheng H, Fu G, Dai T, Huang H. Migration of endothelial progenitor cells mediated by stromal cell-derived factor-1alpha/CXCR4 via PI3K/Akt/eNOS signal transduction pathway. J Cardiovasc Pharmacol 2007;50(3):274–80.

[76] Aiuti A, Webb IJ, Bleul C, Springer T, Gutierrez-Ramos JC. The chemokine SDF-1 is a chemoattractant for human CD34+ hematopoietic progenitor cells and provides a new mechanism to explain the mobilization of CD34+ progenitors to peripheral blood. J Exp Med 1997;185(1):111–20.

[77] Pillarisetti K, Gupta SK. Cloning and relative expression analysis of rat stromal cell derived factor-1 (SDF-1)1: SDF-1 alpha mRNA is selectively induced in rat model of myocardial infarction. Inflammation 2001;25(5):293–300.

[78] Askari AT, Unzek S, Popovic ZB, Goldman CK, Forudi F, Kiedrowski M, et al. Effect of stromal-cell-derived factor 1 on stem-cell homing and tissue regeneration in ischaemic cardiomyopathy. Lancet 2003;362(9385):697–703.

[79] Segers VF, Tokunou T, Higgins LJ, MacGillivray C, Gannon J, Lee RT. Local delivery of protease-resistant stromal cell derived factor-1 for stem cell recruitment after myocardial infarction. Circulation 2007;116(15):1683–92.

[80] Nagata S, Tsuchiya M, Asano S, Kaziro Y, Yamazaki T, Yamamoto O, et al. Molecular cloning and expression of cDNA for human granulocyte colony-stimulating factor. Nature 1986;319(6052):415–8.

[81] Souza LM, Boone TC, Gabrilove J, Lai PH, Zsebo KM, Murdock DC, et al. Recombinant human granulocyte colony-stimulating factor: effects on normal and leukemic myeloid cells. Science 1986;232(4746):61–5.

[82] Ince H, Petzsch M, Kleine HD, Eckard H, Rehders T, Burska D, et al. Prevention of left ventricular remodeling with granulocyte colony-stimulating factor after acute myocardial infarction: final 1-year results of the front-integrated revascularization and stem cell liberation in evolving acute myocardial infarction by granulocyte colony-stimulating factor (FIRSTLINE-AMI) trial. Circulation 2005;112(9 Suppl.):I73–80.

[83] Engelmann MG, Theiss HD, Hennig-Theiss C, Huber A, Wintersperger BJ, Werle-Ruedinger AE, et al. Autologous bone marrow stem cell mobilization induced by granulocyte colony-stimulating factor after subacute ST-segment elevation myocardial infarction undergoing late revascularization: final results from the G-CSF-STEMI (Granulocyte Colony-Stimulating Factor ST-Segment Elevation Myocardial Infarction) trial. J Am Coll Cardiol 2006;48(8):1712–21.

[84] Abdel-Latif A, Bolli R, Zuba-Surma EK, Tleyjeh IM, Hornung CA, Dawn B. Granulocyte colony-stimulating factor therapy for cardiac repair after acute myocardial infarction: a systematic review and meta-analysis of randomized controlled trials. Am Heart J 2008;156(2):216–26.e9.

[85] Harada M, Qin Y, Takano H, Minamino T, Zou Y, Toko H, et al. G-CSF prevents cardiac remodeling after myocardial infarction by activating the Jak-Stat pathway in cardiomyocytes. Nat Med 2005;11(3):305–11.

[86] Boros P, Miller CM. Hepatocyte growth factor: a multifunctional cytokine. Lancet 1995;345(8945):293–5.

[87] Bottaro DP, Rubin JS, Faletto DL, Chan AM, Kmiecik TE, Vande Woude GF, et al. Identification of the hepatocyte growth factor receptor as the c-met proto-oncogene product. Science 1991;251(4995):802–4.

[88] Nakamura T, Mizuno S, Matsumoto K, Sawa Y, Matsuda H, Nakamura T. Myocardial protection from ischemia/reperfusion injury by endogenous and exogenous HGF. J Clin Invest 2000;106(12):1511–9.

[89] Urbanek K, Rota M, Cascapera S, Bearzi C, Nascimbene A, De Angelis A, et al. Cardiac stem cells possess growth factor-receptor systems that after activation regenerate the infarcted myocardium, improving ventricular function and long-term survival. Circ Res 2005;97(7):663–73.

[90] Lemmens K, Doggen K, De Keulenaer GW. Role of neuregulin-1/ErbB signaling in cardiovascular physiology and disease: implications for therapy of heart failure. Circulation 2007;116(8):954–60.

[91] Bersell K, Arab S, Haring B, Kuhn B. Neuregulin1/ErbB4 signaling induces cardiomyocyte proliferation and repair of heart injury. Cell 2009;138(2):257–70.

[92] D'Uva G, Aharonov A, Lauriola M, Kain D, Yahalom-Ronen Y, Carvalho S, et al. ERBB2 triggers mammalian heart regeneration by promoting cardiomyocyte dedifferentiation and proliferation. Nat Cell Biol 2015;17.

[93] Polizzotti BD, Ganapathy B, Walsh S, Choudhury S, Ammanamanchi N, Bennett DG, et al. Neuregulin stimulation of cardiomyocyte regeneration in mice and human myocardium reveals a therapeutic window. Sci Transl Med 2015;7(281):281ra45.
[94] Conway SJ, Molkentin JD. Periostin as a heterofunctional regulator of cardiac development and disease. Curr Genomics 2008;9(8):548–55.
[95] Kuhn B, del Monte F, Hajjar RJ, Chang YS, Lebeche D, Arab S, et al. Periostin induces proliferation of differentiated cardiomyocytes and promotes cardiac repair. Nat Med 2007;13(8):962–9.
[96] Lorts A, Schwanekamp JA, Elrod JW, Sargent MA, Molkentin JD. Genetic manipulation of periostin expression in the heart does not affect myocyte content, cell cycle activity, or cardiac repair. Circ Res 2009;104(1):e1–7.
[97] Sun L, Yu J, Qi S, Hao Y, Liu Y, Li Z. Bone morphogenetic protein-10 induces cardiomyocyte proliferation and improves cardiac function after myocardial infarction. J Cell Biochem 2014;115(11):1868–76.
[98] Chen H, Shi S, Acosta L, Li W, Lu J, Bao S, et al. BMP10 is essential for maintaining cardiac growth during murine cardiogenesis. Development 2004;131(9):2219–31.
[99] Beigi F, Schmeckpeper J, Pow-Anpongkul P, Payne JA, Zhang L, Zhang Z, et al. C3orf58, a novel paracrine protein, stimulates cardiomyocyte cell-cycle progression through the PI3K-AKT-CDK7 pathway. Circ Res 2013;113(4):372–80.
[100] Huang J, Guo J, Beigi F, Hodgkinson CP, Facundo HT, Zhang Z, et al. HASF is a stem cell paracrine factor that activates PKC epsilon mediated cytoprotection. J Mol Cell Cardiol 2014;66:157–64.
[101] Loffredo FS, Steinhauser ML, Jay SM, Gannon J, Pancoast JR, Yalamanchi P, et al. Growth differentiation factor 11 is a circulating factor that reverses age-related cardiac hypertrophy. Cell 2013;153(4):828–39.
[102] Bock-Marquette I, Saxena A, White MD, Dimaio JM, Srivastava D. Thymosin beta4 activates integrin-linked kinase and promotes cardiac cell migration, survival and cardiac repair. Nature 2004;432(7016):466–72.
[103] Shrivastava S, Srivastava D, Olson EN, DiMaio JM, Bock-Marquette I. Thymosin beta4 and cardiac repair. Ann NY Acad Sci 2010;1194:87–96.
[104] Gonzalez A, Rota M, Nurzynska D, Misao Y, Tillmanns J, Ojaimi C, et al. Activation of cardiac progenitor cells reverses the failing heart senescent phenotype and prolongs lifespan. Circ Res 2008;102(5):597–606.
[105] Padin-Iruegas ME, Misao Y, Davis ME, Segers VF, Esposito G, Tokunou T, et al. Cardiac progenitor cells and biotinylated insulin-like growth factor-1 nanofibers improve endogenous and exogenous myocardial regeneration after infarction. Circulation 2009;120(10):876–87.
[106] Jay SM, Lee RT. Protein engineering for cardiovascular therapeutics: untapped potential for cardiac repair. Circ Res 2013;113(7):933–43.
[107] Zhang G, Nakamura Y, Wang X, Hu Q, Suggs LJ, Zhang J. Controlled release of stromal cell-derived factor-1 alpha in situ increases c-kit+ cell homing to the infarcted heart. Tissue Eng 2007;13(8):2063–71.
[108] Ruvinov E, Leor J, Cohen S. The promotion of myocardial repair by the sequential delivery of IGF-1 and HGF from an injectable alginate biomaterial in a model of acute myocardial infarction. Biomaterials 2011;32(2):565–78.
[109] Chiu LL, Reis LA, Radisic M. Controlled delivery of thymosin beta4 for tissue engineering and cardiac regenerative medicine. Ann NY Acad Sci 2012;1269:16–25.
[110] Bastings MM, Koudstaal S, Kieltyka RE, Nakano Y, Pape AC, Feyen DA, et al. A fast pH-switchable and self-healing supramolecular hydrogel carrier for guided, local catheter injection in the infarcted myocardium. Adv Healthc Mater 2014;3(1):70–8.
[111] Scott RC, Rosano JM, Ivanov Z, Wang B, Chong PL, Issekutz AC, et al. Targeting VEGF-encapsulated immunoliposomes to MI heart improves vascularity and cardiac function. FASEB J 2009;23(10):3361–7.
[112] Nguyen J, Sievers R, Motion JP, Kivimae S, Fang Q, Lee RJ. Delivery of lipid micelles into infarcted myocardium using a lipid-linked matrix metalloproteinase targeting peptide. Mol Pharm 2015;12(4):1150–7.
[113] Lui KO, Zangi L, Silva EA, Bu L, Sahara M, Li RA, et al. Driving vascular endothelial cell fate of human multipotent Isl1+ heart progenitors with VEGF modified mRNA. Cell Res 2013;23(10):1172–86.

[114] Zangi L, Lui KO, von Gise A, Ma Q, Ebina W, Ptaszek LM, et al. Modified mRNA directs the fate of heart progenitor cells and induces vascular regeneration after myocardial infarction. Nat Biotechnol 2013;31(10):898–907.

[115] Lui KO, Zangi L, Chien KR. Cardiovascular regenerative therapeutics via synthetic paracrine factor modified mRNA. Stem Cell Res 2014;13(3 Pt B):693–704.

[116] Kariko K, Muramatsu H, Ludwig J, Weissman D. Generating the optimal mRNA for therapy: HPLC purification eliminates immune activation and improves translation of nucleoside-modified, protein-encoding mRNA. Nucleic Acids Res 2011;39(21):e142.

[117] Soonpaa MH, Koh GY, Pajak L, Jing S, Wang H, Franklin MT, et al. Cyclin D1 overexpression promotes cardiomyocyte DNA synthesis and multinucleation in transgenic mice. J Clin Invest 1997;99(11):2644–54.

[118] Pasumarthi KB, Nakajima H, Nakajima HO, Soonpaa MH, Field LJ. Targeted expression of cyclin D2 results in cardiomyocyte DNA synthesis and infarct regression in transgenic mice. Circ Res 2005;96(1):110–8.

[119] Cheng RK, Asai T, Tang H, Dashoush NH, Kara RJ, Costa KD, et al. Cyclin A2 induces cardiac regeneration after myocardial infarction and prevents heart failure. Circ Res 2007;100(12):1741–8.

[120] Shapiro SD, Ranjan AK, Kawase Y, Cheng RK, Kara RJ, Bhattacharya R, et al. Cyclin A2 induces cardiac regeneration after myocardial infarction through cytokinesis of adult cardiomyocytes. Sci Transl Med 2014;6(224):224ra27.

[121] Engel FB, Schebesta M, Duong MT, Lu G, Ren S, Madwed JB, et al. p38 MAP kinase inhibition enables proliferation of adult mammalian cardiomyocytes. Genes Dev 2005;19(10):1175–87.

[122] Lin Z, Pu WT. Harnessing Hippo in the heart: Hippo/Yap signaling and applications to heart regeneration and rejuvenation. Stem Cell Res 2014;13(3 Pt B):571–81.

[123] von Gise A, Lin Z, Schlegelmilch K, Honor LB, Pan GM, Buck JN, et al. YAP1, the nuclear target of Hippo signaling, stimulates heart growth through cardiomyocyte proliferation but not hypertrophy. Proc Natl Acad Sci USA 2012;109(7):2394–9.

[124] Heallen T, Morikawa Y, Leach J, Tao G, Willerson JT, Johnson RL, et al. Hippo signaling impedes adult heart regeneration. Development 2013;140(23):4683–90.

[125] Xin M, Kim Y, Sutherland LB, Murakami M, Qi X, McAnally J, et al. Hippo pathway effector Yap promotes cardiac regeneration. Proc Natl Acad Sci USA 2013;110(34):13839–44.

[126] Eulalio A, Mano M, Dal Ferro M, Zentilin L, Sinagra G, Zacchigna S, et al. Functional screening identifies miRNAs inducing cardiac regeneration. Nature 2012;492(7429):376–81.

[127] Katz EB, Steinhelper ME, Delcarpio JB, Daud AI, Claycomb WC, Field LJ. Cardiomyocyte proliferation in mice expressing alpha-cardiac myosin heavy chain-SV40 T-antigen transgenes. Am J Physiol 1992;262(6 Pt 2):H1867–76.

[128] Daud AI, Lanson Jr NA, Claycomb WC, Field LJ. Identification of SV40 large T-antigen-associated proteins in cardiomyocytes from transgenic mice. Am J Physiol 1993;264(5 Pt 2):H1693–700.

[129] Huh NE, Pasumarthi KB, Soonpaa MH, Jing S, Patton B, Field LJ. Functional abrogation of p53 is required for T-Ag induced proliferation in cardiomyocytes. J Mol Cell Cardiol 2001;33(8):1405–19.

[130] Liang Q, Molkentin JD. Redefining the roles of p38 and JNK signaling in cardiac hypertrophy: dichotomy between cultured myocytes and animal models. J Mol Cell Cardiol 2003;35(12):1385–94.

[131] Engel FB, Hsieh PC, Lee RT, Keating MT. FGF1/p38 MAP kinase inhibitor therapy induces cardiomyocyte mitosis, reduces scarring, and rescues function after myocardial infarction. Proc Natl Acad Sci USA 2006;103(42):15546–51.

[132] Katz MG, Fargnoli AS, Williams RD, Bridges CR. Gene therapy delivery systems for enhancing viral and nonviral vectors for cardiac diseases: current concepts and future applications. Hum Gene Ther 2013;24(11):914–27.

[133] Katz MG, Fargnoli AS, Williams RD, Bridges CR. The road ahead: working towards effective clinical translation of myocardial gene therapies. Ther Deliv 2014;5(1):39–51.

[134] van Rooij E, Olson EN. MicroRNA therapeutics for cardiovascular disease: opportunities and obstacles. Nat Rev Drug Discov 2012;11(11):860–72.

[135] Porrello ER, Johnson BA, Aurora AB, Simpson E, Nam YJ, Matkovich SJ, et al. MiR-15 family regulates postnatal mitotic arrest of cardiomyocytes. Circ Res 2011;109(6):670–9.

[136] Porrello ER, Mahmoud AI, Simpson E, Johnson BA, Grinsfelder D, Canseco D, et al. Regulation of neonatal and adult mammalian heart regeneration by the miR-15 family. Proc Natl Acad Sci USA 2013;110(1):187–92.

[137] Hullinger TG, Montgomery RL, Seto AG, Dickinson BA, Semus HM, Lynch JM, et al. Inhibition of miR-15 protects against cardiac ischemic injury. Circ Res 2012;110(1):71–81.

[138] Takahashi K, Yamanaka S. Induction of pluripotent stem cells from mouse embryonic and adult fibroblast cultures by defined factors. Cell 2006;126(4):663–76.

[139] Takahashi K, Tanabe K, Ohnuki M, Narita M, Ichisaka T, Tomoda K, et al. Induction of pluripotent stem cells from adult human fibroblasts by defined factors. Cell 2007;131(5):861–72.

[140] Mauritz C, Schwanke K, Reppel M, Neef S, Katsirntaki K, Maier LS, et al. Generation of functional murine cardiac myocytes from induced pluripotent stem cells. Circulation 2008;118(5):507–17.

[141] Zhang J, Wilson GF, Soerens AG, Koonce CH, Yu J, Palecek SP, et al. Functional cardiomyocytes derived from human induced pluripotent stem cells. Circ Res 2009;104(4):e30–41.

[142] Addis RC, Epstein JA. Induced regeneration–the progress and promise of direct reprogramming for heart repair. Nat Med 2013;19(7):829–36.

[143] Ieda M, Fu JD, Delgado-Olguin P, Vedantham V, Hayashi Y, Bruneau BG, et al. Direct reprogramming of fibroblasts into functional cardiomyocytes by defined factors. Cell 2010;142(3):375–86.

[144] Chen JX, Krane M, Deutsch MA, Wang L, Rav-Acha M, Gregoire S, et al. Inefficient reprogramming of fibroblasts into cardiomyocytes using Gata4, Mef2c, and Tbx5. Circ Res 2012;111(1):50–5.

[145] Song K, Nam YJ, Luo X, Qi X, Tan W, Huang GN, et al. Heart repair by reprogramming non-myocytes with cardiac transcription factors. Nature 2012;485(7400):599–604.

[146] Protze S, Khattak S, Poulet C, Lindemann D, Tanaka EM, Ravens U. A new approach to transcription factor screening for reprogramming of fibroblasts to cardiomyocyte-like cells. J Mol Cell Cardiol 2012;53(3):323–32.

[147] Jayawardena TM, Egemnazarov B, Finch EA, Zhang L, Payne JA, Pandya K, et al. MicroRNA-mediated in vitro and in vivo direct reprogramming of cardiac fibroblasts to cardiomyocytes. Circ Res 2012;110(11):1465–73.

[148] Addis RC, Ifkovits JL, Pinto F, Kellam LD, Esteso P, Rentschler S, et al. Optimization of direct fibroblast reprogramming to cardiomyocytes using calcium activity as a functional measure of success. J Mol Cell Cardiol 2013;60:97–106.

[149] Christoforou N, Chellappan M, Adler AF, Kirkton RD, Wu T, Addis RC, et al. Transcription factors MYOCD, SRF, Mesp1 and SMARCD3 enhance the cardio-inducing effect of GATA4, TBX5, and MEF2C during direct cellular reprogramming. PLoS One 2013;8(5):e63577.

[150] Fu JD, Stone NR, Liu L, Spencer CI, Qian L, Hayashi Y, et al. Direct reprogramming of human fibroblasts toward a cardiomyocyte-like state. Stem Cell Rep 2013;1(3):235–47.

[151] Nam YJ, Song K, Luo X, Daniel E, Lambeth K, West K, et al. Reprogramming of human fibroblasts toward a cardiac fate. Proc Natl Acad Sci USA 2013;110(14):5588–93.

[152] Qian L, Huang Y, Spencer CI, Foley A, Vedantham V, Liu L, et al. In vivo reprogramming of murine cardiac fibroblasts into induced cardiomyocytes. Nature 2012;485(7400):593–8.

CHAPTER

18

SKIN WOUND HEALING: SKIN REGENERATION WITH PHARMACOLOGICAL MOBILIZED STEM CELLS

Z. Sun, G.M. Williams

The Johns Hopkins University School of Medicine, Baltimore, MD, United States

CHAPTER OUTLINE

In Situ Tissue Regeneration. http://dx.doi.org/10.1016/B978-0-12-802225-2.00018-0

INTRODUCTION

The ability of the skin to repair itself after injury is vital to human survival, and the process of cutaneous wound healing is complex, requiring a coordinated response by immune cells, hematopoietic cells, and resident cells of the skin. While skin wounds heal, they do not regenerate normal human skin. Rather, they heal as a facsimile of normal skin with varying dermal fibrosis, effaced epidermis, and meager or absent sweat glands, oil glands, and hair. This imperfect result causes disfiguration, loss of critical skin functions, and increased vulnerability to late, cosmetic, psychological, and physical defects. More than 70 million surgical procedures are performed in the United States every year [1], with more than one-third resulting in hypertrophic scarring or keloid formation, despite careful and atraumatic techniques. Burn injuries affect >11 million people worldwide annually [2]. The time for burn wound closure is closely correlated with susceptibility to infection, pain duration, length of hospital stay, and incidence of scarring [3]. The fibrosis of large burn wounds across limbs and body parts induces contractures that can limit the mobility and function of the victim. Chronic wounds, such as pressure ulcers and diabetic foot ulcers, represent a significant burden to patients and healthcare professionals, which now affect more than 1% of all people during their lifetime and cost an estimated $20 billion annually in the United States [4]. Despite the advances in last ten years in wound management, up to 50% of chronic wounds still fail to heal [5]. Conventional treatment of chronic wounds does not work well in an aging population in patients with diabetes, obesity, and vascular diseases. Novel approaches for improved wound therapy are badly needed.

Stem cells are the focus of many applications in regenerative medicine because of their extensive ability to self-renew and to generate differentiated progeny. Thus, a current strategy in regenerative medicine is to treat patients by transplanting stem cells or their differentiated derivatives. When stem cells are incorporated into these membranes, more rapid and better repair may occur [6]. Stem cell therapy can improve the quality of burn wound healing, reduce the formation of scars, and reestablish the epidermis and normal function of appendages. A major advance in the treatment of chronic nonhealing wounds (diabetic ulcer) has been made [7] using the patient's bone marrow mesenchymal stem cells (BM-MSCs) in combination with autologous skin fibroblasts on a biodegradable collagen membrane (Coladerm). It has been reported in patients that areas treated with split skin grafts and autologous BM-MSCs were less likely to undergo contraction compared to areas treated with skin grafts alone [8]. The promise of improved wound repair by harnessing stem cells is testified by the existence of 90 clinical trials using mesenchymal stem cell (MSC)-based therapies listed in the National Institutes of Health (NIH) registry [9]. These abundant studies document the importance of stem cells in wound healing and raise the tantalizing possibility that cellular processes can be harnessed to develop practical therapeutic protocols to treat large full-thickness burns and massive soft tissue injuries, which demand immediate therapy.

To avoid the preparation of endogenous stem cells, which is expensive and time-consuming, we proposed to manipulate autochthonous stem cells in vivo by liberating them from their bone marrow (BM) niches pharmacologically. This strategy has the advantage that the regenerated tissue would be self without the need for a donor and immunosuppression. However, many are skeptical of this approach, as it appears unlikely to obtain the quantity of important cell types that will be sufficient to improve healing. As an alternative to growth factors and hormones, many in the field have asked whether new drugs could stimulate and modulate stem cell behavior. Pharmacological agents can be selected or designed to target one aspect of stem cell physiology or function or a signaling pathway; they can be administered by different routes, and they can be modified to reduce toxicity and side effects.

BONE MARROW AND SKIN

There are at least two different lineages of cells in the BM: hematopoietic and mesenchymal cells. Hematopoietic cells are generated from hematopoietic stem cells (HSCs), which reside in the BM stem cell (BMSC) niche. Mesenchymal cells are thought to be derived from MSCs in the BM, although the definitive nature of MSCs is still under investigation [10,11]. MSCs were originally defined as stem cells that could differentiate into mesenchymal lineages, such as osteocytes, chondrocytes, and adipocytes, in culture [12–15]. However, MSCs have also been shown to differentiate into other lineages, including neuronal and epithelial cells [16,17].

Many basic cellular studies have emphasized the plastic relationships between skin and BM. In humans who have undergone BM transplantation (BMT), donor cells that have differentiated into keratinocytes can be detected in the epidermis for at least 3 years [18]. BM cells also contribute to skin development: infusion of green fluorescent protein (GFP) BM cells in utero in mice leads to accumulation of a subpopulation of GFP-positive cells in nonwounded skin dermis, particularly in association with developing hair follicles [19]. With regard to skin repair, BM from both embryonic and postnatal sources has been shown to repair genetic defects in host skin. Mice lacking the skin protein, type VII collagen (Col 7), as well as adult mice lacking type XVII collagen, basement membrane components, are normalized by stem cell infusions [19–21]. Most recently, a clinical trial of allogeneic whole BMT in humans lacking Col 7, which leads to the inherited blistering skin disorder, recessive dystrophic epidermolysis bullosa [22], has demonstrated that BM cells can repair fragile skin and restore Col 7 expression in skin basement membrane [23].

With regard to wound healing, recent studies have demonstrated that systemically administered BM cells migrate to injured skin and contribute to its repair [24–27]. Engineered skin containing BMSCs showed better healing, less wound contraction, and better development of blood vessels when grafted to the burn wounds [28]. Tamai et al. [29] identified specific BM cells that can transform into skin cells to repair damaged skin tissue and discovered a naturally occurring BM cell mobilizer (high-mobility group box 1 protein), which has the ability to attract BM cells expressing the platelet-derived growth factor receptor alpha (PDGFRα). The research showed that around 1 (PDGFRα+) out of 450 BM cells has the capacity to transform into skin cells and regenerate the skin. A more recent study [30] demonstrated that transplanted BM-derived circulating PDGFRα+ cells restore Col 7 in recessive dystrophic epidermolysis bullosa mouse skin graft.

BONE MARROW-DERIVED CELL MOBILIZATION AFTER INJURY

The selective recruitment of BM-derived stem and progenitor cells (herein referred to as BMSCs) may play an important role [31]. BM cells including HSCs, MSCs, endothelial progenitor cells (EPCs), and very small embryonic-like cells are mobilized at varying degrees into the peripheral circulation following injury [32–34]. Subsets of these cells have the ability to migrate from the circulation to a variety of experimentally injured tissues, including muscle, heart, kidney, bone, liver, brain, and skin [32,34–41], where they are likely to contribute to tissue repair through paracrine effects and variable degrees of direct differentiation [32,34,42,43].

During inflammation, monocytes of the hematopoietic lineage are recruited to the wound, where they differentiate into macrophages to clear the wound of debris [44]. In the tissue formation phase, fibroblasts in the newly formed granulation tissue differentiate into myofibroblasts, which express a-smooth muscle actin (a-SMA). These cells are largely responsible for wound contraction and scarring during remodeling [45,46]. Stem cells are involved in the process of wound healing by generating tissue-specific cell types. Circulating BM-derived cells (BMDCs), including fibrocytes, are recruited to wounds [47–50]. Fibrocytes are precursors with both hematopoietic and mesenchymal properties. In mice, up to 37% BMDCs are found in the restored dermis after wounding [48]. Subsequently, these cells differentiate into tissue-specific cell types such as keratinocytes, fibroblasts, and myofibroblasts [46,47,49,51–53].

Despite this knowledge of endogenous stem cell recruitment, the inability of most adult tissues to regenerate flawlessly following injury suggests that these mechanisms are easily overwhelmed. Therapies attempting to augment BMSC involvement by transplanting/injecting cultured cells have proved the principle [54–61], but have generally been ineffective in practice in a variety of preclinical models [62–64]. Poor cellular retention within the harsh injury environment and perhaps the use of inadequate numbers of autochthonous incompletely defined or heterogeneous cellular populations are possible factors limiting the clinical success of stem cell therapies [62,65,66].

DRUGS IN MOBILIZATION OF ENDOGENOUS STEM CELLS

Enhancing a patient's endogenous stem cell response following injury is clinically appealing due to the elimination of time and costs associated with cell harvest, ex vivo processing, and transplantation. Two major stem cell mobilizing agents have shown moderate efficacy in this setting.

AMD3100

AMD3100 (plerixafor or Mozobil), the molecule 1,1′-[1,4-phenylenebis (methylene)] bis [1,4,8,11-tetraazacyclotetradecane], consisting of two cyclam rings linked at the amine nitrogen atoms by a 1,4-xylyl spacer, was first synthesized by Fabbrizzi et al., in 1987 to carry out basic studies on the redox chemistry of dimetallic coordination compounds [67]. In the 1990s, De Clercq proposed that this molecule might be useful in the treatment of HIV because of its role in the blocking of C-X-C chemokine receptor type 4 (CXCR4), a chemokine receptor which acts as a coreceptor for certain strains of HIV [68]. However, it was soon discovered that AMD3100 also mobilized HSCs with high efficiency. BM stromal cells secrete the chemokine, stromal derived factor-1 (SDF-1), which binds to the CXCR4 present on HSCs and anchors them to the BM niche [69–71]. As a highly specific CXCR4 antagonist, AMD3100 can effectively disrupt this axis and release ("mobilize") BMSCs into the peripheral circulation [72]. AMD3100 (plerixafor) was approved by the US Food and Drug Administration (FDA) for the mobilization of HSCs on December 15, 2008. Today, plerixafor is used, often with G-CSF (Neupogen), to mobilize HSCs in lymphoma and multiple myeloma cancer patients for banking prior to myeloablative chemotherapy. Mobilized stem cells are subsequently transplanted back to the patient after cancer treatment. Thus, the drug is well established to be safe and effective. Blockade of the CXCR4/SDF-1 axis with AMD3100 mobilizes not only HSCs, MSCs, and EPCs, but also many other types of stem cells from BM into the peripheral blood, including regulatory T cells [73]. These findings encouraged investigators to test whether increased availability of HSCs, MSCs, EPCs, and other types of stem cells in peripheral blood with AMD3100 treatment will improve healing after injury.

Osteogenesis and bone healing

Within the field of orthopedics and dentistry, bone regeneration strategies utilizing endogenous repair systems are garnering high interest. Wise et al. [74] showed that in a rat model, a single systemic treatment of plerixafor was sufficient to rapidly mobilize MSCs from the BM within an hour. In this model, researchers found that the mobilization by AMD3100, coupled with local treatment to increase SDF-1, led to enhanced concentrations of recombinant human bone morphogenetic protein (BMP)-2–induced ectopic bone formation. After 56 days of treatment, a significant stimulatory effect was found on bone volume and bone mineral content of the plerixafor+SDF-1 treatment compared to saline treatment. This indicates that the AMD3100 plus SDF-1 combination treatment was able to direct MSCs to the ectopic implant site to enhance bone formation.

Kumar and Pannazhagan [75] showed that the combination of insulin-like growth factor 1 (IGF1) and AMD3100 provided significant augmentation of bone growth as determined by dual-energy X-ray absorptiometry (DXA), micro-CT, and histomorphometry in mice bearing segmental fractures. Further, characterization of MSC isolated from mice treated with IGF1 and AMD3100 indicated Akt/PI3K, MEK1/2-Erk1/2, and smad2/3 as key signaling pathways mediating this effect. These studies demonstrate the potential benefit of in vivo stem cell mobilization as a novel alternative for bone healing.

Wound healing in diabetes

Similar therapeutic strategies have found beneficial effects in other wound healing models. In the case of diabetes, neoangiogenesis, a crucial part of the healing process, is impaired. Tepper et al. [76] provided evidence that impaired diabetic wound closure was the result of decreased levels of peripheral BMSCs and that wound healing could be improved significantly with AMD3100. Nishimura et al. [77] confirmed these results in a diabetic wound healing model, showing that wound closure was 2.5-fold better than controls at 14 days after a single high dose topical treatment of AMD3100 (6 mg/kg). The authors observed that AMD3100 was able to promote wound healing through EPC mobilization, enhanced cytokine production, and increased fibroblast and macrophage activity, all of which contributed to neoangiogenesis.

In addition, the provision of AMD3100 to mobilize the endogenous stem cells improved the survival of alcoholic fatty liver grafts in rats [78]. None of the rats survived a whole fatty liver transplant, while 5 of 10 recipients treated with AMD3100 survived long term. AMD3100-mobilized lineage negative Thy-1+CXCR4+CD133+ stem cells played an important role in the survival of fatty liver grafts.

GRANULOCYTE-COLONY STIMULATING FACTOR

G-CSF (Neupogen or Filgrastim), granulocyte-colony stimulating factor, is a glycoprotein that has multiple functions in both physiological and pathophysiological conditions. G-CSF stimulates the BM to produce granulocytes and stem cells and release them into the bloodstream. G-CSF also stimulates the survival, proliferation, differentiation, and function of neutrophil precursors and mature neutrophils via signal transduction pathways. A recombinant form of G-CSF (Neupogen) is used in certain cancer patients to accelerate recovery from neutropenia after chemotherapy [79]. G-CSF is also widely used to increase the number of HSCs in the blood of the donor before collection by leukapheresis for use in HSC transplantation [80].

G-CSF–induced HSC mobilization is also related to disruption of CXCR4/SDF-1 axis [81]. G-CSF reduces the levels of the chemokine SDF-1 while increasing the levels of in its receptor CXCR4 in the BM. The gradual decrease of BM SDF-1 was due mostly to its degradation by neutrophil elastase. Matrix metallopeptidase-9 (MMP-9) was elevated after G-CSF treatment and also was active in the decline of BM SDF-1.

Systemic injection of G-CSF and wound healing effects: The hypothesis that G-CSF mobilized circulating stem cells would be home to the wound site and accelerate healing was tested in a mouse model of tail wounds [82]. G-CSF treatment resulted in migration of bone marrow-derived stem cell (BMDSC) into the wound and a cleared granulating bed. However, there was no improvement in the time of epithelial healing. In a human trial, a 62-year-old male patient with a nonhealing venous ulcer for 3 years was treated with G-CSF. The wound initially responded with an increase in granulation tissue, followed by later improvement in epithelialization [82].

FK506

FK506 (tacrolimus, Prograf) was discovered in 1987 [83]. It is produced by soil bacteria, *Streptomyces tsukubaensis*. FK506 reacts with peptidyl–prolyl isomerase to create a new complex. This FKBP12 (FK binding protein)-FK506 complex interacts with and inhibits calcineurin, thus inhibiting both T lymphocyte signal transduction and interleukin 2 (IL-2) transcription. FK506 was first approved by the FDA in 1994 for use in liver transplantation; this has been extended to include kidney, heart, small bowel, pancreas, lung, trachea, skin, cornea, BM, and limb transplants.

FK506, a well-known immunosuppressant, also exhibits regenerative and wound healing activity. It has been known for two decades that FK506 promoted liver regeneration after partial hepatectomy. Several studies promote different mechanisms to explain liver regeneration by FK506: immunosuppression [84], a reduction of liver resident natural killer (NK) cells [85], and an upregulation of insulin receptor [86]. In a rat model of colon anastomotic healing, FK506 at a dose of 0.01–0.1 mg/kg/day increased anastomotic collagenase activity, which was not changed by treatment with the higher doses (1.0 mg/kg/day). Microscopic examination revealed the presence of the mucosal muscle and a thickened submucosa [87]. Subcutaneous FK506 promoted healing of colonic anastomoses in rats by reducing not only the inflammatory response, but also collagen degradation, resulting in increased anastomotic strength [88]. A case study reported that an oral FK506 given to a 75-year-old Caucasian woman facilitated healing of a lower extremity skin ulcer [89].

FK506 has been shown to display a striking potential to prevent neurodegeneration following both ischemia and chemotoxicity in a variety of species. For example, a low dose of FK506 (0.1–1 mg/kg) reduced cortical damage by approximately 60% in a rat model of middle cerebral artery occlusion. Following spinal cord injury in rats, daily injections of low-dose FK506 (0.2 mg/kg) was able to protect local nerve tissue, promote neural regeneration, reduce neuronal apoptosis, and accelerate the recovery of spinal cord functions [90]. FK506 and nerve growth factor exhibit a synergistic effect in the treatment of spinal cord injury in rats, and the combined treatment can effectively promote neural regeneration and functional recovery following spinal cord injury [91]. Interestingly, the nonimmunosuppressing FKBP ligands (V-10,367, GPI1046, and VX853) do not inhibit calcineurin activity, but are neuroregenerative in models of peripheral neuropathy and following axotomy of central neurons [92,93].

FK506 was found to not only stimulate osteoblastic differentiation, but also to enhance BMP-4 induced osteoblastic differentiation [94]. FK506 at low dose activates bone morphogenetic protein receptor type II (BMPR2), rescues endothelial dysfunction, and reverses pulmonary hypertension [95]. BMP signaling appears to influence the activation of different types of epithelial stem cells because inhibition of BMP signaling by overexpression of Noggin results in induction of hair placode formation as well as de novo formation of intestinal crypts [96–98]. BMP signaling is also required for proper stem cell differentiation, as targeted ablation of Bmpr1a results in the accretion of undifferentiated hair follicle and intestinal epithelial cells [99–101].

These results suggest that FK506 promotes tissue regeneration and wound healing through a variety of signaling pathways, some of which include BMP.

SYNERGY

FK506 HAD A SYNERGISTIC EFFECT WITH AMD3100: LESSONS FROM LIVER TRANSPLANTATION

We have found that liver transplants from Lewis to dark agouti (DA) rats sustain function long term, and that prolonged residence converted most of the parenchyma to the host genotype [102]. Postulating that the provision of more BMSCs might result in the same phenomenon in strongly rejecting Lewis rats (DA into Lewis), we studied the effects of plerixafor (AMD3100). We also provided the hosts with a small dose of tacrolimus (FK506) to "dampen the immune response." To our surprise, FK506 given at one-tenth of the immunosuppressive dose had a synergistic effect with AMD3100 in the mobilization, recruitment, and production of stem cells. In the untreated control group, as expected, liver allografts were all fatally rejected within 12 days after transplantation. Treatment with either AMD3100 or low-dose FK506 (0.1 mg/kg) alone did not significantly prolong graft survival. In contrast, combined treatment with AMD3100 plus low-dose FK506 for only the first week resulted in long-term liver transplant acceptance. This acceptance was associated with host replacement of donor liver tissue and downregulation of the immune response [103]. To explore the mechanisms, we found the percentage of lineage negative (Lin-) Thy-1+, CD34+, CD133+ cells and Lin-Triple positive (Thy1+CD34+CD133+) stem cells were significantly greater in both peripheral blood and cell suspensions made from the liver allografts in the animals receiving dual drug treatment at 7 days after transplantation. Further, these stem cells were derived from the host. Immunohistochemistry staining confirmed the increased recruitment of host BMSCs to rat liver transplants following treatment with dual drug therapy. Essentially, the transplanted graft acted as a scaffold, and the dual drug treatment facilitated host stem cell repopulation of donor graft and modified the allograft response. There was no need for subsequent immunosuppression, enabling normal graft function and survival.

Interestingly, when animals were sacrificed for collecting liver samples, we observed that the incisional wounds healed much better in animals treated with the dual drugs compared to animals treated with AMD3100 or FK506 alone. These findings raised a possibility that pharmacological mobilization of endogenous stem cells may promote skin wound healing. Thus, we applied this combined treatment in wound models and found significantly faster skin wound healing with less scar formation and even regeneration of hair follicles [104]. Lineage tracing demonstrated the critical role of BM-derived CD133 stem cells in enhanced capillary and hair follicle neogenesis, contributing to more rapid and perfect healing.

AMD3100 PLUS LOW-DOSE FK506 ACCELERATED SKIN WOUND HEALING

Full-thickness surgical excisional wound

AMD3100 has been shown to drive endogenous stem cells from the BM to the bloodstream in both animals and man. FK506, in low dosages, proved to have synergistic effects, and combination treatment promised a simple, safe, and rapid means of presenting stem cells to injured sites. We have tested this hypothesis in both mice and rats. Four full-thickness wounds were generated by 5-mm diameter circular excisions on the shaved back of wild-type C57/B6 mice or DA rats. Wounded animals were divided randomly into four experimental groups and received subcutaneous injections of saline or drugs immediately after wounding until complete healing: (1) control group treated with saline; (2) FK506 group treated daily with low dose (0.1 mg/kg); (3) AMD3100 group treated every other day (1.0 mg/kg); and (4) combination group given low-dose FK506 and AMD3100. Each wound site was photographed digitally at the indicated time intervals, and wound areas were calculated using Adobe Photoshop software. Changes in wound areas over time were expressed as the percentage of the initial wound areas. All wound evaluations were double blinded.

In mice treated with saline, wounds reached complete closure on day 12 after surgery ($n=6$), which is consistent with the known healing kinetics in this established model (Fig. 18.1). The mice treated with FK506 or AMD3100 alone exhibited significantly, but only moderately faster healing compared with the saline control group as wounds reached complete closure at day 11. In the mice treated with AMD3100 plus low-dose FK506, the healing time was reduced to 9 days or by 25% compared to the saline control group. The significant effects of dual drug therapy in reducing the size of the skin defect were observed by digital images as early as day 5 postwounding, which was the start of the reepithelialization phase of wound healing. Macroscopically, minimal ulceration and early epithelial ingrowth were observed at the skin boarders on postwounding day 5 in the dual drug-treated group, whereas wounds in the other three groups showed little, if any, epithelialization and continued ulceration.

To exclude the possibility that accelerated healing was caused by contraction, we performed the excisional wound-splinting model using a splinting ring tightly bonded to the skin around the wound (Fig. 18.1G). The wound, therefore, heals through granulation and reepithelialization, a process similar to the healing of most human skin defects. We found that wounds reached complete closure on day 15 after surgery in mice treated with saline controls. Six mice treated with FK506 or AMD3100 alone exhibited significantly faster healing compared with the saline control group (Fig. 18.1D) as wounds reached complete closure at day 13 or 14. The healing time was reduced to 12 days in the mice ($n=6$) treated with AMD3100 plus low-dose FK506. Thus, the therapeutic effects of AMD3100 plus low-dose FK506 were primarily on skin wound epithelialization.

We repeated these studies in rats and found that rats receiving dual drug therapy also showed an equivalent effect, significantly reducing the time for complete healing from 18 to 13 days or by 28%.

To determine the dose-dependent responses, other groups of mice were treated with high-dose AMD3100 (5.0–10 mg/kg) or FK506 (1.0 mg/kg). We found that high dose FK506 impeded skin wound

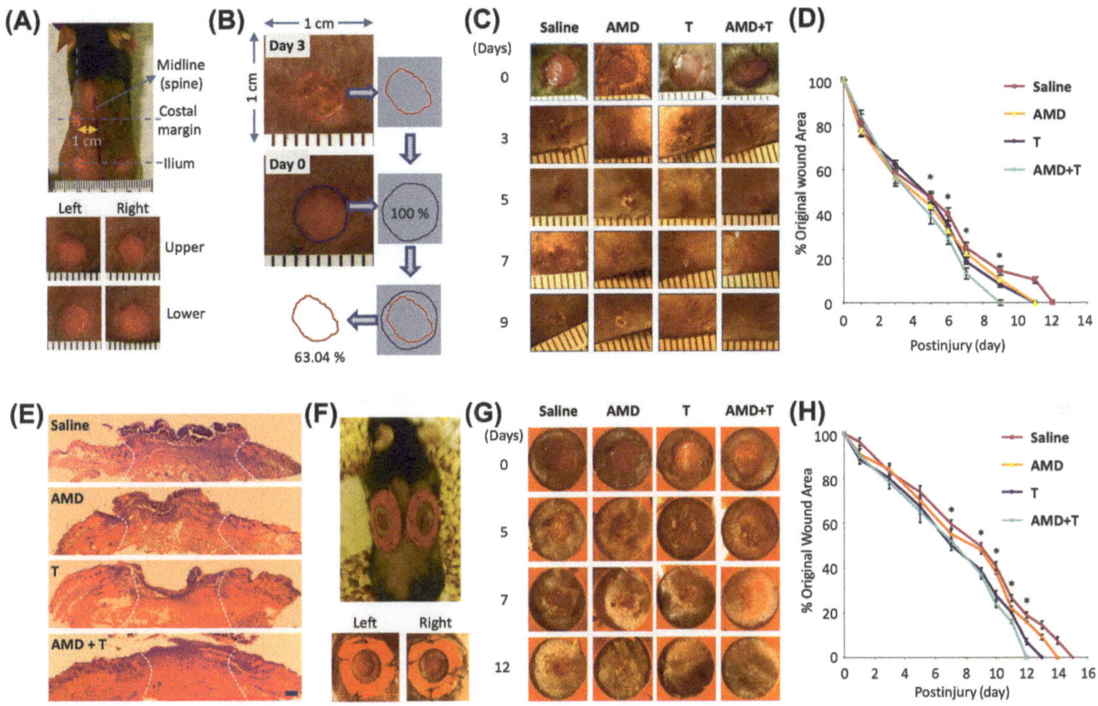

FIGURE 18.1 Accelerated wound healing in mice treated with a combination of low-dose Tacrolimus and AMD3100.

(A) The model: on day 0, four circular excisional wounds were created in C57BL/6 or *CD133+/C-L* mice. (B) Wound measurements. Wound areas were determined using Adobe Photoshop software. (C) Early healing. Representative photographs of wounds in mice (n=6) showing striking differences beginning at day 5. (D) Quantitative analysis of wound closure in mice (n=6). *$p<.05$. (E) Haematoxylin and eosin microphotographs of wounds at day 5. Scale bar: 200 μm. (F) The splinted wound model. (G) Macroscopic analysis of skin wound healing in the splinted mice. (H) Quantitative analysis of wound closure in the splinted mice (n=6). *$p<.05$. All data represent means ±SEM.

healing, whereas increased dosage of AMD3100 showed no significant difference. Thus, AMD3100 and low-dose FK506 are uniquely synergistic and promote more rapid healing.

Burns

Commonly used acute wound models include the incisional, excisional, and burn models. The incisional and excisional wounds fill with a provisional matrix composed of fibrin, fibronectin, and other plasma-derived components that lead to granulation tissue formation and reepithelialization. Chemical, thermal, or radiation burns to the skin or other tissues produce a remarkably different healing response due to their effects on the viability of cells and tissue. Thermal burns, in particular, create an extensive zone of frank necrosis that includes dead cells and denatured or even charred connective tissue. Healing of burns is retarded by the greater need to eliminate necrotic material. Most burns heal with scarring.

The time to burn wound closure is closely correlated with susceptibility to infection, pain duration, length of hospital stay, and incidence of scarring.

Full-thickness burns (12 mm in diameter) were created in the dorsal skin of C57/B6 mice. Burned mice were divided randomly into the same four experimental groups ($n = 10$/group) as described above. Burn wounds reached complete healing (reepithelialization) on day 26 in saline control animals. Low-dose FK506 or AMD3100 treatment alone exhibited moderate faster healing compared with the saline control group as wounds reached complete closure at day 22 or 24. Treatment of AMD3100 plus low-dose FK506 reduced the time of complete healing of full-thickness burn wounds by 25% (19 versus 26 days, $n = 10$/group, $p < .001$). Equally important, healing was accompanied by reduced scar formation (data presented at Congress of Wound Healing Society, 2015).

AMD3100 PLUS LOW-DOSE FK506 IMPROVED THE QUALITY OF HEALING: HAIR FOLLICLE REGENERATION

In both models of surgical excisional wounds and burns, histologically few hair follicles and abundant disorganized collagen fibers were present in animals treated with saline, AMD3100, or FK506 alone. By contrast, the dual drug-treated animals had a thin and well-organized dermis with well-formed hair follicles and much better organized collagen. Not surprisingly, the number of hair follicles in the tissue sections of reepithelialized wound was significantly higher in the dual drug-treated animals compared with the control groups. In surgical excisional wounds, hair growth in the reepithelialized wound was observed in dual drug-treated animals at 15 days after wounding (Fig. 18.2). Similarly, even in the larger burn wounds (12 mm), the size of scars was reduced by 70% in dual drug-treated animals. The combination of AMD3100 and low-dose FK506 improved wound healing by promoting both reepithelialization and differentiation of skin components.

MECHANISMS

AMD3100 AND LOW-DOSE FK506 SYNERGISTICALLY MOBILIZED STEM CELLS

The synergistic activity of low-dose FK506 and AMD3100 was measured by using colony-forming cell (CFC) assays in mobilized peripheral blood samples. Hematopoietic CFC assays have been used extensively for research and clinical applications in humans and animal models as a way of quantifying and assessing the hematopoietic progenitor content of a cell sample. CFCs are able to divide and differentiate into a colony of more mature cells that can be detected by light microscopy. This allows for the quantification of multipotent stem cell lineages mobilized by pharmaceutical agents.

C57/B6 mice were divided into four treatment groups: (1) control group treated with saline; (2) AMD3100 group (1.0 mg/kg); (3) FK506 group treated with low dose (0.1 mg/kg); and (4) AMD3100 plus FK506 group. Animals were sacrificed at 3 h after drug treatment, peripheral blood was collected, and peripheral blood mononuclear cells (PBMC) were isolated. Viable PBBCs were counted and mixed with MethoCult GF methylcellulose medium (STEMCELL Technologies, Vancouver, BC, Canada; Cat.: 03444) containing 100 U/ml penicillin and 100 μg/mL streptomycin to give a final density of 1 X 105 viable PBMCs/1.5 mL of medium. The MethoCult–cell mixture was dispensed into ultra-low cell adherence surface six-well plates (Corning, Lowell, MA), and cultures were incubated at 37°C, 5% CO_2, and 95% humidity for 14 days. Colony-forming units (CFUs) were counted using an inverted microscope (Carl Zeiss Microscopy, Thornwood, NY) at X 4. The number of CFUs was determined by

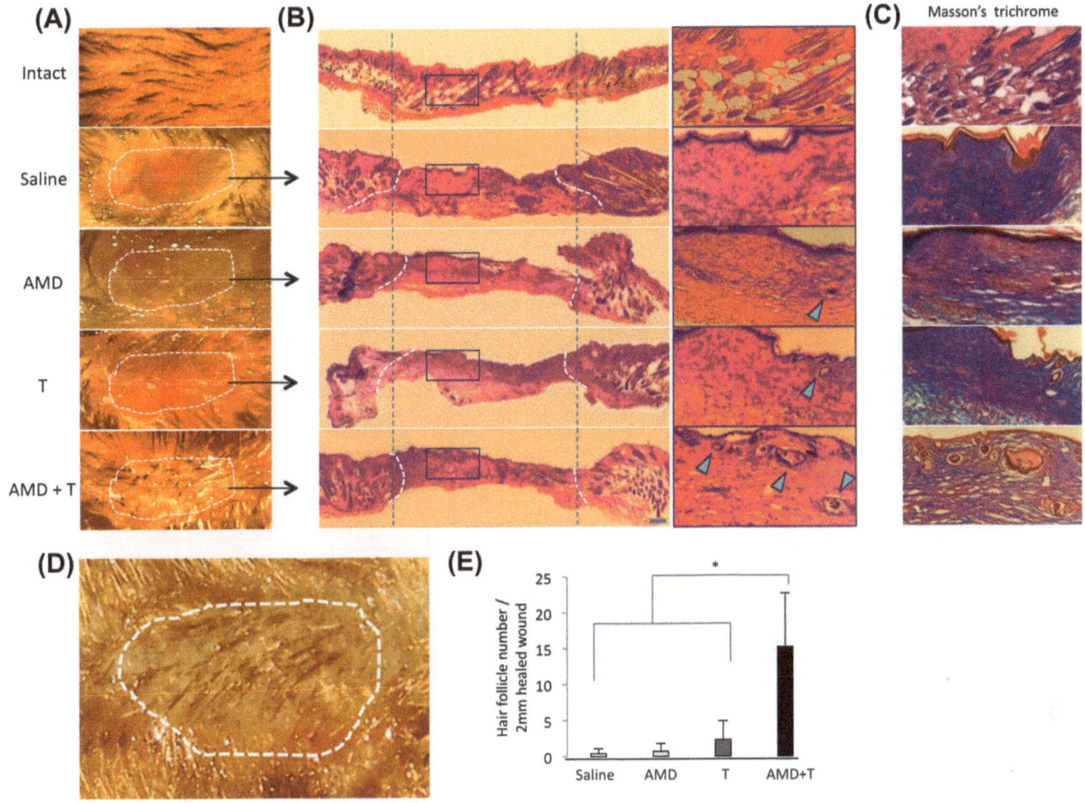

FIGURE 18.2 Increased hair follicle regeneration and diminished scarring in healed skin of mice treated with dual drug therapy.

(A) Representative macroscopic appearance of reepithelialized wounds (day 15). (B) Representative microscopic haematoxylin and eosin-stained sections from the middle of scars show new hair follicles within healed wounds. The scarred area is outlined by broken lines. Two vertical dotted lines help to demarcate the regions with the same length as that of the healed scar area in saline-treated group. Scale bar: 200 μm. (C) Adjacent sections stained with Masson's trichrome. (D) Representative photographs of dual drug-treated animals at 15 days postwounding showing hair growth in the reepithelialized wound. (E) Quantification of follicles within the healed scars (2 mm). Data represent mean ± SEM (n=9). *p<.01.

dividing the number of viable cells per milliliter by the number of plated cells per well and multiplying by the number of counted CFUs/well. The study demonstrated that the number of CFCs was significantly increased in mice treated with AMD3100 alone. Interestingly, the number of CFCs was significantly higher when mice were treated with AMD3100 plus low-dose FK506.

The mechanism responsible for more rapid and better healing in dual-treated animals was associated with increased numbers of lineage-negative, c-Kit+, CD34+, CD133+ cells, and lineage-negative triple-positive (c-Kit+CD34+CD133+) cells in animals receiving dual drug treatment (Fig. 18.3). In vivo stem cell residence and traffic to sites of injury all involve SDF-1/CXCR4 interactions. The SDF-1/CXCR4 axis is the principal mediator for directional stem cell motility. SDF-1 is highly

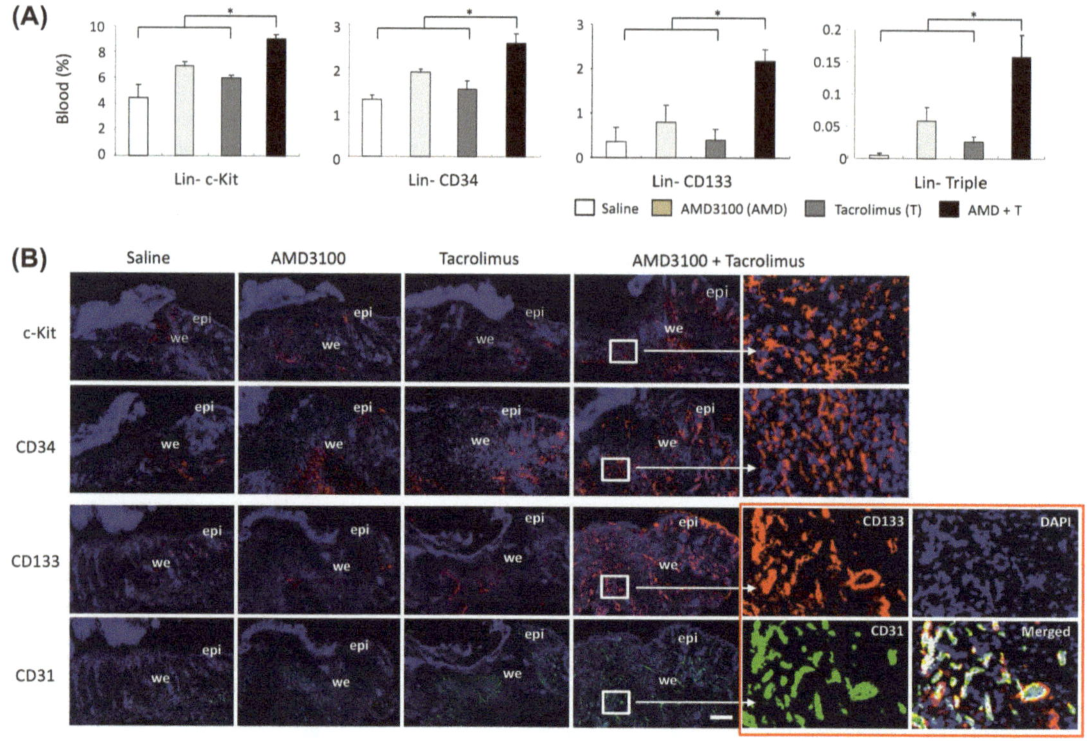

FIGURE 18.3 Recruitment of bone marrow stem cells (BMSCs) with dual drug therapy.

(A) Quantitative analysis of lineage negative (Lin-) c-Kit+, CD34+, and CD133+ cells in peripheral blood by flow cytometry at 5 days after injury. Data represent mean ± SEM (n=3). *p<.05. (B) Immunofluorescence staining for stem cell markers c-Kit, CD34, and CD133 and endothelial cells marker CD31 in tissue sections from wounded mice at 5 days after injury. Boxed areas demonstrate at higher magnification that the mice receiving dual drug treatment had a tubular arrangement of CD133 cells, which costained for CD31. Cell nuclei were stained blue with 4′,6-diamidino-2-phenylindole (DAPI). Representative photographs of n=3 individual injured skin samples per group. *epi*, epidermis; *we*, wound edge. Scale bar: 200 μm.

expressed in the BM by various stromal cells, including osteoblasts, endothelial cells, and perivascular reticular cells. The SDF-1/CXCR4 axis is also essential for both steady state egress and induced mobilization of HSCs from the BM into the circulation, a process required for host defense and repair mechanisms [105]. Decreased BM levels or increased blood levels of SDF-1 (under stress or injury) mobilize BMSCs into the circulation.

The effect of calcineurin inhibitors (CNI), including FK506, on progenitor cell mobilization was mainly attributed to changes in SDF-1 and decreased activity/availability of CD26, a membrane-bound proteinase responsible for the cleavage and inactivation of SDF-1 [106]. It was previously demonstrated that organ recipients receiving immunosuppressant drugs exhibit lower CD26 activity when compared with healthy individuals and that CsA treatment decreases the number of CD26+ cells in the peripheral blood of rats [107]. In a rat model of 5/6 nephrectomy, levels of circulating (stem cell antigen 1) Sca-1+/cKit+ stem cells, as well as blood levels of SDF-1 and stem cell factor (SCF), increase in CNI-treated Nx rats [108]. Thus, FK506 may promote stem cell mobilization through inhibition of CD26 and increased blood levels of SDF-1. The potent synergy in mobilization of BMSCs may be attributed to the CXCR4 blockade by AMD3100, and FK506 induced an increase of SDF-1 levels in peripheral blood.

LOW-DOSE FK506 INCREASED SDF-1-PRODUCING MACROPHAGES

In our mouse surgical excisional wound model, immunofluorescence staining demonstrated that the number of cells having SDF-1 and F4/80 (a marker of macrophages) markers was significantly greater in wound sites in the animals receiving low-dose FK506 alone or those receiving dual drug treatment at 5 days after injury (Fig. 18.4). SDF-1 costained with some of the F4/80 cells, indicating that these macrophages were producing or presenting SDF-1. The increased number of SDF-1-expressing macrophages was associated with the recruitment of stem cells in the wound sites. Immunofluorescence staining of wound tissue sections showed that the number of CD133+ stem cells was increased by the dual drug treatment, as were c-Kit+ and CD34+ cells (Fig. 18.4). These cells were found particularly in newly formed granulation tissues of the wounds. Interestingly, at this 5-day time point, many CD133+ cells costained with CD31, a marker of endothelial cells. The number of CD133+ cells declined at day 7, but remained detectable at day 9 after wound.

To expand on the importance of SDF-1, we inactivated it by local intradermal injection of anti–SDF-1 antibodies. This led to diminished stem cell responses and delayed wound closure in the dual drug-treated mice. Control dual-treated mice injected with equal amounts of isotype controlled IgG healed normally, thereby emphasizing the critical role of SDF-1-mediated stem/progenitor cell mobilization in the improved wound healing. Thus, a strong "push" of stem cells from their BM niches by AMD3100 and a strong "pull" of circulating stem cells by SCF-1 in the wound enhanced by low-dose FK506 best explains why there was a greater accumulation of stem cells in wound sites and more rapid restoration of normal skin with dual drug treatment. The dual drug treatment accelerated the accumulation of stem cells by increasing the numbers of SDF-1-producing macrophages, which led to the recruitment of more stem cells, which produced more SDF-1.

In addition to SDF-1, low-dose FK506 treatment may also influence macrophage polarization. Macrophage polarization is essential to the wound healing process. The macrophages are prominent components of inflammatory cells in wounds, and have many functions in wounds, including host defense, the promotion and resolution of inflammation, the removal of apoptotic cells, and the support of cell proliferation and tissue restoration following injury. Macrophages exist as resident tissue-specific macrophages or are derived from circulating blood monocytes that undergo diapedesis and subsequently differentiate into macrophages. Macrophages in wounds originate mainly from circulating monocytes. Macrophages are a source of growth factors and display various activation states. The two opposite activation states are known as classically activated (M1) and alternatively activated (M2) macrophages [109,110]. M1 macrophages are observed in initial tissue damage responses, are induced by exogenous pathogen-associated molecular patterns or endogenous damage-associated molecular patterns, and exhibit increased phagocytosis and proinflammatory cytokine production, facilitating innate immunity and wound debridement. M2 macrophages predominate later in repair, express vascular endothelial growth factor (VEGF), transforming growth factor beta, and IL-10, are activated by varied stimuli, assist in the resolution of inflammation, and promote tissue formation and remodeling [111].

Proper macrophage polarization is essential to effective wound healing, and distinct phenotypes, such as the angiogenic M2 macrophages, may be of critical importance to this process. Bai et al. [112] showed in vitro that low (20 ng/mL) but not high (2000 ng/mL) dose FK506 treatment skewed BM-derived macrophage polarization toward an active M2 macrophage phenotype. We have studied M2 macrophages in tissue sections from wound sites by using Ym1 (chitinase 3–like 3) antibody staining. The number of Ym1 positive cells was significantly increased by low-dose FK506 or dual drug treatment, as were SDF-1+ and F4/80+ cells at 5 days postinjury. Ym1 costained with not only the majority of F4/80+, but also SDF-1+ cells (unpublished data). These findings suggest (1) low-dose FK506 treatment skewed macrophage polarization toward an active M2 macrophage phenotype during the healing process; and (2) M2 macrophages may produce SDF-1 that acted as an attractor to circulating stem cells.

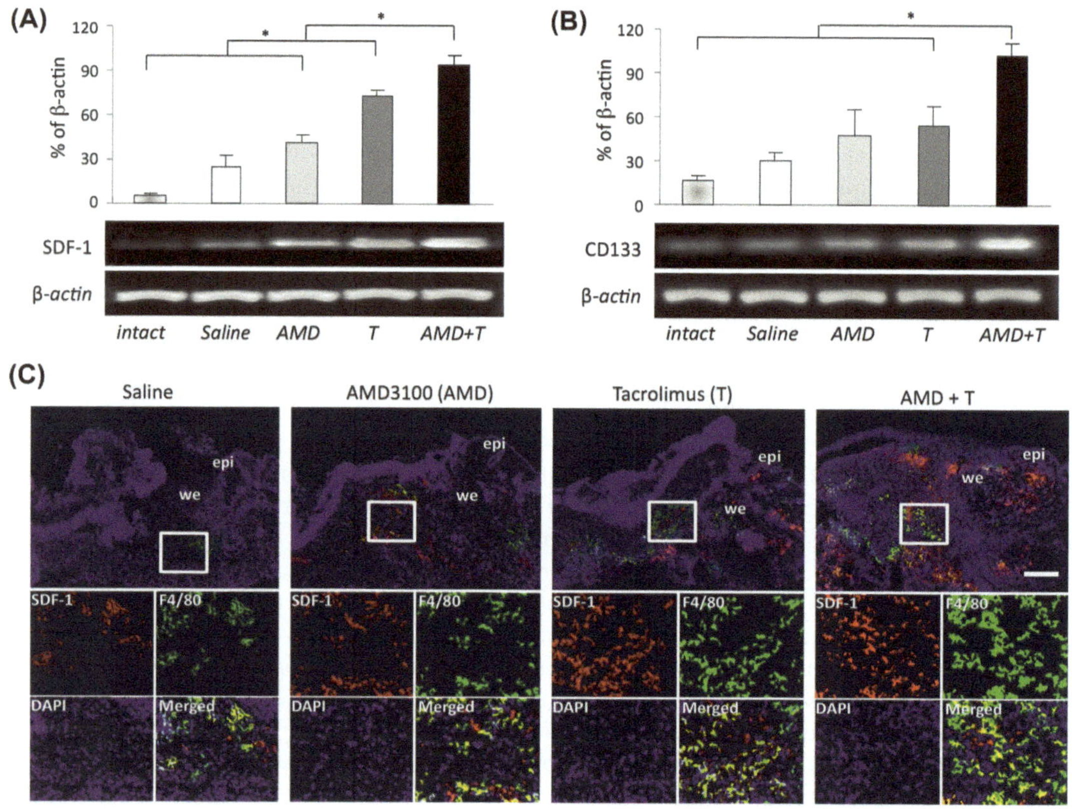

FIGURE 18.4 Increased expression of SDF-1 and CD133 in skin wounds of the mice treated with dual drug therapy.

(A) Semiquantitative reverse transcription-polymerase chain reaction analysis of the granulation tissues in wounded skin at 5 days postinjury. The mRNA expression of the attractor molecule SDF-1 was significantly increased in the low-dose Tacrolimus treatment group, and further elevated in the dual treatment group. (B) The stem cell marker CD133 mRNA level was also significantly higher in wounds in the dual treatment group, paralleling SDF-1 gene expression. All data represent means ±SEM. (n=3). *p<.05. (C) Double immunofluorescence staining for SDF-1 and F4/80 (a marker for macrophages) at 5 days after injury. *epi*, epidermis; *we*, wound edge. Scale bar: 200 μm.

DUAL DRUG TREATMENT INCREASED THE EXPRESSION OF ANGIOGENIC CYTOKINES

The messenger ribonucleic acid (mRNA) expression of the angiogenic cytokines, VEGF, and basic fibroblast growth factor, and an important stem cell mobilizing and homing factor, hepatocyte growth factor (HGF), were all significantly increased in the granulation tissues from mice treated with dual drug compared with mice treated with saline control or single drug (Fig. 18.5). Immunofluorescence staining demonstrated that the number of HGF-positive cells was significantly greater in the granulation tissues recovered from the mice with dual drug therapy 5 days after injury. Similarly, the number of CD31+ endothelial cells in the granulation tissues was markedly increased in the mice treated with dual drug compared with the other groups. Some of these CD31+ cells formed tube-like structures in the granulation tissues, which also stained for HGF, emphasizing the important role of HGF in neovascularization. The tubular structures also costained with CD133, suggesting that HGF may be involved in the differentiation of endothelial cells from CD133 precursors. Immunofluorescence staining

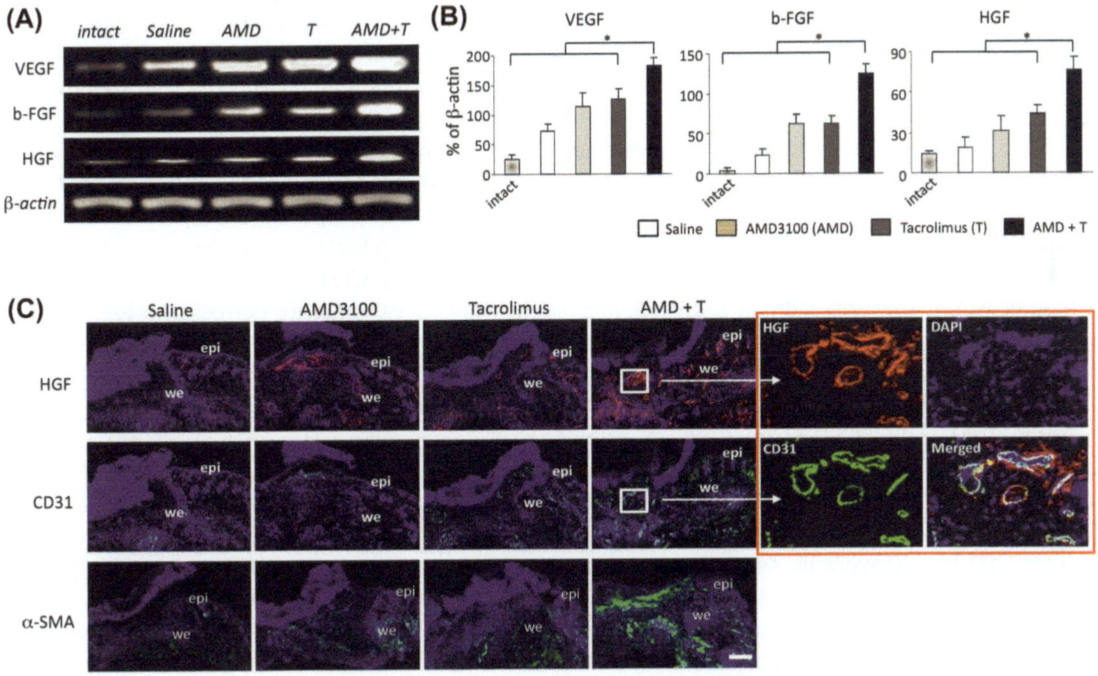

FIGURE 18.5 Increased proangiogenic factor expressions in injured mice treated with dual drug therapy.

(A) Semiquantitative PCR analysis of the granulation tissues (day 5) showing the upregulation of mRNA of vascular endothelial growth factor (VEGF), basic fibroblast growth factor (bFGF), and hepatocyte growth factor (HGF). (B) Graphic representation of increased mRNA expressions determined by calculating growth factor to β-actin ratios. Values represent mean ± SEM ($n=3$). *$p<.05$. (C) Double fluorescence staining shows that the major fraction of HGF-expressing cells costain for the endothelial marker CD31 in granulation tissues (day 5) and that these cells are more abundant in the dual treatment group. Panels in the lower row are stained for α-SMA and show the abundance of these matrix-producing cells, paralleling the findings for CD31. *epi*, epidermis; *we*, wound edge. Scale bar: 200 μm.

demonstrated that the number of a-SMA–positive myofibroblast cells increased in the granulation tissues recovered from the mice treated with AMD3100 or FK506 alone compared with the saline control group, whereas mice with dual drug treatment clearly recruited more myofibroblasts in the granulation tissues at 5 days. These results provide evidence of enhanced production of cells contributing to matrix.

The recruitment of stem cells by dual drugs was associated with elevated expression of VEGF, basic fibroblast growth factor, and HGF mRNA in the wounds. The elaboration of HGF and other autocrine or paracrine mediators produced more proangiogenic factors completing positive feedback loops.

THE CRITICAL ROLE OF CD133 STEM CELLS IN IMPROVING WOUND HEALING

CD133 is the human homologue of mouse prominin-1, a five-transmembrane domain cell surface glycoprotein that has received notable attention because of its expression restricted to various somatic stem cell subpopulations, including HSCs [113], EPCs [114], glioblastoma, and neuronal and glial stem cells [115]. This surface antigen was discovered as a target of a monoclonal antibody defined as Mab AC133, a marker expressed by a subpopulation of CD34-positive HSCs derived from human fetal liver and BM [116–118]. Subsequently, CD133 was detected in various pediatric brain tumors [119] and different human normal tissues, including kidney, prostate, brain, and pancreas, and found to be specifically associated with microvilli and other plasma membrane protrusions [120–122].

CD133 was investigated as a selectable epidermal stem cell marker because it has been widely associated with progenitor status in many organs. It has been reported that antibodies to CD133 recognized a subset of progenitors from the hair follicle bulge [122]. A recent study reported that CD133 is a marker for long-term repopulating murine epidermal stem cells, and CD133þ keratinocytes formed both hair follicles and epidermis after injection into immunodeficient mice [123]. CD133 stem cells also have a vital role in neovascularization and hair follicle regeneration, which is essential for perfect skin regeneration [124]. Such cells have the potential to differentiate along endothelial lineages in vitro [125] and are known to migrate to sites of neovascularization in response to mediators (VEGF and SDF-1).

Lineage tracing studies were performed to confirm the critical role of CD133 stem cells in wound healing [104]. Adult CD133 positive-Cre-nuclear(n) β-galactosidase (lacZ) (CD133 þ/C-L) mice containing the Rosa26GFP reporter allele [CD133 þ/C-L X membrane-targeted tandem dimer Tomato (mT) and membrane-targeted green fluorescent protein (mG) offspring] were used [126]. CreERT2 activity was induced with tamoxifen 7 days before wounding. In this mouse model, progenitor CD133 cells were lacZ positive, whereas the CD133 progeny were GFP positive. LacZ- and GFP-positive cells were observed only in the hair follicles of intact mouse skins as reported by others [123]. Both lacZ- and GFP-positive cells were increased in the granulation tissues at 5 days after wounding [104]. The numbers of lacZ- and GFP-positive cells were significantly higher in the granulation tissues recovered from the group 2 and 3 mice compared with the group 1, but the greatest numbers of lacZ- and GFP-positive cells were found in the granulation tissues of the group 4 mice. Most of the LacZ-positive cells disappeared at 15 days in groups 1, 2, and 3, while their progeny CD133 GFP-positive cells remained in the healed tissues. However, in group 4 mice, newly generated vasculature, epidermis, and hair follicles remained positive for both LacZ and GFP (Fig. 18.6). These results imply that pharmacologically mobilized CD133 stem cells and their progeny are the principle contributors to skin regeneration.

Our lineage tracing studies demonstrated the presence of CD133+ cells in the hair follicles of intact skin. Although it is clear from our lineage tracing studies that increased numbers of CD133 stem cells

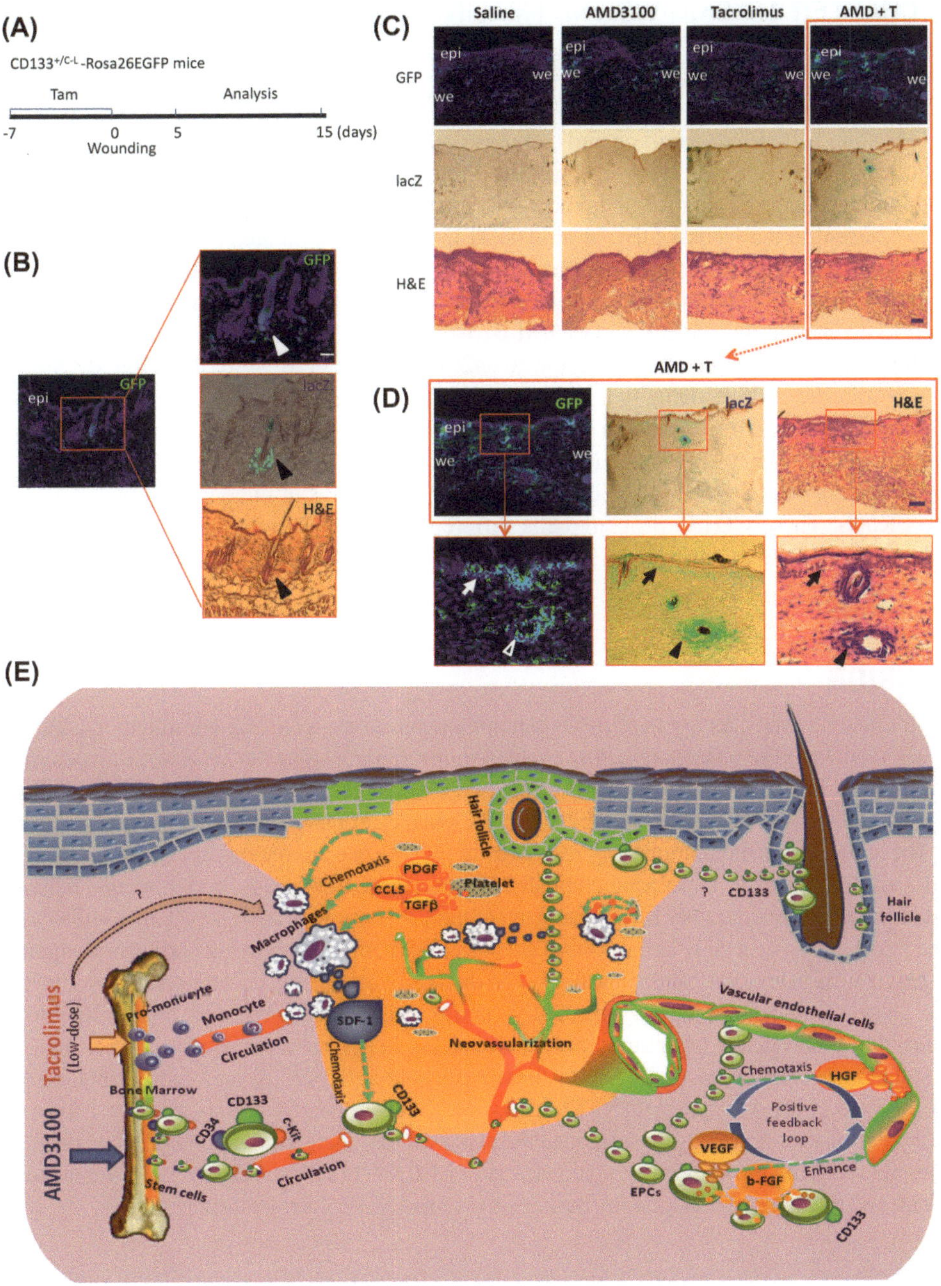

FIGURE 18.6 CD133+ stem cells generate hair follicles and epithelium in the *CD133+/C-L* mice with dual treatment group.

(A) Protocol for analysis of the tamoxifen-induced Cre-dependent green fluorescent protein (GFP) expression in CD133-lineage. (B) Intact mouse skin tissues shows marked GFP and CD133 (lacZ+) expression in the hair follicles. Scale bar: 200 μm. (C) Concurrent GFP fluorescence, β-galactosidase (lacZ), and haematoxylin and eosin staining of the same section of *CD133+/C-L-Rosa26EGFP* wounded skin on day 15 postinjury. Scale bar: 200 μm. (D) Higher power photomicrographs. In the boxed areas, arrowheads marked the hair follicles in the same section stained for GFP+ (left panel), lacZ+ (middle panel), and haematoxylin and eosin (right panel). Arrows point to the GFP and lacZ positive epithelium. *epi*, epidermis; *we*, wound edge. Scale bar: 100 μm. (E) Schematic representation of therapeutic mechanism of combination treatment in skin wound healing.

contributed to hair follicle regeneration and that these cells were liberated from the BM by dual treatment, it is possible that these CD133+ stem cells originate from normal skin. We consider this unlikely for several reasons. Our lineage tracing study did not show the expansion of CD133+ cells in the hair follicles of intact skin adjacent to the wound sites. Instead, CD133+ cells accumulated in the central granulation tissues rather than the wound edges. Further, the number of CD133+ cells in the wound sites correlated with the number of CD133+ cells in peripheral blood. More recently, BMT and lineage tracing approaches were used to determine the critical role of BM-derived CD133 stem cells in wound healing. BM cells from adult CD133 þ/C-L mice containing the Rosa26GFP reporter allele (CD133 þ/C-L X mTmG offspring) were transplanted into lethally irradiated wild-type C57/B6 (syngeneic). At 2 months after BMT, peripheral blood cells were repopulated by donor hematopoietic progenitor-derived cells. Full-thickness burns (12 mm in diameter) were created in the dorsal skin of these transplanted C57/B6 mice. BM-derived CD133+ cells were accumulated in the granulation tissues at 7 days in mice treated with AMD3100 plus low-dose FK506. These CD133 progeny cells differentiated into varieties of skin components. These studies demonstrated the critical role of BM-derived CD133 stem cells in wound healing.

CONCLUSION

In search for better therapy for organ transplantation patients, a new two-drug combination (AMD3100 and FK506) was discovered serendipitously that enabled long-term transplant survival with 1 week of treatment and freedom from immunosuppression. One of the two drugs, AMD3100 is an antagonist of the chemokine receptor CXCR4 and has been used to mobilize BMSCs in cancer patients prior to ablative chemo–radiation therapy. The other drug is the immunosuppressive drug FK506, used to prevent organ rejection and effective only at dosages one-tenth of those used clinically. We tested the dual drugs in skin wound healing models and found FK506 at low dose only had a potent synergistic activity with AMD3100 in mobilization, recruitment, and retention of stem cells in the wound sites. Recruitment of mobilizing endogenous stem cells into skin wounds results in better and faster healing. The dual drug treatment accelerated skin wound healing by 25–28%. The magnitude of both the quantitative and qualitative differences is highly significant and is greater than that found in any other study of wound healing in normal animals. Our studies do not disclose the molecular mechanisms that differentiate these malleable cells into tissue components, such as those reported for Fgf9 [127] or Sept4/ARTS [128]. However, the differentiating steps leading to healing with reestablishment of skin appendages proceeded faultlessly when there were abundant stem cells producing almost normal skin. The profound synergistic effects of AMD3100 and low-dose FK506 in the mobilization, recruitment, and retention of endogenous stem cells promise clinical application [129].

REFERENCES

[1] Sen CK, Gordillo GM, Roy S, Kirsner R, Lambert L, Hunt TK, et al. Human skin wounds: a major and snowballing threat to public health and the economy. Wound Repair Regen November–December 2009;17(6):763–71.

[2] Peck MD. Epidemiology of burns throughout the world. Part I: distribution and risk factors. Burns November 2011;37(7):1087–100.

[3] Butler KL, Goverman J, Ma H, Fischman A, Yu YM, Bilodeau M, et al. Stem cells and burns: review and therapeutic implications. J Burn Care Res November–December 2010;31(6):874–81.

[4] Branski LK, Gauglitz GG, Herndon DN, Jeschke MG. A review of gene and stem cell therapy in cutaneous wound healing. Burns March 2009;35(2):171–80.
[5] Dabiri G, Heiner D, Falanga V. The emerging use of bone marrow-derived mesenchymal stem cells in the treatment of human chronic wounds. Expert Opin Emerg Drugs December 2013;18(4):405–19.
[6] Burd A, Ahmed K, Lam S, Ayyappan T, Huang L. Stem cell strategies in burns care. Burns 2007;33(3):282–91.
[7] Zhang CP, Fu XB. Therapeutic potential of stem cells in skin repair and regeneration. Chin J Traumatol August 2008;11(4):209–21.
[8] Kim WS, Park BS, Sung JH, Yang JM, Park SB, Kwak SJ, et al. Wound healing effect of adipose-derived stem cells: a critical role of secretory factors on human dermal fibroblasts. J Dermatol Sci 2007;48(1):15–24.
[9] Cerqueira MT, Marques AP, Reis RL. Using stem cells in skin regeneration: possibilities and reality. Stem Cells Dev May 20, 2012;21(8):1201–14.
[10] Prockop DJ. Repair of tissues by adult stem/progenitor cells (MSCs): controversies, myths, and changing paradigms. Mol Ther 2009;17:939–46.
[11] Orkin SH, Zon LI. Hematopoiesis: an evolving paradigm for stem cell biology. Cell 2008;132:631–44.
[12] Pittenger MF, Mackay AM, Beck SC, Jaiswal RK, Douglas R, Mosca JD, et al. Multilineage potential of adult human mesenchymal stem cells. Science 1999;284:143–7.
[13] Prockop DJ. Marrow stromal cells as stem cells for nonhematopoietic tissues. Science 1997;276:71–4.
[14] Pereira RF, Halford KW, O'Hara MD, Leeper DB, Sokolov BP, Pollard MD, et al. Cultured adherent cells from marrow can serve as long-lasting precursor cells for bone, cartilage, and lung in irradiated mice. Proc Natl Acad Sci U.S.A. 1995;92:4857–61.
[15] Galmiche MC, Koteliansky VE, Brière J, Hervé P, Charbord P. Stromal cells from human long-term marrow cultures are mesenchymal cells that differentiate following a vascular smooth muscle differentiation pathway. Blood 1993;82:66–76.
[16] Tropel P, Platet N, Platel JC, Noël D, Albrieux M, Benabid AL, et al. Functional neuronal differentiation of bone marrow-derived mesenchymal stem cells. Stem Cells 2006;24:2868–76.
[17] Kang SK, Putnam LA, Ylostalo J, Popescu IR, Dufour J, Belousov A, et al. Neurogenesis of Rhesus adipose stromal cells. J Cell Sci 2004;117:4289–99.
[18] Yamanaka S. Strategies and new developments in the generation of patient-specific pluripotent stem cells. Cell Stem Cell 2007;1(1):39–49.
[19] Takahashi K, Tanabe K, Ohnuki M, Narita M, Ichisaka T, Tomoda K, et al. Induction of pluripotent stem cells from adult human fibroblasts by defined factors. Cell 2007;131(5):861–72.
[20] Shumakov VI, Onishchenko NA, Rasulov MF, Krasheninnikov ME, Zaidenov VA. Mesenchymal bone marrow stem cells more effectively stimulate regeneration of deep burn wounds than embryonic fibroblasts. Bull Exp Biol Med 2003;136(2):192–5.
[21] He L, Nan X, Wang Y, Guan L, Bai C, Shi S, et al. Full-thickness tissue engineered skin constructed with autogenic bone marrow mesenchymal stem cells. Sci China C Life Sci 2007;50(4):429–37.
[22] Kamolz LP, Kolbus A, Wick N, Mazal PR, Eisenbock B, Burjak S, et al. Cultured human epithelium: human umbilical cord blood stem cells differentiate into keratinocytes under in vitro conditions. Burns 2006;32(1):16–9.
[23] Roh C, Lyle S. Cutaneous stem cells and wound healing. Pediatr Res 2006;59(4 Pt 2):100R–3R.
[24] Woodley DT, Remington J, Huang Y, Hou Y, Li W, Keene DR, et al. Intravenously injected human fibroblasts home to skin wounds, deliver type VII collagen, and promote wound healing. Mol Ther 2007;15:628–35.
[25] Chino T, Tamai K, Yamazaki T, Otsuru S, Kikuchi Y, Nimura K, et al. Bone marrow cell transfer into fetal circulation can ameliorate genetic skin diseases by providing fibroblasts to the skin and inducing immune tolerance. Am J Pathol 2008;173:803–14.
[26] Tolar J, Ishida-Yamamoto A, Riddle M, McElmurry RT, Osborn M, Xia L, et al. Amelioration of epidermolysis bullosa by transfer of wild-type bone marrow cells. Blood 2009;113:1167–74.
[27] Fujita Y, Abe R, Inokuma D, Sasaki M, Hoshina D, Natsuga K, et al. Bone marrow transplantation restores epidermal basement membrane protein expression and rescues epidermolysis bullosa model mice. Proc Natl Acad Sci U.S.A. 2010;107:14345–50.

[28] Liu P, Deng Z, Han S, Liu T, Wen N, Lu W, et al. Tissue-engineered skin containing mesenchymal stem cells improves burn wounds. Artif Organs December 2008;32(12):925–31.
[29] Tamai K, Yamazaki T, Chino T, Ishii M, Otsuru S, Kikuchi Y, et al. PDGFRalpha-positive cells in bone marrow are mobilized by high mobility group box 1 (HMGB1) to regenerate injured epithelia. Proc Natl Acad Sci U.S.A. 2011;108:6609–14.
[30] Iinuma S, Aikawa E, Tamai K, Fujita R, Kikuchi Y, Chino T, et al. Transplanted bone marrow-derived circulating PDGFRα+ cells restore type VII collagen in recessive dystrophic epidermolysis bullosa mouse skin graft. J Immunol February 15, 2015;194(4):1996–2003.
[31] Rennert RC, Sorkin M, Garg RK, Gurtner GC. Stem cell recruitment after injury: lessons for regenerative medicine. Regen Med November 2012;7(6):833–50.
[32] Hamou C, Callaghan MJ, Thangarajah H, Chang E, Chang EI, Grogan RH, et al. Mesenchymal stem cells can participate in ischemic neovascularization. Plast Reconstr Surg 2009;123(2 Suppl.):S45–55.
[33] Kucia MJ, Wysoczynski M, Wu W, Zuba-Surma EK, Ratajczak J, Ratajczak MZ. Evidence that very small embryonic-like stem cells are mobilized into peripheral blood. Stem Cells 2008;26(8):2083–92.
[34] Tepper OM, Capla JM, Galiano RD, Ceradini DJ, Callaghan MJ, Kleinman ME, et al. Adult vasculogenesis occurs through in situ recruitment, proliferation, and tubulization of circulating bone marrow-derived cells. Blood 2005;105(3):1068–77.
[35] Xynos A, Corbella P, Belmonte N, Zini R, Manfredini R, Ferrari G. Bone marrow-derived hematopoietic cells undergo myogenic differentiation following a Pax-7 independent pathway. Stem Cells 2010;28(5):965–73.
[36] Deng J, Zou ZM, Zhou TL, Su YP, Ai GP, Wang JP, et al. Bone marrow mesenchymal stem cells can be mobilized into peripheral blood by G-CSF in vivo and integrate into traumatically injured cerebral tissue. Neurol Sci 2011;32(4):641–51.
[37] Qian H, Yang H, Xu W, Yan Y, Chen Q, Zhu W, et al. Bone marrow mesenchymal stem cells ameliorate rat acute renal failure by differentiation into renal tubular epithelial-like cells. Int J Mol Med 2008;22(3):325–32.
[38] Park D, Spencer JA, Koh BI, Kobayashi T, Fujisaki J, Clemens TL, et al. Endogenous bone marrow MSCs are dynamic, fate-restricted participants in bone maintenance and regeneration. Cell Stem Cell 2012;10(3):259–72.
[39] Zhao W, Li JJ, Cao DY, Li X, Zhang LY, He Y, et al. Intravenous injection of mesenchymal stem cells is effective in treating liver fibrosis. World J Gastroenterol 2012;18(10):1048–58.
[40] Schenk S, Mal N, Finan A, Zhang M, Kiedrowski M, Popovic Z, et al. Monocyte chemotactic protein-3 is a myocardial mesenchymal stem cell homing factor. Stem Cells 2007;25(1):245–51.
[41] Hamada H, Kim MK, Iwakura A, Ii M, Thorne T, Qin G, et al. Estrogen receptors α and β mediate contribution of bone marrow-derived endothelial progenitor cells to functional recovery after myocardial infarction. Circulation 2006;114(21):2261–70.
[42] Chen Y, Xiang LX, Shao JZ, Pan RL, Wang YX, Dong XJ, et al. Recruitment of endogenous bone marrow mesenchymal stem cells towards injured liver. J Cell Mol Med 2010;14(6B):1494–508.
[43] Si Y, Tsou CL, Croft K, Charo IF. CCR2 mediates hematopoietic stem and progenitor cell trafficking to sites of inflammation in mice. J Clin Invest 2010;120(4):1192–203.
[44] Verstappen J, Katsaros C, Kuijpers-Jagtman AM, Torensma R, Von den Hoff JW. The recruitment of bone marrow-derived cells to skin wounds is independent of wound size. Wound Repair Regen March–April 2011;19(2):260–7.
[45] Gabbiani G. The myofibroblast in wound healing and fibrocontractive diseases. J Pathol 2003;200:500–3.
[46] Hinz B, Phan SH, Thannickal VJ, Galli A, Bochaton-Piallat M-L, Gabbiani G. The myofibroblast: one function, multiple origins. Am J Pathol 2007;170:1807–16.
[47] Brittan M, Braun KM, Reynolds LE, Conti FJ, Reynolds AR, Poulsom R, et al. Bone marrow cells engraft within the epidermis and proliferate in vivo with no evidence of cell fusion. J Pathol 2005;205:1–13.
[48] Fathke C, Wilson L, Hutter J, Kapoor V, Smith A, Hocking A, et al. Contribution of bone marrow-derived cells to skin: collagen deposition and wound repair. Stem Cells 2004;22:812–22.

[49] Direkze NC, Forbes SJ, Brittan M, Hunt T, Jeffery R, Preston SL, et al. Multiple organ engraftment by bone-marrow-derived myofibroblasts and fibroblasts in bone-marrow-transplanted mice. Stem Cells 2003;21:514–20.
[50] Bucala R, Spiegel LA, Chesney J, Hogan M, Cerami A. Circulating fibrocytes define a new leukocyte subpopulation that mediates tissue repair. Mol Med 1994;1:71–81.
[51] Mori L, Bellini A, Stacey MA, Schmidt M, Mattoli S. Fibrocytes contribute to the myofibroblast population in wounded skin and originate from the bone marrow. Exp Cell Res 2005;304:81–90.
[52] Rea S, Giles NL, Webb S, Adcroft KF, Evill LM, Strickland DH, et al. Bone marrow-derived cells in the healing burn wound–More than just inflammation. Burns 2009;35:356–64.
[53] Jabs A, Moncada GA, Nichols CE, Waller EK, Wilcox JN. Peripheral blood mononuclear cells acquire myofibroblasts characteristics in granulation tissue. J Vasc Res 2005;42:174–80.
[54] Zhao W, Li JJ, Cao DY, Li X, Zhang LY, He Y, et al. Intravenous injection of mesenchymal stem cells is effective in treating liver fibrosis. World J Gastroenterol 2012;18(10):1048–58.
[55] Fan Y, Shen F, Frenzel T, Zhu W, Ye J, Liu J, et al. Endothelial progenitor cell transplantation improves long-term stroke outcome in mice. Ann Neurol 2010;67(4):488–97.
[56] Schuh A, Liehn EA, Sasse A, Hristov M, Sobota R, Kelm M, et al. Transplantation of endothelial progenitor cells improves neovascularization and left ventricular function after myocardial infarction in a rat model. Basic Res Cardiol 2008;103(1):69–77.
[57] Lam CF, Roan JN, Lee CH, Chang PJ, Huang CC, Liu YC, et al. Transplantation of endothelial progenitor cells improves pulmonary endothelial function and gas exchange in rabbits with endotoxin-induced acute lung injury. Anesth Analg 2011;112(3):620–7.
[58] Borlongan CV, Glover LE, Tajiri N, Kaneko Y, Freeman TB. The great migration of bone marrow-derived stem cells toward the ischemic brain: therapeutic implications for stroke and other neurological disorders. Prog Neurobiol 2011;95(2):213–28.
[59] Hara Y, Stolk M, Ringe J, Dehne T, Ladhoff J, Kotsch K, et al. In vivo effect of bone marrow-derived mesenchymal stem cells in a rat kidney transplantation model with prolonged cold ischemia. Transpl Int 2011;24(11):1112–23.
[60] Pati S, Gerber MH, Menge TD, Wataha KA, Zhao Y, Baumgartner JA, et al. Bone marrow derived mesenchymal stem cells inhibit inflammation and preserve vascular endothelial integrity in the lungs after hemorrhagic shock. PLoS One 2011;6(9):e25171.
[61] Dawn B, Tiwari S, Kucia MJ, Zuba-Surma EK, Guo Y, Sanganalmath SK, et al. Transplantation of bone marrow-derived very small embryonic-like stem cells attenuates left ventricular dysfunction and remodeling after myocardial infarction. Stem Cells 2008;26(6):1646–55.
[62] Malliaras K, Kreke M, Marban E. The stuttering progress of cell therapy for heart disease. Review of clinical trials using stem cell therapies for cardiac disease. Clin Pharmacol Ther 2011;90(4):532–41.
[63] Lee JW, Fang X, Krasnodembskaya A, Howard JP, Matthay MA. Concise review. Mesenchymal stem cells for acute lung injury: role of paracrine soluble factors. Stem Cells 2011;29(6):913–9.
[64] Jablonska A, Lukomska B. Stroke induced brain changes: implications for stem cell transplantation. Acta Neurobiol Exp (Wars) 2011;71(1):74–85.
[65] Teng M, Huang Y, Zhang H. Application of stems cells in wound healing–an update. Wound Repair Regen March–April 2014;22(2):151–60.
[66] Phinney DD. Functional heterogeneity of mesenchymal stem cells: implications for cell therapy. J Cell Biochem 2012;113(9):2806–12.
[67] Ciampolini M, Fabbrizzi L, Perotti A, Poggi A, Seghi B, Zanobini F. Dinickel and dicopper complexes with N,N-linked bis(cyclam) ligands. An ideal system for the investigation of electrostatic effects on the redox behavior of pairs of metal ions. Inorg Chem 1987;26(21):3527.
[68] Schols D, Struyf S, Van Damme J, Esté JA, Henson G, De Clercq E. Inhibition of T-tropic HIV strains by selective antagonization of the chemokine receptor CXCR4. J Exp Med 1997;186:1383–8.

[69] Aiuti A, Webb IJ, Bleul C, Springer T, Gutierrez-Ramos JC. The chemokine SDF-1 is a chemoattractant for human CD34+ hematopoietic progenitor cells and provides a new mechanism to explain the mobilization of CD34+ progenitors to peripheral blood. J Exp Med 1997;185:111–20.
[70] Ma Q, Jones D, Springer TA. The chemokine receptor CXCR4 is required for the retention of B lineage and granulocytic precursors within the bone marrow microenvironment. Immunity 1999;10:463–71.
[71] De Clercq E. The AMD3100 story: the path to the discovery of a stem cell mobilizer (Mozobil). Biochem Pharmacol 2009;77:1655–64.
[72] Liles WC, Broxmeyer HE, Rodger E, Wood B, Hübel K, Cooper S, et al. Mobilization of hematopoietic progenitor cells in healthy volunteers by AMD3100, a CXCR4 antagonist. Blood October 15, 2003;102(8):2728–30.
[73] Kean LS, Sen S, Onabajo O, Singh K, Robertson J, Stempora L, et al. Significant mobilization of both conventional and regulatory T cells with AMD3100. Blood December 15, 2011;118(25):6580–90.
[74] Wise JK, Sumner DR, Virdi AS. Modulation of stromal cell-derived factor-1/CXC chemokine receptor 4 axis enhances rhBMP-2-induced ectopic bone formation. Tissue Eng 2012;18:860–9.
[75] Kumar S, Ponnazhagan S. Mobilization of bone marrow mesenchymal stem cells in vivo augments bone healing in a mouse model of segmental bone defect. Bone April 2012;50(4):1012–8.
[76] Tepper OM, Carr J, Allen Jr RJ, Chang CC, Lin CD, Tanaka R, et al. Decreased circulating progenitor cell number and failed mechanisms of stromal cell-derived factor-1alpha mediated bone marrow mobilization impair diabetic tissue repair. Diabetes 2010;59:1974–83.
[77] Nishimura Y, Li M, Qin G, Hamada H, Asai J, Takenaka H, et al. CXCR4 antagonist AMD3100 accelerates impaired wound healing in diabetic mice. J Invest Dermatol 2011;132(3):1–10.
[78] Hisada M, Ota Y, Zhang X, Cameron AM, Gao B, Montgomery RA, et al. Successful transplantation of reduced-sized rat alcoholic fatty livers made possible by mobilization of host stem cells. Am J Transpl December 2012;12(12):3246–56.
[79] Crawford J, Glaspy JA, Stoller RG, Tomita DK, Vincent ME, McGuire BW, et al. Final results of a placebo-controlled study of Filgrastim in small-cell lung cancer: exploration of risk factors for febrile neutropenia. Support Cancer Ther 2005;3(1):36–46.
[80] Thomas J, Liu F, Link DC. Mechanisms of mobilization of hematopoietic progenitors with granulocyte colony-stimulating factor. Curr Opin Hematol May 2002;9(3):183–9.
[81] Jin F, Zhai Q, Qiu L, Meng H, Zou D, Wang Y, et al. Degradation of BM SDF-1 by MMP-9: the role in G-CSF-induced hematopoietic stem/progenitor cell mobilization. Bone Marrow Transpl November 2008;42(9):581–8.
[82] Iwamoto S, Lin X, Ramirez R, Carson P, Fiore D, Goodrich J, et al. Bone marrow cell mobilization by the systemic use of granulocyte colony-stimulating factor (GCSF) improves wound bed preparation. Int J Low Extrem Wounds December 2013;12(4):256–64.
[83] Kino T, Hatanaka H, Hashimoto M, Nishiyama M, Goto T, Okuhara M, et al. FK-506, a novel immunosuppressant isolated from a Streptomyces. I. Fermentation, isolation, and physico-chemical and biological characteristics. J Antibiot (Tokyo) 1987;40(9):1249–55.
[84] Tanaka N, Yamamoto H, Tatemoto A, Urabe T, Orita K. Regulation of liver regeneration by interleukin-2 and its inhibitors: cyclosporine A and FK 506. Int J Immunopharmacol February 1993;15(2):211–8.
[85] Tamura F, Masuhara A, Sakaida I, Fukumoto E, Nakamura T, Okita K. FK506 promotes liver regeneration by suppressing natural killer cell activity. J Gastroenterol Hepatol July 1998;13(7):703–8.
[86] Escribano O, Fernández-Moreno MD, Piña MJ, Fueyo J, Menor C, Román ID, et al. Pretreatment with FK506 up-regulates insulin receptors in regenerating rat liver. Hepatology September 2002;36(3):555–61.
[87] Kiyama T, Tajiri T, Tokunaga A, Yoshiyuki T, Barbul A. Tacrolimus enhances colon anastomotic healing in rats. Wound Repair Regen September–October 2002;10(5):308–13.
[88] Raptis D, Mantzoros I, Pramateftakis MG, Despoudi K, Zaraboukas T, Koliakos G, et al. The effects of tacrolimus on colonic anastomotic healing in rats. Int J Colorectal Dis March 2012;27(3):299–308.

[89] Miller S. The effect of tacrolimus on lower extremity ulcers: a case study and review of the literature. Ostomy Wound Manage April 2008;54(4):36–42.
[90] López-Vales R, García-Alías G, Forés J, Udina E, Gold BG, Navarro X, et al. FK 506 reduces tissue damage and prevents functional deficit after spinal cord injury in the rat. J Neurosci Res September 15, 2005;81(6):827–36.
[91] Chen G, Zhang Z, Wang S, Lv D. Combined treatment with FK506 and nerve growth factor for spinal cord injury in rats. Exp Ther Med October 2013;6(4):868–72.
[92] Gold BG, Zeleny-Pooley M, Wang MS, Chaturvedi P, Armistead DM. A nonimmunosuppressant FKBP-12 ligand increases nerve regeneration. Exp Neurol October 1997;147(2):269–78.
[93] Herdegan T, Fischer G, Bold BG. Immunophilin ligands as a novel treatment of neurological disorders. Trends Pharmacol Sci January 2000;21(1):3–5.
[94] Tang L, Ebara S, Kawasaki S, Wakabayashi S, Nikaido T, Takaoka K. FK506 enhanced osteoblastic differentiation in mesenchymal cells. Cell Biol Int 2002;26(1):75–84.
[95] Spiekerkoetter E, Tian X, Cai J, Hopper RK, Sudheendra D, Li CG, et al. FK506 activates BMPR2, rescues endothelial dysfunction, and reverses pulmonary hypertension. J Clin Invest August 2013;123(8):3600–13.
[96] Botchkarev VA, Botchkareva NV, Nakamura M, Huber O, Funa K, Lauster R, et al. Noggin is required for induction of the hair follicle growth phase in postnatal skin. FASEB J October 2001;15(12):2205–14.
[97] Haramis AP, Begthel H, van den Born M, van Es J, Jonkheer S, Offerhaus GJ, et al. De novo crypt formation and juvenile polyposis on BMP inhibition in mouse intestine. Science March 12, 2004;303(5664):1684–6.
[98] He XC, Zhang J, Tong WG, Tawfik O, Ross J, Scoville DH, et al. BMP signaling inhibits intestinal stem cell self-renewal through suppression of Wnt-beta-catenin signaling. Nat Genet October 2004;36(10):1117–21.
[99] Andl T, Ahn K, Kairo A, Chu EY, Wine-Lee L, Reddy ST, et al. Epithelial Bmpr1a regulates differentiation and proliferation in postnatal hair follicles and is essential for tooth development. Development May 2004;131(10):2257–68.
[100] Kobielak K, Pasolli HA, Alonso L, Polak L, Fuchs E. Defining BMP functions in the hair follicle by conditional ablation of BMP receptor IA. J Cell Biol November 10, 2003;163(3):609–23.
[101] Sancho E, Batlle E, Clevers H. Signaling pathways in intestinal development and cancer. Annu Rev Cell Dev Biol 2004;20:695–723.
[102] Sun Z, Zhang X, Locke JE, Zheng Q, Tachibana S, Diehl AM, et al. Recruitment of host progenitor cells in rat liver transplants. Hepatology February 2009;49(2):587–97.
[103] Okabayashi T, Cameron AM, Hisada M, Montgomery RA, Williams GM, Sun Z. Mobilization of host stem cells enables long-term liver transplant acceptance in a strongly rejecting rat strain combination. Am J Transpl October 2011;11(10):2046–56.
[104] Lin Q, Wesson RN, Maeda H, Wang Y, Cui Z, Liu JO, et al. Pharmacological mobilization of endogenous stem cells significantly promotes skin regeneration after full-thickness excision: the synergistic activity of AMD3100 and tacrolimus. J Invest Dermatol September 2014;134(9):2458–68.
[105] Hopman RK, DiPersio JF. Advances in stem cell mobilization. Blood Rev January 2014;28(1):31–40. http://dx.doi.org/10.1016/j.blre.2014.01.001.
[106] Wang CH, Cherng WJ, Yang NI, Hsu CM, Yeh CH, Lan YJ, et al. Cyclosporine increases ischemia-induced endothelial progenitor cell mobilization through manipulation of the CD26 system. Am J Physiol Regul Integr Comp Physiol March 1, 2008;294(3):R811–8.
[107] Korom S, De Meester I, Maas E, Stein A, Wilker S, Jung F, et al. CD26 expression and enzymatic activity in recipients of kidney allografts. Transpl Proc August 2002;34(5):1753–4.
[108] Di Marco GS, Reuter S, Kentrup D, Ting L, Ting L, Grabner A, et al. Cardioprotective effect of calcineurin inhibition in an animal model of renal disease. Eur Heart J August 2011;32(15):1935–45.
[109] Gordon S, Taylor PR. Monocyte and macrophage heterogeneity. Nat Rev Immunol 2005;5(12):953–64.
[110] Mosser DM, Edwards JP. Exploring the full spectrum of macrophage activation. Nat Rev Immunol 2008;8(12):958–69.

[111] Ploeger DT, Hosper NA, Schipper M, Koerts JA, de Rond S, Bank RA. Cell plasticity in wound healing: paracrine factors of M1/M2 polarized macrophages influence the phenotypical state of dermal fibroblasts. Cell Commun Signal April 19, 2013;11(1):29.

[112] Bai L, Gabriels K, Wijnands E, Rousch M, Daemen MJ, Tervaert JW, et al. Low- but not high-dose FK506 treatment confers atheroprotection due to alternative macrophage activation and unaffected cholesterol levels. Thromb Haemost 2010;104:143–50.

[113] Horn PA, Tesch H, Staib P, Kube D, Diehl V, Voliotis D. Expression of AC133, a novel hematopoietic precursor antigen, on acute myeloid leukemia cells. Blood 1999;93(4):1435–7.

[114] Corbeil D, Röper K, Hellwig A, Tavian M, Miraglia S, Watt SM, et al. The human AC133 hematopoietic stem cell antigen is also expressed in epithelial cells and targeted to plasma membrane protrusions. J Biol Chem 2000;275(8):5512–20.

[115] Sanai N, Alvarez-Buylla A, Berger MS. Neural stem cells and the origin of gliomas. N Engl J Med 2005;353(8):811–22.

[116] Bauer N, Fonseca A–V, Florek M, Freund D, Jaszai J, Bornhauser M, et al. New insights into the cell biology of hematopoietic progenitors by studying prominin-1 (CD133). Cells Tissues Organs 2008;188(1–2):127–38.

[117] Miraglia S, Godfrey W, Yin AH, Atkins K, Warnke R, Holden JT, et al. A novel five-transmembrane hematopoietic stem cell antigen: isolation, characterization, and molecular cloning. Blood 1997;90(12):5013–21.

[118] Yin AH, Miraglia S, Zanjani ED, Almeida-Porada G, Ogawa M, Leary AG, et al. AC133, a novel marker for human hematopoietic stem and progenitor cells. Blood 1997;90(12):5002–12.

[119] Singh SK, Clarke ID, Terasaki M, Bonn VE, Hawkins C, Squire J, et al. Identification of a cancer stem cell in human brain tumors. Cancer Res 2003;63(1):5821–8.

[120] Shmelkov SV, St Clair R, Lyden D, Rafii S. AC133/CD133/Prominin-1. Int J Biochem Cell Biol 2005;37(4):715–9.

[121] Mizrak D, Brittan M, Alison M. CD133: molecule of the moment. J Pathol 2008;214(1):3–9.

[122] Nam-Cha SH, Serrano-Vargas R, Escario E, Azaña JM, Calero-Oliver R, Martín AG, et al. CD133 expression in normal skin and in epithelial cutaneous tumors. Biomed Res Int 2013;2013:385604.

[123] Charruyer A, Strachan LR, Yue L, Toth AS, Cecchini G, Mancianti ML, et al. CD133 is a marker for long-term repopulating murine epidermal stem cells. J Invest Dermatol 2012;132:2522–33.

[124] Sun G, Zhang X, Shen YI, Sebastian R, Dickinson LE, Fox-Talbot K, et al. Dextran hydrogel scaffolds enhance angiogenic responses and promote complete skin regeneration during burn wound healing. Proc Natl Acad Sci U.S.A. 2011;108:20976–81.

[125] Hollemann D, Yanagida G, Rüger BM, Neuchrist C, Fischer MB. New vessel formation in peritumoral area of squamous cell carcinoma of the head and neck. Head Neck 2012;34:813–20.

[126] Zhu L, Gibson P, Currle DS, Tong Y, Richardson RJ, Bayazitov IT, et al. Prominin 1 marks intestinal stem cells that are susceptible to neoplastic transformation. Nature 2009;457:603–7.

[127] Gay D, Kwon O, Zhang Z, Spata M, Plikus MV, Holler PD, et al. Fgf9 from dermal γδ T cells induces hair follicle neogenesis after wounding. Nat Med 2013;19:916–23.

[128] Fuchs Y, Brown S, Gorenc T, et al. Sept4/ARTS regulates stem cell apoptosis and skin regeneration. Science 2013;341:286–9.

[129] Tolar J, McGrath JA. Augmentation of cutaneous wound healing by pharmacologic mobilization of endogenous bone marrow stem cells. J Invest Dermatol September 2014;134(9):2312–4.

CHAPTER

IN SITU RENAL REGENERATION 19

H.J. Wang[1], S.J. Lee[2], A. Atala[2], J.J. Yoo[2]

[1]Chang Gung Memorial Hospital, Kaohsiung County, Taiwan; [2]Wake Forest School of Medicine, Winston-Salem, NC, United States

CHAPTER OUTLINE

INTRODUCTION

Chronic renal diseases are common conditions that elevate the risk of complete renal failure as well as cardiovascular diseases and other complications [1]. The prevalence of chronic renal failure has continuously increased in the United States in the last decade [2]. The current treatment options for end-stage renal disease (ESRD) are dialysis or kidney transplantation; however, both options are associated with limited organ donors, potential organ rejection, and considerable medical costs. Dialysis, usually performed three times per week, is a costly and tedious procedure that decreases the patient's quality of life and does not replace renal functions such as erythropoietin and vitamin D synthesis [3]. The 5-year survival rates between 1995 and 1999 were under 35% for both hemodialysis and peritoneal dialysis [3]. Kidney transplantation, on the other hand, could replace all renal functions, but the rising prevalence of ESRD in the United States continues to outpace the rate of organ donation, as reflected by the fact that the waiting list continues to grow by 3000 to 4000 people per year [4]. Furthermore, long-term results of kidney transplantation remain unsatisfactory, mainly because of chronic rejection and complications associated with immunosuppressive medications [5,6]. Except for the chronic condition, acute renal failure (ARF) remains common and affects 5–7% of total hospitalized patients. Despite the progress achieved in medical care in these patients, ARF remains a significant problem with a high mortality rate ranging from 20% to 70%, depending on the studies' populations. The incidence of ARF and its sequel remain unchanged during the past 50 years due to older population [7,8].

In Situ Tissue Regeneration. http://dx.doi.org/10.1016/B978-0-12-802225-2.00019-2

The strategy of in situ renal regeneration is to mobilize the host renal stem/progenitor cells or adjacent stem cells to target the renal injury sites. The recruiting stem or progenitor cells could be differentiated into the renal-related cells and formed typical renal structures, including glomerular and tubular structures for in site renal regeneration. This chapter will review the current status of in situ renal regeneration using host biologic resources and environmental conditions.

IN SITU RENAL REGENERATION: STRATEGY

In mammals, kidney development originates from the interaction of ureteric bud (UB) and metanephric mesenchyme (MM). The UB is an epithelial outgrowth of the Wolffian duct, while MM arises from the intermediate mesoderm. The permanent kidney develops through complex and reciprocal interactions, which begin from the invasion of the UB into an undifferentiated MM [9]. The UB undergoes branching and finally forms the collecting ducts and ureter. As the UB branching reaches the MM, the tip of the UB induces the adjacent MM to aggregate and differentiates into epithelium, which is known as mesenchymal–epithelial transformation (MET) [10]. Each MET event forms a new glomerulus and tubular nephron at the center of MM. The peripheral area of MM, which has not undergone MET, is referred to as the nephrogenic zone. In rodent, nephrogenesis is completed 1–2 weeks after birth, whereas it ends by 36 weeks of gestation age in humans [11]. For in situ renal regeneration, it will be a key to the development of regenerative therapies for renal injury via understanding the molecular and normal development process of kidney.

During the past decade, several studies have focused on the understanding of cellular and molecular underpinnings of the renal regeneration after either acute or chronic renal injuries. Through the lineage tracing results, we have perceived in some studies concerning the renal regeneration that several cellular interactions have participated in the renal regeneration after injury. These cells elicit the renal function recovery from recruitment of bone marrow–derived cells (BMDCs) [12], renal tubular cell dedifferentiation and migration [13,14], interstitial cell transdifferentiation [15], or the endogenous renal stem cell population [16]. However, which cell is primarily involved in tissue repair has not been definitively proved. The kidney recovery after renal injury in mammals has only been shown at the level of cellular repair, whereas the structure repair or "real" regeneration is very limited. In some species like elasmobranchs, their nephrogenesis can take place after partial excision to replace the missing kidney [17]. However, in mammals, resection of parts of the kidney leads to hypertrophy of remaining tissues and contralateral kidney but not the regeneration as we observe in the resection of liver. In another study, regeneration of renal medulla tubules without forming new nephrons is noted after release from the obstructive renal injury [18]. Actually, the development of new nephrons has never been observed at the time of or shortly after birth in any circumstance [11]. Chronic injury of the kidney will only result in severe glomerular and renal tubular damage and results in tissue fibrosis, scarring, and irreversible loss of renal function.

Recently, a number of cell-based therapeutic approaches using cells and/or biomaterials have been attempted for restoring the tissue or organ function [19–26]. These approaches have shown functional recovery of the damaged or diseased tissues or organs by implementing biomaterial scaffolds with preseeded desirable cells to generate functional tissue structure and progressive maturation. By using this strategy, several clinical conditions, such as cardiovascular diseases, osteoarthritic cartilage defects, urethral stricture, or bladder dysfunction, have been treated [27–30]. One of the most critical initial steps is the choice of an appropriate cell source. Although these approaches have been successful in various preclinical or clinical trials, a tissue biopsy followed by isolating and expanding these cells in large quantities is typically necessitated while maintaining uniform activity and remaining pathogen free [31]. However, in complex tissues or organs, including kidney, obtaining an appropriate cell source might meet extreme challenges. Kidney is a complex organ, which consists of at least 26 terminally differentiated cell types, including tubular epithelial cells, interstitial cells, glomerular cells, and vascular cells [32]. Isolating all these different cell types and integrating in a biomaterial scaffold to form a de novo functional structure may not be clinically feasible.

Recent advances in cellular and molecular biology have expanded the potential applications of this approach. Although a variety of therapeutic proteins such as human erythropoietin and insulin using recombinant genetic engineering can be produced, these proteins are unable to completely correct or reverse disease states because most common disease processes are not due to the deficiency of a single protein but develop due to alterations in the complex interactions of a variety of cell components [23]. By providing a dynamic and interactive therapeutic approach, cell-based therapy may be a more successful strategy that responds to the pathophysiological condition of the patient. In this regard, cells may provide novel and innovative methods for in situ modulation of biologics, immunotherapy, and tissue regenerative or replacement engineering [23,33,34].

Potential cell-based therapeutic options for the treatment of renal disease could be delivered in situ or ex vivo. The ex vivo approach might involve autologous renal or nonrenal stem cells and nonautologous stem cells from a variety of sources. These cells can be cultured and expanded ex vivo for redelivery into the damaged kidney. In situ renal regeneration involves the delivery of biomaterials or soluble reparative factors that would facilitate renal tissue repair (Fig. 19.1). This approach involves the recruitment of stem cells from bone marrow and from kidney itself for the repair of injured tissue [35]. It has

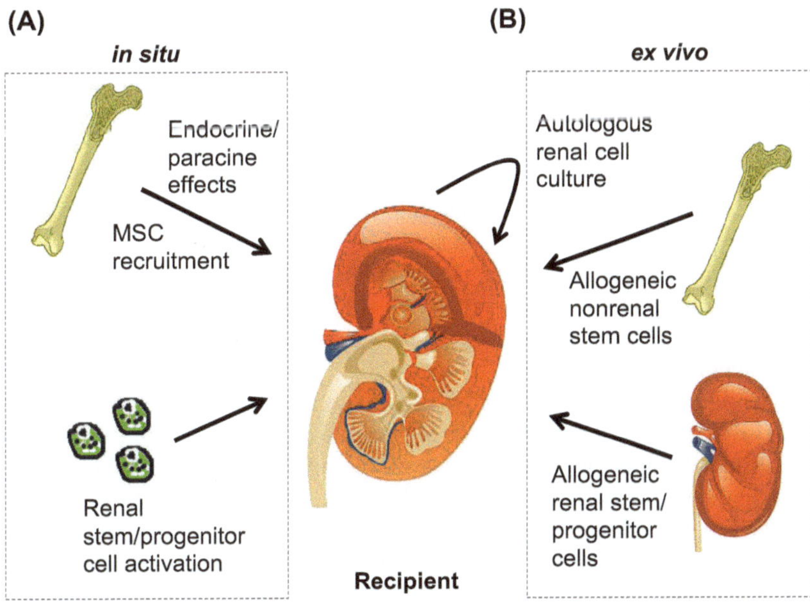

FIGURE 19.1

Strategies for renal regeneration. (A) In situ renal regeneration to utilize host stem/progenitor cells; and (B) ex vivo cell manipulation for cell injection therapy.

been widely accepted that in the body, almost every tissue contains certain types of stem or progenitor cells, including skin, fat, muscle, liver, and heart [36–39]. In our previous study, we demonstrated that host cells expressing several stem cell markers can be mobilized into an implanted biomaterial and that these cells are capable of differentiating into multiple cell lineages if appropriate conditions are provided [40]. This suggests that it may be possible to control tissue morphogenesis in vivo by providing the appropriate cues to infiltrating multipotent stem cells. This novel strategy could lead to the production of functional tissues in situ, which is in contrast to conventional tissue engineering strategies that focus on in vitro manipulation of cells.

STEM CELLS CONTRIBUTE TO RENAL REGENERATION

In stem cell–based approaches, resident stem or progenitor cells within the kidney or neighboring stem cells have been identified to investigate their regenerative potential for repairing renal injury (Table 19.1). Although most of these cells do not fulfill the criteria of true stem cells such as self-renewal and differentiation potential, several studies have attempted to understand their contribution to the renal regeneration [41].

RENAL STEM OR PROGENITOR CELLS

Several researchers have reported the existence of resident renal stem or progenitor cells, which can contribute to the renal regeneration in the kidney. Recently, it has been demonstrated that stem or progenitor cells derived from neonatal or fetal kidneys have regenerative potential in acute and chronic renal injury, acting either by paracrine mechanisms or by permanent engraftment [42,43]. Many attempts and efforts have been made to identify such populations; however, to date, no definitive data proves the existence of a distinct cell in adult kidney which process long-term self-renewing character with the capability to generate distinct daughter cells with renal regenerative potential. Langworthy et al. demonstrated that a subpopulation of proximal tubular cells express the transcription factor Nfatc1 [44]. These Nfatc1-labeled cells survived to apoptosis and proliferated to repair the damaged proximal tubule segment after mercuric chloride–induced injury. These outcomes could provide evidence for a resident progenitor proximal tubular cell population. However, Humphreys et al. evaluated if a population of intratubular adult progenitor cells are responsible for this epithelial repair after acute kidney injury via an unbiased DNA analog-based approach. They found no evidence of a population of specialized progenitor cells that respond to injury, but scattered resident injured tubular cells that had survived the injury mediated the repair [45].

Oliver et al. identified a population of slow cycling cells within the papilla of kidney [46]. They administered a pulse of the nucleotide bromodeoxyuridine (BrdU) to rat and mouse pups at the first postnatal week, during which the nephrogenesis is still going in rodents. After 2 months of monitoring, numerous low-cycling cells were identified at renal papilla. These cells were able to form a group of nestin-positive cells in vitro, which was also seen in other stem cells. During the repair phase of transient renal ischemia, these cells entered the cell cycle and mitosis rapidly, especially within the outer medulla. Another study also described the presence of BrdU-labeled cells located at adult rat renal tubules. These cells are able to reenter mitosis in response to renal injury and differentiate into epithelial structures [47]. Furthermore, the number of these cells significantly increased after ureteral

Table 19.1 Renal Stem/Progenitor Cells for Renal Regeneration

Cell Types	Species	Specific Markers	Description	References
Renal progenitor-like cells	Wistar rat	BrdU, PCNA targeting to proliferating cells	Increased in the number of label-retaining cells (LRC) in the kidneys after renal ischemia	Maeshima et al. [47]
Renal progenitor cells	Human	Pax2, CD133	Isolation of renal progenitor cells from adult human kidney	Bussolati et al. [50]
Renal highly proliferating cells	SD rat	Pan-cytokeratin, aquaporin-1, vimentin, c-met	Isolated from S3 segment of proximal tubule in rat kidney, self-renewal and multipotency	Kitamura et al. [49]
Renal progenitor cells	Human	CD133, CD24	Parietal epithelial cells isolated from Bowman's capsule, glycerol-induced acute renal failure SCID mice	Sagrinati et al. [52]
Mesenchymal stem cells	C57BL/6 mouse	CD44	CD44-mediated HA binding to recruit MSCs, glycerol-induced acute tubular injury mouse model	Herrera et al. [69]
Renal progenitor cells	Human	CD133, CD24	Isolated from embryonic kidneys, human CD133+CD24+ cells injected into SCID mice after glycerol-induced acute kidney injury	Lazzeri et al. [85]
Renal progenitor cells	Human	Pax2, CD133	Located in Bowman's capsule and proximal tubules	Loverre et al. [86]
Kidney epithelial progenitor cells	Human	Pax2, CD133, CD24, CD29, CD44	Isolated from fetal kidney, developed long-term cultures (more than 60 population doublings)	Loo et al. [57]
Renal progenitor cells	Human	CD133, CD24, PDX, nestin	Located in Bowman's capsule, hyperplastic lesions of podocytopathies, and crescentic glomerulonephritis	Smeets et al. [87]
Glomerular mesenchymal stem cells	Human	CD146, not CD133	Multipotency, potential to differentiate into mesangial cells	Bruno et al. [79]
Renal progenitor cells	Human	CD133, CD24, PDX	PDX- cells differentiated into both tubular cells and potocytes, PDX+ cell differentiated into only potocytes	Ronconi et al. [88]
Renal progenitor-like cells	Human	CD133, CD24	Aldehyde dehydrogenase (ALDH)-based cell sorting	Lindgren et al. [89]
Renal progenitor cells	Human	CD133/1	Isolated from renal papillary loops of Henle, differentiated into neural- and epithelial-like lineages to undergo tubulogenesis	Ward et al. [90]
Renal progenitor cells	Human	CD133, CD24, not CD106	Located in proximal tubule and distal convoluted tubule, SCID mice with acute tubular injury	Angelotti et al. [91]
Renal progenitor cells	Human	Pax2, CD133, CD24	Located in Bowman's capsule, miR-1915 and miR-1225 seem to regulate adult renal progenitor cell activation	Sallustio et al. [92]
Renal progenitor cells	Human	NCAM1	Isolated from fetal kidney, nephrectomy model in NOD/SCID mice	Harari-Steinberg et al. [43]
Renal progenitor cells	C57BL/6 mouse	Oct-4, Pax2, α-SMA, vimentin	Combination with erythropoietin or suramin, I/R-induced acute kidney injury mice	Han et al. [93]
Renal progenitor cells	Human	CD133, CD24, NCAM1	Isolated from human kidney epithelial cells, human NCAM1+ cells injected into NOD/SCID mice after glycerol-induced acute kidney injury	Buzhor et al. [58]
Parietal epithelial cells and podocyte progenitors	B6129SV/j mouse	Pax2, *p*-ERK and WT-1, *p*-ERK	Located in Bowman's capsule, focal segmental glomerulosclerosis (FSGS) in mice	Zhang et al. [94]

obstruction, and most of them were positive for proliferating cell nuclear antigen (PCNA) as well as vimentin, heat shock protein 47, or α-smooth muscle actin [48]. Kitamura et al. dissected a postnatal murine kidney to various nephron segments and cultured after dissociation to a single cell [49]. They defined a cell line from the S3 segment of the proximal tubules. This cell line can be maintained as long as 300 days without transformation and differentiated into mature tubular cells under different culture conditions. These cells also expressed Sca-1 and c-kit, markers of progenitor cells, and Pax-2, GDNF, WT-1, and Wnt-4, which are essential molecules involved in nephrogenesis. Under ischemia/reperfusion injury, they seem to contribute to renal tubular regeneration.

In another study, CD133+ cells from the adult kidney were isolated and characterized to identify their progenitor characteristic as renal stem cells [50–53]. CD133+ cells were subsequently identified in different segments of nephron, which were localized in the Bowman's capsule of the glomeruli, in the proximal tubules as well as in the inner medullary papilla region, including Henle's loop and the S3 limb segment. These cells express several mesenchymal stem cell (MSC) markers such as CD29, CD73, and CD90, with embryonic renal markers Pax-2, Six1, and Six2 but not the hematopoietic markers CD34 or CD45 [50–53]. Different populations of these progenitor cells from different nephron segments exhibit different properties and possibly different functions. CD133+ cells isolated from the Henle's loop had higher differentiation ability as compared with those in the tubules. The hypoxic environment of the inner medulla induces the expression of stem cell transcription factor Oct4A under the control of hypoxia inducible factor-1 [53]. The CD133+ cells isolated from a subset of parietal epithelial cells in Bowman's capsule of adult human kidney also express positive CD24 marker and the stem cell–specific transcription factors Oct-4 and BmI-1. These cells unveiled the multipotent differentiation ability, being able to generate mature, functional, tubular cells with phenotypic features of proximal or distal tubules, osteogenic cells, adipocytes, and cells that exhibited phenotypic and functional features of neuronal cells. Treatment of ARF induced by glycerol with these cells significantly improved the morphologic and functional renal damage [52].

Gupta et al. isolated a unique population of multipotent, self-renewal, spindle-shaped cells with expression of vimentin, CD90, Pax-2, and Oct4 but not cytokeratin in the rat kidney [54]. After delivering intraarterially into an ischemia/reperfusion–injured kidney, the cells were able to differentiate into renal tubules, suggesting that these cells may be candidate renal stem cells. Another population of cell was identified throughout the renal capsule at the density of 10 cells/mm^2. These cells expressed MSC markers (CD29, vimentin, Sca-1, nestin) without expressing any hematopoietic or endothelial stem cell marker [55]. With the ability to differentiate and self-renew, these cells can migrate from renal capsule to the ischemia renal parenchyma in vivo at the speed of 30 μm/h. The protective effect against ischemic injury was relative lower in the decapsulated kidney compared with intact ischemic kidney. These demonstrated that renal capsule could be a stem cell niche, providing renal stem cells to participate in renal repair [55]. In another study, an MSC population has also been identified in the glomeruli of mice [56]. These cells were shown to be multipotent and express smooth muscle myosin, like the mesangial cells, and express mesenchymal markers, including CD29, CD90, CD73, and CD44. Finally, Loo et al. isolated and cultured highly homogeneous human fetal kidney epithelial progenitor cells. The cells express the embryonic kidney mesenchyme/epithelial marker Pax-2, the stem cell protein CD133, the kidney embryonic progenitor protein CD24, as well as CD29 and CD44. The cells are negative for E-cadherin when grown under low calcium conditions (<0.05 mM), but the expression is induced when cells are cultured under normal calcium conditions (1.2 mM). This suggests that the calcium level in the environment may play a role in modulation of epithelial progenitor cell differentiation [57].

Recently, neural cell adhesion molecule 1 (NCAM1) has been discovered in the mature kidney epithelia [43,58] because NCAM1+ cells in kidney uniformly expressed CD24 and CD133. Buzhor et al. injected NCAM1+ and NCM1− cells subcutaneously into nonobese diabetic (NOD)/severe combined immunodeficiency (SCID) mice and analyzed at 2 weeks after injection [58]. The injected NCAM1+ cells reconstituted differentiated cytokeratin+ tubules and generated both *Lotus tetragonolobus* agglutinin+ (LTA+) and *Dolichos biflorus* agglutinin+ (DBA+) proximal and distal tubules (Fig. 19.2A). After NCAM1+ cell injection at 3 days, blood urea nitrogen (BUN) and creatinine levels were reduced at 3 days after injection compared with the saline-injected group (Fig. 19.2B).

BONE MARROW–DERIVED CELLS

It has been widely accepted that a subpopulation of cells derived from bone marrow can transdifferentiate into mesangial cell [59,60], tubular epithelial cells [12], and glomerular endothelial cells [61,62]. Research studies demonstrate the presence of Y chromosome–bearing cells in female kidneys after receiving a male bone marrow transplant. By using the in situ hybridization technique to detect Y chromosomes, it has been demonstrated that circulating BMDCs frequently engraft into the kidney and differentiate into renal parenchymal cells [12]. However, only a small amount of total cells presented in the proliferated kidney tissue was bone marrow origin. Lin et al. used transgenic mice that express enhanced green fluorescent protein (GFP) significantly in mature renal tubular epithelial cells [63]. After ischemia/reperfusion injury, bone marrow cells were transplanted into the mice. Only 11% of proliferated epithelial cells originated from donor BMDCs, while 89% originated from host cells, and the level does decline over time. Twenty-eight days after ischemia/reperfusion injury, the kidneys contained 8% donor-derived cells, of which 8.4% were epithelial cells, 10.6% were glomerular cells, and 81% were interstitial cells. Duffield et al. reported an even lower percentage (0.06%) of proliferated epithelial cells originated from BMDC transplantation in ischemia/reperfusion injury mice [64]. Both of these two studies [63,64] conclude that BMDCs do not make significant contributions to the restoration of epithelial integrity. The repair is elicited via recruitment and proliferation of endogenous renal cells. The injected BMDCs might contribute a cytokine environment or immunomodulatory effects that may be important in functional tissue regeneration, which reduces the severity of renal injury following ischemia/reperfusion injury [64]. It has not been completely investigated whether BMDCs' mobilization and recruitment improve or worsen the renal damage. Togel et al. tested whether further increment in circulating stem cell numbers, induced by mobilization from the bone marrow, would improve renal function and outcome in ischemic injured mice [65]. However, with their protocol high numbers of activated granulocytosis obscure the positive effect of hematopoietic stem cells and have potential detrimental effects on renal regeneration. In contrast, Fang et al. demonstrated that the renal tubular epithelium regeneration in a mouse folic acid-induced acute renal injury model was achieved by transplantation of BMDCs with granulocyte colony-stimulating factor (G-CSF) [66]. This renoprotective effect has also been observed in the other studies [64].

NONRENAL STEM CELLS

MSCs are typically isolated from bone marrow, and they possess the ability to differentiate into multiple cell lines with therapeutic behavior mainly in mesodermal tissues in vivo [67]. However, MSCs are also sourced from other tissues, including adipose tissue, placenta, umbilical cord, or amniotic fluid, and they share similar properties and phenotypes. MSCs are identified by the expression of many

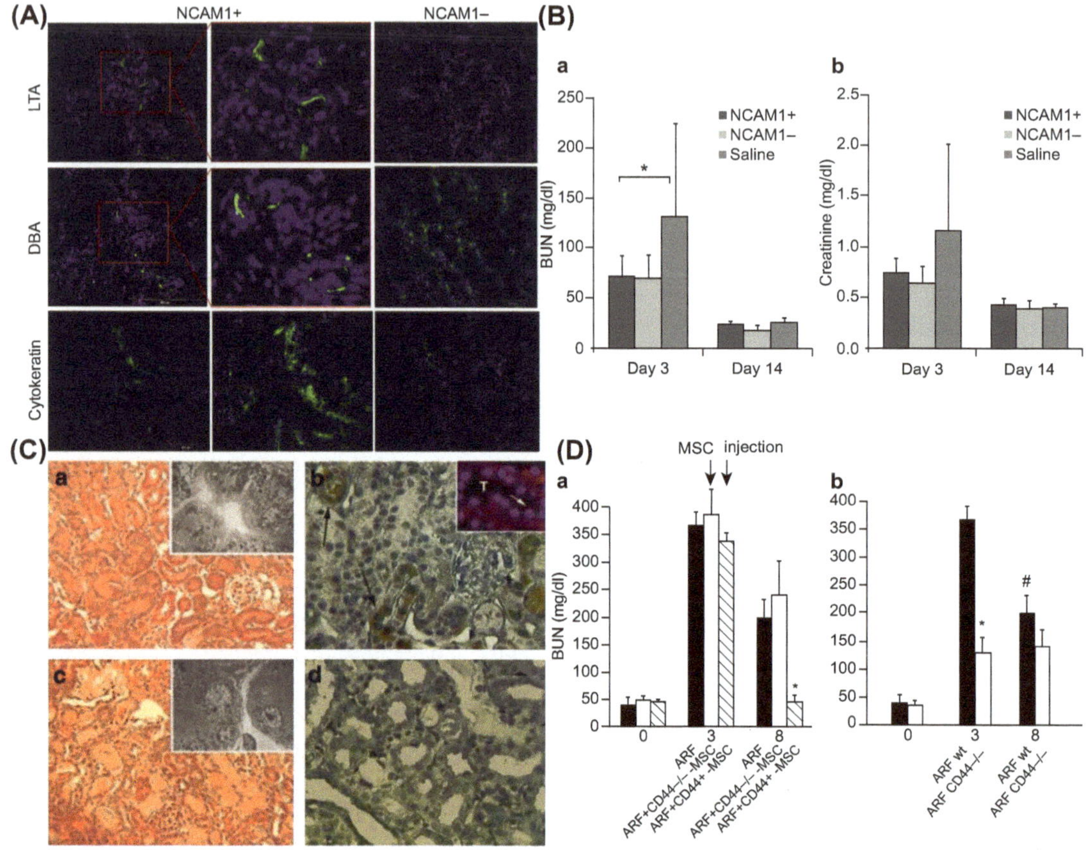

FIGURE 19.2

(A,B) Renal stem or progenitor cells: (A) NCAM1+ cells contributed the renal tubule formation after injection subcutaneously into NOD/SCID mice at 2 weeks. (B) Renal functional assessment: (a) BUN and (b) creatinine levels after NCAM1+ or NCAM1− cells injection. *(Reproduced with permission from Buzhor E, Omer D, Harari-Steinberg O, Dotan Z, Vax E, Pri-Chen S, et al. Reactivation of NCAM1 defines a subpopulation of human adult kidney epithelial cells with clonogenic and stem/progenitor properties. Am J Pathol 2013;183:1621–33.)* (C, D) Nonrenal stem cells: (C) CD44+ MSC in mice ARF induction: (a and b) CD44+ MSC renal localization at 5 days after injection. (a) Hematoxylin and eosin (H&E) (×250) and electron microscopy (×4000). (b) Fluorescein-labeled CD44+-MSC (×250) and detection of Y chromosome by FISH (×600) (*arrows*; T = tubule). (c and d) CD44−/− MSC renal localization at 5 days after injection. (c) H&E (×250) and of electron microscopy (×4000). (d) Absence of localization of fluorescein-labeled CD44−/−-MSC (×250). (D) Evaluation of renal function in wild-type mice injected with CD44+ or CD44−/−-MSC and in CD44−/− mice at 3 and 8 days after glycerol-induced ARF: (a) evaluation of BUN in CD44+-MSC, CD44−/−-MSC, and MSC untreated mice before, 3 and 8 days after glycerol injection; and (b) comparison of the BUN levels in wild-type (wt) or CD44−/− mice before, 3 and 8 days after glycerol injection. *(Reproduced with permission from Herrera MB, Bussolati B, Bruno S, Fonsato V, Romanazzi GM, Camussi G. Mesenchymal stem cells contribute to the renal repair of acute tubular epithelial injury. Int J Mol Med 2004;14:1035–41.)*

molecules, including CD105 and CD73, and are negative for the hematopoietic markers CD34, CD45, and CD14 expression [67]. It has been shown that intravenously-injected exogenous MSC expressing GFP homed to the glycerol-induced acute renal injury but not to the normal kidney in mice [68]. Treatment with MSCs enhanced renal tubular proliferation and preserved microvascular integrity [68,69]. The homing effect of MSCs to the injured kidney is correlated with CD44 and hyaluronic acid interaction (Fig. 19.2C and D) [69]. It is believed that protease induced matrix degeneration may release hyaluronic acid in injured kidney. The CD44 receptor is upregulated in renal cortex after injury. In vitro, hyaluronic acid can induce dose-dependent stem cell migration, and the injected MSCs migrate to the injured kidney, where hyaluronic acid expression is increased. This homing ability of MSC was blocked by preincubation with the CD44 blocking antibody or by soluble hyaluronic acid. Morigi et al. investigated the renotropic and renoprotective capacity of MSC using a cisplatin-induced renal failure model [70]. MSCs differentiated into epithelial cells and integrated into renal tubules, which were not elicited by hematopoietic stem cells. Several recent studies confirmed the beneficial effect of MSCs with some differences related to the source of origin. Higher efficacy of renal protective effect was noted in the cord blood–derived MSCs [71].

Homing is not a mandatory need for the beneficial effect of MSCs-related therapy. Imberti et al. examined the protective effect of MSCs in the murine model of cisplatin-induced kidney injury [72]. Administering insulin-like growth factor-1 (IGF-1), gene-silenced MSC limited their protective effect on renal function and tubular structure. These findings indicate that MSCs exert beneficial effects on tubular cell repair in acute kidney injury by producing the factor IGF-1. Bi et al. collected conditioned media of MSCs and successfully induced migration and proliferation of renal tubular epithelial cells, which diminished cisplatin-induced proximal tubular cell death in vitro. Intraperitoneal injection of this conditioned medium in mice treated with cisplatin diminished tubular cell apoptosis and decreased renal injury [73]. It has been demonstrated that the secreting factors that limit apoptosis and enhance proliferation of the endogenous tubular cells, which suggests that transplantation of the cells themselves may not be necessary. Therefore MSCs may protect the kidney from acute injury though the release of mediators such as IGF-1, epidermal growth factor, hepatocyte growth factor, and other mediators that modify the microenvironment, reduce the recruitment of inflammatory cells, and enhance the differentiation and expansion of the residual progenitor cells into tubules [72,74–76].

Currently research studies involving endocrine and paracrine effects of MSCs have been focused on extracellular microvesicles (MVs) released by various cells types, including stem cells and progenitors [77]. MVs are known to be involved in cell-to-cell communication via interaction with target cells with surface expressed ligands and receptors as well as delivery of proteins and bioactive lipids [77,78]. Bruno et al. characterized these MVs derived from MSCs and showed spheroid morphology with mean size of 135 nm. Several adhesion molecules, including CD44, CD29, α4-and α5 integrins, and CD73, have been identified in these vesicles. MVs accelerated the proliferation of tubular cells in glycerol-induced renal injury in mice and achieved functional and morphologic recovery. This renoprotective effect was similar to that of direct MSC injection in vivo but is abolished by RNase, suggesting the existence of RNA-dependent biologic effects [79]. Further in vitro studies established that MVs upregulated antiapoptotic genes, such as Bcl-xL, Bcl2, and BIRC8 in cisplatin-treated human tubular epithelial cells and downregulated genes that are involved in the execution phase of cell apoptosis, such as Casp1, Casp8, and LTA [80]. MVs injected into cisplatin induced acute kidney injury further protect the renal function and morphologic normalization in a dose-dependent effect [80]. All these preclinical data suggest a new prospect of stem cell therapy. Through administrating of MVs, we may be able to provoke the localized progenitor cell activation without the potential risk associated with stem cell therapy, such as tumor development or maldifferentiation. Therapeutic effects of MSC-derived MVs have proved not only in acute renal injury but also in some other pathological conditions in endocrine, pulmonary, and neurological fields [81–84]. Further studies regarding the biodistribution, efficacy, and safety of MV administration should be completed before clinical application.

SUMMARY AND FURTHER DIRECTIONS

Research studies have shown that the concept of in situ tissue regeneration can be applied to kidneys. The presence of resident renal stem or progenitor cells indicates that these cells are able to contribute to renal tissue regeneration, and recent studies have demonstrated functional recovery in ARF. Stem and progenitor cells, including MSCs, have shown expression of factors that are involved in tissue development, repair, and regeneration. Studies indicate that host stem or progenitor cells can be mobilized and recruited into the injured renal tissue by controlling microenvironment. In our previous study, we explored this hypothesis by introducing a biomaterial into normal kidneys and kidneys damaged by ischemia/reperfusion. Our results suggest that it is possible to recruit a predominance of cells with renal regenerative potential into a scaffolding system. This approach eliminates the need for harvesting tissues for cell isolation and ex vivo handling of cells for implantation. Furthermore, a new therapeutic strategy could be developed to generate pharmacological approaches to enhance renal repair through the understanding of the molecular mechanisms and cellular interactions involved in their proliferation and differentiation. Importantly, the identification of renal stem cell markers that participate in the renal regenerative machinery and in situ renal regeneration by antibodies, small molecules, growth factors, and peptides would be a novel therapeutic strategy for renal injury. In addition, bioproducts from stem or progenitor cells, such as MVs or newly developed biomaterials, may play a role in recruitment and reprogramming the endogenous cells involved in the renal regeneration. The presence of an underlying regenerative mechanism in the form of tissue-specific stem or progenitor cells suggests that there might be a potential opportunity to bias the host response toward repair of renal injury.

REFERENCES

[1] Foley RN, Collins AJ. End-stage renal disease in the United States: an update from the United States Renal Data System. J Am Soc Nephrol 2007;18:2644–8.

[2] Coresh J, Selvin E, Stevens LA, Manzi J, Kusek JW, Eggers P, et al. Prevalence of chronic kidney disease in the United States. JAMA 2007;298:2038–47.

[3] Meyer TW, Hostetter TH. Uremia. N Engl J Med 2007;357:1316–25.

[4] Danovitch GM, Cohen DJ, Weir MR, Stock PG, Bennett WM, Christensen LL, et al. Current status of kidney and pancreas transplantation in the United States, 1994–2003. Am J Transplant 2005;5:904–15.

[5] Pascual M, Theruvath T, Kawai T, Tolkoff-Rubin N, Cosimi AB. Strategies to improve long-term outcomes after renal transplantation. N Engl J Med 2002;346:580–90.

[6] Sayegh MH, Carpenter CB. Transplantation 50 years later–progress, challenges, and promises. N Engl J Med 2004;351:2761–6.

[7] Singri N, Ahya SN, Levin ML. Acute renal failure. JAMA 2003;289:747–51.

[8] Nash K, Hafeez A, Hou S. Hospital-acquired renal insufficiency. Am J Kidney Dis 2002;39:930–6.

[9] Pohl M, Bhatnagar V, Mendoza SA, Nigam SK. Toward an etiological classification of developmental disorders of the kidney and upper urinary tract. Kidney Int 2002;61:10–9.
[10] Pohl M, Stuart RO, Sakurai H, Nigam SK. Branching morphogenesis during kidney development. Annu Rev Physiol 2000;62:595–620.
[11] Saxen L, Sariola H. Early organogenesis of the kidney. Pediatr Nephrol 1987;1:385–92.
[12] Poulsom R, Forbes SJ, Hodivala-Dilke K, Ryan E, Wyles S, Navaratnarasah S, et al. Bone marrow contributes to renal parenchymal turnover and regeneration. J Pathol 2001;195:229–35.
[13] Bonventre JV. Dedifferentiation and proliferation of surviving epithelial cells in acute renal failure. J Am Soc Nephrol 2003;14(Suppl. 1):S55–61.
[14] Witzgall R, Brown D, Schwarz C, Bonventre JV. Localization of proliferating cell nuclear antigen, vimentin, c-Fos, and clusterin in the postischemic kidney. Evidence for a heterogenous genetic response among nephron segments, and a large pool of mitotically active and dedifferentiated cells. J Clin Invest 1994;93:2175–88.
[15] Strutz F, Okada H, Lo CW, Danoff T, Carone RL, Tomaszewski JE, et al. Identification and characterization of a fibroblast marker: FSP1. J Cell Biol 1995;130:393–405.
[16] Cantley LG. Adult stem cells in the repair of the injured renal tubule. Nat Clin Pract Nephrol 2005;1:22–32.
[17] Elger M, Hentschel H, Litteral J, Wellner M, Kirsch T, Luft FC, et al. Nephrogenesis is induced by partial nephrectomy in the elasmobranch *Leucoraja erinacea*. J Am Soc Nephrol 2003;14:1506–18.
[18] Cochrane AL, Kett MM, Samuel CS, Campanale NV, Anderson WP, Hume DA, et al. Renal structural and functional repair in a mouse model of reversal of ureteral obstruction. J Am Soc Nephrol 2005;16:3623–30.
[19] Abbattista MR, Schena FP. Stem cells and kidney diseases. Minerva Med 2004;95:411–8.
[20] Blattmann A, Denk L, Strehl R, Castrop H, Minuth WW. The formation of pores in the basal lamina of regenerated renal tubules. Biomaterials 2008;29:2749–56.
[21] Fang TC, Poulsom R. Cell-based therapies for birth defects: a role for adult stem cell plasticity? Birth Defects Res C Embryo Today 2003;69:238–49.
[22] Hammerman MR. Tissue engineering the kidney. Kidney Int 2003;63:1195–204.
[23] Humes HD, Szczypka MS. Advances in cell therapy for renal failure. Transpl Immunol 2004;12:219–27.
[24] Humes HD, Weitzel WF, Fissell WH. Renal cell therapy in the treatment of patients with acute and chronic renal failure. Blood Purif 2004;22:60–72.
[25] Perin L, Giuliani S, Sedrakyan S, Da Sacco S, De Filippo RE. Stem cell and regenerative science applications in the development of bioengineering of renal tissue. Pediatr Res 2008;63:467–71.
[26] Steer DL, Nigam SK. Developmental approaches to kidney tissue engineering. Am J Physiol Renal Physiol 2004;286:F1–7.
[27] Atala A, Bauer SB, Soker S, Yoo JJ, Retik AB. Tissue-engineered autologous bladders for patients needing cystoplasty. Lancet 2006;367:1241–6.
[28] El-Kassaby AW, Retik AB, Yoo JJ, Atala A. Urethral stricture repair with an off-the-shelf collagen matrix. J Urol 2003;169:170–3. discussion 3.
[29] Ossendorf C, Kaps C, Kreuz PC, Burmester GR, Sittinger M, Erggelet C. Treatment of posttraumatic and focal osteoarthritic cartilage defects of the knee with autologous polymer-based three-dimensional chondrocyte grafts: 2-year clinical results. Arthritis Res Ther 2007;9:R41.
[30] Shin'oka T, Matsumura G, Hibino N, Naito Y, Watanabe M, Konuma T, et al. Midterm clinical result of tissue-engineered vascular autografts seeded with autologous bone marrow cells. J Thorac Cardiovasc Surg 2005;129:1330–8.
[31] Langer R, Vacanti JP. Tissue engineering. Science 1993;260:920–6.
[32] Al-Awqati Q, Oliver JA. Stem cells in the kidney. Kidney Int 2002;61:387–95.
[33] Dove A. Cell-based therapies go live. Nat Biotechnol 2002;20:339–43.
[34] Gage FH. Cell therapy. Nature 1998;392:18–24.
[35] Little MH. Regrow or repair: potential regenerative therapies for the kidney. J Am Soc Nephrol 2006;17:2390–401.

[36] Bartsch G, Yoo JJ, De Coppi P, Siddiqui MM, Schuch G, Pohl HG, et al. Propagation, expansion, and multilineage differentiation of human somatic stem cells from dermal progenitors. Stem Cells Dev 2005;14:337–48.

[37] Deasy BM, Huard J. Gene therapy and tissue engineering based on muscle-derived stem cells. Curr Opin Mol Ther 2002;4:382–9.

[38] Pfister O, Mouquet F, Jain M, Summer R, Helmes M, Fine A, et al. CD31− but Not CD31+ cardiac side population cells exhibit functional cardiomyogenic differentiation. Circ Res 2005;97:52–61.

[39] Zhang Y, Bai XF, Huang CX. Hepatic stem cells: existence and origin. World J Gastroenterol 2003;9:201–4.

[40] Lee SJ, Van Dyke M, Atala A, Yoo JJ. Host cell mobilization for in situ tissue regeneration. Rejuvenation Res 2008;11:747–56.

[41] Biancone L, Camussi G. Stem cells in 2013: potential use of stem or progenitor cells for kidney regeneration. Nat Rev Nephrol 2014;10:67–8.

[42] Rangel EB, Gomes SA, Dulce RA, Premer C, Rodrigues CO, Kanashiro-Takeuchi RM, et al. C-kit(+) cells isolated from developing kidneys are a novel population of stem cells with regenerative potential. Stem Cells 2013;31:1644–56.

[43] Harari-Steinberg O, Metsuyanim S, Omer D, Gnatek Y, Gershon R, Pri-Chen S, et al. Identification of human nephron progenitors capable of generation of kidney structures and functional repair of chronic renal disease. EMBO Mol Med 2013;5:1556–68.

[44] Langworthy M, Zhou B, de Caestecker M, Moeckel G, Baldwin HS. NFATc1 identifies a population of proximal tubule cell progenitors. J Am Soc Nephrol 2009;20:311–21.

[45] Humphreys BD, Czerniak S, DiRocco DP, Hasnain W, Cheema R, Bonventre JV. Repair of injured proximal tubule does not involve specialized progenitors. Proc Natl Acad Sci USA 2011;108:9226–31.

[46] Oliver JA, Maarouf O, Cheema FH, Martens TP, Al-Awqati Q. The renal papilla is a niche for adult kidney stem cells. J Clin Invest 2004;114:795–804.

[47] Maeshima A, Yamashita S, Nojima Y. Identification of renal progenitor-like tubular cells that participate in the regeneration processes of the kidney. J Am Soc Nephrol 2003;14:3138–46.

[48] Yamashita S, Maeshima A, Nojima Y. Involvement of renal progenitor tubular cells in epithelial-to-mesenchymal transition in fibrotic rat kidneys. J Am Soc Nephrol 2005;16:2044–51.

[49] Kitamura S, Yamasaki Y, Kinomura M, Sugaya T, Sugiyama H, Maeshima Y, et al. Establishment and characterization of renal progenitor like cells from S3 segment of nephron in rat adult kidney. FASEB J 2005;19:1789–97.

[50] Bussolati B, Bruno S, Grange C, Buttiglieri S, Deregibus MC, Cantino D, et al. Isolation of renal progenitor cells from adult human kidney. Am J Pathol 2005;166:545–55.

[51] Bussolati B, Tetta C, Camussi G. Contribution of stem cells to kidney repair. Am J Nephrol 2008;28:813–22.

[52] Sagrinati C, Netti GS, Mazzinghi B, Lazzeri E, Liotta F, Frosali F, et al. Isolation and characterization of multipotent progenitor cells from the Bowman's capsule of adult human kidneys. J Am Soc Nephrol 2006;17:2443–56.

[53] Bussolati B, Moggio A, Collino F, Aghemo G, D'Armento G, Grange C, et al. Hypoxia modulates the undifferentiated phenotype of human renal inner medullary CD133+ progenitors through Oct4/miR-145 balance. Am J Physiol Renal Physiol 2012;302:F116–28.

[54] Gupta S, Verfaillie C, Chmielewski D, Kren S, Eidman K, Connaire J, et al. Isolation and characterization of kidney-derived stem cells. J Am Soc Nephrol 2006;17:3028–40.

[55] Park HC, Yasuda K, Kuo MC, Ni J, Ratliff B, Chander P, et al. Renal capsule as a stem cell niche. Am J Physiol Renal Physiol 2010;298:F1254–62.

[56] da Silva Meirelles L, Chagastelles PC, Nardi NB. Mesenchymal stem cells reside in virtually all post-natal organs and tissues. J Cell Sci 2006;119:2204–13.

[57] Loo D, Beltejar C, Hooley J, Xu X. Primary and multipassage culture of human fetal kidney epithelial progenitor cells. Methods Cell Biol 2008;86:241–55.

[58] Buzhor E, Omer D, Harari-Steinberg O, Dotan Z, Vax E, Pri-Chen S, et al. Reactivation of NCAM1 defines a subpopulation of human adult kidney epithelial cells with clonogenic and stem/progenitor properties. Am J Pathol 2013;183:1621–33.
[59] Ito T, Suzuki A, Imai E, Okabe M, Hori M. Bone marrow is a reservoir of repopulating mesangial cells during glomerular remodeling. J Am Soc Nephrol 2001;12:2625–35.
[60] Ito T, Suzuki A, Okabe M, Imai E, Hori M. Application of bone marrow-derived stem cells in experimental nephrology. Exp Nephrol 2001;9:444–50.
[61] Hayakawa M, Ishizaki M, Hayakawa J, Migita M, Murakami M, Shimada T, et al. Role of bone marrow cells in the healing process of mouse experimental glomerulonephritis. Pediatr Res 2005;58:323–8.
[62] Ikarashi K, Li B, Suwa M, Kawamura K, Morioka T, Yao J, et al. Bone marrow cells contribute to regeneration of damaged glomerular endothelial cells. Kidney Int 2005;67:1925–33.
[63] Lin F, Moran A, Igarashi P. Intrarenal cells, not bone marrow-derived cells, are the major source for regeneration in postischemic kidney. J Clin Invest 2005;115:1756–64.
[64] Duffield JS, Park KM, Hsiao LL, Kelley VR, Scadden DT, Ichimura T, et al. Restoration of tubular epithelial cells during repair of the postischemic kidney occurs independently of bone marrow-derived stem cells. J Clin Invest 2005;115:1743–55.
[65] Togel F, Isaac J, Westenfelder C. Hematopoietic stem cell mobilization-associated granulocytosis severely worsens acute renal failure. J Am Soc Nephrol 2004;15:1261–7.
[66] Fang TC, Alison MR, Cook HT, Jeffery R, Wright NA, Poulsom R. Proliferation of bone marrow-derived cells contributes to regeneration after folic acid-induced acute tubular injury. J Am Soc Nephrol 2005;16:1723–32.
[67] Chamberlain G, Fox J, Ashton B, Middleton J. Concise review: mesenchymal stem cells: their phenotype, differentiation capacity, immunological features, and potential for homing. Stem Cells 2007;25:2739–49.
[68] Herrera MB, Bussolati B, Bruno S, Fonsato V, Romanazzi GM, Camussi G. Mesenchymal stem cells contribute to the renal repair of acute tubular epithelial injury. Int J Mol Med 2004;14:1035–41.
[69] Herrera MB, Bussolati B, Bruno S, Morando L, Mauriello-Romanazzi G, Sanavio F, et al. Exogenous mesenchymal stem cells localize to the kidney by means of CD44 following acute tubular injury. Kidney Int 2007;72:430–41.
[70] Morigi M, Imberti B, Zoja C, Corna D, Tomasoni S, Abbate M, et al. Mesenchymal stem cells are renotropic, helping to repair the kidney and improve function in acute renal failure. J Am Soc Nephrol 2004;15:1794–804.
[71] Morigi M, Rota C, Montemurro T, Montelatici E, Lo Cicero V, Imberti B, et al. Life-sparing effect of human cord blood-mesenchymal stem cells in experimental acute kidney injury. Stem Cells 2010;28:513–22.
[72] Imberti B, Morigi M, Tomasoni S, Rota C, Corna D, Longaretti L, et al. Insulin-like growth factor-1 sustains stem cell mediated renal repair. J Am Soc Nephrol 2007;18:2921–8.
[73] Bi B, Schmitt R, Israilova M, Nishio H, Cantley LG. Stromal cells protect against acute tubular injury via an endocrine effect. J Am Soc Nephrol 2007;18:2486–96.
[74] Baer PC, Schubert R, Bereiter-Hahn J, Plosser M, Geiger H. Expression of a functional epidermal growth factor receptor on human adipose-derived mesenchymal stem cells and its signaling mechanism. Eur J Cell Biol 2009;88:273–83.
[75] Birchmeier C, Gherardi E. Developmental roles of HGF/SF and its receptor, the c-Met tyrosine kinase. Trends Cell Biol 1998;8:404–10.
[76] Zhuang S, Dang Y, Schnellmann RG. Requirement of the epidermal growth factor receptor in renal epithelial cell proliferation and migration. Am J Physiol Renal Physiol 2004;287:F365–72.
[77] Ratajczak J, Miekus K, Kucia M, Zhang J, Reca R, Dvorak P, et al. Embryonic stem cell-derived microvesicles reprogram hematopoietic progenitors: evidence for horizontal transfer of mRNA and protein delivery. Leukemia 2006;20:847–56.
[78] Schorey JS, Bhatnagar S. Exosome function: from tumor immunology to pathogen biology. Traffic 2008;9:871–81.
[79] Bruno S, Grange C, Deregibus MC, Calogero RA, Saviozzi S, Collino F, et al. Mesenchymal stem cell-derived microvesicles protect against acute tubular injury. J Am Soc Nephrol 2009;20:1053–67.

[80] Bruno S, Grange C, Collino F, Deregibus MC, Cantaluppi V, Biancone L, et al. Microvesicles derived from mesenchymal stem cells enhance survival in a lethal model of acute kidney injury. PLoS One 2012;7:e33115.

[81] Chen JY, An R, Liu ZJ, Wang JJ, Chen SZ, Hong MM, et al. Therapeutic effects of mesenchymal stem cell-derived microvesicles on pulmonary arterial hypertension in rats. Acta Pharmacol Sin 2014;35:1121–8.

[82] Mokarizadeh A, Rezvanfar MA, Dorostkar K, Abdollahi M. Mesenchymal stem cell derived microvesicles: trophic shuttles for enhancement of sperm quality parameters. Reprod Toxicol 2013;42:78–84.

[83] Monsel A, Zhu YG, Gennai S, Hao Q, Hu S, Rouby JJ, et al. Therapeutic effects of human mesenchymal stem cell-derived microvesicles in severe pneumonia in mice. Am J Respir Crit Care Med 2015;192:324–36.

[84] Raisi A, Azizi S, Delirezh N, Heshmatian B, Farshid AA, Amini K. The mesenchymal stem cell-derived microvesicles enhance sciatic nerve regeneration in rat: a novel approach in peripheral nerve cell therapy. J Trauma Acute Care Surg 2014;76:991–7.

[85] Lazzeri E, Crescioli C, Ronconi E, Mazzinghi B, Sagrinati C, Netti GS, et al. Regenerative potential of embryonic renal multipotent progenitors in acute renal failure. J Am Soc Nephrol 2007;18:3128–38.

[86] Loverre A, Capobianco C, Ditonno P, Battaglia M, Grandaliano G, Schena FP. Increase of proliferating renal progenitor cells in acute tubular necrosis underlying delayed graft function. Transplantation 2008;85:1112–9.

[87] Smeets B, Angelotti ML, Rizzo P, Dijkman H, Lazzeri E, Mooren F, et al. Renal progenitor cells contribute to hyperplastic lesions of podocytopathies and crescentic glomerulonephritis. J Am Soc Nephrol 2009;20:2593–603.

[88] Ronconi E, Sagrinati C, Angelotti ML, Lazzeri E, Mazzinghi B, Ballerini L, et al. Regeneration of glomerular podocytes by human renal progenitors. J Am Soc Nephrol 2009;20:322–32.

[89] Lindgren D, Bostrom AK, Nilsson K, Hansson J, Sjolund J, Moller C, et al. Isolation and characterization of progenitor-like cells from human renal proximal tubules. Am J Pathol 2011;178:828–37.

[90] Ward HH, Romero E, Welford A, Pickett G, Bacallao R, Gattone 2nd VH, et al. Adult human CD133/1(+) kidney cells isolated from papilla integrate into developing kidney tubules. Biochim Biophys Acta 2011;1812:1344–57.

[91] Angelotti ML, Ronconi E, Ballerini L, Peired A, Mazzinghi B, Sagrinati C, et al. Characterization of renal progenitors committed toward tubular lineage and their regenerative potential in renal tubular injury. Stem Cells 2012;30:1714–25.

[92] Sallustio F, Serino G, Costantino V, Curci C, Cox SN, De Palma G, et al. miR-1915 and miR-1225-5p regulate the expression of CD133, PAX2 and TLR2 in adult renal progenitor cells. PLoS One 2013;8:e68296.

[93] Han X, Zhao L, Lu G, Ge J, Zhao Y, Zu S, et al. Improving outcomes of acute kidney injury using mouse renal progenitor cells alone or in combination with erythropoietin or suramin. Stem Cell Res Ther 2013;4:74.

[94] Zhang J, Pippin JW, Krofft RD, Naito S, Liu ZH, Shankland SJ. Podocyte repopulation by renal progenitor cells following glucocorticoids treatment in experimental FSGS. Am J Physiol Renal Physiol 2013;304:F1375–89.

CHAPTER

20 REGULATORY ASPECTS: REGULATION OF CELL-FREE BIOMATERIAL IMPLANTS

N. Zhang[1], A. Baume[2], R. Payne[2], J. Allickson[2]

[1]National Institutes for Health, Bethesda, MD, United States;
[2]Wake Forest School of Medicine, Winston-Salem, NC, United States

CHAPTER OUTLINE

In Situ Tissue Regeneration. http://dx.doi.org/10.1016/B978-0-12-802225-2.00020-9

INTRODUCTION

In general, biomaterials used in medicine are regulated as medical devices. Regulation of devices has become an area of difficulty for product developers and regulatory bodies alike. For regulators, it poses challenges to properly ensure these complex devices are safe and effective for patients by creating new regulatory frameworks. For product developers, the difficulty becomes navigating this regulatory framework correctly and in the most efficient manner.

In tissue engineering (TE) applications, biomaterials are commonly used as scaffolds, which are necessary for recruiting cells and delivering other bioactive components. In some cases, they may be implanted together with cells as combination products; however, there is great variability in the manner in which TE products employ biomaterials. Some TE products will use natural biomaterials that eventually integrate with patient tissue. In other instances, TE products use bioactive biomaterials to recruit cells or elicit a metabolic response in much the same way as a drug.

This chapter aims to summarize the regulatory pathways for TE products and provide specific guidance for the development of biomaterials from research to clinical studies.

MEDICAL DEVICES

Biomaterials are defined as any materials that are in contact with human or any animal biologic systems to perform their intended function and are usually identified as "nonviable material used in a medical device, intended to interact with biological systems [1]." In the United States, the Food and Drug Administration (FDA) regulates the design, manufacturing, and marketing of medical devices. The Center for Devices and Radiological Health (CDRH) is the branch of the FDA with oversight of medical devices. Regulation involves manufacturing, repackaging, relabeling, and importation of medical devices sold in the United States.

A medical device is: "an instrument, apparatus, implement, machine, contrivance, implant, in vitro reagent, or other similar or related article, including a component part, or accessory, which is:

- intended for use in the diagnosis of disease or other conditions, or in the cure, mitigation, treatment, or prevention of disease, in man or other animals, OR
- intended to affect the structure or any function of the body of man or other animals, and which does not achieve any of its primary intended purposes through chemical action within or on the body of man or other animals and which is not dependent upon being metabolized for the achievement of any of its primary intended purposes [2]."

CLASSIFICATION OF MEDICAL DEVICES

A medical device is distinct from a drug in that its primary mechanism of action is not chemical or requiring metabolism of the product. Broad classification of medical devices is risk based and dependent on the final application. In the United States, medical devices are either Class I, II, or III, where Class III products pose the most significant risks (SRs). For example, a synthetic polymer scaffold may be classified as a Class II device for use as a skin substitute; however, if the same biomaterial is applied for bladder augmentation, then the FDA would deem this a higher-risk application and could reassign as a Class III device. For the most part, TE products will be implanted in the patient and directly interact with the host tissue; therefore, they are classified as Class II or III products.

Class I medical devices, such as external wound dressings, tongue depressors, and surgical gloves, are deemed to be the lowest risk and require only general controls to demonstrate safety and efficacy. General controls relate to labeling, current good manufacturing practices (cGMP), postmarket surveillance, adulteration, misbranding, device registration, and reporting [3].

For Class II medical devices, general and special controls are usually adequate to justify the safety and efficacy of the device. Special controls include, but may not be limited to, special labeling requirements, premarket data requirements, and performance standards [3]. Special controls include product-specific controls that the FDA deems necessary to mitigate the increased risks of Class II devices. For biomaterials, this usually involves biocompatibility data as well as characterization of the device according to FDA-recognized standards. For example, the FDA requires the developers of dental amalgam to provide data on compressive strength, creep, chemical composition, and other important performance characteristics [4]. Class II devices require FDA approval of a premarket application [510(k)] before the device can be marketed in the United States. For the 510(k) application, the developer must demonstrate "substantial equivalence" to a "predicate," which is a similar device marketed in the United States. This includes: a device that has been recently cleared through the 510(k) process, a legally marketed device approved before 1976, a Class III device that was later downclassified to Class II or I. or a 510(k) exempt device [5]. Substantial equivalence can usually be demonstrated with in vitro and animal testing alone. Typically, no clinical trials in a target population are required for 510(k) approval; however, if no substantial equivalence to a marketed product exists, then the new product may require clinical demonstration of safety and efficacy for 510(k) premarket notification.

For Class III medical devices, general and special controls alone are not adequate to demonstrate safety and efficacy, and clinical trials are required for PMA. An Investigational Device Exemption (IDE) must be submitted to the FDA for approval to conduct the clinical studies. An IDE should include a full product description, including manufacturing methods and surgical protocols. All nonclinical data should be included to fully characterize the final product, and the methods used in the characterization must follow recognized standards and guidelines. A definitive study should be included, which is usually an animal model that must follow Good Laboratory Practices (GLP). Any early positive clinical data available should be included with the IDE to provide strong justification for clinical approval.

Biomaterials have historically been classified by the FDA as Class II medical devices. As biomaterials increase in sophistication and novelty, they must be classified as Class III devices. Furthermore, there are some bioactive materials currently in development that no longer meet the FDA definition of a medical device [6,7].

COMBINATION PRODUCTS

For TE products, a large proportion of the final products include cells with scaffolds. These TE products are recognized as a combination product composed of two or more components that would normally be regulated under different authorities (ie, drug–device, device–biologic, drug–biologic, and drug–device–biologic). For biomaterials, the most relevant FDA divisions to regulate combination products are the Center for Biologics Evaluation and Research (CBER), Center for Drug Evaluation and Research (CDER), and CDRH.

- Drug: "articles intended for use in the diagnosis, cure, mitigation, treatment, or prevention of disease in man or other animals; and articles (other than food) intended to affect the structure or any function of the body of man or other animals" [2].
- Biological products: These products are defined as drugs under the Federal Food, Drug, and Cosmetic (FD&C) Act. They are further clarified by the Public Health Services Act as "virus, therapeutic serum, toxin, antitoxin, vaccine, blood, blood component or derivative, allergenic product, or analogous product, ...applicable to the prevention, treatment, or cure of a disease or condition of human beings." [2].

In the US, biomaterials/devices are usually regulated by CDRH; drugs are regulated by CDER; and biologics are regulated by CBER. It is critical to have the formal process for the jurisdiction of combination products based on determination of the primary mode of action. The analysis scientifically identifies the most important therapeutic effect of the product and dictates the appropriate center to lead in the review process in the regulatory pathway. To evaluate a cell/scaffold product, it is critical to access both impacts of one upon the other. For device–biologic combinations, cells are usually evaluated for survival rate and genotypic/phenotypic changes to avoid potential risks of immune rejection and transmission of adventitious agents. Biologic–device combinations are similar to device only, where degradation and biocompatibility issues are evaluated. This chapter focuses on biomaterials only that are regulated as devices. Thus the focus will be on the regulation of medical devices by CDRH.

QUALITY SYSTEM REGULATIONS

Quality System Regulations (QSR) provide direction to medical device manufacturers for the manufacturing, packaging, and distribution of the final device. Detailed information can be found at the FDA website [8]. These requirements were established by the FDA to ensure that safe and effective products are used in the marketplace. The FDA conducts periodic inspections of manufacturers to assure their quality systems meet the QSR standards. Manufacturers are also expected to meet cGMP standards.

REGULATORY SCOPE

The regulation of a device applies not only to an unapproved device but also to the use of an approved device in a population or manner that has not been approved. There are generally three types of device studies: (1) studies exempt from IDE regulation; (2) nonsignificant risk (NSR) studies with an abbreviated IDE; and (3) significant risk (SR) studies with full requirements of IDE application. The following flowchart illustrates the general regulation pathway for medical devices (Fig. 20.1) [9].

INVESTIGATIONAL DEVICE EXEMPTION

Under FDA exemption criteria, certain devices can be exempt from IDE regulation [10]. These devices include those that were marketed before 1976 or transitional devices, 510(k)-cleared, Humanitarian Device Exemption, or a PMA-approved device with an approved label, basic physiological research, in vitro diagnostic devices, or combinations of legally marketed devices.

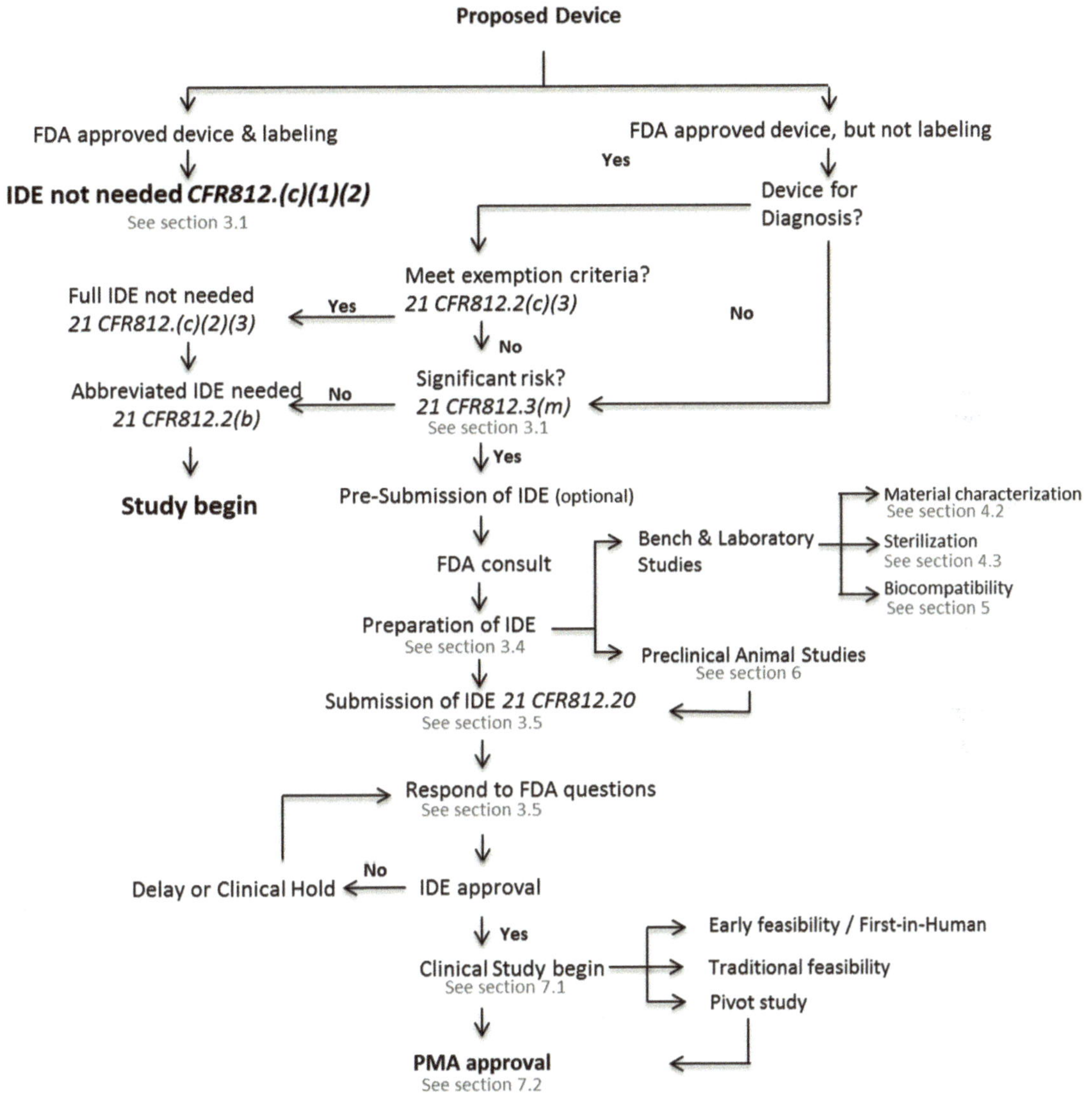

FIGURE 20.1

Flowchart for a medical device regulatory pathway.

SIGNIFICANT RISK STUDY

If a study does not meet exemption criteria, then a risk evaluation is required for the device.

Approval of a Premarket Approval (PMA) application is based on the criteria established in the SR study and depends on whether the device is "*intended as an implant and presents a potential for serious risk to the health, safety, or welfare of a subject; purported or represented to be for use supporting or sustaining human life and presents a potential for serious risk to the health, safety, or welfare of a subject; for a use of substantial importance in diagnosing, curing, mitigating, or treating disease, or otherwise preventing impairment of human health and presents a potential for serious risk to the health, safety, or welfare of a subject; or otherwise presents a potential for serious risk to the health, safety, or welfare of a subject*" (21 CFR 812.3). In most cases, the local Institutional Review Board (IRB) will make this assessment, and the FDA may assist with the final determination. If a device study is recognized as NSR, then an abbreviated IDE is required with information such as labeling of an IDE, prohibitions regarding promotion of the investigational device, meeting the general investigator obligation for IRB approval, and the agreement of an NSR device, documentation, monitoring, and recordkeeping.

More information can be found at Information Sheet Guidance for IRBs, Clinical Investigators, and Sponsors [11,12].

FDA REVIEW PROCESS

In the United States, FDA approval of an IDE is required for human studies using a device that poses an SR and has not been approved for the indication being studied [10]. For a PMA device, there are usually four stages of the review process [13] (Fig. 20.2).

IDE PREPARATION

The IDE submission includes a cover letter and the application.

The cover letter should include the following:

- a statement that this is an original IDE application;
- device information: name and intended use;
- sponsor contact information (all correspondence from the FDA is sent via email);
- manufacturer information;
- correspondent information;
- presubmission/presubmission meetings with the FDA;
- waiver requests; and
- referenced files, such as referenced premarket approval, premarket notification 510(k), IDE, or device master files (MFs).

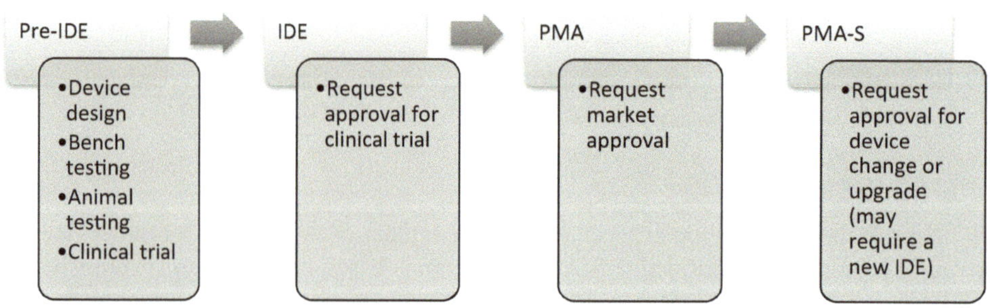

FIGURE 20.2

Overview of the review process for a PMA device.

Unlike investigational new drug (IND) applications, no preprinted forms are available for IDE applications; however, the FDA requires information to be submitted in the order specified in Table 20.1. Bold sections will be explained in further detail later in the chapter. More information can be found at the FDA website [14].

INVESTIGATIONAL DEVICE EXEMPTION SUBMISSION AND FDA RESPONSES

Since January 1, 2013, the FDA requires manufacturers to submit two paper copies and one electronic copy (eCopy) for IDE applications [15]. The file must include the statement that "eCopy is an exact duplicate of paper copies." The eCopy must contain a compact disc, digital video disk, or a flash drive.

An IDE application is considered approved 30 days after it has been received unless the FDA informs the sponsor otherwise. Based on the supporting information, the FDA may approve the investigation as

Table 20.1 IDE Application Form

Table of Contents	
Sponsor Information	
Report of prior investigations	**All prior clinical, preclinical, and laboratory testing of the device necessary to justify the proposed research**
	References for all publication
	All published and unpublished adverse effects
	Other significant information, if requested by an IRB or the FDA
	Summary of all information that is relevant to the evaluation of safety and efficacy of the device
	Statement that nonclinical studies were performed in compliance with GLP or reason for noncompliance, if nonclinical data are provided
Investigational plan	Purpose: name, intended use of the device, objectives, and duration of the investigation
	Protocol: methodology to be used and analysis of scientific soundness
	Risk analysis: all increased risks and how to be minimized; justification of the investigation; inclusion and exclusion criteria of patient population
	Description of the device: each component, ingredient, property, and principle of operation of the device and any anticipated changes during the investigation
	Monitoring procedures
	Additional records and reports
Manufacturing information	**Methods, facilities, controls of manufacture, processing, packing, storage, and installation**
Example of the agreement to be signed and investigator information	
Certification from above	
IRB information	
All relevant institution information	
Amount charged and explanation	
Labeling	
Informed consent materials	
Other information as pertinent	

proposed with conditions or disapprove it. According to 21 CFR 812.30(b) [4], the FDA will disapprove an IDE when foreseeable risks to the study subjects do not outweigh the anticipated benefits and the importance of the knowledge to be gained. When approved with conditions, sponsors can begin the trial if they agree to address the deficiency outlined in the conditional approval letter within 45 days.

PMA approval is based on a benefit–risk assessment of the outcome of primary safety and effectiveness endpoints. Due to the challenging trial design process, it is advisable to initiate communication with the FDA early in the presubmission process. The FDA Guidance document, "Guidance for the Preparation of a Premarket Notification Application for a Surgical Mesh," outlines the different types of characterization required for synthetic materials (polymers, metals, ceramics) versus collagen and other animal-derived materials for meshes and scaffolds [16,17].

BENCH AND LABORATORY TESTING

TYPES OF BIOMATERIALS

Synthetic materials

One of the main driving forces in the regulation of biomaterials is the type and source of the materials to be used. Scaffolds are often fabricated from bioabsorbable polymers such as polyglycolic acid, polylactic acid, polycaprolactone (PCL), and their various copolymers. These materials have a long history of use as medical devices for drug delivery, suture materials, and a number of other clinical applications. Therefore regulators will be more concerned with potentially harmful residuals introduced during the manufacturing process, such as organic solvents. For novel synthetic biomaterials, additional laboratory testing may be required prior to beginning clinical investigations to demonstrate safety. Owing to their more controlled manufacture and lack of disease-related risks, the regulatory bar may be lower for synthetic biomaterials than for animal-derived materials, which could reduce the time and cost of development.

Animal-derived materials

Due to the limited supply of human donor tissue and incidence of donor site morbidity, there are increasing numbers of devices using cells and organs derived from animal sources as xenotransplantation. For example, many scaffolds are composed of extracellular matrix proteins, such as collagen, that are derived from animal tissue. Xenogeneic tissues may have potential risks, such as transmission of zoonotic diseases and introduction of new pathogenic entities to the public. Additional guidance documents and standards regarding the use of animal-derived materials can be found on the FDA website [18–21].

If a product intended for use in humans is made using animal tissue-derived materials or chemical reagents, then the FDA requires that Certificates of Analysis and Materials Safety Data Sheets be submitted and include information such as control of animal tissue collection, manufacturing, and sterilization techniques [22]. In addition, the FDA focuses on other specific issues, such as transmissible bovine spongiform encephalopathy. Depending on the nature and body contact of the device, the FDA may require thorough characterization of the product before any clinical trials may proceed. For permanent implants, detailed biochemical characterization may be needed, such as residual cellular material, growth factors, extracellular matrix proteins, glycosaminoglycans, and proteoglycans. Appropriate cell-based assays should be developed to quantitate these biological materials and their activity level. Due to the nature of tissue, batch-to-batch variations need to be adequately addressed. It may be helpful to compare the product characterization to the targeted tissue and further establish acceptance criteria for animal tissue collection.

The use of these materials is heavily scrutinized by regulators due to the possibility of harboring disease and causing immune reactions in patients. Animal-derived tissue, in particular, has additional regulatory challenges due to the potential risk for the introduction of new pathogens and transmission of zoonotic diseases [23]. Overcoming these challenges may be crucial for future TE, as animals represent a more available tissue source than humans.

MATERIAL CHARACTERIZATION

The physical properties of the scaffold will ultimately determine the functional properties and its general manufacturability (Table 20.2).

As shown in Table 20.2, there are a variety of tests available to characterize biomaterial/scaffolds; however, not all methods are relevant or possible in every case. FDA guidance documents can provide some recommendations for the testing required for specific applications. It is possible that innovative TE biomaterials will necessitate developers to design new methods or adapt existing methods, such as American Society for Testing and Materials (ASTM) standards, for testing performance parameters. Certain general scaffold parameters are often important and include those listed below (Table 20.3).

Mechanical properties: TE scaffolds must often provide mechanical support to allow proper regeneration. The type of mechanical performance of the biomaterial depends on its application and the corresponding physiological conditions [25]. For example, a bone scaffold must possess high compressive strength to prevent crushing, whereas a vascular scaffold must have high burst strength. FDA guidance documents for medical devices with similar applications may serve as a starting point in understanding the level of mechanical characterization expected. For instance, the FDA guidance

Table 20.2 Testing for Biomaterial Characterization [24]

	Testing
Mechanical/thermal	Stress–strain
	Strain to failure
	Flex fatigue testing over time
	Viscoelastic properties
	Dynamic scanning calorimetry/thermogravimetric analysis
Morphological	Light microscopy
	Scanning electron microscopy
	Atomic force microscopy
	Permeation of aqueous fluids
	Brunauer, Emmett, and Teller
Chemical	Electron spectroscopy for chemical analysis
	Static secondary ion mass spectrometry
	Contact angle
	Infrared surface studies
	Infrared spectroscopy
	Nuclear magnetic resonance spectroscopy
Chemical stability	In aqueous media
	In enzyme solutions
	In oxidant solutions
Biological	Cell attachment/proliferation
	Endotoxin

Table 20.3 Parameters for Biomaterial Characterization

Characterization	Parameters
Mechanical properties	Flexing or static environment, how comparable to native tissue
Chemical properties	Molecular weight, polydispersity, cross-linkers, initiators, catalysts, inhibitors
Physical properties	Pore size, geometry, distribution, interconnectivity, porosity, degree of cross-linking, surface structure, controlled release of bioactive factors
Biodegradation	Rate, mechanics versus time

document, "Non-Clinical Engineering Tests and Recommended Labeling for Intravascular Stents and Associated Delivery Systems," provides good indication on the level of mechanical analysis expected for a vascular scaffold, [26]. For bioabsorbable materials, the mechanical properties should be characterized as the material degrades over time [17].

Chemical properties: Biomaterial chemistry must be fully characterized. This is mainly a safety issue, as certain chemical species may be toxic, carcinogenic, or immunogenic [17]. The concentration of all such chemicals must be detailed and validated as being within safe levels for human exposure. Chemical property characterization can also be linked to the efficacy of the material. For example, polymer molecular properties, such as molecular weight and polydispersity, may change during biomaterial manufacturing, sterilization, and storage. Changes in these properties may indicate alterations in the material performance from those intended.

Physical properties: The physical structure must be characterized. For scaffolds, this relates to the porosity, pore size, fiber diameter, pore architecture, and interconnectivity [17,25]. These properties must be characterized using approved standard methods and shown to be reliable batch-to-batch. There are a number of methods that can be used to measure the porosity of scaffolds. Of these, mercury porosimetry is a cost-effective method that will provide the porosity, median pore size, and surface area of the scaffold. Other physical properties will need to be determined depending on the scaffold type. For example, glass transition temperature should be determined and controlled for hydrogels.

Biodegradation: There must be detailed analysis of the degradation profile of all degradable materials. This includes degradation kinetics as well as characterization and quantification of degradation products [25]. Sterilization can affect degradation profile, particularly in polymers; thus the testing should apply to the final manufactured scaffold poststerilization [27,28]. The mechanism for degradation should also be included, and corresponding test conditions should be modeled in the degradation testing. Furthermore, the test conditions should mimic the applicable physiological milieu. For slow-degrading biomaterials, accelerated degradation testing may be used, but the applicability of the testing must be justified.

STERILIZATION

Sterility of biomaterials, which is crucial to ensure patient safety upon implantation, alludes to the absolute nonexistence of viable pathogenic organisms on a product. In reality and from a regulatory perspective, sterility is conceptualized as the probability that a single pathogenic organism will be present on the product. The safe sterility assurance level is 10^{-6}, meaning one out of one million devices may contain a single organism [27].

Sterility is often achieved by terminal sterilization processes such as gamma irradiation, ethylene oxide sterilization, or steam autoclaving. Many biomaterial scaffolds are sensitive to the harsh environments generated by terminal sterilization methods that may cause irreversible changes to the product.

Developers may utilize terminal sterilization to impart favorable properties such as increased mechanical properties; however, the changes often will decrease the efficacy of the biomaterial. This is especially the case in scaffolds containing natural biomaterials such as collagen or chitosan [29,30]. As such, terminal sterilization may not be suitable, and aseptic manufacturing must be demonstrated to ensure sterility [31]. It is important to note that terminal sterilization alone does not ensure a product is clean or will not harm the patient. Microorganisms that are killed during the process can leave behind pyrogens that can trigger a host immune response [27]. Furthermore, dust particles in the air, if allowed to contact and adhere to the product, could jeopardize product safety. The FDA will likely require a biomaterial that will be terminally sterilized to be manufactured in a certified clean room and for the raw material sourcing and storage to be controlled.

When terminal sterilization is considered, so too must be a sterile packaging system. The packaging must facilitate the sterilizing process while maintaining the integrity of the sterile barrier during storage and transportation so the device can be implanted aseptically [27]. There are usually two separate components to product packaging: (1) the sterile barrier; and (2) the physical barrier. The sterile barrier maintains an aseptic environment inside the package after sterilization by blocking the entry of microorganisms and allergenic particles. The physical barrier protects both the sterile barrier and the product from damage. Both the physical and sterile barriers must be permeable to the sterilant. For example, if a PCL scaffold is to be sterilized by ethylene oxide treatment, the packaging must be porous to allow the intrusion of ethylene oxide gas so that it can enter the packaging and permeate the scaffold.

Since an aseptic product is essential for its safety and efficacy, regulators will require validation of the sterilization process and the packaging system. Sterilization validation will be dependent upon the sterilization method chosen. Generally, requirements include:

- equipment qualification
- bioburden testing
- sterility testing

The equipment qualification requires Installation Qualification (IQ), Operational Qualification (OQ), and, in many instances, Performance Qualification (PQ). The IQ and OQ ensure that the equipment was installed according to the manufacturer's instructions and in the proper working conditions and that the equipment is functioning correctly. The PQ is more complex and device-specific to test a biological indicator (BI) against the sterilization process in the worst-case packaging and loading scenario [27]. A BI is a self-contained assay comprising 1 million viable bacterial spores physically separated from media and an indicator. If the BI is cultured under the correct conditions, then the bacteria will grow and produce metabolic products. If the BI is adequately sterilized, then there will be no viable spores, and consequently, no bacterial growth will be seen.

Bioburden testing is used to enumerate and characterize the opportunistic microbial load on the device after manufacturing but prior to sterilization [31]. If a biomaterial is not processed aseptically, some microorganisms from the manufacturing environment are expected to be present. Bioburden testing is described in the standard International Organization for Standardization (ISO) 11737. A key part on the process is to validate the microbe removal technique chosen such that the method does not kill the microbes being retrieved and to establish the removal efficiency. TE scaffolds provide a particular challenge in this regard, as the complex porous or hydrogel structure can interfere with the removal of microbes [27].

Sterility testing usually involves seeding a quantified bacterial load onto the device and validating that no colony-forming units are present poststerilization. For biomaterial scaffolds that have antibacterial properties, extra validation may be required to confirm that the sterilization is responsible for the asepsis. *United States Pharmacopeia* (USP) chapter 71 is the most accepted guidance for sterility testing, and includes a number of different methods to suit the wide range of drugs and devices [32].

BIOLOGICAL EVALUATION: BIOCOMPATIBILITY

The biocompatibility of a final device depends not only on the materials but also on the manufacturing methods (including the sterilization process). It is usually required as a basic safety test prior to clinical investigation. The FDA has a draft guidance for industry and the agency itself, ISO 10993, "Biological Evaluation of Medical Devices Part 1: Evaluation and Testing" to replace ODE General Program Memorandum #G95-1 (1995). The document focuses on evaluation of the final finished device including material or materials, processing of the materials, manufacturing methods (including the sterilization process), and the manufacturing residuals that may be present on the final device [33].

ISO 10993 discusses the following issues:

- test selection;
- general testing considerations, including sample preparation;
- specific considerations for the following testing: cytotoxicity, sensitization, hemocompatibility, pyrogenicity, implantation, genotoxicity, carcinogenicity, reproductive and developmental toxicity, and biodegradation;
- use of animal safety studies to justify omission of specific biocompatibility tests;
- assessment of known or potentially toxic chemical entities; and
- contents of a biocompatibility test report.

Medical devices can be classified based on both the nature and duration of body contact. Both categories need to be considered to select appropriate tests. Duration of body contact is categorized into three time points, including single or multiple use (Table 20.4). When the exposure time is less than 24 h, limited tests will be needed for biocompatibility. When duration exceeds 30 days, the device is considered as permanent contact. Duration between 24 h and 30 days is considered as prolonged exposure. Nature of contact is listed in Table 20.4. A biocompatibility flowchart is shown in Fig. 20.3.

Table 20.4 Types and Examples of Medical Devices

Nature of Contact	Types	Examples
Surface	Skin	Electrodes, tapes, external orthopedic braces
	Mucous membranes	Feeding tubes, endoscopes, oral swabs
	Breached or compromised surface	Dressings/bandages for wounds, burns, ulcers
External communicating	Blood path	IV sets, extension sets, transfer sets
	Tissue/bone/dentin	Dental cements, skin sutures, arthroscopes
	Circulating blood	Extracorporeal tubing, filters, intravascular catheters
Implantable	Tissue/bone	Orthopedic pins, plates, pacemakers
	Blood	Heart valves, vascular grafts, internal delivery catheters

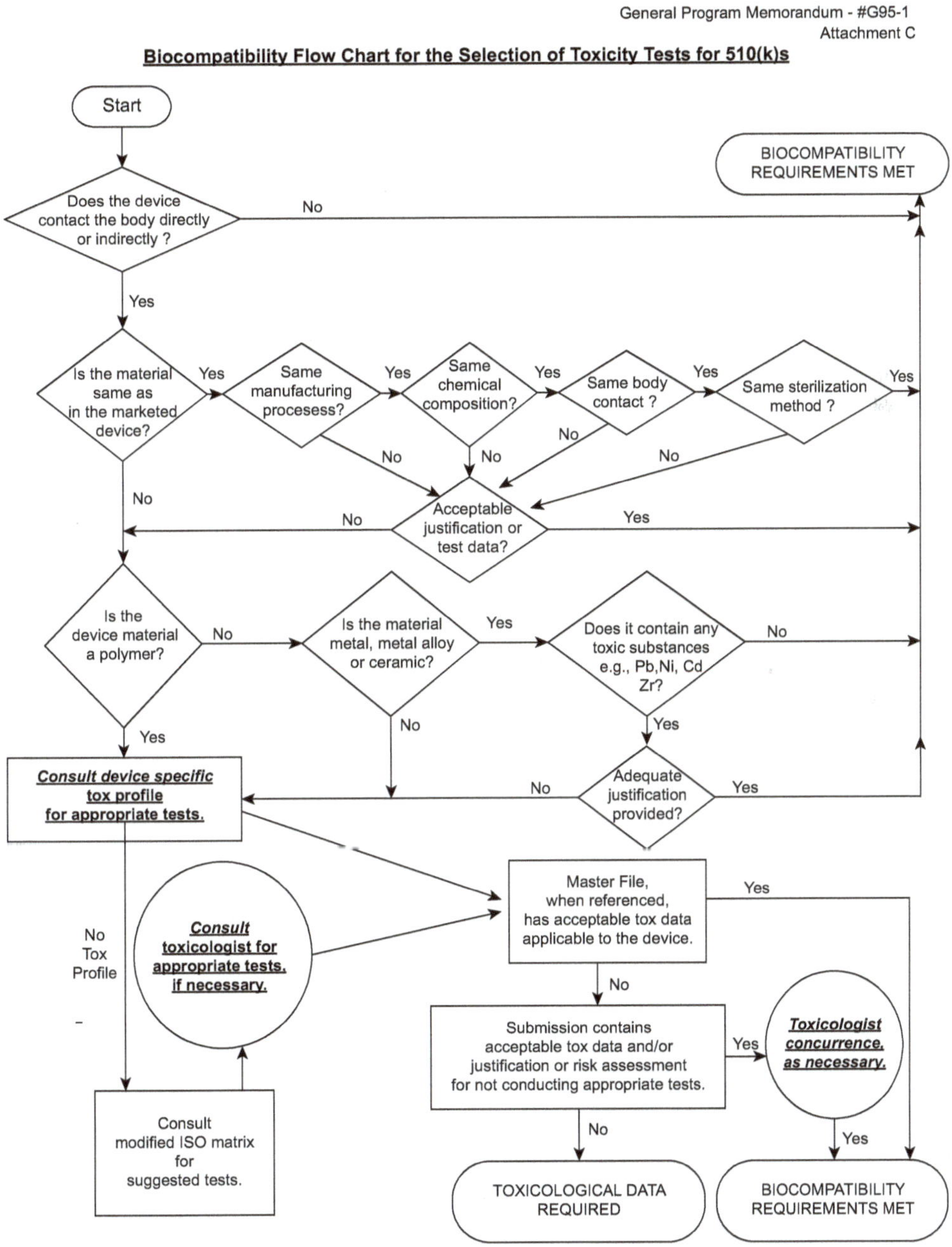

FIGURE 20.3

Biocompatibility flowchart [33].

TEST SELECTION

If the following items are changed, then the device or final product must be reevaluated or related risk assessment must be conducted (Table 20.5).

BIOCOMPATIBILITY TESTING

A full set of biocompatibility testing may not be required by the FDA. Depending on the intended use and the category of the device, different biocompatibility testing may be assigned. Detailed information can be found at the FDA website [33].

In this chapter, a general explanation of each testing is provided, and a list of guidance or documents that may be followed when certain testing is required by the FDA is outlined in Table 20.6.

Extract preparation and test material selection have significant impacts on the result and testing sensitivity. Whenever practicable or possible, the sterilized final product should be used to conduct biocompatibility testing. If this is not possible, then the appropriate sample preparation should be selected using representative portions or materials processed in the same manner as the final product. When using a portion of the final product, then the test sample must have maximum exposure of the test system to the components of the device. If the extract method is selected, then multiple factors need to be considered, including intended use, chemical and physical nature, type of tests, and extraction media.

When using representative samples, additional testing may be necessary to justify the differences between test samples and the final sterilized product, such as the type and quantity of chemical leachables that are eluted, exhaustive extraction, and surface characterization techniques. If the material is in situ polymerizing and bioabsorbable, then it is recommended that toxicity of the final sterilized product, as well as various time points over the course of polymerization and/or degradation, are assessed. Appropriate chemical analytical testing of the extract may determine whether single or multiple tests are necessary. The endpoint of in vivo tests is usually when the polymer is no long present in the tissue or the biological tissue response is stable.

Cytotoxicity test is used to determine the cell death, cell growth inhibition, and other adverse effects on cells caused by the device or its extracts. For materials that have not been used in the market with the same nature and duration of contact, both direct contact and dilution methods will be required.

Table 20.5 Examples of Changes That May Require Additional Biocompatibility Testing

Changes	Examples
Source or specification of the materials used in the manufacture of the product	Supplier, animal origin source to vegetable-derived material, molecular mass, pore size
Formulation, processing, primary packaging, sterilization	Addition of BaSO4, additives, process aids, laser marking, chemical etching, ink jet marking, polyethylene (PE) or glass vials, ethylene oxide (EO) or irradiation
Storage	Degradation during shelf-life, improper storage, catastrophes, substances leaching from packaging materials
Intended use	Body contact, contact duration
Adverse effects	Postmarket surveillance data, reprocessing of single-use devices

Table 20.6 References for Biocompatibility Testing

	Standard
Cytotoxicity	ISO 10993-5: 2010 Biological evaluation of medical devices – Part 5: Tests for in vitro cytotoxicity.
	ISO 10993-12: 2007 Biological evaluation of medical devices – Part 12: Sample preparation and reference materials.
Acute systemic toxicity	ISO 10993-1: 2009 Evaluation and testing in the risk management process.
Sensitization	ISO 10993-1:2009 Evaluation and testing in the risk management process.
	ASTM F2148 Standard Practice for Evaluation of Delayed Contact Hypersensitivity Using the Murine Local Lymph Node Assay (LLNA).
	ISO 10993-12: 2007 Biological evaluation of medical devices – Part 12: Sample preparation and reference materials.
	ISO 10993-10: 2010 Biological evaluation of medical devices – Part 10: Tests for irritation and skin sensitization.
	OECD 429 Skin Sensitization: Local Lymph Node Assay.
	OECD 442A Skin Sensitization: Local Lymph Node Assay: DA.
	OECD 442B Skin Sensitization: Local Lymph Node Assay: Brdu-ELISA.
Hemocompatibility	ASTM F756-08 Standard Practice for Assessment of Hemolytic Properties of Materials.
	ASTM F2065-00 (2010) Standard Practice for Testing for Alternative Pathway Complement Activation in Serum by Solid Materials.
	ASTM F1984-99 (2008) Standard Practice for Testing for Whole Complement Activation in Serum by Solid Materials.
	Autian J. Toxicological evaluation of biomaterials: Primary Acute Toxicity Screening Program. Artif Organs August 1977;1(1):53–60.
	National Institute of Arthritis, Metabolism, and Digestive diseases. Report of a Study Group for the Artificial Kidney – Chronic Uremia Program: Evaluation of Hemodialyzers and Dialysis Membranes (NIH Publication No. 77-1294). Washington, DC: U.S. Government Printing Office; 1977.
Pyrogenicity	ISO 10993-12: 2007 Biological evaluation of medical devices – Part 12: Sample preparation and reference materials.
Implantation	Buchen SY, Cunanan CM, Gwon A, et al. Assessing intraocular lens calcification in an animal model. J Cataract Refract Surg 2001;27:1473–84.
Genotoxicity	OECD 471 (1997) Bacterial Gene Mutation Assay.
	OECD 473 (1997) In Vitro Genotoxicity Chromosomal Aberration Assay.
	OECD 474 (1997) In Vivo Bone Marrow Micronucleus Assay.
	OECD 475 (1997) In Vivo Bone Marrow Chromosomal Aberration Test.
	OECD 476 (1997) In Vitro Genotoxicity Mouse Lymphoma Gene Mutation Assay.
	OECD 487 (2010) In Vitro Micronucleus Assay.
Carcinogenicity	OECD 451 (2009) Guidelines for the Testing of Chemicals – Carcinogenicity Studies.
	OECD 453 (2009) Guidelines for the Testing of Chemicals – Combined Chronic Toxicity/Carcinogenicity Studies.
	Buchen SY, Cunanan CM, Gwon A, et al. Assessing intraocular lens calcification in an animal model. J Cataract Refract Surg 2001;27:1473–84.
Reproductive and developmental toxicity	ISO 10993-1: 2009 Evaluation and testing in the risk management process.

Sensitization test is used to determine the delayed-type hypersensitivity of a material or device. There are three methods available: (1) guinea pig maximization test (GPMT); (2) guinea pig closed patch method; and (3) local lymph node assay (LLNA). According to the FDA, GPMT and LLNA are usually submitted for devices.

Irritation test is used to determine irritant effects of a device, materials, and its extracts of tissues such as skin, eye, and mucosal membranes.

Systemic toxicity test is used to address the evaluation of generalized systemic toxicity and not specific target organ or organ system toxicity, even though these effects may result from the systemic absorption and distribution of toxicants. Time points include acute (<24 h), subacute (24 h–28 day), subchronic (28–90 day), and chronic (6–12 months).

Genotoxicity test is used to determine gene mutations, changes in chromosome structure and number, and other DNA or gene toxicities caused by the device, material, and its extracts. ISO 10993, Part 3 describes two options. The first option includes a test for gene mutations in bacteria, a test for gene mutations in mammalian cells, and a test for clastogenicity in mammalian cells. The second option is similar except for the mammalian assays, where two endpoints are covered in one test. According to ISO, requirements can be met using in vitro assays, and in vivo assays are only indicated in the case when positive genotoxic results are observed in the in vitro assays. The FDA, however, has a specific requirement of in vivo testing as part of a battery of tests.

Implantation test is used to determine the local effect of the test material after implantation by comparing the tissue response to the test material with control materials. Evaluation of results includes macroscopic, microscopic, and semiquantitative assessment of responses.

Hemocompatibility is used to determine the compatibility of devices or components with circulating blood. It is applicable to external communicating devices and implant devices. Tests will evaluate thrombosis, coagulation, platelets, hematology, and complement system.

Early detection of a product failing any of these biocompatibility tests generally leads to an IDE not being accepted. Due to the duration of some of the tests, it is recommended that they be initiated as soon as the product composition is finalized to eliminate the need for modification of the biomaterial after animal testing has begun. If issues with the biocompatibility results do emerge, options include repeating the tests with less sensitive methods and/or using a different test to verify the results.

CROSS-REFERENCING OTHER DOCUMENTS

If the device follows certain pathways according to the flowchart, it is possible to cross-reference the data from other INDs, IDEs, and MFs (Table 20.7). It is the sponsor's responsibility to obtain

Table 20.7 Cross-Reference an Existing IND/IDE

Existing application IND/IDE or existing marketing application new drug application (NDA)/biologic license application (BLA)/PMA/510(k)	• Letter of cross-reference • Letter of authorization
Previous human experience	• Letter of cross-reference • Include a rationale for use of the drug outside the current labeled dose, duration, or in combination with other drugs • Copies of published materials

permission to cross-reference in support of the file. The file under review must contain a signed letter by the person who submitted the file (21 CFR 312.23(b)) Fig. 20.4.

In general, IDEs on clinical hold, inactive, or withdrawn cannot be cross-referenced [33–37].

- Hold: An order issued by the FDA to delay a proposed clinical investigation or suspend an ongoing investigation (21 CFR 312.42).
- Inactivated: IDE is subject to no activity but may be reactivated (21 CFR 312.45).
- Withdrawal: Sponsor requests to end IDE; IDE cannot be reactivated (21 CFR 312.38).

PRECLINICAL STUDIES

In vivo animal studies may be required to support the initiation of an early feasibility study. It can provide unique anatomic and clinical pathologic information on the local and systemic responses of the device use, which is very relevant to biomaterials. It is not considered as an alternative to adequate bench testing.

First, the animal model should be validated, as results are likely to predict risks in humans. If no model is available, then a focused animal study may be conducted to address a limited range of safety issues. Sample size should be large enough to generate consistent results and is usually dependent on the device and how comparable the animal model is to humans. Short-term studies may be sufficient for the initiation of an early feasibility study; however, additional animal studies may be needed to support a larger clinical study with a near final or final device design. According to the specificity of biomaterials, the authors recommend that the device design be finalized as early as possible to avoid further issues such as biocompatibility and chemistry testing.

Generally, GLP studies are required to assure the quality and integrity of safety data to support IDE applications; however, in the early feasibility study, a non-GLP study may also be acceptable with identified and justified deviations.

CLINICAL INVESTIGATION

SCOPE OF CLINICAL STUDY

It is critical to determine what types of clinical studies are needed for a medical device. There are generally three types of clinical studies for IDEs: (1) early feasibility study or First in Human study; (2) traditional feasibility study; and (3) pivotal study. Determining the type of clinical study will depend upon certain factors, such as the novelty of the device, intended clinical use, stability, and the amount

Investigator requests LOA from IND/IDE holder
IND/IDE holder submits LOA to investigator (Also referred to as the "Authorized Party")
Authorized Party includes copy of LOA in IND/IDE submission and references same in appropriate sections
Authorized party submits IND/IDE to FDA
FDA reviews holder's IND/IDE in support of Authorized Party's IND/IDE

FIGURE 20.4

Letter of authorization process.

Table 20.8 Stages of Clinical Studies

	Early Feasibility Study/First in Human Study	Traditional Feasibility Study	Pivotal Study
Timeline	Before the design has been finalized for the specific indication/when the device for a specific indication is evaluated for the first time in human subjects	Near final or final device	Final design
Purpose	To identify appropriate modifications to the procedure or device; to evaluate device design concept of clinical safety and functionality; to establish deliver/implant/use procedure for the device; to provide information that is not available by nonclinical assessments or tests, such as device failures, intended use population, and therapeutic parameters	To capture preliminary safety and effectiveness information; to plan an appropriate pivotal study	To collect definitive evidence of the safety and effectiveness of the device for a marketing application with endpoints and sample size statistically driven
Necessity	Not mandated	Either traditional feasibility study or pivotal study are required	
Number of subjects	Usually less than 10	10–40 but may be larger	In a statistically justified number of subjects

of test data (Table 20.8). Note that not all novel devices or uses warrant an early feasibility study, nor would the FDA mandate that an early feasibility study be conducted [38]. It is advisable to contact the FDA to determine whether the proposed investigation can be classified as an early feasibility study prior to IDE submission. Additionally, the FDA recommends that sponsors use the presubmission process to optimize the preparation and quality of early feasibility study IDE applications. More detailed information regarding presubmission can be found at the FDA website [38].

To improve the likelihood of IDE approval, the FDA listed the following factors that should be addressed in the original early feasibility study IDE application [38]:

- clinical condition to be treated or assessed by the device;
- standard of care for the clinical condition and expected clinical outcomes;
- anticipated benefits;
- does report of prior investigations have adequate information to support initiation of the study;
- risk analysis, sufficient risk mitigation strategies, adequate human subject protection measures, clinical study protocol; and
- are the potential risks likely to be outweighed by the anticipated benefits?

Device trials are unique and tend to not be as large as drug trials; moreover, device trials may be highly dependent on a physician's technique. Modification of the device is allowed to occur; however, they are usually difficult to render blind, randomize, and control and may yield highly variable endpoints [13]. Generally, less nonclinical data in the Report of Prior Investigations will be needed for an early feasibility study compared to a traditional feasibility or pivotal study. Additional bench and animal testing may be necessary to support a larger clinical study of a near final or final device design [38].

For early feasibility studies, certain information needs to be included in the Report of Prior Investigations, including the expectation of acceptable clinical use (successful placement and function of the device using a benchtop model that simulates clinical conditions or a suitable animal model); basic device safety (sterility, biocompatibility, software verification and validation, electromagnetic compatibility, chemical compatibility); characterization of catastrophic failure modes; and identification of risk mitigation approaches.

A pivotal study is generally intended as the primary clinical support of a marketing application. The relevant FDA review is much more complex compared to feasibility studies. The IDE application generally focuses on safety and the plan for collecting and evaluating study data, with additional information such as trial endpoints, trial design, study conduct and monitoring, and statistical analysis plan. Pivotal IDEs usually contain primary and secondary endpoints, a discussion of appropriate endpoint parameters, hypothesis, and success criteria. Primary endpoint design should evaluate safety, effectiveness, and durability of the device in the intended population. The trial would be considered successful if endpoints for both safety and effectiveness are met. When primary endpoints are successful, secondary endpoints are used to support claims [38].

PMA APPLICATION

Approval of a PMA application is based on a benefit–risk assessment of the outcome of primary safety and effectiveness endpoints. Due to the challenging trial design process, it is advisable to initiate communication with the FDA early through the presubmission process [13,38].

CONCLUSION

In the United States, it is mandatory to meet FDA regulatory requirements in order to market and manufacture biomaterials as medical devices. These requirements have presented challenges for those seeking to move their products toward clinical use. Extensive studies with appropriate quality management are required during this process and include material characterization, safety, preclinical animal testing, and clinical studies. Process development plays a role as a bridge from bench to clinic, facilitating the translational period within feasible budgets, timelines, and workloads. It is recommended to base decisions according to risk analysis, regulatory expertise, as well as communications with the FDA. With proper guidance and direction, regulatory requirements should not be an obstacle to successfully bringing innovative science to patients.

REFERENCES

[1] Amato SF, Ezzell RM. Regulatory affairs for biomaterials and medical devices. 2014.
[2] Federal Food, Drug, and Cosmetic Act, 21 U.S.C. Subchapter II – definitions. 2010. Edition.
[3] FDA. Regulatory controls. 2014.
[4] FDA. Class II special controls guidance document: dental amalgam, mercury, and amalgam alloy – Guidance for Industry and FDA Staff. 2009.
[5] FDA. How to find and effectively use predicate devices. 2014. Available from: http://www.fda.gov/MedicalDevices/DeviceRegulationandGuidance/HowtoMarketYourDevice/PremarketSubmissions/PremarketNotification510k/ucm134571.htm. [09.03.2015].

[6] Amato SF. 3-Regulatory strategies for biomaterials and medical devices in the USA: classification, design, and risk analysis. In: Amato SF, Ezzell RM, editors. Regulatory affairs for biomaterials and medical devices. Woodhead Publishing; 2015. p. 27–46.
[7] Amato SF. 4-Clinical development and endpoint strategies for biomaterials and medical devices. In: Amato SF, Ezzell RM, editors. Regulatory affairs for biomaterials and medical devices. Woodhead Publishing; 2015. p. 47–66.
[8] FDA. In: Design control guidance for medical device manufacturers. CDRH; 1997.
[9] Blair Holbein ME, Berglund JP. Understanding FDA regulatory requirements for an investigational device exemption (IDE) for sponsor-investigators. J Investig Med 2012;60(7):987–94.
[10] Medical devices. Title 21 C.F.R. Part 812 Subchapter H. 2011.
[11] FDA. Information sheet guidance for IRBs, clinical investigators, and sponsors significant risk and nonsignificant risk medical device studies. 2006.
[12] FDA. Information sheet guidance for IRBs, clinical investigators, and sponsors frequently asked questions about medical devices. 2006.
[13] Faris O. Clinical trials for medical devices: FDA and the IDE process, 2013. Available from: http://www.fda.gov/downloads/training/clinicalinvestigatortrainingcourse/ucm378265.pdf.
[14] FDA. IDE application. Available from: http://www.fda.gov/MedicalDevices/DeviceRegulationandGuidance/HowtoMarketYourDevice/InvestigationalDeviceExemptionIDE/ucm046706.htm.
[15] FDA. eCopy Program for medical device submissions guidance for industry and food and drug administration staff. 2013.
[16] Witten C. FDA perspective/review of cell scaffold products. In: FDA/NIST sponsored workshop on in vitro analyses of cell/scaffold products. 2007.
[17] FDA. Guidance for the preparation of a premarket notification application for a surgical mesh. CDRH; 1999.
[18] FDA. Medical devices containing materials derived from animal sources (except for in vitro diagnostic devices) – draft guidance for industry and food and drug administration staff. 2014.
[19] FDA. Guidance for industry: source animal, product, preclinical, and clinical issues concerning the use of xenotransplantation products in humans. 2003.
[20] FDA. PHS guideline on infectious disease issues in xenotransplantation. 2001.
[21] FDA. Guidance for industry: Public health issues posed by the use of non-human primate xenografts in humans. 1999.
[22] FDA. Draft guidance for industry and food and drug administration staff – medical devices containing materials derived from animal sources (except for in vitro diagnostic devices). 2014.
[23] Lee MH, Arcidiacono JA, Bilek AM, Wille JJ, Hamill CA, Wonnacott KM, et al. Considerations for tissue-engineered and regenerative medicine product development prior to clinical trials in the United States. Tissue Eng Part B Rev 2010;16(1):41–54.
[24] Bandhyopadhya A, Bose S, editors. Characterization of Biomaterials. 2013.
[25] ASTM. ASTM F2150–13. Standard guide for characterization and testing of biomaterial scaffolds used in tissue-engineered medical products. West Conshohocken, PA: ASTM International; 2013.
[26] FDA. Non-clinical engineering tests and recommended labeling for intravascular stents and associated delivery systems. 2010.
[27] Baume A, Coleman N, Boughton P. Methods for achieving soft tissue scaffold sterility. J Biomim Biomater Tissue Eng 2009;4:59–69.
[28] Cottam E, Hukins DW, Lee K, Hewitt C, Jenkins MJ. Effect of sterilization by gamma irradiation on the ability of polycaprolactone (PCL) to act as a scaffold material. Med Eng Phys 2009;31(2):221–6.
[29] Gorham SD, Srivastava S, French DA, Scott R. The effect of gamma-ray and ethylene oxide sterilization on collagen-based wound-repair materials. J Mater Sci Mater Med 1993;4(1):40–9.
[30] Noah EM, Chen J, Jiao X, Heschel I, Pallua N. Impact of sterilization on the porous design and cell behavior in collagen sponges prepared for tissue engineering. Biomaterials 2002;23(14):2855–61.

[31] Baume AS, Boughton PC, Coleman NV, Ruys AJ. Sterilization of tissue scaffolds. Characterization and design of tissue scaffolds. 2015.
[32] Richter SG. A white paper. Microtest Laboratories, Inc.; 2014.
[33] FDA. Use of ISO 10993 biological evaluation of medical devices 1 evaluation and testing. Draft Guid Industry Food Drug Administration Staff. 2013.
[34] Frey JL. Reliance on information not developed by the applicant. Guidance for industry and FDA staff: early development considerations for innovative combination products. 2006.
[35] Frey JL. Overview of the IND process, 2004. Available from: https://secure.emmes.com/pactweb/system/files/cber101032204jf.pdf.
[36] Henley L. Clinical Investigator: how to put together an IDE application?. 2013.
[37] Navigators JHI. Letter of Authorization: IND right of reference guidance and template. 2013.
[38] FDA. IDE for early feasibility medical device clinical studies, including certain FIH studies. Guidance for Industry and Food and Drug Administration Staff. 2011.

CHAPTER

21 BUSINESS PERSPECTIVE: CASE STUDY: COMMERCIALIZED CELL-FREE CARDIOVASCULAR IMPLANT

A. Sheehy, B. Lambert, R. Rapoza
Abbott Vascular, Santa Clara, CA, United States

CHAPTER OUTLINE

In Situ Tissue Regeneration. http://dx.doi.org/10.1016/B978-0-12-802225-2.00021-0

INTRODUCTION

Regenerating failed tissue and organs through tissue engineering offers hope of treating disease and revolutionizing the practice of medicine in ways as significant as the introduction of antibiotics. However, major technological success is only one leg of the race. Commercializing technology with a viable business model in a rapidly changing healthcare system requires not just the successful development of technology but also a consideration of the investment required to scale manufacturing and meet regulatory requirements, integration within today's standard care delivery models, and demonstration of clinical and health economic value necessary to provide a return on investment.

Various techniques in tissue engineering therapy naturally lend themselves to certain commercialization pathways. The commonality is that the more the technology minimizes disruption to the existing models of care and sales, the lower the barrier to adoption and the easier the commercialization. For instance, cell harvesting and culturing to create a new tissue layer or organ lends itself to designing and commercializing tools that facilitate the process of culturing, decellularizing, or immune pacifying the therapeutic product. In these situations, the harvested and/or cultured cell is a unique product customized for the patient. The commercialized tools are technologies that enable this customization to be performed with minimal additional overhead from the healthcare delivery system. In contrast, in situ scaffolds for tissue engineering focus on developing a consistent and scalable implant that engineers the tissue in situ, where the customization steps are performed by the body itself. This approach focuses on using precise manufacturing processes to commercialize a scalable off-the-shelf implant that can be implanted/administered to a patient with minimal disruption to the healthcare delivery system.

Development and clinical and regulatory dynamics are intrinsically related to the business of investment. The value that any therapy brings to patients and society ultimately drives the approach to how the technology can eventually reach patients. This value starts with the clinical need. The value of addressing that clinical need must offset the cost and complexity of getting the therapy to market. Beyond just treating a disease, however, therapies must be cost-effective, not just from a risk–benefit perspective, but from a cost adjusted risk–benefit perspective. As governments and societies across the globe recognize the skyrocketing cost of healthcare, a margin of improvement in patients' disease status must be valued by society at large (or at least by established and agreed upon criteria) as delivering sufficient improvement to be worth the cost of both the technology/device/product as well as its implementation (eg, any disruption to the standard care delivery model). Through addressing the latter and integrating an understanding of healthcare system costs, in situ tissue regeneration devices can become viable commercialized health technology.

Commercialization of bioresorbable vascular scaffolds within interventional cardiology is a case study in both the business challenges and pathway forward for in situ tissue engineering scaffolds. Absorb BVS (BVS) is the first commercialized bioresorbable vascular scaffold and serves as the basis for this case study. BVS is a temporary implant designed to maintain patency of a coronary artery following angioplasty, much like a stent. It functions as an in situ tissue engineering device by serving as a scaffold upon which the artery can repopulate healthy cells of the artery. As the device degrades and loses mechanical strength, it mechanically conditions the repopulated cells with physiologic cyclic strain and fluid shear stress. Over time, as the device is completely resorbed, the artery is restored to a functional state. Through mapping the business factors involved in the development and commercialization of BVS, we can understand the challenges that in situ tissue regenerative medicine technology faces from a business perspective.

PRODUCT AND MARKET DYNAMICS

Interventional cardiology advanced through the 1990s and 2000s with exceptional technological investment, adoption, and advances in patient care. Typical business factors all pointed to success:

1. The market was large and growing; cardiovascular disease and specifically coronary artery disease affects millions of people worldwide, leading to worsening quality of life, increased healthcare costs, and increased morbidity and mortality.
2. Interventional cardiologists were increasing in number, increasing in hospital influence, and ready adopters of technology.
3. Competition was fierce, leading to rapid technological advancement.

In this market, technologic solutions to improving clinical problems, coupled with increased ease of use for physicians, resulted in rapid advancement of the field.

THE HISTORY OF PERCUTANEOUS CORONARY INTERVENTION

The beneficial clinical and societal impact of Gruentzig's invention of balloon angioplasty is considered a major revolution in the field of cardiology. In successful cases, angioplasty restores blood flow back to the heart while drastically reducing both in-hospital and off-work patient recuperation time relative to that for patients undergoing coronary artery bypass graft surgery for treatment of a blocked coronary artery. However, in a significant number of cases, balloon angioplasty has had its own complications [1–3], including artery dissection and acute occlusions due to vessel recoil, which ultimately result in patients undergoing coronary artery bypass grafting. In addition, 30–60% of patients develop restenosis in the first year requiring revascularization.

These problems led to the second wave of new products in the 1990s, bare metal stents (BMS) [4]. The sturdy metal stents placed in the clogged artery following balloon angioplasty solved the acute occlusion problem by stabilizing dissection flaps and by preventing arteries from acute recoil and later constrictive negative remodeling. This significantly reduced revascularization rates [5] to 15–30%; the second revolution had arrived. A good portion of the residual restenosis was from a new problem of in-stent restenosis [6] resultant from neointimal hyperplasia. Undesired tissue proliferation within the stented artery leading to vascular blockage was not, however, the only complication of these permanent implants. The presence of a rigid metallic implant can restrict vascular motion and/or result later in strut malapposition [7–9]. In addition, the residual metallic stent hinders both future revascularization as well as noninvasive imaging, such as MRI and multislice CT [8]. When placed near a bifurcation, the metal stent may also impair access to and flow to side branches, resulting in "jailed" side branches on the vascular tree [10,11].

While other technologies were tried and failed to address [12] the 15–30% restenosis rate, a third wave of products emerged in the 2000s, metallic drug-eluting stents (metallic DES) [13–17]. The healthcare system and patients around the world have adopted this new procedure, which suppresses in-stent restenosis rates consistently below 10%, leading to a marked reduction in the need for revascularization. These clinical gains are the result of the targeted release of an antiproliferative and/or anti-inflammatory drug (eg, sirolimus, everolimus, paclitaxel) from a polymer coating on the stent in order to reduce neointimal hyperplasia.

ABSORB BVS

From the perspective of percutaneous coronary intervention (PCI) technologies, BVS is designed to achieve the original intent of balloon angioplasty: percutaneous revascularization of an atherosclerotic artery that restores the patency of the vessel while maintaining the natural physiologic environment. The evolution of BMS and DES has been instructive on the mechanical and pharmacological characteristics necessary to achieve this vision. BVS behaves mechanically like a metallic stent in the critical initial months after implantation to avoid acute occlusion and constrictive remodeling of the arteries. Similar to a DES, it releases an antiproliferative drug to suppress neointimal hyperplasia and restenosis. Finally, over time, the scaffold transitions the biomechanics of the vessel back to the vessel wall and disappears over time as the scaffold benignly bioresorbs [18]. In this context, it represents the next revolution of PCI technology. Taken from another viewpoint, BVS is an in situ tissue engineering device masquerading as the next-generation stent and represents one of the first commercial applications of in situ tissue regeneration.

Intuitively, in situ tissue regeneration via a bioresorbable scaffold that could address the clinical problems of previous technologies would be readily adopted. However, key factors need to be addressed:

1. The clinical barrier to "improvement" with DES is high. Demonstrating clinical success is not as easy as when improving upon the benefits of angioplasty.
2. Competition is high. After 20 years of investment and consolidation, competition is high from large stent companies with much to lose from disruptive technologies. Additional competition exists from alternatives, such as medical therapy or coronary artery bypass grafting, both of which continue to improve.
3. Dynamics of rising healthcare costs and concerns of overuse in medical treatments create headwinds for new technologies.

All of these factors influence the balance between investment cost/risk and potential commercial opportunity. Balancing this investment cost and commercial opportunity extends through all phases of product cycle planning: technical optimization during development and regulatory approvals, clinical trial design, full-scale production, and global commercialization.

COST AND COMPLEXITY OF GETTING A HIGHLY TECHNICAL IN SITU SCAFFOLD TO MARKET

Successfully getting an in situ scaffold for tissue engineering to market has two major components. The first is product development; associated costs and complexities are the focus of this section. The second is market development, ie, getting patients, administrators, healthcare systems, insurance companies, and reimbursement bodies to support adoption of the product. This is addressed in the next section, Changing Dynamics of Healthcare, although aspects of product development that can limit or facilitate market acceptance are highlighted in this section.

As discussed previously, there is a spectrum of regeneration products that have vastly different development challenges. The scope of this chapter is limited to in situ scaffolds, a product illustrative of those having development challenges related to producing a scalable off-the-shelf system that takes regenerative medicine concepts and enables an in situ approach that is minimally disruptive to the existing healthcare infrastructure and models of care delivery. Challenges inherent to this model include technical challenges of scaling highly reproducible processes for complex technology and market competition from existing products.

BVS is an in situ tissue engineering device designed to be implanted like a traditional stent, leveraging the existing commercialization and healthcare delivery system, but providing the value and promise of regenerating a diseased, occluded coronary artery. The design, development, manufacturing, and evaluation of BVS illustrate the major factors that any scalable in situ regenerative scaffold would need to consider. One of the critical challenges to any in situ regenerative medicine technology is to understand where to build upon the existing development and manufacturing standards and where to develop brand new modes of operation.

After extensively illustrating the design, development, and manufacturing objectives and challenges associated with commercialization of a scalable in situ product, BVS, the associated preclinical evaluation and clinical evaluation objectives and challenges are discussed in this section.

DESIGN, DEVELOPMENT, AND MANUFACTURING

In situ scaffolds for tissue engineering are designed as a replacement for drug-eluting metallic stents, a mature multibillion dollar market. To understand the design, development, and manufacturing challenges of scaffolds, it is important to understand the related metallic DES challenges. This provides a foundation from which specific deviations from the metallic world related to in situ bioabsorbable scaffold can be discussed. A key component of this foundation is related to the inclusion of a pharmaceutical in the device. As experienced by second wave bare metallic stent catheter manufacturers, the addition of a drug product in the stent polymeric coating increased the cost and complexity of manufacturing and regulatory approval significantly.

Similar to a metallic DES, the BVS system is comprised of:

1. a balloon catheter delivery system;
2. a bioresorbable scaffold (replaces metallic stent);
3. a polymeric scaffold coating from which an active agent or drug elutes; and
4. a sterile barrier package.

In brief, manufacturing processes for these systems include manufacture of a balloon catheter, with a focus on deliverability; manufacture of the BVS in situ scaffold, with a focus on scaffold material and design; coating of the scaffold with the drug/active agent embedded in a polymer; crimping the coated scaffold onto the balloon catheter; sealing the device into a sterile barrier package; and terminal sterilization of the finished product. These devices must be manufactured in accordance with regulatory guidance and standards, eg, ISO 13485:2003 Medical devices—Quality management systems—Requirements for regulatory purposes; and CFR (Code of Federal Regulations) Title 21, Part 820: Quality System Regulations; CFR 21 Part 210: Current Good Manufacturing Practice (cGMP) in Manufacturing, Processing, Packaging, or Holding of Drugs, General; and Part 211: cGMP for Finished Pharmaceuticals. These standards ensure consistency of product, process, equipment, and operations. Key features and desired attributes for such metallic product with associated pharmaceutical and processes are highlighted in the following sections, together with issues specific to bioabsorbable materials that facilitate tissue regeneration.

Balloon catheter and scaffold deliverability

This dimension of product development, seemingly far removed from the value of tissue regeneration in situ, can be market limiting to in situ PCI scaffolds if not addressed responsibly. An important lesson learned from the battle for market share with the first three generations of PCI products is that intact deliverability of the balloon, metallic stent, or metallic DES to the diseased vessel is extremely important. If the physician cannot easily get the device to access lesions in the coronary anatomy, he does not want the product. Crossing profiles of catheters, balloons and stents, together with their steerability and flexibility, are very important in achieving ease of deliverability to complex anatomies.

Scaffold material and design

The heart of the BVS system is the scaffold. Material and design decisions and considerations, including stent/scaffold geometrical design for optimum acute mechanical support of the vasculature in the first 3 months, are similar to those for metallic stents. However, there are also questions related to aspects unique to bioabsorbable materials used for tissue regeneration, for example:

1. Which bioabsorbable material should be utilized? Some have been shown to trigger inflammation within the vessel wall [19]. The source of vascular inflammation is not limited to the material used; it may also result from the degradation profile, which is related to the bioabsorbable polymer's molecular weight, molecular weight distribution, and many facets of how it is processed. The choice of raw material also influences availability and quality of suppliers, which can be important for meeting regulatory standards as well as supply chain strategy.
2. How will the biomaterials be processed to create metallic-like properties in the initial 3 months when revascularization is the key priority? After intentional loss of mechanical integrity, scaffold degradation profiles must be optimized to facilitate regeneration of vascular motion and integrity while not leading to inflammatory pathways. Processes in scaffold manufacture may include extrusion, expansion, and lasing. Inherent with biomaterials is their sensitivity to thermal processing, which complicates both the processing and the storage of the scaffolds. Both bulk and minute details of the scaffold are thermally sensitive, and maintaining thermal control is challenging, especially during product commercialization to high volumes.

Coating the scaffold

Following PCI product iterations from balloon catheters to permanent implant stents (BMS), DES became the third generation and standard of care in PCI. It is on this foundation that bioresorbable in situ scaffolds build. A common design, and the one most germane to this case study, uses an antiproliferative drug in a thin biocompatible polymer coating over the stent. The fourth-generation BVS in situ regenerative scaffold uses this same technology. Essentially all of the lessons learned from DES stent coating can be applied to regenerative scaffold coating. One has to pause, however, and appreciate that coating the scaffold with a drug, like coating a permanent implant stent with a drug, introduces enormous development complexity. This is a huge lesson learned for PCI manufactures of metallic stents as they transitioned into the world of drug-coated stents a decade or more ago. The drug development industry has an extensively rigorous regulatory process, which is difficult and time-consuming to navigate.

One of the key aspects of drug development, again identical to that of DES, is managing the drug release profile from the scaffold coating. Drug release profiles from successful metallic DES products currently on the market are emulated and/or new release profiles are demonstrated to be safe and effective through the development process with bench, animal, and clinical data. In either case, this is another component of development that is seemingly far removed from in situ regeneration but which requires significant focus and resources to successfully bring a product to market with worldwide regulatory approvals.

Crimping the scaffold onto the delivery system

Another lesson learned from earlier PCI product generations is the importance of successfully crimping the scaffold onto the delivery system. Bare metallic stents, as well as metallic DES, have been challenged with this important attribute. Losing a stent or scaffold in the vasculature such that the patient is sent to surgery for device recovery is exceedingly problematic. In the case of fully bioresorbable scaffolds, successful attachment of the scaffold to the delivery system to achieve an appropriate diameter (profile) for adequate deliverability without damaging the coating or the backbone is technically challenging. This manufacturing unit operation will continue to be an important consideration in the design of all bioresorbable products.

Packaging and sterilization

Sterile barrier packaging must be designed and validated [20] to:

1. properly identify the product with appropriate labeling;
2. protect the product from mechanical damage during shipment and storage;
3. maintain the environment within the package if control is required, eg, products may require inert environment for radiation sterilization to minimize drug or scaffold degradation;
4. allow for ingress and egress of sterilization gases, such as ethylene oxide, and humidity if gas sterilization is used; and
5. maintain sterility of the product throughout the intended life time of the product.

The terminal sterilization process must be designed and validated [21] to:

1. reduce the initial microbial contamination level of the product (typically 10 to 100 colony-forming contaminants) to the very secure sterility assurance level of, typically, one nonsterile unit in 1 million devices; and
2. accomplish this formidable sterilization goal while not negatively affecting the delicately engineered properties of the bioabsorbable scaffold, the delivery system, the drug coating, or the active pharmaceutical agent, if applicable. Ethylene oxide and radiation sterilization are the workhorses of the medical device industry and represent significant material compatibility challenges to materials for regenerative scaffolds. EO sterilization involves alkylation chemistry, and significant thermal stresses and radiation chemistry effects are significant in radiation-sterilized products. The terminal sterilization scientific community is taking steps to develop and optimize effective and sustainable high-volume sterilization procedures and other creative solutions that will be applicable to regenerative devices and other sensitive combination products [22–25].

PRECLINICAL EVALUATION

BVS built upon the preexisting foundation of safety assessment of predecessor PCI BMS and DES products, which have preexisting regulatory and academic guidance. Model selection (porcine coronary and rabbit iliac artery models), study objectives (safety, pharmacokinetics), study design, and study endpoints are similar for BVS as for BMS and DES. Importantly, any preclinical evaluation of medical technology should reflect the same ultimate clinical objectives and applications [26–29]. Working from this foundation, the following aspects are unique to BVS and require careful consideration in establishing a comprehensive preclinical program. In particular, evaluation deviated in the evaluation and timing of loss of structural integrity and degradation. The preclinical focus and resources required to lay the foundations for commercialization are summarized below.

Study objectives

Safety and pharmacokinetics are shared study objectives between bioresorbable scaffolds and metallic stents, but additionally, in vitro and in vivo degradation studies are needed in order to characterize the degradation profile and to align with the scaffold's safety and performance. There are two critical aspects to be considered with respect to the degradation of scaffolds. First, degradation studies should be aligned with safety studies so that critical time points within the life of the implant can be appropriately evaluated, eg, biocompatibility during and following the most rapid phase of degradation. Second, additional and more stringent pharmacologic and biocompatibility requirements should be addressed with respect to contaminants or leachables, degradation products, and subsequent metabolites derived from the scaffold. Special attention is required if the scaffold results in degradation products that are to be excreted from the body (eg, polyanhydrides) as opposed to being assimilated or metabolized [eg, polylactic acid (PLA) and polyglycolic acid].

Study duration

Preclinical studies should evaluate critical performance intervals and include a temporal duration that extends the entirety of the scaffold's lifespan. These intervals include acute (<7 days), subchronic (28 and 90 days), and chronic durations (≥180 days). Chronic phase evaluations should be based on (1) the expected pharmacokinetic and degradation profile for the appropriate number of time intervals selected (at least three suggested); and (2) the projected total lifespan, with lifespan being defined as the duration in which there is arterial wall and/or systemic exposure to degradant products.

Scaffold integrity

While the integrity of metallic devices has been routinely evaluated angiographically in vivo and with high-resolution radiography postmortem, the integrity of biodegradable scaffolds requires an alternate modality. Micro-CT or 3-D optical coherence tomography (OCT) reconstruction may be used to assess scaffold integrity. As a decline in scaffold integrity is an inherent design feature to allow for restoration of arterial function and vasomotion, the integrity of a BVS is a transient feature and is pertinent only during the phase of revascularization.

CLINICAL EVALUATION

Clinical trials are a major necessary investment for new technologies but also offer opportunities to demonstrate meaningful value to support global commercialization efforts. The nature of the market opportunity and the potential clinical value of the device are critical to balancing the risk, reward, and investment decisions of a technology like BVS.

Global versus regional clinical strategy

Coronary artery disease is a worldwide disease with growing prevalence. As countries and their respective regulatory policies and agencies have continued to develop, the need for clinical trial data from patient populations representative of that country is increasingly demanded. This can be designed into a worldwide clinical program through adaptive clinical trial design, integrated multicountry strategies, such as pooling across geographies, and individualized randomized trials.

Noninferiority, superiority, and differentiated endpoints

Additionally, deciding whether to demonstrate noninferiority to existing technologies, superiority to existing technologies, or to advance different trial endpoints that better capture the value of the technological solution is critical to the investment required. Each of these options and permutations in between require incremental investment. For instance, BMS and DES trials have evaluated endpoints that focus on device failure (mostly restenosis and myocardial infarction) at 1 year. Most of these trials have compared to a predicate device for noninferiority, meaning that within a prespecified margin, the new device demonstrates itself not to be better but to be no worse than the previous device. From a regulatory and investment perspective, this makes sense. A company investing in an iterative technology that is expecting to bring little to no additional value to patients, but to just compete with the previous iteration, would have little probability of "winning" a superiority trial. Likewise, a regulatory agency is not in the business of ensuring that the first technology to market has a regulatory monopoly over competing equivalent technology. They want to help bring competition that has demonstrated safety and effectiveness to the market to the benefit of all.

In contrast, a revolutionary technology that is expected to bring superior benefit to patients and healthcare systems has both the expected opportunity to justify as well as the burden of proof to demand the investment in trials to demonstrate superiority and/or differentiated value compared to existing technology.

Absorb clinical trial program

The BVS clinical trial program illustrates the way a company can incrementally increase this clinical trial investment balanced against a scaling down of risk as the clinical program moves toward larger more expensive trials. As illustrated in Table 21.1 below, an incremental clinical trial program steadily advances a therapy from feasibility and design evaluation phases to enable larger clinical trial design. Along the way, the investment profile of trials increases, but the commercial opportunity that success within each trial offers increases as well.

Table 21.1 Absorb BVS Clinical Trial Program

Trial	Purpose	Investment	Opportunity
Absorb Cohort A	Feasibility/design evaluation	Low	Low
Absorb Cohort B	Feasibility/redesign evaluation; European (CE mark) approval	Low	Medium
Absorb extend	Continued access registry; increased patient complexity	Low	Medium
Absorb II	First randomized trial; evaluation of unique endpoints (angina, vasomotion); supportive clinical adoption; cost effectiveness	Moderate	Moderate
Absorb III	US approval; large randomized clinical trial; cost effectiveness	Large	High
Absorb Japan	Japan approval	Moderate	High
Absorb China	China approval	Moderate	High
Absorb IV	Superiority; postapproval	Large	High

The Absorb clinical program conducted initial feasibility in a small trial referred to as Cohort A. This trial extensively followed a small cohort of patients with multiple invasive imaging diagnostics. Key learnings from this trial fed into a design iteration, following which another small trial, Cohort B, was conducted using a similar approach. The sequence of trials thereafter has incorporated increased patient complexity, increased rigor, worldwide geographic expansion, as well as unique clinical endpoints aimed at establishing the value of the product.

The scope of this chapter is not to explain in detail the process by which a clinical program should be designed but rather to reflect the underlying business need to balance the investment cost, risk, and opportunity. New technology evaluations and appropriate design of the clinical trial must strategically maximize the investment in the technology with the long-term commercial success firmly in mind.

For instance, the incremental investment in the Absorb Cohort A trial to include invasive imaging such as intravascular ultrasound (IVUS), OCT, and angiography allowed the program to (1) identify that the inherent technology was both feasible and safe; (2) to begin establishing safety with long-term follow-up on a small number of patients with PLA-based scaffold in their arteries; and (3) to identify that short-term performance could be optimized with a scaffold redesign. These learnings were tremendously valuable to an early program and set it on a path to success by mitigating long-term commercial risks and still making progress with the clinical and regulatory questions that needed to be answered.

Importantly, the totality of clinical evaluation of Absorb BVS extends beyond studies sponsored by the manufacturer. Investigator sponsored studies are an important tool for evaluating new indications and/or patient populations. A strategy that maximizes investment in investigator sponsored studies to focus on areas of strategic commercial opportunity is important to the overall clinical strategy.

In summary, clinical trials can no longer simply demonstrate safety but must demonstrate meaningful value of a new technology to support global commercialization. Strategic incremental investment can optimize technology refinement and clinical trial design and balance investment risk with opportunity.

CHANGING DYNAMICS OF HEALTHCARE

Innovative technologies must address the changing dynamics of the healthcare environment by delivering superior outcomes that improve costs for the system. As summarized in Fig. 21.1, historically, medical technologies generated success by creating products that were just as safe as the competition. After products were approved, sales and marketing channels created awareness, stimulated demand, and drove product adoption. Within this framework, technological and regulatory hurdles were the primary barriers to entry. For innovative technologies of the future, such as scaffolds for in situ tissue regeneration, the technological and regulatory hurdles are just the beginning. In situ tissue engineering devices must deliver superior value to the hospitals, payers, and patients to meet the needs of a rapidly evolving healthcare system. Value in this context focuses on value for patients measured by outcomes per dollar spent [30].

In the United States, as well as internationally, the healthcare technology stakeholder environment is evolving. Hospitals are consolidating, increasing both purchasing power and administrator influence over treatment decisions. Governments are scrutinizing healthcare costs, as these costs become an ever increasingly large proportion of their budgets. At the same time, citizens are demanding access to the best health care available. Patients are increasingly involved in healthcare decision-making and in some

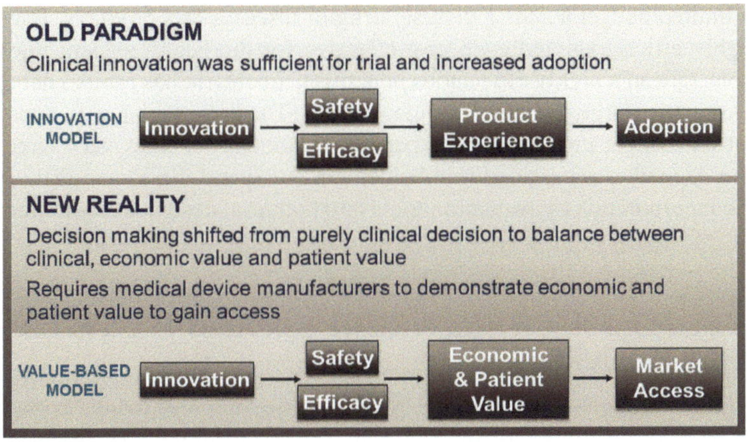

FIGURE 21.1

Changing paradigm of medical innovation adoption.

Table 21.2 Stakeholder Needs and Concerns

Stakeholders	Needs	Key Concerns
Regulators	Safe and efficacious	Clinical trial endpoints
Patients	Improved health Convenient Affordable	Predicted morbidity/mortality Quality of life Out-of-pocket costs
Physicians	Safe and efficacious Easy to administer	Unmet clinical needs Supportive clinical data Addressing hurdles in care delivery (procedural complexity, need for patient compliance, etc.)
Payers	Better value for money Affordable	Comparative effectiveness Budget impact

countries are responsible for the payment or premium payment of their care. Table 21.2 outlines some of the critical needs and concerns that regenerative medicine needs to address for each stakeholder [31].

MARKET ACCESS AND REIMBURSEMENT

While many stakeholders are important in the decision process for adopting a new technology or treatment, payers deserve specific attention. Developers of in situ regenerative scaffolds must look ahead to the market access and reimbursement challenges that commercialization will encounter and incorporate rigorous mechanisms into both trial design and early commercialization activities to demonstrate the added value of their technologies. Governments and private payers incorporate a broad array of systems and tools into spending decisions. Many of these are designed to control spending, but some are designed to provide patients, particularly patients with high unmet needs, with access to superior technologies.

Payers allocate a limited budget across a diverse array of diseases and products. For this reason, even drugs that are highly efficacious and even cost-effective for the health system may encounter challenges. For example, Gilead's highly efficacious hepatitis C treatment has ignited debate, despite a 90% cure rate in a disease with a large untreated population [32]. The large at-risk patient population of hepatitis C means that the budget impact of an expensive treatment becomes very large very quickly. A detailed discussion of market access and reimbursement is beyond the scope of this text. It is simply noted that strategic incorporation of evaluation tools into both trial design and commercialization activities to demonstrate the added value is critical to a successful long-term commercialization strategy.

CASE STUDY: ABSORB: FOLLOW THE PATIENT THROUGH THE SYSTEM—SYMPTOMS DRIVE RESOURCES

The technological advantages of Absorb BVS have been discussed in detail throughout its development. Advantages include: restoration of vascular function or vasomotion, ability to utilize noninvasive diagnostics, normalization of vascular compliance and wall shear stress, and improved vascular endothelial function. The translation of these unique technical benefits to value for all stakeholders has required a methodical understanding of the healthcare system and incorporation into clinical trials.

Traditionally, PCI had focused on discrete points in the continuum of care that pertained to evaluating the clinical performance of a given revascularization technology. Clinical trial endpoints were refined over time to enable precise measurement of technological success or failure in well-defined patient populations. To understand the true value of a new technology for all stakeholders, a rethinking of the scope of measurement was required. As illustrated in Fig. 21.2 below, the true cost of care for either a healthcare

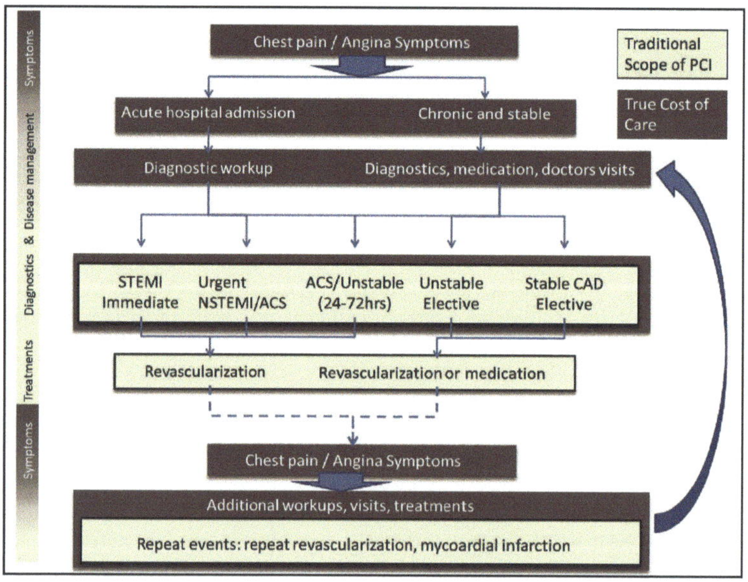

FIGURE 21.2

Cost of care in coronary artery disease.

system or a patient's burden of disease incorporates a host of hospital admissions, doctor's office visits, symptom management, and diagnostics. Understanding the value of BVS required a focus on the key drivers of cost (dollars to the system or patient burden) throughout the continuum of care.

Based on this reorientation, symptoms of angina/chest pain are the central node driving resource consumption. This is true both prior to PCI as well as after PCI. Interestingly, the clinical literature on PCI had not discussed angina as a trial endpoint for a decade or more because it is hard to measure and considered a "soft" endpoint. But it is this very measurement difficulty that makes it such a burden on the healthcare system. Patients often can undergo multiple diagnostics and medication changes before being sent to the catheterization laboratory and revascularized. Addressing the challenge of understanding the impact on the "soft" (hard to measure) endpoint was key to elucidating the total value of BVS for all stakeholders.

Investigators working on BVS oriented several analyses from Absorb clinical trials and real-world insurance databases to:

1. understand the resource and quality of life burden of angina post-PCI;
2. comprehensively evaluate the impact of Absorb BVS on angina; and
3. understand the impact of BVS on angina-related resources and quality of life.

Initial data suggests that post-PCI angina is a fruitful target to reduce the burden to patients and the health system, and that it may be improved with BVS. Regardless of the success or failure of Absorb BVS as a technology in this regard, this approach illustrates the need and challenges that in situ scaffolds will have in demonstrating value to all stakeholders. Reorienting the scope of focus of an industry away from traditional clinical endpoints may seem outside the immediate domain of tissue engineering. Successful commercialization of regenerative medicine technologies will benefit from the foresight of understanding, from establishing where the technology can provide value to the healthcare system, and from a willingness take on new health economic challenges.

CONCLUSION AND VIEW TO THE FUTURE

The applications of in situ tissue regeneration toward preventing major clinical events or altering the course of disease treatment present a compelling solution for patients and payers. These types of clinical opportunities, combined with a large market opportunity, are compelling propositions for the large investment required to develop and commercialize the technology. However, it is important to realize that not all of these factors need to be understood or central to the value proposition on day 1. Both the healthcare business environment and the clinical environment will evolve throughout the development of the technology. Recognizing opportunity and capitalizing on that value during concurrent development is necessary for business success in an inherently risky research and development process.

With BVS, the development of the technology has paralleled concurrent technological advancements in diagnostics that may enable additive benefits beyond those designed into the clinical and economic superiority. Coronary computed tomography angiography (CCTA) is increasingly well recognized as a noninvasive diagnostic that offers similar utility as a traditional catheterization angiography with the added benefits of being less costly and more patient friendly while leading to less complications. Due to its polymeric design, BVS is uniquely capable of being imaged by CCTA.

Though BVS is highly effective at reducing angina compared to DES [33], some patients continue to experience symptoms. Diagnostic evaluation of these patients with a cheaper tool saves the healthcare system money.

A second development in care that has coincided with BVS development is that of evaluating vulnerable plaques. Vulnerable plaques are lesions of the coronary artery that have a high propensity for causing future patient symptoms or clinical events such as myocardial infarction. During the past decade that BVS has been under development, diagnostics attempting to predict which lesions of a diseased coronary artery are vulnerable plaques have been advancing. The intersection of these diagnostic technologies with an in situ regenerative technology offers the potential to "cap" the plaque, pacifying it and then returning the vessel to a more native, healthy state. Preventing disease rather than just treating it would represent a major breakthrough in regenerative medicine. In the development of a scaffold, recognizing the valuable intersections of adjacent technologies, particularly diagnostics, that offer the ability to maximize clinical and healthcare system value is necessary to build a business model around an in situ tissue regeneration technology.

Commercializing in situ regenerative scaffolds with a viable business model in a rapidly changing healthcare system requires upfront consideration of the business factors involved and nimble adaptation along the way. By carefully balancing the opportunity with the associated technical, stakeholder, and societal needs, regenerative medicine can meet its promise of transforming the practice of medicine by changing the course of disease.

REFERENCES

[1] Meier B, Rutishauser W. Transluminal coronary angioplasty-state of the art 1984. Acta Med Scand Suppl 1985;701:142–7.

[2] Mintz GS, et al. Arterial remodeling after coronary angioplasty: a serial intravascular ultrasound study. Circulation 1996;94:35–43.

[3] Serruys PW, et al. Coronary-artery stents. N Engl J Med 2006;354:483–95.

[4] Serruys PW, et al. A comparison of balloon-expandable-stent implantation with balloon angioplasty in patients with coronary artery disease. Benestent Study Group. N Engl J Med 1994;331:489–95.

[5] Pocock SJ, et al. Angiographic surrogate end points in drug-eluting stent trials: a systematic evaluation based on individual patient data from 11 randomized, controlled trials. J Am Coll Cardiol 2008;51:23–32.

[6] van Beusekom HM, et al. Histology after stenting of human saphenous vein bypass grafts: observations from surgically excised grafts 3 to 320 days after stent implantation. J Am Coll Cardiol 1993;21:45–54.

[7] Cook S, et al. Correlation of intravascular ultrasound findings with histopathological analysis of thrombus aspirates in patients with very late drug-eluting stent thrombosis. Circulation 2009;120:391–9.

[8] Khattab AA, Windecker S. Vascular restoration therapy: what should the clinical and angiographic measures for success be? EuroIntervention 2009;5(Suppl. F):F49–53.

[9] Shah V, et al. Background incidence of late malapposition after bare-metal stent implantation. Circulation 2002;106(14):1753–5.

[10] Vorpahl M, et al. The bioabsorption process: tissue and cellular mechanisms and outcomes. EuroIntervention 2009;5(Suppl. F):F28–35.

[11] Waksman R, Pakala R. Coating bioabsorption and chronic bare metal scaffolding versus fully bioabsorbable stent. EuroIntervention 2009;5(Suppl. F):F36–42.

[12] Waksman R, Weinberger J. Coronary brachytherapy in the drug-eluting stent era. Circulation 2003;108:386.

[13] Sousa JE, et al. Sustained suppression of neointimal proliferation by sirolimus-eluting stents: one-year angiographic and intravascular ultrasound follow-up. Circulation 2001;104:2007–11.
[14] Morice MC, et al. A randomized comparison of a sirolimus-eluting stent with a standard stent for coronary revascularization. N Engl J Med 2002;346:1773–80.
[15] Moses JW, et al. Sirolimus-eluting stents versus standard stents in patients with stenosis in a native coronary artery. N Engl J Med 2003;349:1315–23.
[16] Stone GW, et al. A polymer-based, paclitaxel-eluting stent in patients with coronary artery disease. N Engl J Med 2004;350:221–31.
[17] Stone GW, et al. Comparison of a polymer based paclitaxel-eluting stent with a bare metal stent in patients with complex coronary artery disease: a randomized controlled trial. JAMA 2005;294:1215–23.
[18] Vert M. Bioabsorbable polymers in medicine: an overview. EuroIntervention 2009;5(Suppl. F):F9–14.
[19] van der Giessen WJ, et al. Marked inflammatory sequelae to implantation of biodegradable and nonbiodegradable polymers in porcine coronary arteries. Circulation 1996;94:1690–7.
[20] International Standards Organization. ISO 11607–1:2006, Packaging for terminally sterilized medical devices Part 1: requirements for materials, sterile barrier systems and packaging.
[21] International Standards Organization. ISO 11137–1:2006, Sterilization of health care products—radiation—Part 1: requirements for the development validation and routine control of a sterilization process for medical devices. International standards are available to provide requirements and guidance for the validation and routine control of many sterilization modalities. The most common for bioabsorbable materials are radiation sterilization (ISO 11137-1, above) and ethylene oxide sterilization (ISO 11135-1).
[22] Association for the Advancement of Medical Instrumentation. AAMI TIR17:2008, compatibility of materials subject to sterilisation.
[23] The range of solutions being explored to provide terminal sterilization solutions includes providing guidance to the industry on using alternative sterility assurance levels that are applicable to sensitive combination products such as regenerative scaffolds. See ISO TC198, recent new work item proposal, document N1112, "Guidance on aspects of a risk-based approach to assuring sterility of terminally-sterilized, single-use health care products".
[24] Lambert BJ, et al. Radiation and ethylene oxide terminal sterilization experiences with drug eluting stent products. AAPS PharmSciTech 2011;12(No. 4).
[25] Lambert B, Martin J. Sterilization of implants and devices. In: Ratner BD, Hoffman AS, Schoen FJ, editors. Biomaterials science. Elsevier Inc., Academic Press; 2013. p. 1339–53.
[26] Schwartz RS, et al. Drug-eluting stents in preclinical studies: updated consensus recommendations for preclinical evaluation. Circ Cardiovasc Interv 2008;1:143–53.
[27] Perkins LEL. Preclinical models of restenosis and their application in the evaluation of drug-eluting stent systems. Vet Pathol 2010;47:58–76.
[28] USDHHS. In: Guidance for industry and FDA staff: general considerations for animal studies for cardiovascular devices. Rockville, MD: CDRH FDA; 2010.
[29] Schwartz RS, et al. Drug-eluting stents in preclinical studies: recommended evaluation from a consensus group. Circulation 2002;106:1867–73.
[30] Porter M. What is value in health care? N Engl J Med 2010;363(26):2477–81.
[31] Saadi R, Grima D, Ferko N. The science of commerce: succeeding in the changed medical device market. ECON Publishing; 2012. p. 19.
[32] Rockoff JD. Hepatitis C Pill Rockets Gilead into Big Leagues. Wall St J October 10, 2014:20–1.
[33] Serruys PW, et al. A bioresorbable everolimus-eluting scaffold versus a metallic everolimus-eluting stent for ischaemic heart disease caused by de-novo native coronary artery lesions (ABSORB II): an interim 1-year analysis of clinical and procedural secondary outcomes from a randomised controlled trial. Lancet 2015;385(9962):43–54.

Index

'*Note*: Page numbers followed by "f" indicate figures and "t" indicate tables.'

C

D

F

G

K

N

O

P

Q

R

S

T

U

V

W

X

Kolibri 360 GmbH
Ferdinand-Jühlke-Straße 7
99095 Erfurt, Deutschland
produktsicherheit@kolibri360.de